Radiation Oncology

Radiation Oncology

A Case-Based Review

Gokhan Ozyigit · Ugur Selek

Editors

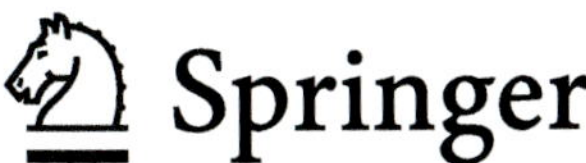

Springer

Editors
Gokhan Ozyigit
Chair and Professor
Department of Radiation Oncology
Faculty of Medicine, Hacettepe University
Ankara
Turkey

Ugur Selek
Chair and Professor
Department of Radiation Oncology
School of Medicine, Koç University
Istanbul
Turkey

Adjunct Professor
Department of Radiation Oncology
The University of Texas MD Anderson
Cancer Center
Houston, TX
USA

ISBN 978-3-319-97144-5   ISBN 978-3-319-97145-2   (eBook)
https://doi.org/10.1007/978-3-319-97145-2

Library of Congress Control Number: 2018967706

This Springer imprint is published by the registered company Springer Nature Switzerland AG
The registered company address is: Gewerbestrasse 11, 6330 Cham, Switzerland

*To our parents Gülcan and Bekir Özyiğit and
Hacer and Hasan Hüseyin Selek.*

Preface

Radiation Oncology: A Case-Based Review provides residents, fellows, and practicing radiation oncologists with an evidence-based guide to the current management of cases in major tumor sites to appropriately decide, delineate, and prescribe tumor volumes/fields for intensity-modulated radiation therapy (IMRT) including volumetric modulated arc therapy (VMAT) and stereotactic radiosurgery (SRS) or stereotactic body radiotherapy (SBRT). Each section with an academic expert's perspective includes the most commonly seen cases to clarify different stages and specific clinical concepts in an order of case presentation, literature review, patient preparation, simulation, contouring, treatment planning, image-guided delivery, and follow-up. Every chapter offers practical step-by-step question and answer-based guidelines on clinical target volume (CTV) selection and treatment planning, accompanied with illustrations from slice-by-slice delineations on planning CT images to finalized plan evaluations based on detailed acceptance criteria. We will also provide acute and late toxicity management for each specific tumor site. Each individual chapter will begin with a representative case presentation. Then, we provided evidence-based review for each case from their diagnostic evaluation to radiotherapy. We also provided several high-quality figures for each case.

Case-based approach will prepare the reader for real-time clinical discussion environment in multidisciplinary setting. Furthermore, evidence-based guidance per case from scratch to evaluate the treatment planning and to follow up for toxicity management will provide self-confidence in a great spectrum of tumor sites. Case-based cutting-edge histopathological findings will equip the reader with tumor-specific adaptive immune classifications for future discussions in future oncological environment, along with the standard treatment approaches.

This comprehensive book will support knowledge- and guideline-based confidence, especially to manage the common cancers without outside referral, as well as to help in clinical challenges seen in practice. We hope *Radiation Oncology: A Case-Based Review* will meet the need for a practical and up-to-date review of major tumors for residents, fellows, and clinicians of radiation, medical, and surgical oncology, as well as for medical students, physicians, and medical physicists.

Ankara, Turkey
Istanbul, Turkey
Gokhan Ozyigit
Ugur Selek

Acknowledgments

The editors are indebted to Gesa Frese and Wilma McHugh from Springer DE and Samantha Sharmine Steven and SwarnaDivya Chokkalingam from SPi Global/ Springer Nature for their assistance in preparing *Radiation Oncology: A Case-Based Review*. We extend our most sincere gratitude to our colleagues and friends at Hacettepe University, Koç University, and Baskent University as well as our families.

Contents

Contributors

Fadil Akyol Department of Radiation Oncology, Faculty of Medicine, Hacettepe University, Ankara, Turkey

Fatih Biltekin Department of Radiation Oncology, Faculty of Medicine, Hacettepe University, Ankara, Turkey

Yasemin Bolukbasi Department of Radiation Oncology, Faculty of Medicine, Koç University, Istanbul, Turkey

Department of Radiation Oncology, The University of Texas MD Anderson Cancer Center, Houston, TX, USA

Mustafa Cengiz Department of Radiation Oncology, Faculty of Medicine, Hacettepe University, Ankara, Turkey

Ozan Cem Guler Department of Radiation Oncology, Faculty of Medicine, Karadeniz Technical University, Trabzon, Turkey

Melis Gultekin Department of Radiation Oncology, Faculty of Medicine, Hacettepe University, Ankara, Turkey

Murat Gurkaynak Department of Radiation Oncology, Faculty of Medicine, Hacettepe University, Ankara, Turkey

Pervin Hurmuz Department of Radiation Oncology, Faculty of Medicine, Hacettepe University, Ankara, Turkey

Cem Onal Department of Radiation Oncology, Faculty of Medicine, Başkent University, Adana, Turkey

Gokhan Ozyigit Department of Radiation Oncology, Faculty of Medicine, Hacettepe University, Ankara, Turkey

Yucel Saglam Department of Radiation Oncology, School of Medicine, Koç University, Istanbul, Turkey

Sezin Yuce Sari Department of Radiation Oncology, Faculty of Medicine, Hacettepe University, Ankara, Turkey

Ugur Selek Department of Radiation Oncology, School of Medicine, Koç University, Istanbul, Turkey

Department of Radiation Oncology, The University of Texas MD Anderson Cancer Center, Houston, TX, USA

Duygu Sezen Department of Radiation Oncology, School of Medicine, Koç University, Istanbul, Turkey

Gozde Yazici Department of Radiation Oncology, Faculty of Medicine, Hacettepe University, Ankara, Turkey

Ferah Yildiz Department of Radiation Oncology, Faculty of Medicine, Hacettepe University, Ankara, Turkey

Faruk Zorlu Department of Radiation Oncology, Faculty of Medicine, Hacettepe University, Ankara, Turkey

Central Nervous System Tumors

1

Gozde Yazici, Melis Gultekin, Pervin Hurmuz,
Sezin Yuce Sari, Faruk Zorlu, and Gokhan Ozyigit

1.1 Medulloblastoma

Overview

Medulloblastoma accounts for approximately 20% of all primary tumors of the central nervous system among children <19 years of age. The peak incidence is between 5 and 9 years of age, and nearly 70% of patients are diagnosed before 20 years of age.

These tumors occur exclusively in the posterior fossa. Patients with medulloblastoma present with symptoms of increased intracranial pressure, including headaches, nausea, vomiting, and altered mental status. Gait ataxia or truncal instability is seen in midline lesions, whereas tumors in the lateral cerebellar lesions cause limb clumsiness or incoordination.

One third of patients will have evidence of tumor dissemination through the subarachnoid space either by imaging or cerebrospinal fluid (CSF) examination. Magnetic resonance imaging (MRI) of the craniospinal axis and CSF examination are complementary techniques for diagnosis of dissemination and both should be performed at diagnosis unless contraindicated. In that case lumbar puncture should be delayed for 2 weeks to avoid potential contamination of the specimen with surgical debris. Medulloblastomas rarely metastasize outside of the nervous system, and systemic staging is not required unless there are findings of bone metastases.

G. Yazici (✉) · M. Gultekin · P. Hurmuz · S. Y. Sari · F. Zorlu · G. Ozyigit
Department of Radiation Oncology, Faculty of Medicine, Hacettepe University, Ankara, Turkey
e-mail: yazicig@hacettepe.edu.tr

© Springer Nature Switzerland AG 2019
G. Ozyigit, U. Selek (eds.), *Radiation Oncology*,
https://doi.org/10.1007/978-3-319-97145-2_1

Maximal safe resection is the first step in treatment of medulloblastoma, there is no role for a biopsy if the medulloblastoma diagnosis is supported by imaging studies. The differential diagnosis of a posterior fossa mass in a child includes pilocytic astrocytoma, ependymoma, and atypical teratoid/rhabdoid tumors (ATRT). Metastatic tumors should be kept in mind in an adult patient with a posterior fossa lesion.

Treatment includes a combination of surgery, radiation therapy (in patients >3 years old). Craniospinal irradiation (CSI) plays a critical role in providing long-term disease control. Patients >3 years old are stratified based on the volume of postoperative residual tumor, the presence or absence of metastases, and the presence or absence of diffuse anaplasia into "standard risk" and "high risk" categories. Recent trials treating standard-risk medulloblastoma using reduced-dose CSI and adjuvant chemotherapy have produced EFS rates of 81–86%. However the survival rates for high risk disease is 70%, respectively. Outcomes are inferior in infants and children younger than 3 years with exception of those patients with the MBEN histologic subtype. Treatment for medulloblastoma is associated with significant morbidity, especially in the youngest patients. Recent molecular subclassification of medulloblastoma has potential prognostic and therapeutic implications. Future incorporation of molecular subgroups into treatment protocols will hopefully improve both survival outcomes and post-treatment quality of life.

Key Words: Medulloblastoma; Radiotherapy

1.1.1 Case Presentation

Sixteen year old boy admitted to the hospital with complaints of headache and vomiting. His headache started a week prior to his admission. His physical examination revealed loss of motor strength in his left arm and leg (4/5). A cranial magnetic resonance imaging (MRI) was performed. The MRI showed a left heterogeneous contrast enhancing cerebellar lesion 5 × 4 cm in diameter (Fig. 1.1). There was cerebellar tonsillar herniation due to mass effect. Cranial MRI suggested that the lesion was highly suspicious of medulloblastoma so he underwent spinal MRI. The spinal MRI was normal with no signs of nodular seeding or leptomeningeal infiltration. The cerebrospinal fluid (CSF) examination was planned after surgery due to tonsillar herniation. A gross total resection was performed and in the postoperative MRI performed in the first 24 h there was no residual disease (Fig. 1.2). The pathological diagnosis was medulloblastoma. Histopathologically it was anaplastic large cell and genetically it was SHH active and p53 mutated. The CSF examination performed 2 weeks after the surgery was normal.

He had high risk disease so he underwent craniospinal irradiation to a total dose of 36 Gy with 1.8 Gy/fraction, and a posterior fossa boost of 18 Gy with 1.8 Gy/

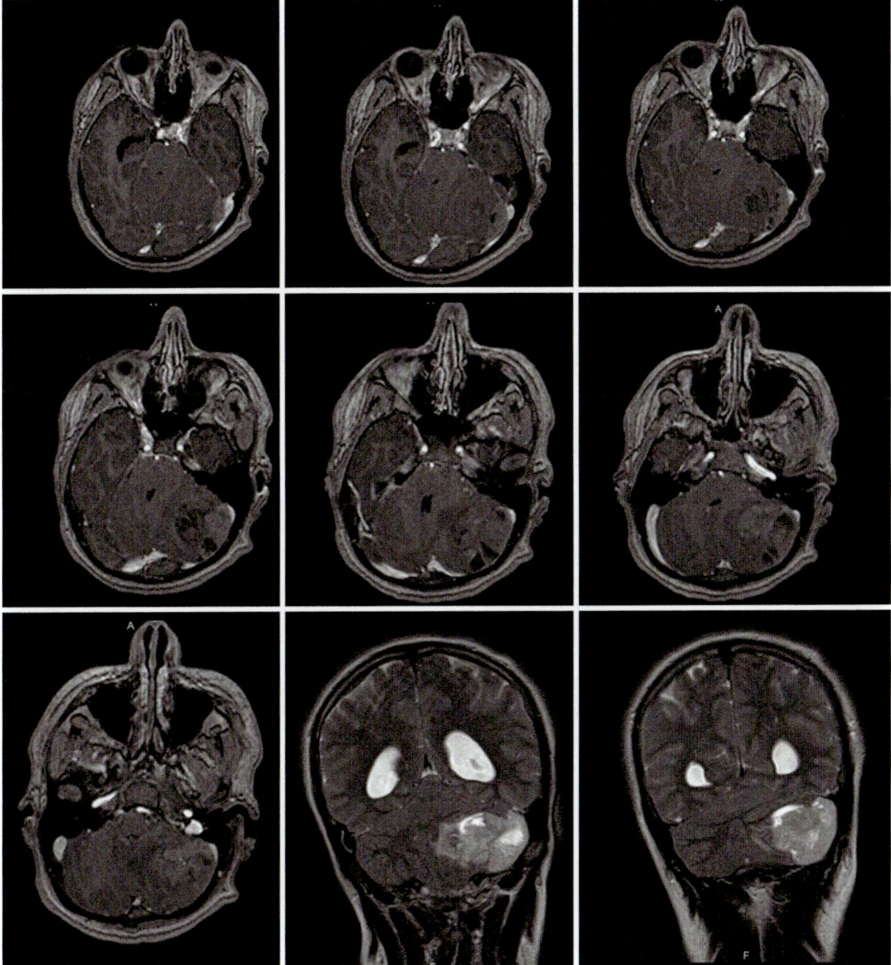

Fig. 1.1 Preoperative magnetic resonance images showing left cerebellar lesion

fraction. He received three cycles of cisplatin and etoposide after radiation, and consolidation chemotherapy consisting of vincristine and cyclophosphamide.

1.1.2 Evidence Based Treatment Recommendations

1.1.2.1 Risk Stratification

Chang et al. proposed an operative staging system for medulloblastomas in 1969 [1]. The Chang Staging system for medulloblastoma is given in Table 1.1.

T stage of the Chang system, relating to tumor size and extent of local invasion at surgery, does not seem to demonstrate prognostic significance and is no longer used. Instead of the initial T stage the presence of residual tumour >1.5 cm^2 confer an increased risk for local recurrence.

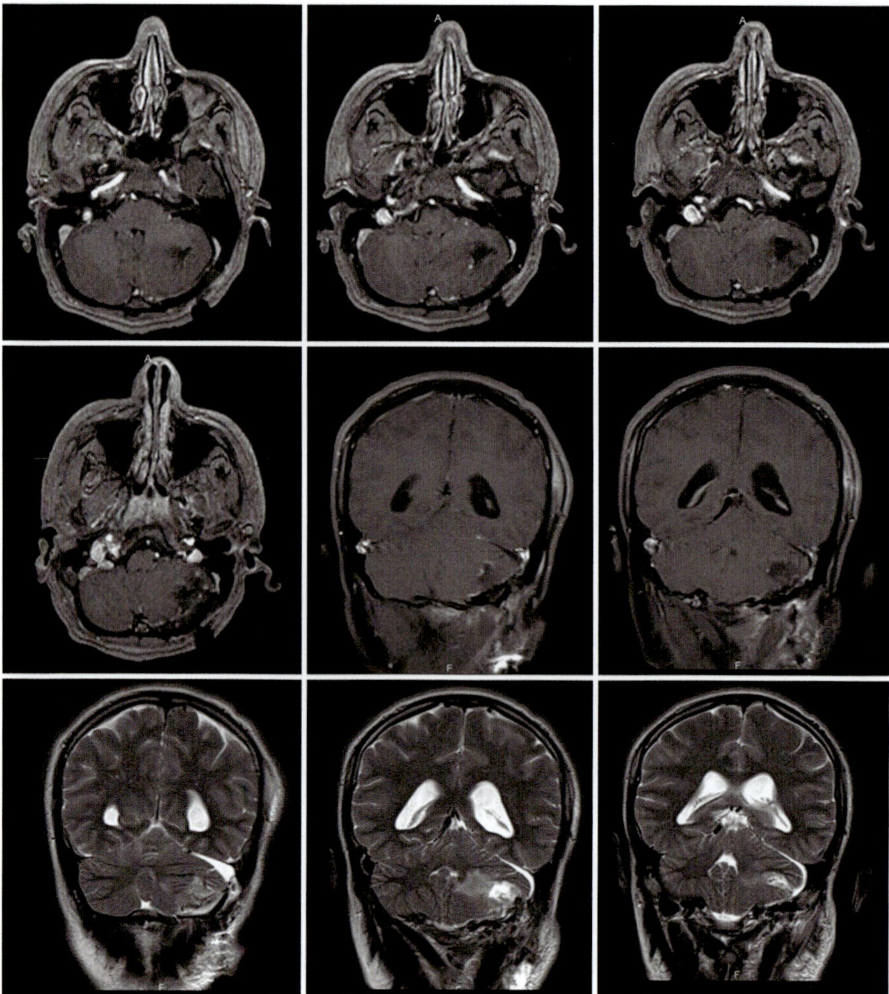

Fig. 1.2 Postoperative magnetic resonance images showing gross total excision of the left cerebellar lesion

The most important factors affecting outcome have been the extent of disease, the residual tumour volume and the age of the patient at diagnosis. There is a non-linear relationship between age and prognosis in patients with medulloblastoma. Those younger than 3 years old and adults do worse.

Historically the treatment decisions were based on these three factors. CSI causes severe neurologic impairment if performed in patients younger than 3 years of age. In this specific group aim is not just to improve disease control but also to prevent progressively worse neurologic outcome.

Children ≥3 years of age are stratified to average-risk disease and high-risk disease groups.

Table 1.1 Chang staging system for medulloblastoma

T stage

T1	Tumor <3 cm in diameter and limited to the classic midline position in the vermis, the roof of the fourth ventricle, and less frequently to the cerebellar hemispheres
T2	Tumor more than 3 cm in diameter, further invading one adjacent structure or partially filling the fourth ventricle
T3	T3a: Tumor further invading two adjacent structures or completely filling the fourth ventricle with extension into the aqueduct of Sylvius, foramen of Magendie, or foramen of Luschka, thus producing marked internal hydrocephalus T3b: Tumor arising from the floor of the fourth ventricle or brain stem and filling the fourth ventricle.
T4	Tumor further spreading through the aqueduct of Sylvius to involve the third ventricle or midbrain, or tumor extending to the upper cervical cord

M stage

M0	No evidence of gross subarachnoid or hematogenous metastasis
M1	Microscopic tumor cells found in cerebrospinal fluid
M2	Gross nodular seedings demonstrated in the cerebellar, cerebral subarachnoid space, or in the third or lateral ventricles
M3	Gross nodular seeding in spinal subarachnoid space
M4	Extraneuroaxial metastasis

Standard risk disease was defined as total or near-total resection (<1.5 cm^2 residual disease) at the time of surgery and no evidence of disseminated disease by brain and spine magnetic resonance imaging (MRI) and cerebrospinal fluid (CSF) analysis [2].

High-risk disease was defined as the presence of ≥ 1.5 cm^2 of residual tumor after surgery and/or evidence of metastatic disease.

However there is an evolving understanding other prognostic factors such as molecular markers and histopathology in determining prognosis.

The 2007 WHO classification system recognizes classic medulloblastoma, desmoplastic/nodular medulloblastoma, medulloblastoma with extensive nodularity (MBEN), anaplastic medulloblastoma, and large cell medulloblastoma as histopathologic variants of medulloblastoma, and all are categorized as grade IV neoplasms. The desmoplastic/nodular and MBEN variants are associated with an improved prognosis, and large cell and anaplastic medulloblastomas have a distinctly poor prognosis when compared to the classic variant [3]. Large cell and anaplastic variants are differentiated by the degree of anaplasia, Significantly inferior outcomes have been observed in patients with increasing degrees of anaplasia [3].

Current risk stratification includes the presence of diffuse anaplasia as high risk (Table 1.2).

In 2010, in Boston, a consensus on the molecular subgrouping was developed between experts of medulloblastoma. Four distinct subgroups were identified [4]. Wingless (Wnt), sonic hedgehog (Shh), Group 3, and Group 4 subgroups were characterized which have divergent cell histology, genetics, clinical behavior. These subgroups predict outcome more accurately than the histopathological or clinical staging. Tumors that show activation of the Wingless (WNT) pathway have

Table 1.2 Medulloblastoma risk stratification in patients older than 3 years of age

Risk group	Characteristics
Standard risk	Total or near-total resection with <1.5 cm^2 residual disease and M0 disease and No diffuse anaplasia
High risk	Residual disease more than 1.5 cm^2 or M+ disease or Diffuse anaplasia

Table 1.3 2016 WHO classification of medulloblastoma based on genetics

2016 WHO classification of medulloblastoma
Medulloblastoma, WNT-activated
Medulloblastoma, SHH-activated
TP53-mutant
TP53-wildtype
Medulloblastoma, non-WNT/non-SHH
Medulloblastoma, Group 3
Medulloblastoma, Group 4

excellent prognosis with the standard therapeutic approaches. Whereas, tumors with amplification of the MYC proto-oncogene ("group 3") have the worst prognosis. The sonic hedgehog (SHH) pathway activated group and those in group 4 have an intermediate prognosis, with the exception of SHH tumors containing TP53 mutations, which are associated with a particularly poor prognosis.

In the last update of WHO classification (2016) besides the histopathological features the molecular characteristics are used in the classification of medulloblastoma. The molecular classification is based on the transcriptome or methylome profiling (Table 1.3).

These subgroups are being integrated into clinical trial designs. In 2015, a consensus conference was held in Heidelberg and the risk stratification based on molecular subgroups was defined in childhood medulloblastoma [5]. The consortium reached a consensus on the following risk groups: low risk (>90% survival), average (standard) risk (75–90% survival), high risk (50–75% survival) and very high risk (<50% survival) disease (Table 1.4).

1.1.2.2 Treatment Recommendations for Standard Risk Patients Older than 3 Years of Age

The term "medulloblastoma" was first introduced by Harvey Cushing and Percival Bailey in 1925. In this era no children with this diagnosis survived until craniospinal irradiation was used potoperativelly. Paterson and Farr, in 1953, reported a 65% of

Table 1.4 Proposed risk stratification for non-infant childhood medulloblastoma

Risk group	Characteristics
Low risk	Non-metastatic WNT patients under the age of 16 Non-metastatic Group 4 patients with chromosome 11 loss
Standard risk	SHH: Non-metastatic, TP53-wild type, no MYCN amplification Group 3: Non metastatic, no MYC amplification Group 4: Non-metastatic, no chromosome 11 loss
High risk	SHH: Metastatic or MYCN amplification Group 4: Metastatic
Very high risk	SHH: TP53 mutation Group 3: Metastatic
Indeterminate groups, unanswered questions	Non-metastatic MYC amplified group 3 patients Cut-off for MYC or MYCN amplification Melanotic medulloblastoma and medullomyoblastoma Anaplastic and/or large cell histology in Group 3 and Group 4 Isochromosome 17q in Group 3 Metastatic WNT patients

3 year survival rate with 35 Gy craniospinal irradiation and a 15 Gy posterior fossa boost [6]. In the subsequent multicenter randomized trials chemotherapy was integrated to surgical resection and RT with the purpose of increasing the overall survival and decreasing the long term toxicity related to high dose craniospinal irradiation.

In standard risk patients several strategies were used to decrease the craniospinal radiation (CSI) dose and to increase overall survival. Deutsch *et al.* decreased the CSI dose to 23.4 Gy but in their early report they observed an increased rate of CNS failure compared to 36 Gy [7, 8]. With longer follow-up there were no differences between the two groups [8]. Packer et al. combined chemotherapy with 23.4 Gy CSI and reported a 5 year event free survival rate of 90% [9]. Studies conducted by the International Society of Pediatric Oncology (SIOP) and the Children's Oncology Group supported the use of 23.4–24 Gy CSI with adjuvant chemotherapy [10, 11].

In Children's Oncology Group (COG) phase III study, published in 2006 and updated in 2012, 379 patients with M0 medulloblastoma between the ages of 3 and 21 years were treated with 2340 cGy of craniospinal and 5580 cGy of posterior fossa irradiation and concomitant weekly vincristine [2, 9]. Patients were randomized between postradiation cisplatin and vincristine plus either CCNU or cyclophosphamide. Five- and 10-year event-free survivals were 81% and 76%; overall survivals were 87% and 81%. Event-free survival was not impacted by the chemotherapeutic regimen.

A COG (ACNS0331) study investigated further CSI dose-reduction to 18 Gy in young children (aged 3–7 years) with standard risk disease [12]. However the preliminary results showed worse outcomes with the reduced (18 Gy) dose of CSI, and therefore 23.4 Gy CSI remains the standard of care in this group.

A retrospective study analyzing pattern of recurrence in patients treated with a CSI and a posterior fossa boost showed that isolated failures in the PF but outside the tumor bed is rare (1 out of 27 pts) [13]. Other studies also confirmed that posterior fossa failures are primarily in the tumor bed and are often associated with leptomeningeal failure [14]. Current protocols use a tumour bed boost instead of a posterior fossa boost to further decrease the neurological side effects of radiotherapy by decreasing the total dose to the temporal lobes [10].

In a study analyzing the impact of neoadjuvant approach on survival as compared to maintenance chemotherapy after completion of radiotherapy, delays in the initiation of radiation therapy was associated with inferior outcomes [15–17].

1.1.2.3 High–Risk Disease in Children Older than 3 Years

The optimal treatment for children with high risk disease is unknown. There is an increased risk for recurrence and death even with intensified treatments.

In a Pediatric Oncology Group Randomized Trial (POG 9031) 224 patients with high-risk medulloblastoma were randomly assigned to receive either chemotherapy entailing three cycles of cisplatin and etoposide before radiation or the same chemotherapy regimen after radiation; both groups received consolidation chemotherapy consisting of vincristine and cyclophosphamide [18]. CSI dose for patients with M0-1 disease was 35.2 Gy. Patients with M2-3 disease received 40.0 Gy CSI. Five-year EFS and OS rates for initial chemotherapy arm were 66.0% and 73%, in the radiotherapy first arm these values were 70.0% and 76% respectively.

In a phase II COG study, 161 children ≥3 years of age with high-risk medulloblastoma were treated with postoperative craniospinal RT with concurrent carboplatin and vincristine, followed by six maintenance cycles of cyclophosphamide and vincristine with or without cisplatin. The five-year progression-free and overall survival rates for patients treated with the cisplatin-containing regimen were 59% and 68%; for those not treated with cisplatin, progression-free and overall survival rates were similar (71 and 82%) [19].

Treatment modifications to improve outcomes in high risk medulloblastoma patients are being studied. High-dose chemotherapy and autologous hematopoietic cell transplantation (HCT) following RT or hyperfractionated accelerated RT with increased dose have been shown to be feasible but long term results are needed [11, 20].

1.1.2.4 Infants and Children Younger than 3 Years of Age

Children younger than 3 years of age are at high risk of severe neurologic impairment if treated with craniospinal RT. The studies focused on intensifying chemotherapy at the postoperative setting to delay or omit CSI. However survival outcomes have been poor with 1 and 2 year progression free survival rates of 42% and 34% [21, 22].

Studies using intensive five-drug chemotherapy regimen and intraventricular methotrexate reported five-year overall survival and progression-free survival rates were 66% and 58%, respectively [23]. In patients without postoperative residual tumor or evidence of metastatic disease, five-year progression-free survival and overall survival rates were up to 82% and 92%, respectively. Unfortunately, the use intraventricular methotrexate was shown to be associated with significantly lower age-matched IQ scores, but the impairment was less severe than in children in who received RT.

Totally resected M0 desmoplastic nodular medulloblastoma or medulloblastoma with extensive nodularity (MBEN) histological subtypes are an exception. The HIT-SKK'92 trial showed five-year progression-free and overall survival of 85% and 95% in this group [22]. Outcomes were significantly inferior in patients with other histologic variants.

1.1.3 Target Delineation and Treatment

Craniospinal radiotherapy is a critical component in the management of medulloblastoma. The goal is to treat the entire intracranial volume and the subarachnoid space throughout the spinal axis.

During target delineation attention should be paid to the cribriform plate, inferior border of the theca sac, lateral sacral nerve roots, and the subdural space extending alone the nerve roots. An example of target delineation for craniospinal irradiation is given in Fig. 1.3.

When the posterior fossa volume is considered as boost CTV, one should cover the tentorium superiorly and C1 inferiorly. Laterally the posterior fossa volume includes the entire cerebellum and anteriorly it includes the brainstem and lower midbrain. The involved field volume GTV should include the tumor bed (anything in contact with the initial tumor before surgery) and any residual gross disease. Care should be taken to account for anatomical shifts following surgery. An expansion of 1–1.5 cm is typically used to form the CTV for the involved field boost. An example of target delineation for posterior fossa boost and involved field boost are given in Figs. 1.4 and 1.5.

Most CSI treatments are delivered with the patient in the prone position, and most techniques involve field matching with fields matched anterior to the spinal cord, which creates a small area of underdosing in the cord but avoids any areas of overlap (Fig. 1.6). The use of IMRT and scanning proton techniques allow for treatment without matching of fields (Figs. 1.7 and 1.8). Protons have a theoretical advantage because of the lack of exit dose which avoids dose to the thyroid, heart, lungs, abdominal organs and ovaries. However in a recent report no difference in patterns of failure, recurrence free survival, or overall survival was found according to radiotherapy modality.

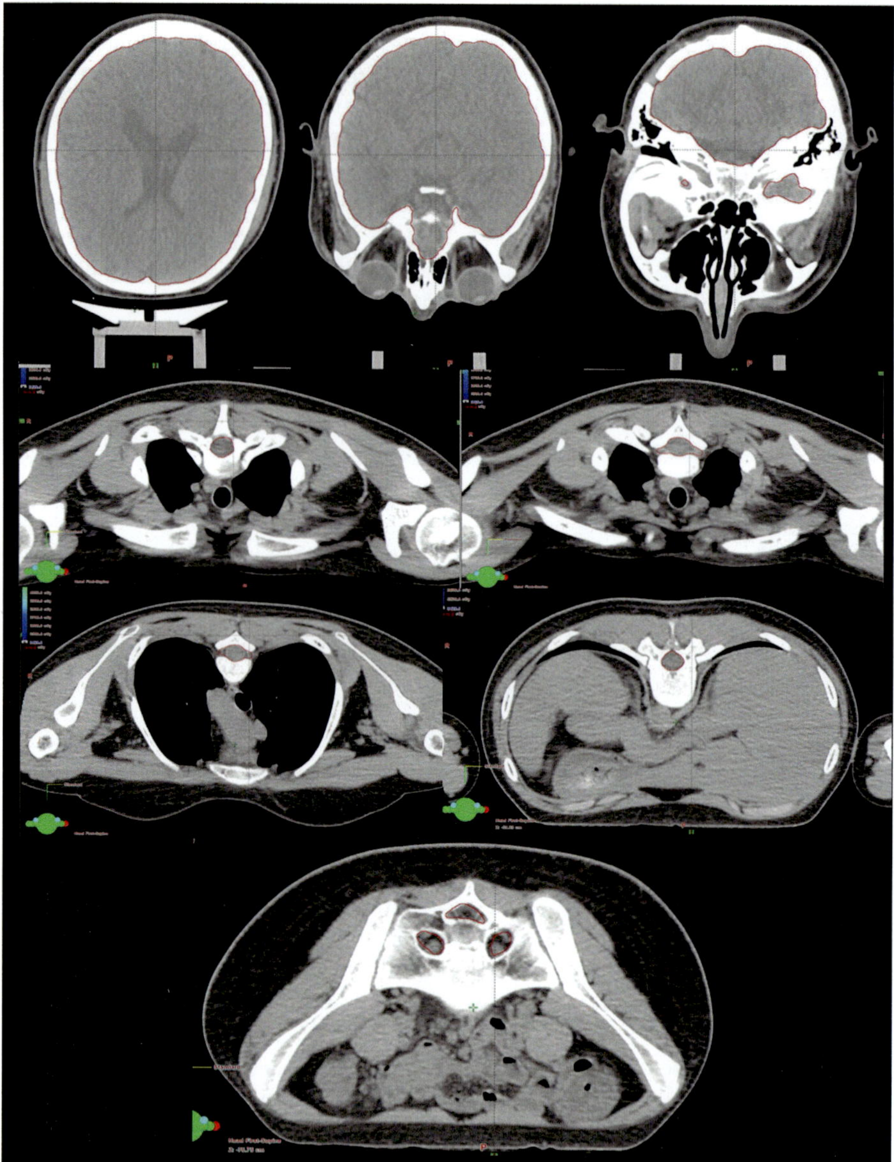

Fig. 1.3 Target delineation for cranispinal irradiation

1.1.4 Follow-Up

Patients should be followed at regular intervals to monitor for treatment complications and disease recurrence. The recommended follow-up periods are every 3 months for the first 1–2 years, then every 6–12 months thereafter. Recurrence after

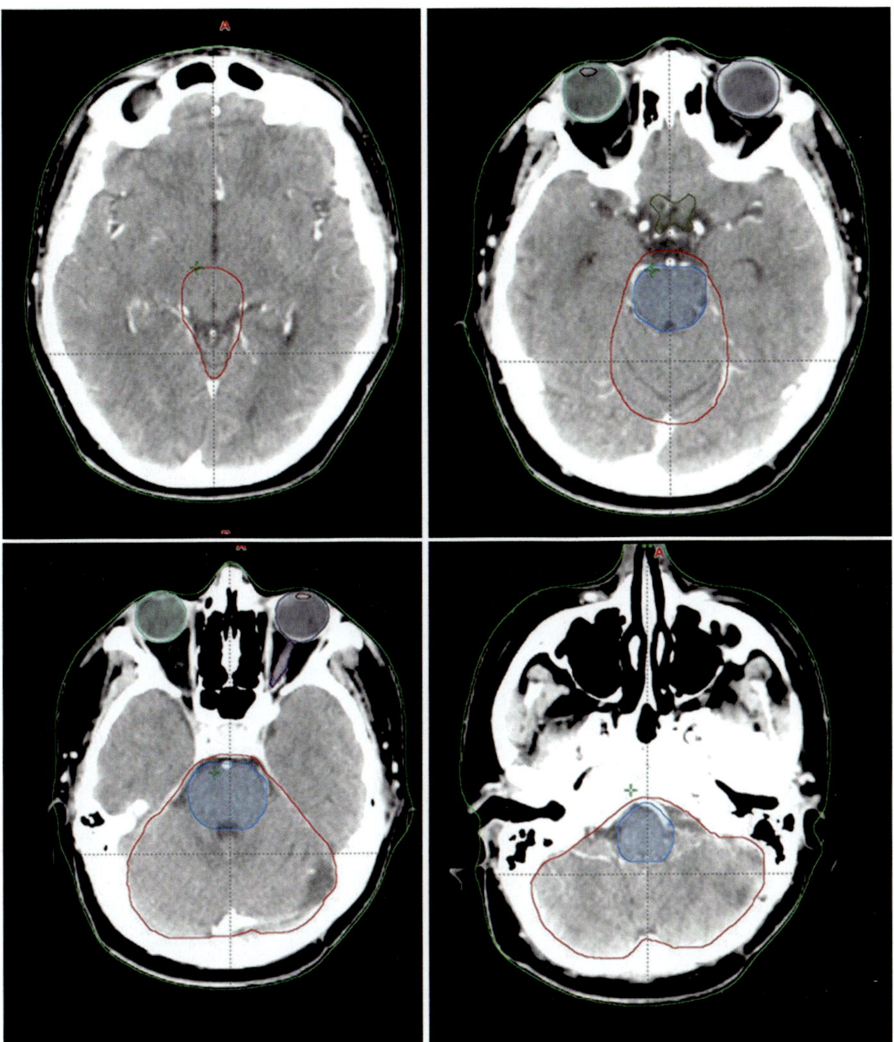

Fig. 1.4 Target delineation for posterior fossa boost

7 years is uncommon but the follow-up should continue to evaluate treatment related complications.

Isolated spinal relapse are less frequent than brain or combined brain and spine relapses. The imaging of the brain should be performed in all patients. However spinal imaging can be restricted to patients with M+ disease at diagnosis.

Endocrinopathies such as GH, adrenocorticotrophic hormone (ACTH), and thyroid-stimulation hormone (TSH) deficiencies, neurocognitive and neurosensory impairment, primary hypothyroidism and cerebrovascular disease can be observed in survivors of medulloblastoma. We should be aware of these side effects during the follow up.

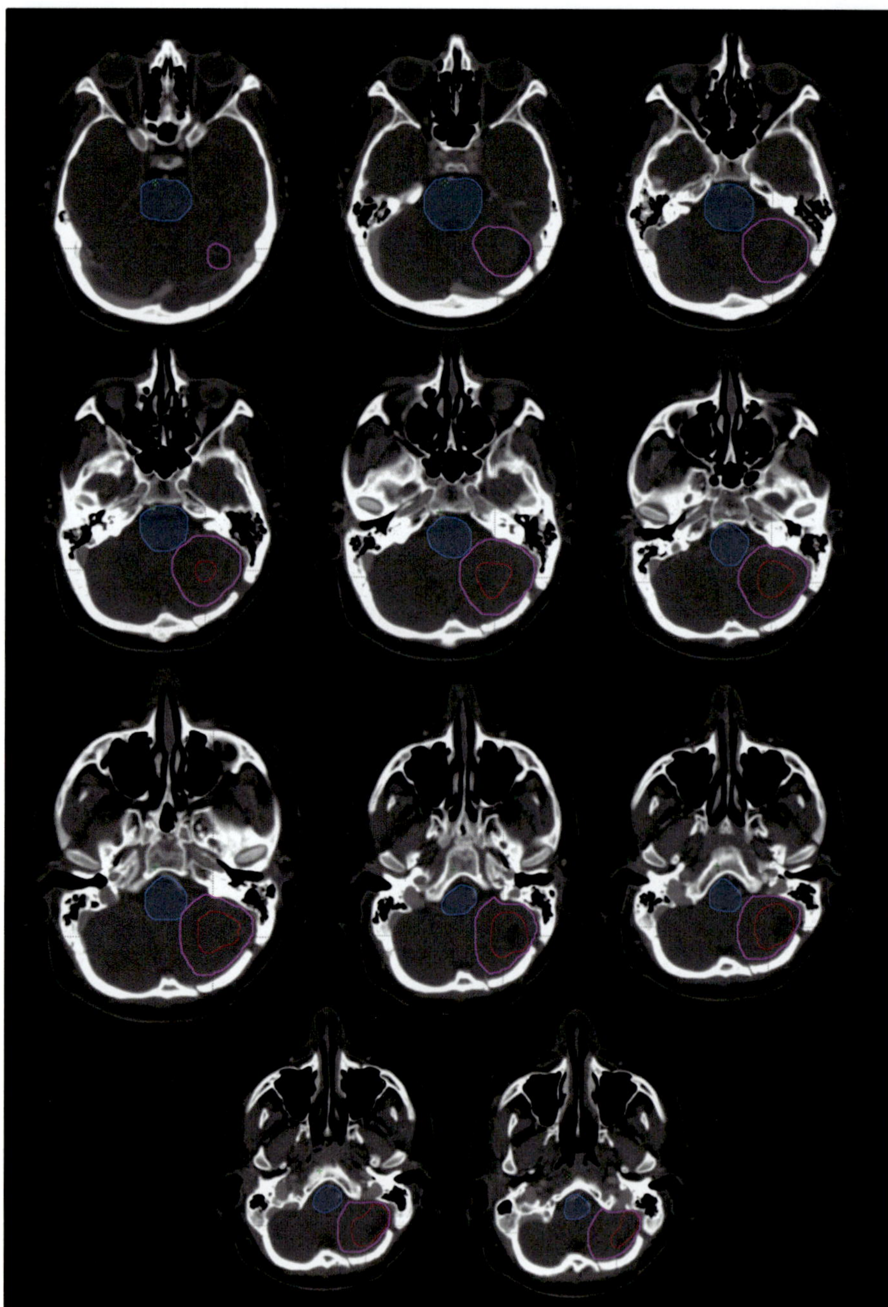

Fig. 1.5 Target delineation for tumor bed boost. Gross tumor volume (GTV) is delineated as red, and clinical target volume (CTV) is formed by defining 1 cm margin around GTV. Gross tumor volume (GTV) is delineated as magenda

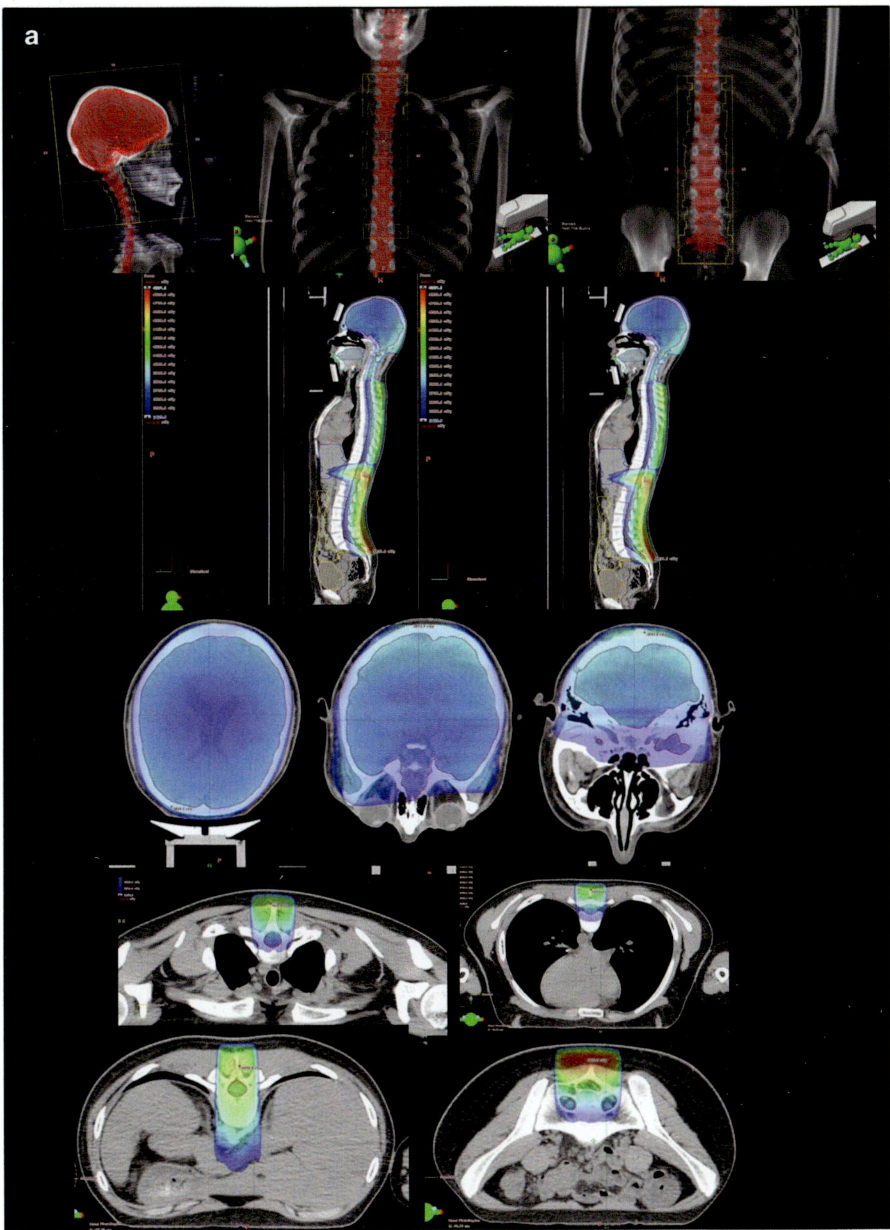

Fig. 1.6 (**a**) 3D conformal plan of craniospinal irradiation with coach angle. Notice the overdose is in abdomen. (**b**) 3D conformal plan of craniospinal irradiation with asymetric collimation. Notice the overdose is in heart

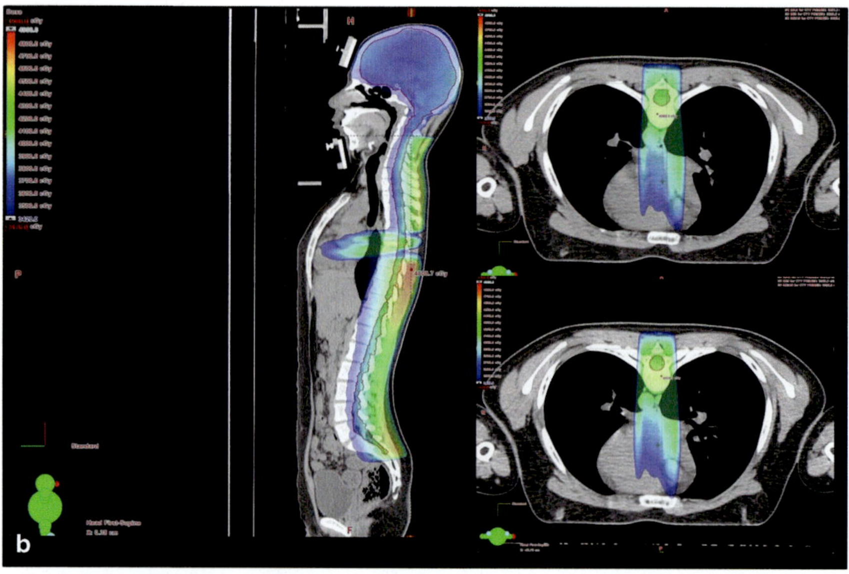

Fig. 1.6 (continued)

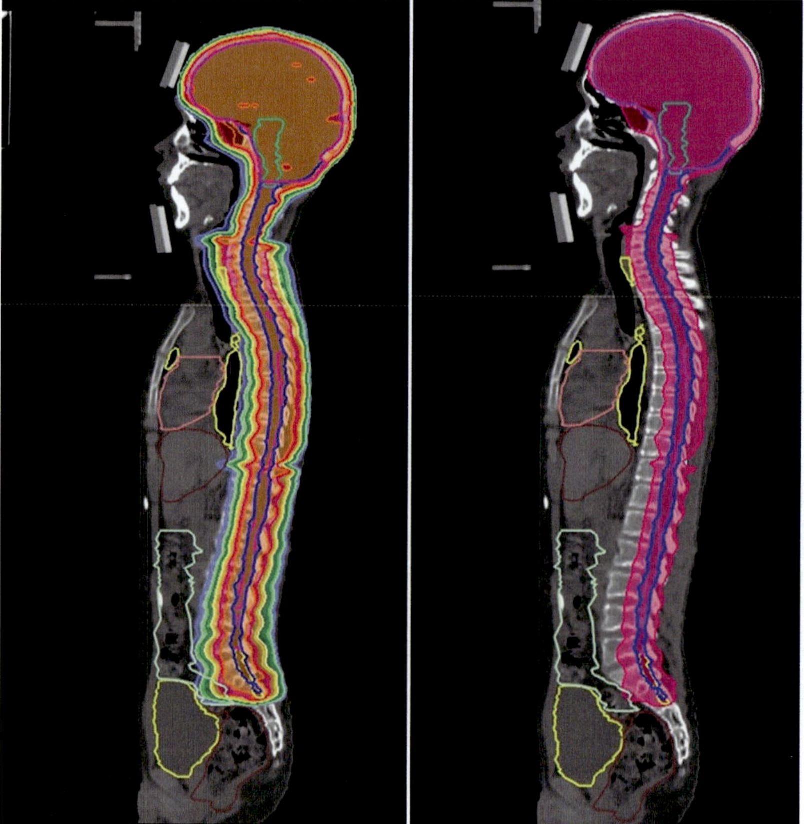

Fig. 1.7 VMAT plan for the cranispinal radiotherapy

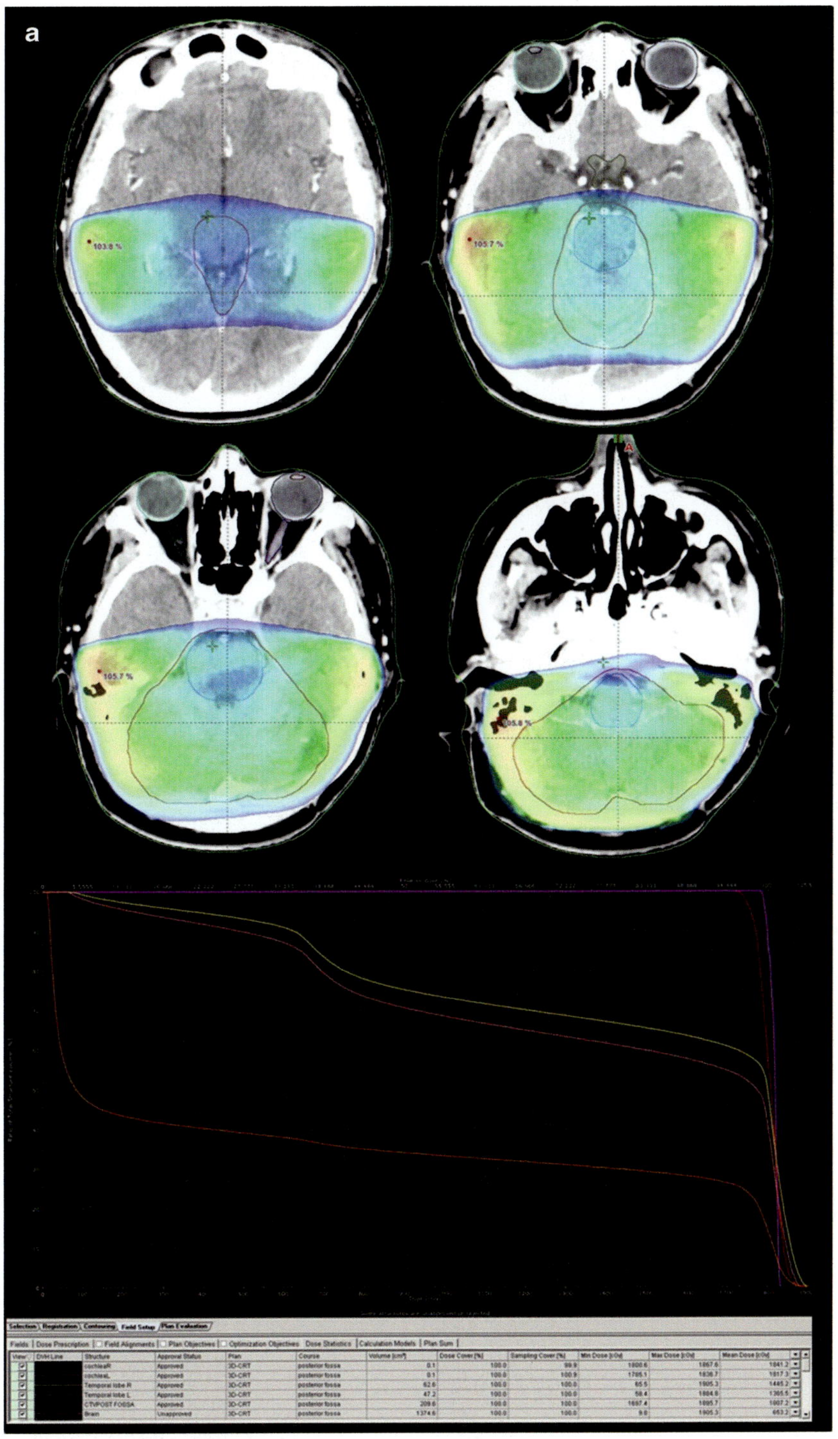

Fig. 1.8 (a) 3D plan for the posterior fossa boost, (b) IMRT plan for the posterior fossa boost, (c) IMRT plan for the tumor bed boost

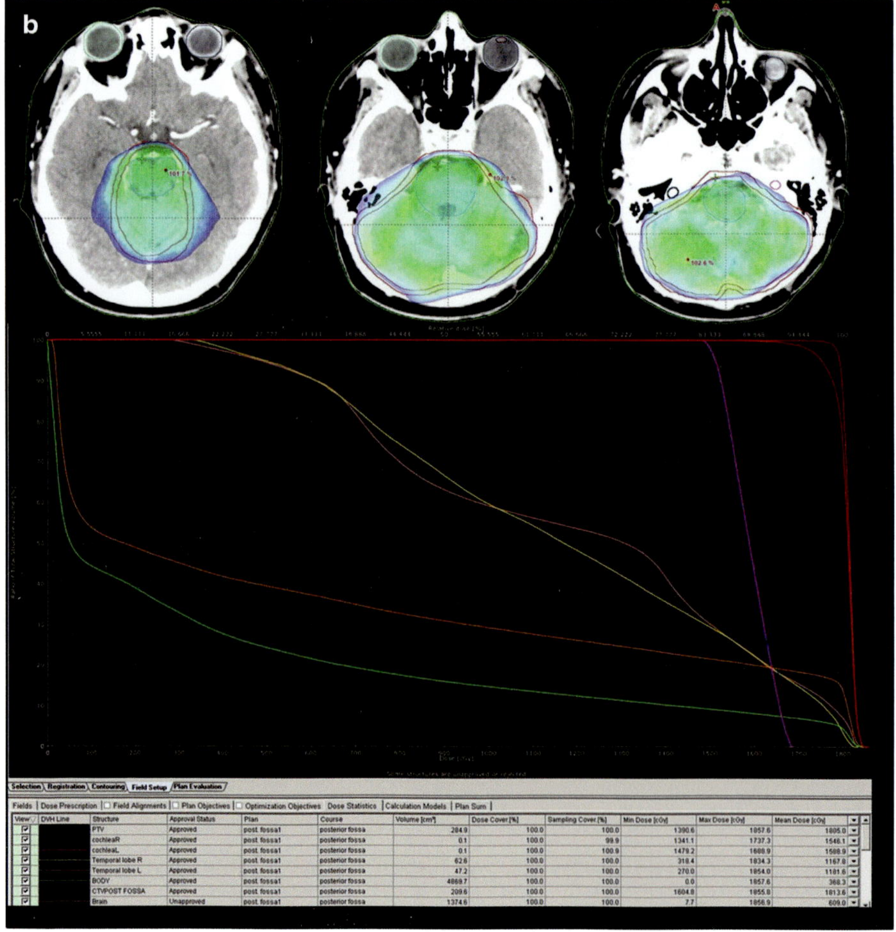

Fig. 1.8 (continued)

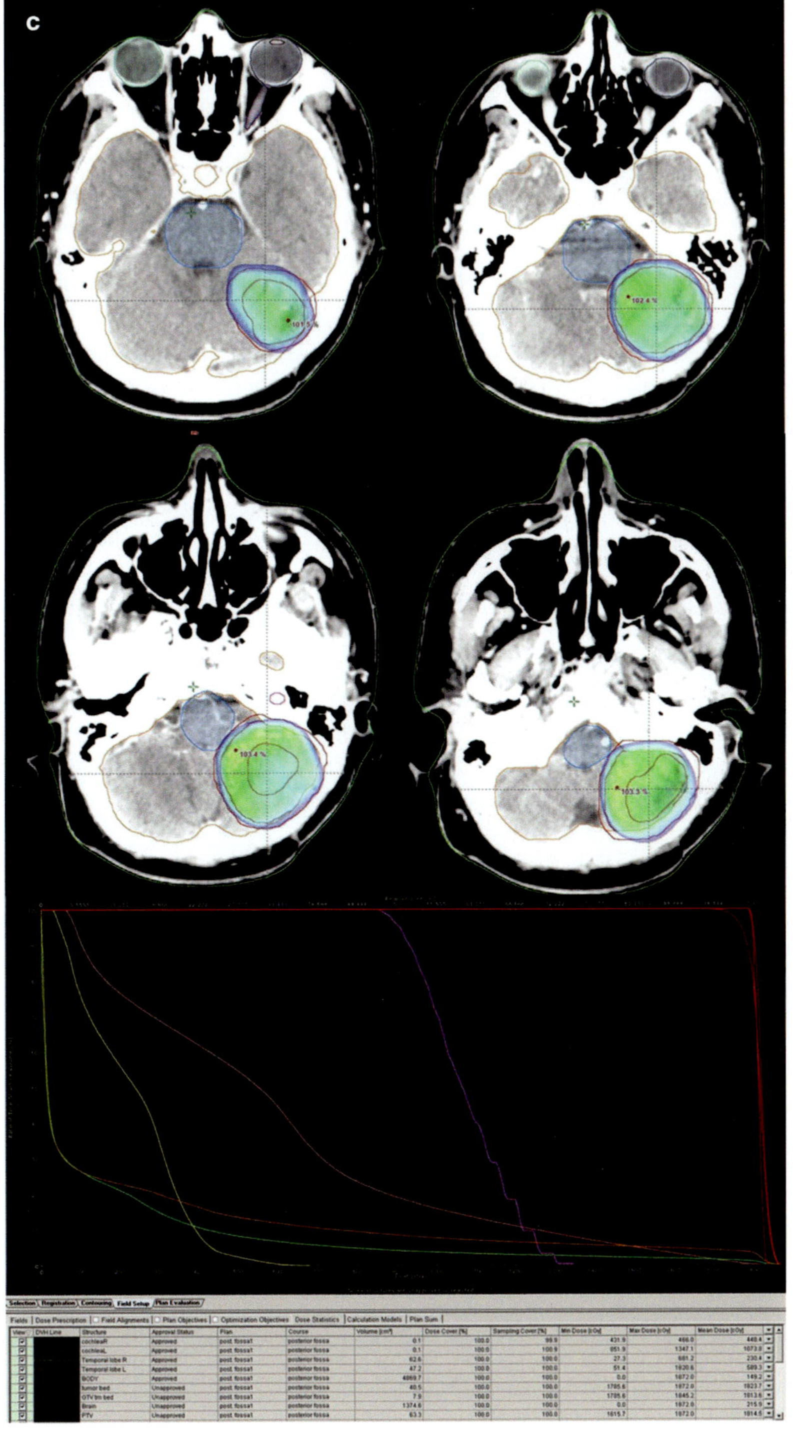

Fig. 1.8 (continued)

1.2   High Grade Glioma

Overview

High-grade gliomas are malignant, rapidly progressive brain tumors. Historically, the subgroups consisted of anaplastic astrocytoma, anaplastic oligodendroglioma, anaplastic oligoastrocytoma and glioblastoma based on histopathologic features. However, the 2016 update of glioma World Health Organization (WHO) classification is not only based on histopathologic appearance but also on molecular parameters, and both WHO classification and International Society of Neuropathology-Haarlem guidelines encourage the use of integrated and layered diagnoses 1 [24]. Astrocytic and oligodendroglial tumors are now grouped as diffuse gliomas. Nuclear atypia and increased mitotic activity characterize anaplastic, grade III tumors, while microvascular proliferation and necrosis define grade IV tumors. The two key molecular parameters used in glioma diagnosis are isocitrate dehydrogenase (IDH) mutation status and the presence or absence of 1p/19q-codeletion. Both tumor type and histologic grade continue to hold prognostic value in the absence of molecular data.

Patients present with headache, seizures, memory loss, cognitive changes, motor weakness, etc. which are dependent upon the location and size of the lesion. Seizures, as a presenting symptom, occur less frequently in patients with glioblastoma than with lower-grade gliomas.

Brain magnetic resonance imaging (MRI) with contrast is often the only study required preoperatively. Patients with a contraindication to brain MRI should undergo head computed tomography (CT) with contrast. Screening for systemic malignancy is not necessary when the clinical and radiographic suspicion for high-grade glioma is high.

A tissue diagnosis is essential. A biopsy, either at the time of surgical resection or with a stereotactic biopsy, is required for diagnosis. Maximal surgical resection is the preferred treatment option. Although gross total resection is preferred whenever possible, subtotal resection or biopsy alone may be required depending upon the location and extent of the tumor.

The median overall survival of patients with glioblastoma is approximately 10–12 months. Patients with anaplastic astrocytoma, IDH-wildtype, have a median overall survival of 2–3 years. Whereas this value is 8–10 years for IDH-mutant anaplastic astrocytoma. The median overall survival is 15–20 years for IDH-mutant 1p/19q-codeleted anaplastic oligodendroglioma.

IDH-mutant glioblastomas make up approximately 10% of all glioblastomas. They are histologically similar to IDH-wildtype glioblastoma. IDH-mutant glioblastomas occur in younger adults (mean age 45 years) and have a more favorable prognosis, with a median survival approximately two times longer than that of IDH-wildtype tumors.

IDH-wildtype glioblastoma is the most common malignant primary brain tumor in adults. Histologic variants include giant cell glioblastoma, gliosarcoma, and epithelioid glioblastoma. The prognosis for all glioblastoma variants is poor, with survival commonly <2 years.

A designation of not otherwise specified (NOS) is possible in new 2016 WHO classification system and signifies that a complete, integrated histopathologic and molecular diagnosis is not available because genetic testing was not performed or was inconclusive.

The most important prognostic factors affecting outcome in patients with high-grade glioma are age, Karnofsky performance status (KPS), tumor grade (glioblastoma versus anaplastic glioma), isocitrate dehydrogenase (IDH) status, and several additional molecular genetic alterations. The extent of initial surgical resection also influences the prognosis.

There are nomograms incorporating patient age at diagnosis, gender, KPS, extent of resection, and O6-methylguanine-DNA methyltransferase (MGMT) status to estimate 6-, 12-, and 24-month survival probability.

Adjuvant radiation therapy is a standard component of therapy for glioblastoma that has been shown to improve local control and survival after resection. Temozolomide, an oral alkylating agent, also improves progression-free and overall survival when given in combination with radiation. In addition, a device that delivers alternating electric fields (TTFields) may also improve survival when used in patients with newly diagnosed glioblastoma.

Key Words: High-grade glioma; Radiotherapy

1.2.1 Case Presentation

A 60 year old man admitted to the hospital with complaints of confusion and hallucination. He had complaints of headache for the past 3 weeks. His physical examination was normal. His MRI revealed a left temporal 4.5 × 4.6 cm contrast enhancing lesion (Fig. 1.9). The lesion had a necrotic center and there was peripheral edema. The MRI was highly suspicious of a malign glial lesion. He had no history of smoking and had no known illnesses. He underwent surgery. His postoperative MRI performed in the first 24 h after surgery showed early operative changes in the left temporal lobe. There was a 12 × 10 mm residual lesion in the inferior part of the resection cavity (Fig. 1.10). The pathological examination was consistent with glioblastoma, IDH wild type. He had no complications after surgery and he received concomitant chemoradiotherapy (60 Gy in 2 Gy/fraction) with temozolomide. He also received adjuvant temozolomide for six cycles.

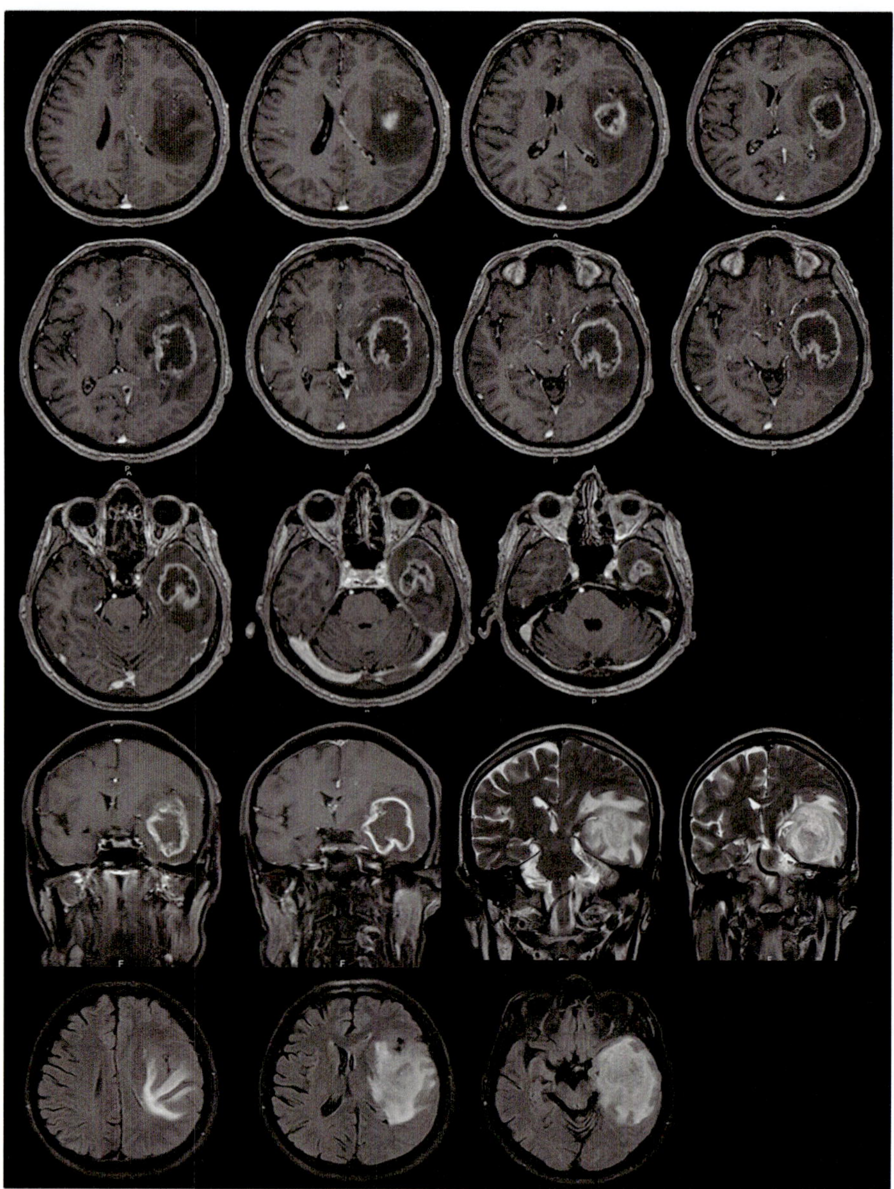

Fig. 1.9 MRI revealed a left temporal 4.5 × 4.6 cm contrast enhancing lesion

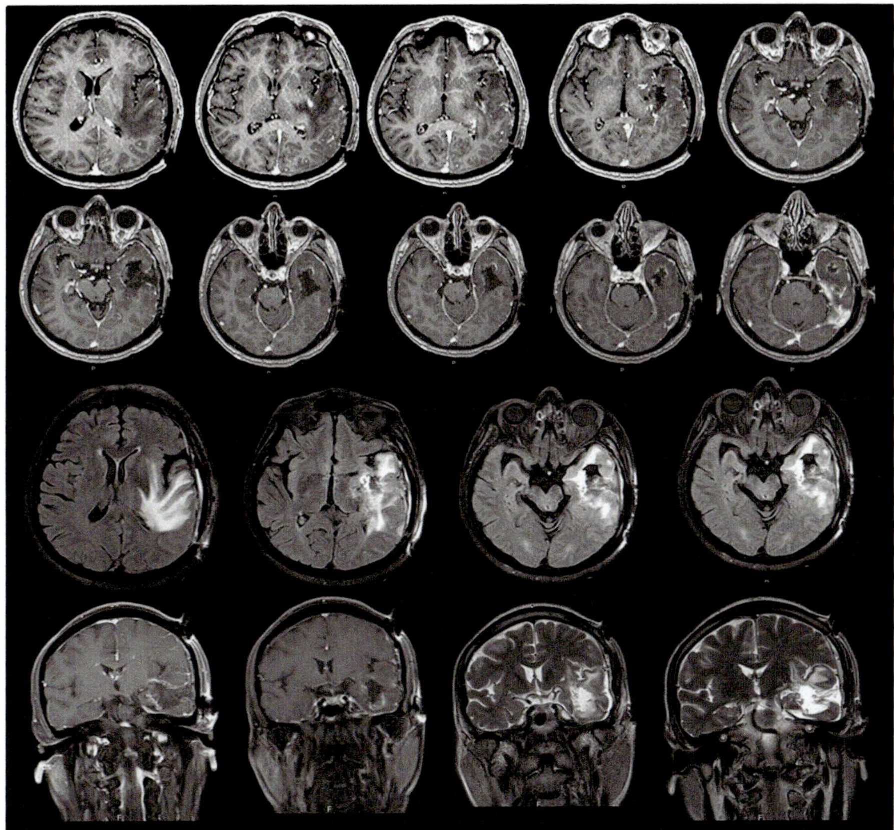

Fig. 1.10 His postoperative MRI performed in the first 24 h after surgery showed early operative changes in the left temporal lobe. There was a 12 × 10 mm residual lesion in the inferior part of the resection cavity

1.2.2 Evidence Based Treatment Recommendations

1.2.2.1 Radiotherapy

The effect of post operative radiotherapy was shown in a randomised trial published in 1978 [25]. In this study patients were randomised to four arms:

1. 1,3-bis(2-chloroethyl)-l-nitrosourea (BCNU) as a single chemotherapeutic agent,
2. Radiotherapy
3. Combination of BCNU and radiotherapy
4. Best conventional care (supportive care).

Radiotherapy was given to the entire cranial fossa, and the dose was 50 Gy with a fraction dose of 1.71–2 Gy. Ten months after the initiation of the study, the dose of radiotherapy was increased from 50 to 60 Gy. A total of 303 patients with a median age of 57 years (range: 6 to 79 years) entered the study. The diagnosis was glioblastoma in 90% of the patients and 10% had anaplastic glioma. Patients who had best conventional care but no radiotherapy or BCNU had a median survival of 14 weeks, while those who had BCNU only had a median survival of 18.5 weeks ($p = 0.119$). Radiotherapy on the other hand provided a clear-cut improvement with a median survival of 36 weeks ($p = 0.001$) and radiotherapy plus BCNU had a median survival of 34.5 weeks ($p = 0.001$). Patients who received at least two cycles of BCNU had a modest (47%) increase in median survival time which was, however, highly significant ($p = 0.002$). This study demonstrated a modest value for BCNU in those patients who received two or more courses. The role of radiotherapy in the treatment of anaplastic glioma was clearly demonstrated, and in this study it increases median survival by approximately 150%.

The dose effect relationship was established in 1979 by Walker et al. [26]. Data from three protocols were collected. For the purpose of analysis, the 621 study patients were divided into subgroups of

1. No radiotherapy
2. 45 Gy
3. 50 Gy
4. 55 Gy
5. 60 Gy of radiotherapy.

The group of patients who received 45 Gy of was quite ill and had a lower performance status, frequently succumbing to their disease prior to receiving all of their radiotherapy. Patients who received no radiotherapy had a median survival of 18 weeks from randomization. Those who had 45 Gy had a median survival of 13.5 weeks. However, there was a progressive increase in median survival consistent with a dose-effect relationship seen in the groups of patients who received 50 Gy, 55 Gy, and 60 Gy.

Dose escalation has remained an important investigational option because the pattern of failure is characterized by local progression or recurrence. However, dose escalation above 60 Gy using conventionally fractionated RT, hyperfractionation, brachytherapy, or stereotactic radiosurgical boost has not been shown to provide further benefit [27–30].

1.2.2.2 Chemotherapy

Until the Stupp trial the chemotherapy trials gave conflicting results. The meta-analysis showed a survival advantage with adjuvant chemotherapy [31]. The Stupp trial changed the practice [32, 33]. Patients 18–70 years of age with newly diagnosed glioblastoma were randomly assigned to receive radiotherapy (286 patients) or radiotherapy plus temozolomide (287 patients). The results indicated a 37% relative reduction in the risk of death for patients treated with radiotherapy plus temozolomide, compared to those who received radiotherapy alone. The median survival benefit was 2.5 months; the median survival was 14.6 months with radiotherapy plus temozolomide and 12.1 months with radiotherapy alone. The two-year survival rates were 26.5% and 10.4% in the groups given radiotherapy plus temozolomide, and radiotherapy alone, respectively. Patients in the experimental group received the alkylating agent temozolomide at a dose of 75 mg per square meter of body-surface area daily during standard fractionated radiotherapy (60 Gy) for 6–7 weeks and at a dose of 150–200 mg per square meter per day for 5 days of every 28-day cycle after radiotherapy, for up to six cycles. Radiotherapy plus temozolomide was associated with a significant improvement in median overall survival in nearly all subgroups of patients; except the two small subgroups one of which was 93 patients who underwent biopsy only and the other was 70 patients with a poor performance status.

With this study concomitant temozolomide with radiotherapy and adjuvant 6 cycles of temozolomide became the standard of care for glioblastoma patients.

Monika E. Hegi et al. evaluated the patients enrolled in the European Organisation for Research and Treatment of Cancer (EORTC) and the National Cancer Institute of Canada (NCIC) trial according to their MGMT (O^6-methylguanine–DNA methyltransferase) status [34]. Epigenetic silencing of the MGMT gene by promoter methylation has been associated with longer overall survival in patients with glioblastoma who, in addition to radiotherapy, received alkylating chemotherapy with carmustine or temozolomide [35]. High levels of MGMT activity in cancer cells create a resistant phenotype by blunting the therapeutic effect of alkylating agents. For the entire population of 206 patients for whom MGMT status could be evaluated, there was a significant difference, irrespective of treatment assignment, in overall survival between patients whose tumors had MGMT promoter methylation and those whose tumors did not. The median overall survival among patients with methylation was 18.2 months, as compared with 12.2 months among those without methylation. Their two-year survival rate was 46%, as compared with 22.7% among those with MGMT promoter methylation who were assigned to radiotherapy alone.

By contrast, among patients whose tumors were not MGMT methylated, the difference in overall survival was only marginally significant; the median survival was 12.7 months among those assigned to temozolomide and radiotherapy and 11.8 months among those assigned to radiotherapy, with 2-year survival rates of 13.8% and <2%, respectively. In the group of patients whose tumors contained a methylated MGMT promoter, those who received temozolomide and radiotherapy had a median PFS of 10.3 months, as compared with 5.9 months for patients who received radiotherapy alone ($p = 0.001$). Among the patients whose tumors contained an unmethylated MGMT promoter, those who received temozolomide and radiotherapy had a median progression-free survival of 5.3 months, as compared with 4.4 months for patients who were treated with radiotherapy alone ($p = 0.02$).

In the 5 year follow up of the EORTC/NCIC trial a benefit of combined therapy was recorded in all subgroups, including patients aged 60–70 years [33]. Methylation of the MGMT promoter was the strongest predictor for outcome and also benefit from temozolomide chemotherapy.

Stupp et al. published a recent article evaluating the effect of Tumor-Treating Fields (TTFields) in patients with glioblastoma [36, 37]. After the completion of treatment with temozolomide and radio-therapy, patients were randomized at a ratio of 2 to 1 to receive standard maintenance temozolomide chemotherapy with or without the addition of TTFields. After a median follow-up of 38 months the median progression-free survival from randomization was 7.1 months in the TTFields plus temozolomide group compared with 4.0 months in the temozolomide alone group. Median overall survival in the per-protocol population was 20.5 months in the TTFields plus temozolomide group ($n = 196$) compared with 15.6 months in the temozolomide alone group ($n = 84$).

A variety of therapies like carmustine polymer wafers and bevacizumab have been studied but none have been shown to increase survival in a randomized trial [38–42].

1.2.2.3 Elderly

The EORTC/NCIC trial was limited to patients 18–70 years of age, and 170 of the 573 patients (30%) were aged 61–70 years [33]. For these patients the median overall survival was 10.9 versus 11.8 months for the combined treatment group and radiotherapy group respectively. Two and 5 year survival rates were 22% versus 6% and 7% versus 0%, in favor of combined treatment.

In Surveillance, Epidemiology, and End Results (SEER) based analysis there was a significant heterogeneity in the management of elderly patients with GBM, and 86% of patients received some form of treatment and only 46% of patients underwent both surgery and radiation [43].

In NOA-08 trial patients with de-novo anaplastic astrocytoma or glioblastoma, age older than 65 years, and a Karnofsky performance score of 60 or more were assigned to temozolomide alone or to radiotherapy alone [44]. Temozolomide was administered according to a 1 week on, 1 week off schedule, with 100 mg/m^2 given on days 1–7. Radiotherapy was administered to the gross tumour volume plus a 2 cm margin, to a total 60.0 Gy. After a minimum follow-up of 12 months overall survival at 6 months was 66.7% in the temozolomide group and 71.7% in the radio-therapy group, and at 1 year, it was 34.4% (27.6–41.4) in the temozolomide group and 37.4% (30.1–44.7) in the radiotherapy group. Median overall survival was 8.6 months in the temozolomide group and 9.6 months in the radiotherapy group which indicated that temozolomide was non-inferior to radiotherapy. MGMT promoter methylation was associated with improved EFS in the temozolomide group, where median was 8.4 months compared with 3.3 months for patients with an unmethylated MGMT. Methylation status did not affect EFS in the radiotherapy group. Methylated MGMT was also associated with differences in EFS between treatment groups, and a trend was seen for overall survival. MGMT methylation was associated with better EFS only in the temozolomide group, but not in the radiotherapy group, and the opposite was true for an unmethylated MGMT promoter status.

For the Nordic trial patients with newly diagnosed aged 60 years or older were eligible [45]. After 2004, patients younger than 65 years who were deemed fit to receive combined treatment were excluded. Patients were randomized to

1. Hypofractionated radiotherapy schedule: 34 Gy in ten fractions
2. Standard radiotherapy: 60 Gy in 30 fractions
3. Temozolomide

Survival did not differ between treatments for patients aged 60–70 years. By contrast, for patients older than 70 years, survival was better with temozolomide and with hypofractionated radiotherapy than with standard radiotherapy. Of patients who received temozolomide, those with MGMT promoter methylated tumours had better survival than did those with unmethylated MGMT status.

In a recent trial by Perry et al. [46], 65 years of age or older patients with glioblastoma who were deemed by their physicians not to be suitable to receive conventional radiotherapy were randomized to:

1. Radiotherapy alone (40.05 Gy in 15 fractions)
2. Radiotherapy plus temozolomide.

The median age was 73 years, with 29.5% of the patients older than 75 years of age. The risk of death was lower by 33% with radiotherapy plus temozolomide than with radiotherapy alone. In subgroup analyses, the benefit of chemoradiotherapy was particularly evident in patients with methylated MGMT status, but benefit was also observed in patients with unmethylated MGMT status.

1.2.2.4 Anaplastic Astrocytoma

Molecularly anaplastic astrocytomas are evaluated as two distinct groups, anaplastic astrocytomas with IDH mutation, and anaplastic astrocytoma IDH-wildtype. They differ in clinical behaviour and the IDH-wildtype astrocytoma may follow a course more similar to that of glioblastoma. IDH-mutant anaplastic oligoastrocytomas with 1p/19q co-deletion, correspond molecularly and prognostically with anaplastic oligodendroglioma, thus eliminating the category of mixed gliomas.

Common practice of care for patients with anaplastic astrocytoma (AA) is surgery followed by radiotherapy alone or radiochemotherapy. The survival benefit achieved with radiochemotherapy in glioblastoma are extrapolated to AA.

The NOA-04 trial for patients with newly diagnosed anaplastic gliomas compared the efficacy of initial RT, followed by chemotherapy (procarbazine, lomustine and vincristine (PCV) or temozolomide (TMZ)) at progression with the inverse sequence [47, 48]. Molecular classification of samples based on IDH and 1p/19q status into three subgroups was prognostically superior to histological classification for PFS, TTF, and OS. There was a superior PFS with RT compared with TMZ, while RT and PCV conferred a similar outcome. MGMT promoter methylation was associated with improved PFS in chemotherapy-treated patients only in the subgroup of patients with IDH wild-type tumors. In patients with IDH-mutant tumors (with or without 1p/19q codeletion), an unmethylated MGMT promoter was rare.

There was no statistically significant difference in the median time to treatment failure between those given radiation first and those initially managed with chemotherapy (4.6 vs. 4.4 years). In subgroup analyses, patients with 1p/19q-codeleted tumors who were assigned to receive PCV had improved progression-free survival compared with those assigned to temozolomide (9.4 vs. 4.5 years) and similar progression-free survival compared with those assigned to radiation (9.4 vs. 8.7 years).

In the CATNON intergroup trial patients with non-co-deleted anaplastic gliomas were assigned to receive

1. Radiotherapy alone
2. Radiotherapy with adjuvant temozolomide
3. Radiotherapy with concurrent temozolomide
4. Receive radiotherapy with concurrent temozolomide and adjuvant temozolomide.

At the time of the interim analysis adjuvant temozolomide was associated with a significant survival benefit in patients with newly diagnosed non-co-deleted anaplastic glioma [49]. We need mature results from the CATNON study to determine whether use of concurrent temozolomide during radiation provides any benefit.

1.2.2.5 Anaplastic Oligodendroglioma

Both PCV (procarbazine, lomustine, and vincristine) and temozolomide are reasonable options. However use of PCV is supported by two large randomized trials in patients with anaplastic oligodendroglial tumors, in which the addition of PCV to RT was associated with improved progression-free and overall survival compared with RT alone in those with 1p19q co-deleted tumors [50–53].

In the EORTC 26951 trial, 368 patients were randomly assigned to immediate RT only or RT followed by six cycles of PCV [50, 51]. At a median follow-up of 60 months, progression-free was significantly prolonged with adjuvant PCV compared to RT alone. With more prolonged follow-up, the survival benefit from combined treatment was seen primarily in patients with the 1p/19q co-deletion.

In the RTOG 9402 trial, 291 patients with anaplastic oligodendrogliomas or anaplastic oligoastrocytomas were randomized to either four cycles of intensified PCV followed by RT or immediate RT without chemotherapy [52, 53]. With 11.3 years follow-up overall survival was significantly prolonged in patients with 1p/19q codeletion and treated with PCV followed by RT compared with those given only RT.

1.2.3   Simulation and Target Delineation

To ensure accurate positioning the patient should be immobilized using a thermoplastic mask system. The head in neutral position is the most widely accepted practice. A CT scan with 1–3 mm slice thickness from the vertex to the lower border of C3 is used for treatment planning. To help with the countering planning CT should be fused with pre and postoperative MR images. Relatively new MR images (up to 2 weeks prior to radiotherapy) are preferred for target delineation. However if new MR imaging is not possible IV contrast should be performed during the planning CT.

Instead of treatment with chemoradiotherapy almost all patients recur, and over 80% of recurrences within a 2 cm margin of the contrast enhanced lesion on CT- or MRI scans [54, 55]. Mainly there are two protocols for target delineation, and are actively used in ongoing trials. One is the European Organization for Research and Treatment of Cancer (EORTC) and the other is the Radiotherapy and Oncology Group (RTOG) recommendations. In two recent multicenter trials (CENTRIC and RTOG 0525) both protocols were used according to the institution preferences [56, 57]. When the results were evaluated according to radiotherapy technique there was no difference in progression-free or overall survival. ESTRO-ACROP guidelines for target delineation of glioblastoma is recently reported [58].

1.2.3.1 EORTC Guidelines

Gross Tumor Volume (GTV): the resection cavity plus any residual enhancing tumor on contrast-enhanced T1 weighted MRI. Peri-tumoral edema is not included in GTV. An exception is for patients with a secondary glioblastoma where non-enhancing areas may be a component of the tumor. Hyperintensity on T2/FLAIR can be included in the GTV in these patients and CTV margin can be modified accordingly.

Clinical Target Volume (CTV): GTV plus a 20 mm margin to account for microscopic spread is defined as CTV. Anatomical barriers should be taken into account (Fig. 1.11).

Planning Target Volume (PTV): CTV to PTV margin is usually defined as 3–5 mm. Ideally each department should define their margins according to their stabilization system and daily imaging techniques. This volume is treated to a total dose of 60 Gy in 2 Gy per fractions.

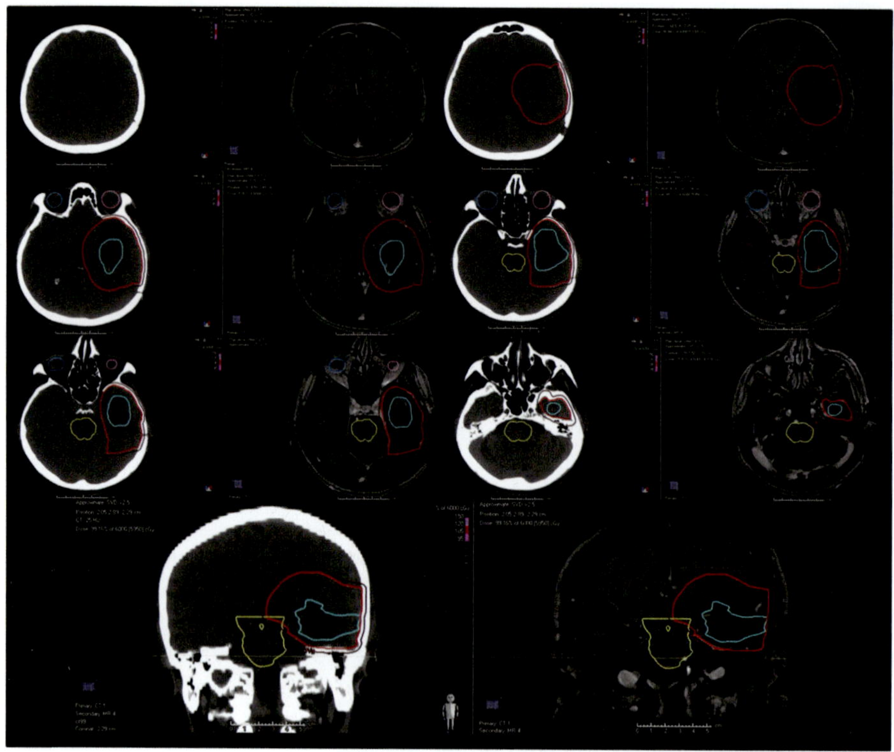

Fig. 1.11 GTV plus a 20 mm margin to account for microscopic spread is defined as CTV. Anatomical barriers should be taken into account

1.2.3.2 RTOG Guidelines

The initial GTV includes the contrast enhancing lesion and surrounding edema (if it exists) demonstrated on CT/MRI. The initial CTV is defined by a 2 cm margin around GTV. If no surrounding edema is present, the initial CTV should include the contrast-enhancing lesion plus a 2.5 cm margin. This volume is treated to 46.0 Gy in 23 fractions, 2.0 Gy per fraction. After 46 Gy, the cone-down target volumes are defined.

Cone-down GTV includes the contrast-enhancing lesion only. Cone-down CTV is defined by a 2.5 cm margin around this GTV. This volume is treated to an additional dose of 14 Gy in 2 Gy per fractions.

While 3D-CRT remains standart for the majority of GBM, IMRT/VMAT is increasingly being used for spatially challenging tumors (Figs. 1.12 and 1.13).

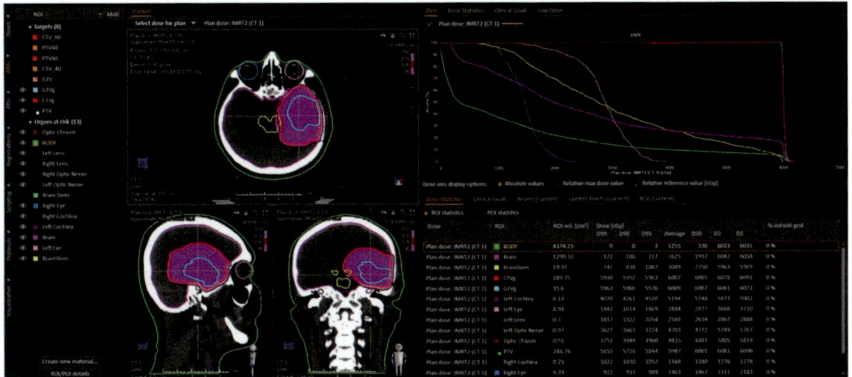

Fig. 1.12 IMRT plan of the patient

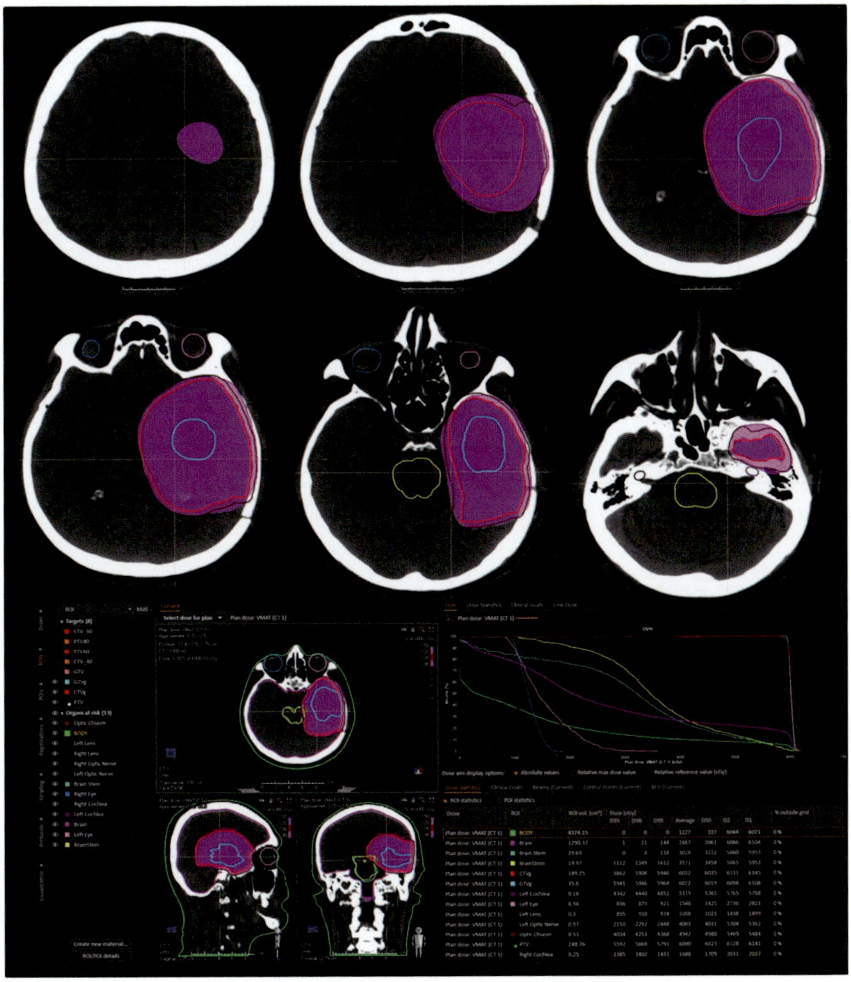

Fig. 1.13 VMAT plan of the patient

1.3   Diffuse Low Grade Glioma

Overview

In the 2016 edition of the WHO classification, gliomas are classified based on histopathologic and molecular parameters. Historically defined 'low-grade glioma' (LGG) includes a heterogenous groups of tumours such as grade II diffuse astrocytoma, oligodendroglioma, and grade I pilocytic astrocytoma, and the updated WHO classification recommends avoiding the term 'low-grade glioma'. Grade II diffuse gliomas consist of diffuse astrocytoma and oligodendroglioma. The diagnosis of oligoastrocytoma no longer exists for fully characterised tumours. IDH wild-type LGGs frequently present a much more malignant phenotype.

Surgery is generally required to establish diagnosis and to debulk the tumour for symptomatic patients presenting with a large mass. However the timing of surgery for patients with a small tumour and minimal symptoms is controversial. Extensive resection rather than partial resection or biopsy in amenable tumours is the preferred treatment. There are no randomised trials evaluating the effect of the extent of surgery on outcome, but retrospective studies and reviews suggest a benefit.

Surgery alone is not curative but the optimal timing of additional therapy a topic under investigation. İndividualized treatment based on risk factors like age ≥40 years, large preoperative tumor size (e.g., ≥5 cm), incomplete resection, astrocytic histology, elevated MIB-1 index (>3%), absence of an isocitrate dehydrogenase (IDH) mutation, and absence of a 1p/19q-codeletion is preferred.

When radiotherapy is delivered a dose of 50–54 Gy is offered in 1.8 Gy per fraction. Survival increases with adjuvant PCV after radiotherapy compared to radiation alone.

Key Words: Low grade glioma; Radiotherapy

1.3.1   Case Presentation

A 38 year old man admitted to the hospital with the complaint of headache for the past 2 months. His physical examination was normal and he had no known illnesses. The cranial MRI revealed a left temporal lobe lesion, 4.9 × 5 cm in size (Fig. 1.14). He underwent surgery and the postoperative MRI performed in the first 24 h revealed a 1.5 cm residual lesion at the anteroinferior part of the resection cavity (Fig. 1.15). The pathologic examination was reported as diffuse astrocytoma, IDH mutant, ATRX mutant. Ki-67 proliferation index was 5%. He underwent postoperative radiotherapy to a total dose of 54 Gy. After he completed his radiation treatment he received 6 cycles of PCV chemotherapy.

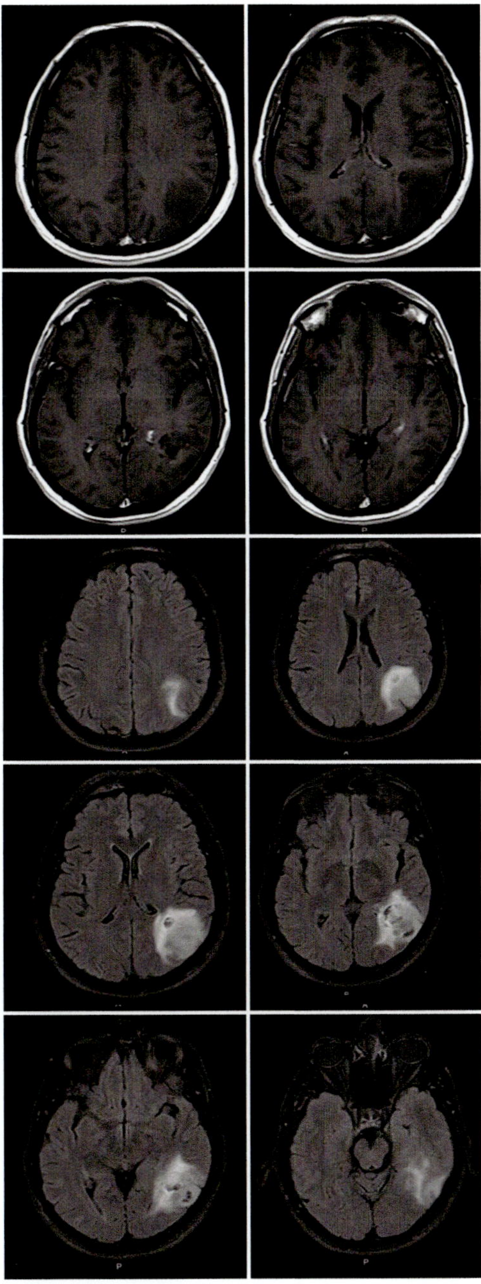

Fig. 1.14 Cranial MRI revealed a left temporal lobe lesion, 4.9 × 5 cm in size

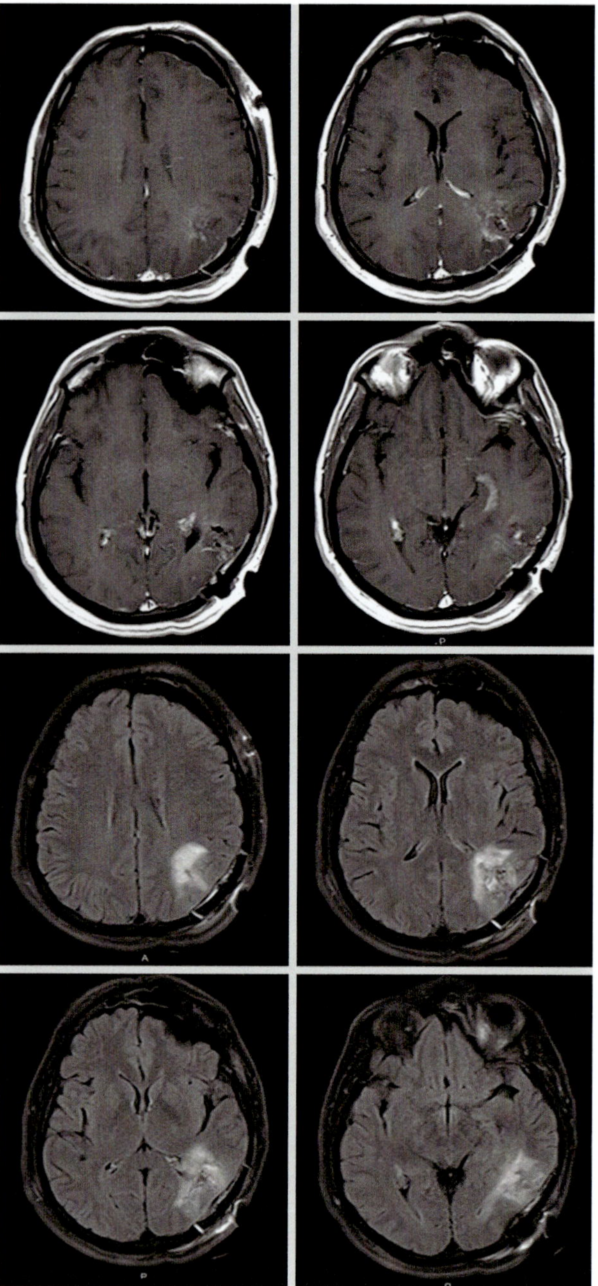

Fig. 1.15 Postoperative MRI performed in the first 24 h revealed a 1.5 cm residual lesion at the anteroinferior part of the resection cavity

1.3.2 Evidence Based Treatment Recommendations

1.3.2.1 Surgery

In patients with a suspicion of low-grade gliomas, surgery provides tissue for histopathologic diagnosis and molecular characterization as imaging cannot establish grade or histology. But the timing of surgery is under debate. For patients presenting with a large mass or extensive neurologic symptoms immediate surgery is the preferred treatment.

In a retrospective cohort study from Norway early versus delayed surgery in LGG was assessed based on two adjacent regional referral centers one of which favored early surgical resection (Hospital A) and the other favored biopsy and watchful waiting (Hospital B) [59]. Initial biopsy alone was carried out in 47 (71%) patients served by Hospital B and in 12 (14%) patients served by the Hospital A. The groups were comparable with respect to baseline parameters. Median survival was 5.9 years (95% CI, 4.5–7.3) in the Hospital B, and the median survival was not reached in Hospital A. This benefit likely reflected the extent of resection rather than the timing of resection. Overall survival was significantly better with early surgical resection ($p = 0.01$). Estimated 5-year survival was 60% and 74% for biopsy and watchful waiting and early resection, respectively.

In a recent analysis the investigators provided long-term survival data and assess molecular markers in their cohorts of LGG [60]. The patients were assigned to one of three molecular groups: (1) the low-risk group (IDH mutated, 1p19q codeleted), (2) the intermediate-risk group (IDH mutated and 1p19q non-codeleted), and (3) the high-risk group (IDH wild-type).

Seventy percent of patients had an IDH mutated tumors. They demonstrated that early resection resulted in a clinical relevant survival benefit, and the effect on survival persisted after adjustment for molecular markers.

There are no randomized trials evaluating the effect of the extent of surgery on outcome. Observational studies provide support for a more extensive resection [61, 62].

In a study consisting of 216 adults undergoing initial resection for LGG, the tumour volumes were evaluated on fluid-attenuated inversion-recovery (FLAIR) imaging series [61]. Patients with at least 90% extent of resection had 5- and 8-year overall survival rates of 97% and 91%. These values were 76% and 60% for patients with <90% extent of resection.

Wijnenga et al. evaluated the impact of surgery in molecularly defined LGG [62]. They showed that the postoperative volume was associated with OS, with a hazard ratio of 1.01 per cm^3 increase in volume. The impact of postoperative volume was particularly strong in IDH mutated astrocytoma patients.

1.3.2.2 Radiotherapy

Radiotherapy is a standard component of therapy for patients with low-grade glioma, but the optimal timing is uncertain. Early versus delayed radiotherapy is associated with symptomatic improvement and prolonged progression-free but not overall survival. Factors effecting the early versus delayed treatment include presence of tumor associated symptoms and risk factors for worse outcome. The defined poor prognostic factors are age $\geq$40 years, large preoperative tumor size (e.g., $\geq$5 cm), incomplete resection, astrocytic histology, elevated MIB-1 index (>3%), absence of an isocitrate dehydrogenase (IDH) mutation, and absence of a 1p/19q-codeletion. However these risk factors are not agreed on completely and the definition of low versus high risk has been variably defined across trials.

In the European Organization for Research and Treatment of Cancer (EORTC) 22,845 trial 311 patients with low-grade gliomas were randomly assigned to receive either immediate RT (54 Gy, 1.8 Gy per fraction) or observation until progression following initial biopsy or resection [63]. At a median follow-up of almost 8 years, median progression-free survival was 5.3 years in the early radiotherapy group and 3.4 years in the control group. Overall survival was similar between groups. In the control group, 65% of patients received radiotherapy at progression. Seizures were better controlled in the early radiotherapy group at 1 year.

RT dose is 50–54 Gy with 1.8 Gy per fraction. Two multicenter randomized trials failed to show a survival benefit from dose escalation. In EORTC trial 22,844 [64], patients with low-grade gliomas were randomized to two different radiotherapy dose arms following surgery or biopsy:

1. 59.4 Gy in 33 treatments
2. 45 Gy in 25 treatments.

At a minimum follow-up of 50 months, there were no significant differences in progression free or overall survival.

In a trial reported by Shaw et al. 203 patients with supratentorial low-grade gliomas were randomised to 64.8 Gy or 50.4 Gy [65]. A higher rate of severe radiation necrosis was seen with the higher dose of RT without an improvement in survival.

Hyperfractionated radiotherapy, proton radiotherapy, and fractionated stereotactic radiotherapy were studied to increase the effectiveness of treatment [66–69]. However, none has been shown to increase the results compared to conventional RT.

1.3.2.3 Chemotherapy

In the RTOG 9802 trial patients with low-grade glioma were randomly assigned to postoperative radiotherapy with or without six cycles of adjuvant PCV chemotherapy [70]. Patients were eligible for this trial if they had supratentorial grade 2 astrocytoma, oligodendroglioma, or oligoastrocytoma. Patients who were 18–39 years of age were eligible if they had undergone a subtotal resection or biopsy, and those who were 40 years of age or older were eligible if they had undergone biopsy or resection. The radiation dose was 54 Gy. Patients assigned to receive chemotherapy received the treatment after they completed radiation therapy. Chemotherapy consisted of six cycles of procarbazine, CCNU, and vincristine. One hundred and twenty eight patients were assigned to radiation therapy alone, and 126 to radiation therapy plus combination chemotherapy with procarbazine, CCNU, and vincristine. With a median follow-up time of 11.9 years there was a survival benefit among patients who were treated with radiation therapy plus chemotherapy, as compared with those who received radiation therapy alone. The treatment effect appeared to be largest in patients with oligodendroglioma or oligoastrocytoma and in patients with IDH1 mutations.

It is also unclear whether temozolomide is equally effective as PCV, and there are no trials that have compared these two regimens.

1.3.3   Simulation and Target Delineation

To ensure accurate positioning the patient should be immobilized using a thermoplastic mask system. The head in neutral position is the most widely accepted practice. A CT scan with 1–3 mm slice thickness from the vertex to the lower border of C3 is used for treatment planning. To help with the countering planning CT should be fused with pre and postoperative MR images.

GTV is the surgical cavity plus the MRI FLAIR or T2 abnormality (Fig. 1.16). CTV is obtained by expanding the GTV isotropically by 1–1.5 cm and then editing

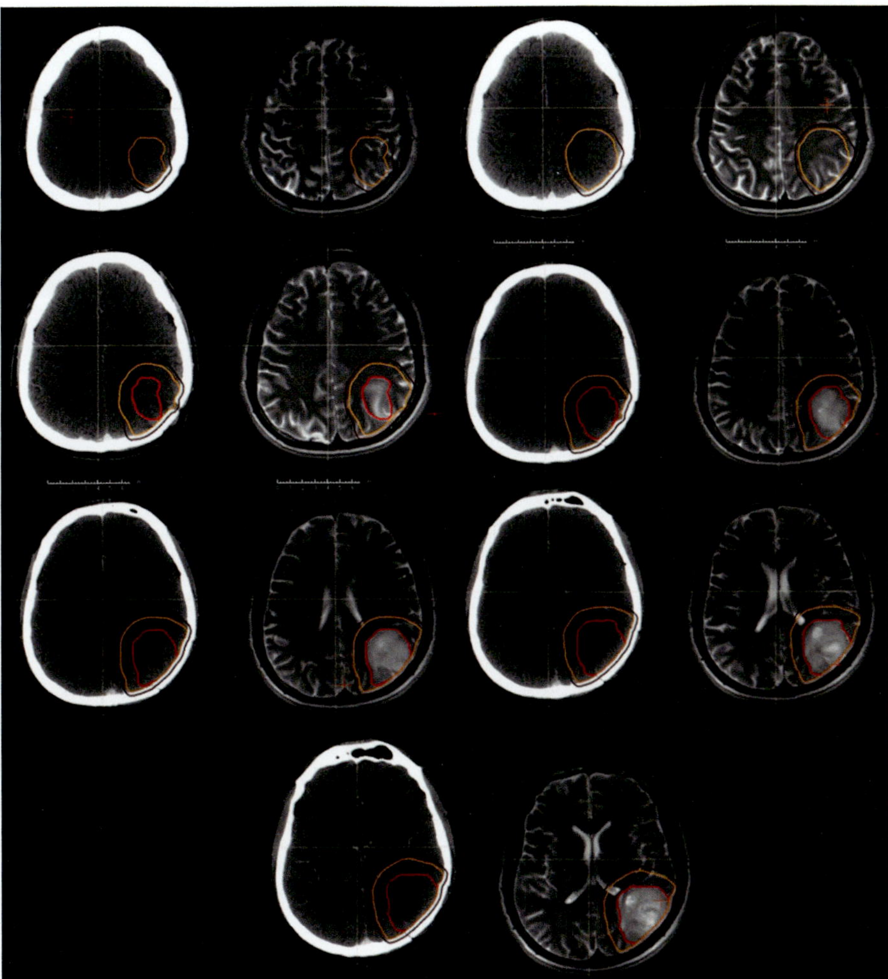

Fig. 1.16 GTV is the surgical cavity plus the MRI FLAIR or T2 abnormality. CTV is obtained by expanding the GTV isotropically by 1–1.5 cm and then editing this, taking into account anatomical boundaries

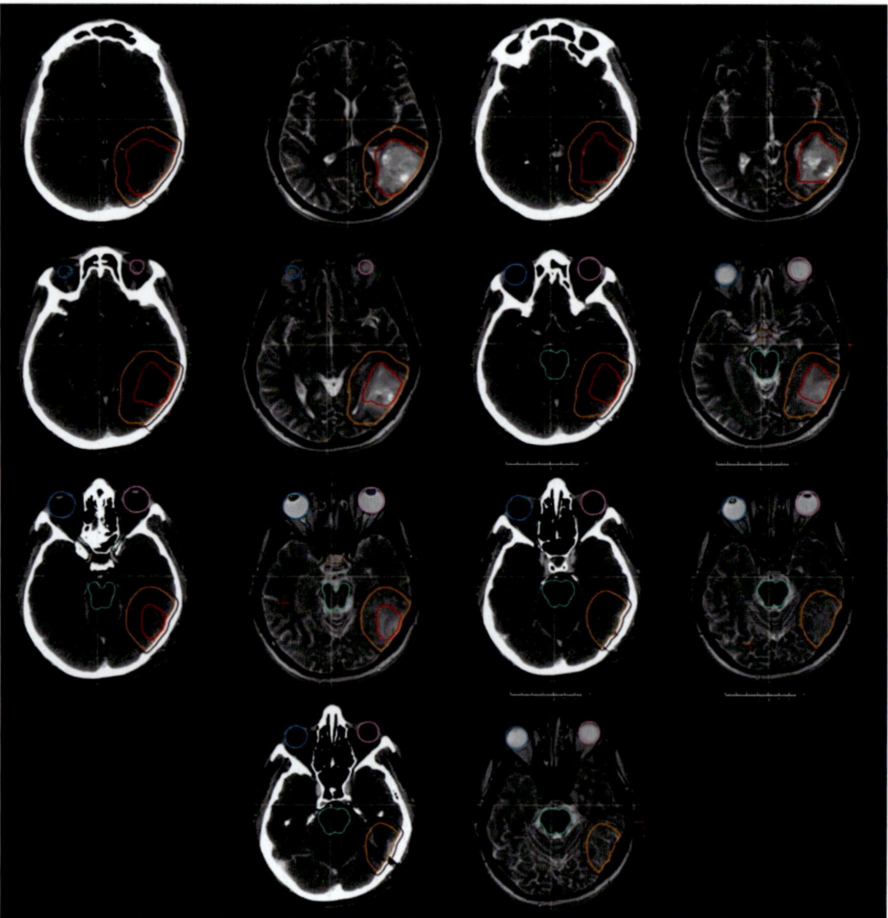

Fig. 1.16 (continued)

this, taking into account anatomical boundaries. Every centre should define their PTV margin according to the immobilization system and daily imaging modality they use.

While 3D-CRT remains standard for the majority of GBM, IMRT/VMAT is increasingly being used for spatially challenging tumors (Fig. 1.17).

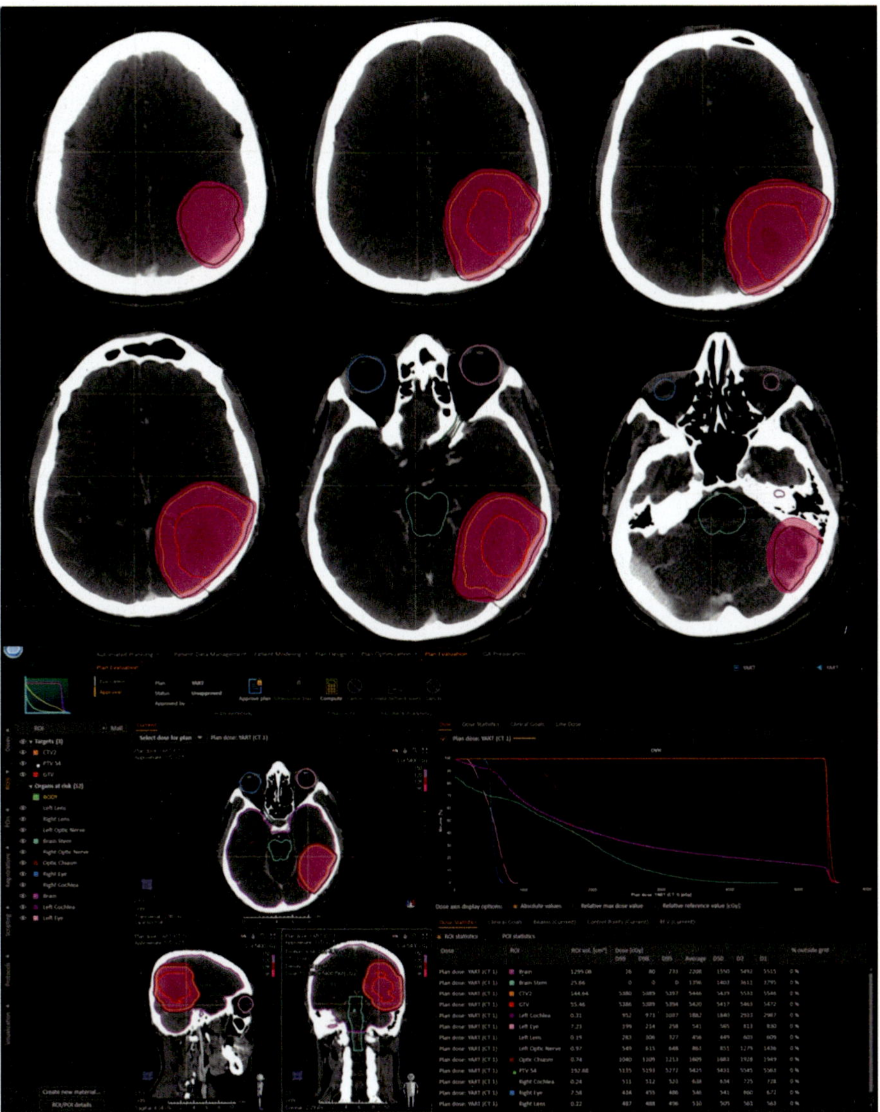

Fig. 1.17 Treatment plan of the patient

References

1. Chang CH, Housepian EM, Herbert C Jr. An operative staging system and a megavoltage radiotherapeutic technic for cerebellar medulloblastomas. Radiology. 1969;93(6):1351–9.
2. Packer RJ, Gajjar A, Vezina G, et al. Phase III study of craniospinal radiation therapy followed by adjuvant chemotherapy for newly diagnosed average-risk medulloblastoma. J clin oncol. 2006;24(25):4202–8.
3. Rutkowski S, von Hoff K, Emser A, et al. Survival and prognostic factors of early childhood medulloblastoma: an international meta-analysis. J clin oncol. 2010;28(33):4961–8.
4. Taylor MD, Northcott PA, Korshunov A, et al. Molecular subgroups of medulloblastoma: the current consensus. Acta Neuropathol. 2012;123(4):465–72.
5. Ramaswamy V, Remke M, Bouffet E, et al. Risk stratification of childhood medulloblastoma in the molecular era: the current consensus. Acta Neuropathol. 2016;131(6):821–31.
6. Paterson E, Farr RF. Cerebellar medulloblastoma: treatment by irradiation of the whole central nervous system. Acta Radiol. 1953;39(4):323–36.
7. Deutsch M, Thomas PR, Krischer J, et al. Results of a prospective randomized trial comparing standard dose neuraxis irradiation (3,600 cGy/20) with reduced neuraxis irradiation (2,340 cGy/13) in patients with low-stage medulloblastoma. A combined children's cancer group-pediatric oncology group study. Pediatr Neurosurg. 1996;24(4):167–76. discussion 76–7.
8. Thomas PR, Deutsch M, Kepner JL, et al. Low-stage medulloblastoma: final analysis of trial comparing standard-dose with reduced-dose neuraxis irradiation. J Clin Oncol. 2000;18(16):3004–11.
9. Packer RJ, Zhou T, Holmes E, Vezina G, Gajjar A. Survival and secondary tumors in children with medulloblastoma receiving radiotherapy and adjuvant chemotherapy: results of Children's Oncology Group trial A9961. Neuro-Oncology. 2013;15(1):97–103.
10. Merchant TE, Kun LE, Krasin MJ, et al. Multi-institution prospective trial of reduced-dose craniospinal irradiation (23.4 Gy) followed by conformal posterior fossa (36 Gy) and primary site irradiation (55.8 Gy) and dose-intensive chemotherapy for average-risk medulloblastoma. Int J Radiat Oncol Biol Phys. 2008;70(3):782–7.
11. Gajjar A, Chintagumpala M, Ashley D, et al. Risk-adapted craniospinal radiotherapy followed by high-dose chemotherapy and stem-cell rescue in children with newly diagnosed medulloblastoma (St Jude Medulloblastoma-96): long-term results from a prospective, multicentre trial. Lancet Oncol. 2006;7(10):813–20. Erratum: Lancet Oncol. 2006 Oct;7(10):797.
12. Michalski JM, Janss A, Vezina G, et al. Results of COG ACNS0331: a phase III trial of involved-field radiotherapy (IFRT) and low dose craniospinal irradiation (LD-CSI) with chemotherapy in average-risk medulloblastoma: a report from the children's oncology group. Int J Radiat Oncol Biol Phys. 2016;96(5):937–8.
13. Fukunaga-Johnson N, Lee JH, Sandler HM, Robertson P, McNeil E, Goldwein JW. Patterns of failure following treatment for medulloblastoma: is it necessary to treat the entire posterior fossa? Int J Radiat Oncol Biol Phys. 1998;42(1):143–6.
14. Wolden SL, Dunkel IJ, Souweidane MM, et al. Patterns of failure using a conformal radiation therapy tumor bed boost for medulloblastoma. J Clin Oncol. 2003;21(16):3079–83.
15. Taylor RE, Bailey CC, Robinson K, et al. Results of a randomized study of preradiation chemotherapy versus radiotherapy alone for nonmetastatic medulloblastoma: the International Society of Paediatric Oncology United Kingdom Children's Cancer Study Group PNET-3 study. J Clin Oncol. 2003;21(8):1581–91.
16. Oyharcabal-Bourden V, Kalifa C, Gentet JC, et al. Standard-risk medulloblastoma treated by adjuvant chemotherapy followed by reduced-dose craniospinal radiation therapy: a French Society of Pediatric Oncology study. J Clin Oncol. 2005;23(21):4726–34.
17. Kortmann RD, Kuhl J, Timmermann B, et al. Postoperative neoadjuvant chemotherapy before radiotherapy as compared to immediate radiotherapy followed by maintenance chemotherapy in the treatment of medulloblastoma in childhood: results of the German prospective randomized trial HIT '91. Int J Radiat Oncol Biol Phys. 2000;46(2):269–79.

18. Kortmann RD. Chemotherapy before or after radiation therapy does not influence survival of children with high-risk medulloblastomas results of the multicentric randomized study of the pediatric oncology group (POG 9031). Strahlenther Onkol. 2014;190(1):106–8.
19. Jakacki RI, Burger PC, Zhou TN, et al. Outcome of children with metastatic medulloblastoma treated with carboplatin during craniospinal radiotherapy: a children's oncology group phase I/II study. J Clin Oncol. 2012;30(21):2648–53.
20. Gandola L, Massimino M, Cefalo G, et al. Hyperfractionated accelerated radiotherapy in the Milan strategy for metastatic medulloblastoma. J Clin Oncol. 2009;27(4):566–71.
21. Geyer JR, Sposto R, Jennings M, et al. Multiagent chemotherapy and deferred radiotherapy in infants with malignant brain tumors: a report from the children's cancer group. J Clin Oncol. 2005;23(30):7621–31.
22. Rutkowski S, Gerber NU, von Hoff K, et al. Treatment of early childhood medulloblastoma by postoperative chemotherapy and deferred radiotherapy. Neuro-Oncology. 2009;11(2):201–10.
23. Rutkowski S, Bode U, Deinlein F, et al. Treatment of early childhood medulloblastoma by postoperative chemotherapy alone. N Engl J Med. 2005;352(10):978–86.
24. Louis DN, Perry A, Reifenberger G, et al. The 2016 World Health Organization classification of tumors of the central nervous system: a summary. Acta Neuropathol. 2016;131(6):803–20.
25. Walker MD, Alexander E Jr, Hunt WE, et al. Evaluation of BCNU and/or radiotherapy in the treatment of anaplastic gliomas. A cooperative clinical trial. J Neurosurg. 1978;49(3):333–43.
26. Walker MD, Strike TA, Sheline GE. An analysis of dose-effect relationship in the radiotherapy of malignant gliomas. Int J Radiat Oncol Biol Phys. 1979;5(10):1725–31.
27. Souhami L, Seiferheld W, Brachman D, et al. Randomized comparison of stereotactic radio-surgery followed by conventional radiotherapy with carmustine to conventional radiotherapy with carmustine for patients with glioblastoma multiforme: report of radiation therapy oncology group 93-05 protocol. Int J Radiat Oncol Biol Phys. 2004;60(3):853–60.
28. Laperriere NJ, Leung PM, McKenzie S, et al. Randomized study of brachytherapy in the initial management of patients with malignant astrocytoma. Int J Radiat Oncol Biol Phys. 1998;41(5):1005–11.
29. Selker RG, Shapiro WR, Burger P, et al. The Brain Tumor Cooperative Group NIH Trial 87-01: a randomized comparison of surgery, external radiotherapy, and carmustine versus surgery, interstitial radiotherapy boost, external radiation therapy, and carmustine. Neurosurgery. 2002;51(2):343–55. discussion 55–7.
30. Nelson DF, Diener-West M, Horton J, Chang CH, Schoenfeld D, Nelson JS. Combined modality approach to treatment of malignant gliomas--re-evaluation of RTOG 7401/ECOG 1374 with long-term follow-up: a joint study of the Radiation Therapy Oncology Group and the Eastern Cooperative Oncology Group. NCI Monogr. 1988;1998(6):279–84.
31. Stewart LA. Chemotherapy in adult high-grade glioma: a systematic review and meta-analysis of individual patient data from 12 randomised trials. Lancet. 2002;359(9311):1011–8.
32. Stupp R, Mason WP, van den Bent MJ, et al. Radiotherapy plus concomitant and adjuvant temozolomide for glioblastoma. N Engl J Med. 2005;352(10):987–96.
33. Stupp R, Hegi ME, Mason WP, et al. Effects of radiotherapy with concomitant and adjuvant temozolomide versus radiotherapy alone on survival in glioblastoma in a randomised phase III study: 5-year analysis of the EORTC-NCIC trial. Lancet Oncol. 2009;10(5):459–66.
34. Hegi ME, Diserens AC, Gorlia T, et al. MGMT gene silencing and benefit from temozolomide in glioblastoma. N Engl J Med. 2005;352(10):997–1003.
35. Hegi ME, Liu L, Herman JG, et al. Correlation of O6-methylguanine methyltransferase (MGMT) promoter methylation with clinical outcomes in glioblastoma and clinical strategies to modulate MGMT activity. J Clin Oncol. 2008;26(25):4189–99.
36. Stupp R, Taillibert S, Kanner AA, et al. Maintenance therapy with tumor-treating fields plus temozolomide vs temozolomide alone for glioblastoma: a randomized clinical trial. JAMA. 2015;314(23):2535–43.
37. Stupp R, Taillibert S, Kanner A, et al. Effect of tumor-treating fields plus maintenance temozolomide vs maintenance temozolomide alone on survival in patients with glioblastoma: a randomized clinical trial. JAMA. 2017;318(23):2306–16.

38. Dixit S, Hingorani M, Achawal S, Scott I. Retrospective comparison of chemoradiotherapy followed by adjuvant chemotherapy, with or without previous gliadel implantation (carmustine) after initial surgery in patients with newly diagnosed high-grade gliomas: in regard to Noel et al. (Int J Radiat Oncol Biol Phys 2011; https://doi.org/10.1016/j.ijrobp.2010.11.073). Int J Radiat Oncol Biol Phys. 2011;81(5):1593.
39. Pallud J, Audureau E, Noel G, et al. Long-term results of carmustine wafer implantation for newly diagnosed glioblastomas: a controlled propensity-matched analysis of a French multicenter cohort. Neuro-Oncology. 2015;17(12):1609–19.
40. Burri SH, Prabhu RS, Sumrall AL, et al. BCNU wafer placement with temozolomide (TMZ) in the immediate postoperative period after tumor resection followed by radiation therapy with TMZ in patients with newly diagnosed high grade glioma: final results of a prospective, multi-institutional, phase II trial. J Neuro-Oncol. 2015;123(2):259–66.
41. Chinot OL, Wick W, Mason W, et al. Bevacizumab plus radiotherapy-temozolomide for newly diagnosed glioblastoma. N Engl J Med. 2014;370(8):709–22.
42. Gilbert MR, Dignam JJ, Armstrong TS, et al. A randomized trial of bevacizumab for newly diagnosed glioblastoma. N Engl J Med. 2014;370(8):699–708.
43. Iwamoto FM, Reiner AS, Nayak L, Panageas KS, Elkin EB, Abrey LE. Prognosis and patterns of care in elderly patients with glioma. Cancer. 2009;115(23):5534–40.
44. Wick W, Platten M, Meisner C, et al. Temozolomide chemotherapy alone versus radiotherapy alone for malignant astrocytoma in the elderly: the NOA-08 randomised, phase 3 trial. Lancet Oncol. 2012;13(7):707–15.
45. Malmstrom A, Gronberg BH, Marosi C, et al. Temozolomide versus standard 6-week radiotherapy versus hypofractionated radiotherapy in patients older than 60 years with glioblastoma: the Nordic randomised, phase 3 trial. Lancet Oncol. 2012;13(9):916–26.
46. Perry JR, Laperriere N, O'Callaghan CJ, et al. Short-course radiation plus temozolomide in elderly patients with glioblastoma. N Engl J Med. 2017;376(11):1027–37.
47. Wick W, Hartmann C, Engel C, et al. NOA-04 randomized phase III trial of sequential radiochemotherapy of anaplastic glioma with procarbazine, lomustine, and vincristine or temozolomide. J Clin oncol. 2009;27(35):5874–80.
48. Wick W, Roth P, Hartmann C, et al. Long-term analysis of the NOA-04 randomized phase III trial of sequential radiochemotherapy of anaplastic glioma with PCV or temozolomide. Neuro-Oncology. 2016;18(11):1529–37.
49. van den Bent MJ, Baumert B, Erridge SC, et al. Interim results from the CATNON trial (EORTC study 26053-22054) of treatment with concurrent and adjuvant temozolomide for 1p/19q non-co-deleted anaplastic glioma: a phase 3, randomised, open-label intergroup study. Lancet. 2017;390(10103):1645–53.
50. Kouwenhoven MC, Gorlia T, Kros JM, et al. Molecular analysis of anaplastic oligodendroglial tumors in a prospective randomized study: a report from EORTC study 26951. Neuro-Oncology. 2009;11(6):737–46.
51. van den Bent MJ, Brandes AA, Taphoorn MJ, et al. Adjuvant procarbazine, lomustine, and vincristine chemotherapy in newly diagnosed anaplastic oligodendroglioma: long-term follow-up of EORTC brain tumor group study 26951. J Clin Oncol. 2013;31(3):344–50.
52. Intergroup Radiation Therapy Oncology Group Trial 9402, Cairncross G, Berkey B, et al. Phase III trial of chemotherapy plus radiotherapy compared with radiotherapy alone for pure and mixed anaplastic oligodendroglioma: Intergroup Radiation Therapy Oncology Group Trial 9402. J Clin Oncol. 2006;24(18):2707–14.
53. Cairncross G, Wang M, Shaw E, et al. Phase III trial of chemoradiotherapy for anaplastic oligodendroglioma: long-term results of RTOG 9402. J Clin Oncol. 2013;31(3):337–43.
54. Aydin H, Sillenberg I, von Lieven H. Patterns of failure following CT-based 3-D irradiation for malignant glioma. Strahlenther Onkol. 2001;177(8):424–31.
55. Chang EL, Akyurek S, Avalos T, et al. Evaluation of peritumoral edema in the delineation of radiotherapy clinical target volumes for glioblastoma. Int J Radiat Oncol Biol Phys. 2007;68(1):144–50.

56. Gilbert MR, Wang M, Aldape KD, et al. Dose-dense temozolomide for newly diagnosed glioblastoma: a randomized phase III clinical trial. J Clin Oncol. 2013;31(32):4085–91.
57. Stupp R, Hegi ME, Gorlia T, et al. Cilengitide combined with standard treatment for patients with newly diagnosed glioblastoma with methylated MGMT promoter (CENTRIC EORTC 26071-22072 study): a multicentre, randomised, open-label, phase 3 trial. Lancet Oncol. 2014;15(10):1100–8.
58. Niyazi M, Brada M, Chalmers AJ, et al. ESTRO-ACROP guideline "target delineation of glioblastomas". Radiother Oncol. 2016;118(1):35–42.
59. Jakola AS, Myrmel KS, Kloster R, Torp SH, Lindal S, Unsgård G, Solheim O. Comparison of a strategy favoring early surgical resection vs a strategy favoring watchful waiting in low-grade gliomas. JAMA. 2012;308(18):1881–8.
60. Jakola AS, Skjulsvik AJ, Myrmel KS, Sjåvik K, Unsgård G, Torp SH, Aaberg K, Berg T, Dai HY, Johnsen K, Kloster R, Solheim O. Surgical resection versus watchful waiting in low-grade gliomas. Ann Oncol. 2017;28(8):1942–8.
61. Smith JS, Chang EF, Lamborn KR, Chang SM, Prados MD, Cha S, Tihan T, Vandenberg S, McDermott MW, Berger MS. Role of extent of resection in the long-term outcome of low-grade hemispheric gliomas. J Clin Oncol. 2008;26(8):1338.
62. Wijnenga MMJ, French PJ, Dubbink HJ, Dinjens WNM, Atmodimedjo PN, Kros JM, Smits M, Gahrmann R, Rutten GJ, Verheul JB, Fleischeuer R, Dirven CMF, Vincent AJPE, van den Bent MJ. The impact of surgery in molecularly defined low-grade glioma: an integrated clinical, radiological, and molecular analysis. Neuro-Oncology. 2018;20(1):103.
63. van den Bent MJ, Afra D, de Witte O, Ben Hassel M, Schraub S, Hoang-Xuan K, Malmström PO, Collette L, Piérart M, Mirimanoff R, Karim AB, EORTC Radiotherapy and Brain Tumor Groups and the UK Medical Research Council. Long-term efficacy of early versus delayed radiotherapy for low-grade astrocytoma and oligodendroglioma in adults: the EORTC 22845 randomised trial. Lancet. 2005;366(9490):985–90.
64. Karim AB, Maat B, Hatlevoll R, Menten J, Rutten EH, Thomas DG, Mascarenhas F, Horiot JC, Parvinen LM, van Reijn M, Jager JJ, Fabrini MG, van Alphen AM, Hamers HP, Gaspar L, Noordman E, Pierart M, van Glabbeke M. A randomized trial on dose-response in radiation therapy of low-grade cerebral glioma: European Organization for Research and Treatment of Cancer (EORTC) Study 22844. Int J Radiat Oncol Biol Phys. 1996;36(3):549.
65. Shaw E, Arusell R, Scheithauer B, O'Fallon J, O'Neill B, Dinapoli R, Nelson D, Earle J, Jones C, Cascino T, Nichols D, Ivnik R, Hellman R, Curran W, Abrams RJ. Prospective randomized trial of low- versus high-dose radiation therapy in adults with supratentorial low-grade glioma: initial report of a north central cancer treatment group/radiation therapy oncology group/eastern cooperative oncology group study. Clin Oncol. 2002;20(9):2267.
66. Jeremic B, Shibamoto Y, Grujicic D, Milicic B, Stojanovic M, Nikolic N, Dagovic A. Hyperfractionated radiation therapy for incompletely resected supratentorial low-grade glioma. A phase II study. Radiother Oncol. 1998;49(1):49.
67. Shih HA, Sherman JC, Nachtigall LB, Colvin MK, Fullerton BC, Daartz J, Winrich BK, Batchelor TT, Thornton LT, Mancuso SM, Saums MK, Oh KS, Curry WT, Loeffler JS, Yeap BY. Proton therapy for low-grade gliomas: results from a prospective trial. Cancer. 2015;121(10):1712–9. Epub 2015 Jan 13.
68. Sherman JC, Colvin MK, Mancuso SM, Batchelor TT, Oh KS, Loeffler JS, Yeap BY, Shih HA. Neurocognitive effects of proton radiation therapy in adults with low-grade glioma. J Neuro-Oncol. 2016;126(1):157.
69. Plathow C, Schulz-Ertner D, Thilman C, Zuna I, Lichy M, Weber MA, Schlemmer HP, Wannenmacher M, Debus J. Fractionated stereotactic radiotherapy in low-grade astrocytomas: long-term outcome and prognostic factors. Int J Radiat Oncol Biol Phys. 2003;57(4):996.
70. Buckner JC, Shaw EG, Pugh SL, Chakravarti A, Gilbert MR, Barger GR, Coons S, Ricci P, Bullard D, Brown PD, Stelzer K, Brachman D, Suh JH, Schultz CJ, Bahary JP, Fisher BJ, Kim H, Murtha AD, Bell EH, Won M, Mehta MP, Curran WJ Jr. Radiation plus Procarbazine, CCNU, and Vincristine in Low-Grade Glioma. N Engl J Med. 2016;374(14):1344.

Head and Neck Cancers

2

Ugur Selek, Duygu Sezen, Yucel Saglam,
and Yasemin Bolukbasi

2.1 Nasopharynx

Overview

Epidemiology

The distribution exhibits rare prevalence in United States and Europe while high incidence in Southern China, Southeast Asia, North Africa and the Middle East. Early infection with EBV results in developing NPC after EBV re-activation. EBV latent integral membrane proteins (EBNA-1, LMP-1 and LMP-2), and BamHI-A genome fragment are commonly expressed.

High incidence might be related with nitrosamines and/or potential EBV activators such as salt-cured foods, preserved or fermented foods, rancid butter and sheep's fat. Smoking is related with keratinizing NPC.

Pathological and Biological Features

WHO Type I: sporadic, keratinizing squamous cell carcinoma, high risk of local regional recurrence,

U. Selek (✉) · Y. Bolukbasi
Department of Radiation Oncology, Koç University, Istanbul, Turkey

Department of Radiation Oncology, The University of Texas MD Anderson Cancer Center, Houston, TX, USA

D. Sezen · Y. Saglam
Department of Radiation Oncology, School of Medicine, Koç University, Istanbul, Turkey
e-mail: yucels@amerikanhastanesi.org

© Springer Nature Switzerland AG 2019
G. Ozyigit, U. Selek (eds.), *Radiation Oncology*,
https://doi.org/10.1007/978-3-319-97145-2_2

WHO Type IIA/B: endemic, EBV related, non-keratinizing/undifferentiated carcinoma, high risk of distant metastasis

Lymphoepithelioma: High lymphoid component, high risk of distant metastasis, good local control.

Definitive Therapy

Radiation therapy is the backbone of treatment for all stages, sufficient alone in stage I, concurrent with chemotherapy for stages II–IVB. Neoadjuvant/Induction chemotherapy with platinum/5FU ± taxane followed by concurrent chemoradiotherapy is also an investigated option for stages II–IVB. Induction chemotherapy followed by response evaluation with definitive radiotherapy if complete response; if incomplete, then palliative radiotherapy to metastatic sites.

Adjuvant Therapy

Adjuvant chemotherapy is a standard approach following concurrent chemoradiotherapy.

Key Words: Nasopharynx cancer, Radiotherapy

2.1.1 Case Presentation

Forty years old female with no nonsmoking or significant past medical history admitted with a left neck swelling, a congested nose and epistaxis. She had no dysphagia, odynophagia, or swallowing, and chewing problems. Cranial nerves II–XII are grossly intact without any facial numbness. Her physical exam was normal for ears and nose. Exam with visualization or palpation showed no dental problems, no lesions of the gingiva, buccal mucosa, floor of mouth, oral tongue, base of tongue, hard palate, soft palate, tonsillar fossa or posterior oropharyngeal wall. Palate elevation and tongue protrusion were normal. There was approximately 1.5–2 cm hardly palpable, mobile nodes in bilateral level II. The fiberoptic scope through left nasal cavity revealed a left erythematous nasopharyngeal mass centered on the left fossa of Rosenmuller, superiorly to the roof of the nasopharynx, and inferiorly to the level of the soft palate, without any extention into the posterior aspect of the nasal cavity, oropharynx, larynx (mobile vocal cords), and hypopharynx. MRI defined a left nasopharyngeal lesion filling the Rosen Muller fossa with intact pharyngobasilar fascia and parapharyngeal space. (Figs. 2.1, 2.2, 2.3, and 2.4). The lesion was touching the carotid space posterolaterally without any invasion, as there was no invasion to clivus. The longus colli posterior to the lesion showed blurred enhancement with no direct invasion. No intracranial extension was defined. The imaging also revealed bilateral retropharyngeal nodal disease with central necrosis (one on right, two on left side), largest on left measuring 1.5 cm. Bilateral nodal disease was documented as left 13 × 12 mm and 7 × 4 mm at level IIA, 10 × 5 mm at level VA, right largest

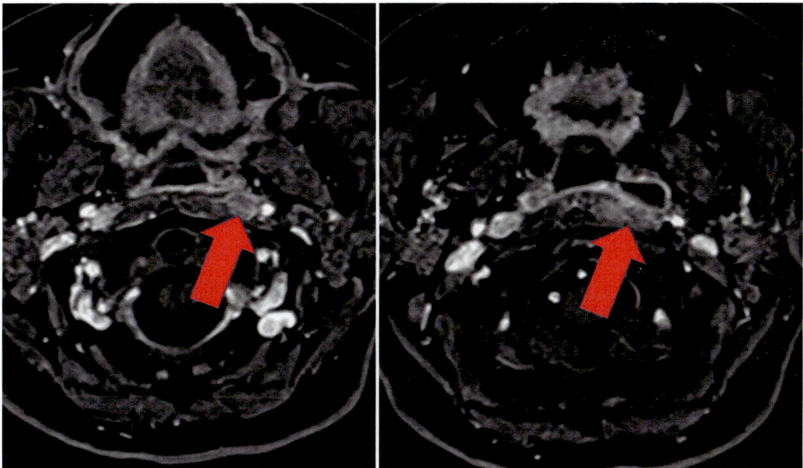

Fig. 2.1 Axial MRI images displaying retropharyngeal nodes

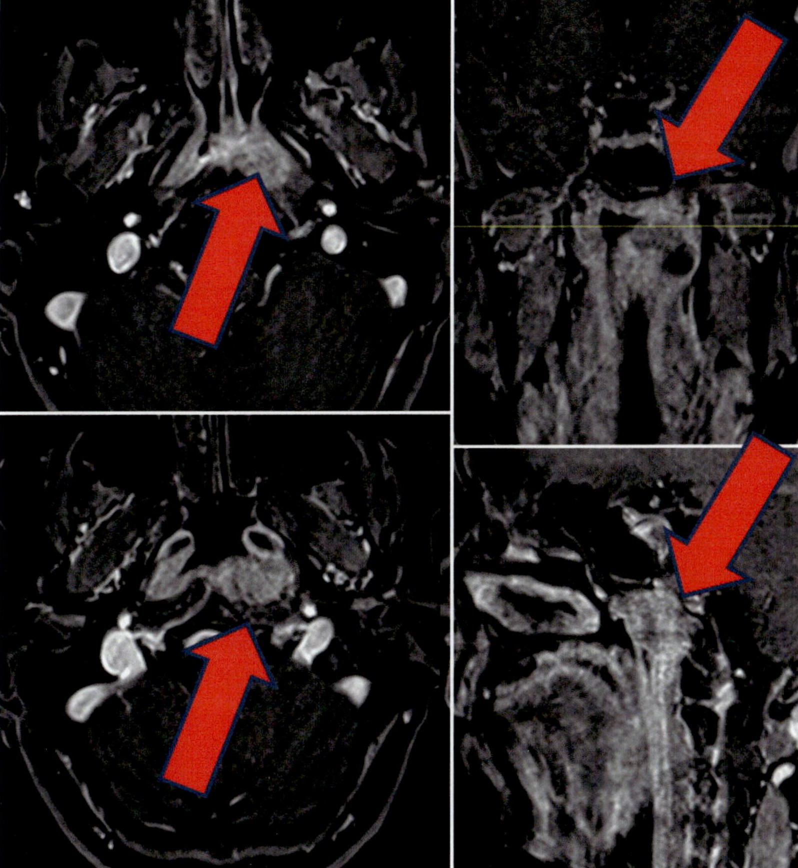

Fig. 2.2 Axial and coronal and sagittal MRI images showing left nasopharyngeal lesion filling the Rosen Muller fossa

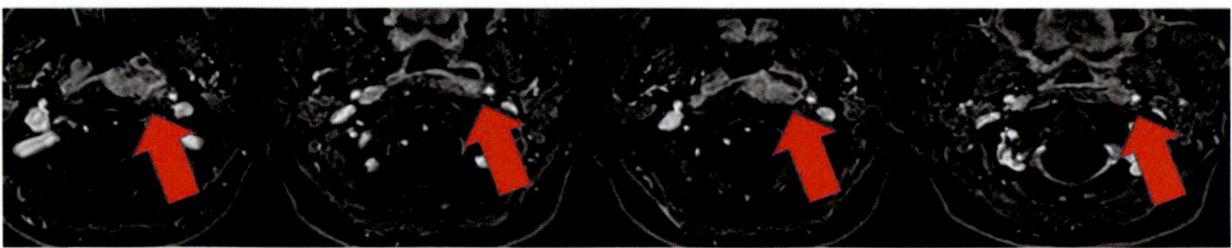

Fig. 2.3 Axial MRI images showing left nasopharyngeal lesion craniocaudally

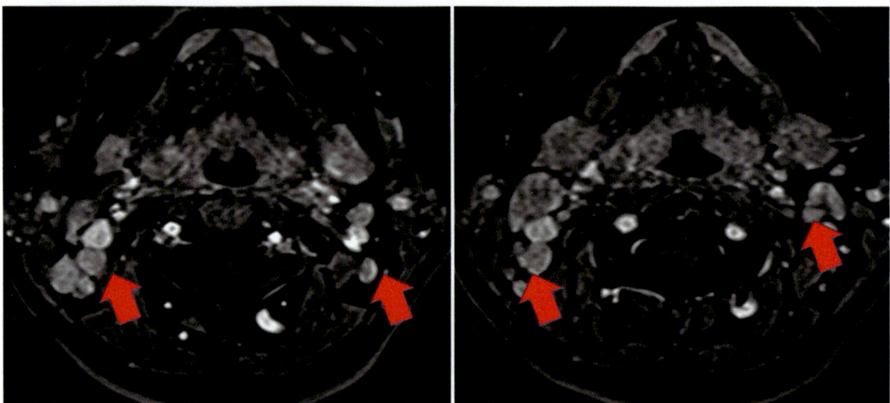

Fig. 2.4 Axial MRI images showing bilateral nodal involvement

20 × 13 mm at Level IIA, largest 12 × 6 mm at level VA in addition to multiple small levels II A, II B and VA nodes.

A biopsy from the left nasopharyngeal lesion confirmed the undifferentiated nonkeratinizing carcinoma (WHO Type IIB).

She was staged as T2N2M0, advanced stage nasopharyngeal cancer.

2.1.2 Staging

Physical examination ± fiberoptic examination is crucial. Head and neck MRI with contrast is encouraged for skull base invasion and soft tissue extension, while contrast enhanced CT might add cortical bone invasion details.

Systemic staging requires FDG PET/CT scan (preferred) or chest CT with upper abdomen. Pre-RT functional examination could require dental, speech and swallow, and audiology evaluation in addition to nutritional assesment.

The 8th Edition of AJCC Cancer Staging Manual Has Recent Changes (Tables 2.1 and 2.2)

T2 includes adjacent muscle involvement of medial, lateral pterygoid and prevertebral muscles.

T4 covers specific description of soft tissue involvement.

N3a and N3b are now in N3.

Table 2.1 AJCC Staging for Nasopharynx

Primary tumor (T)	
TX	Primary tumor cannot be assessed
	No tumor identified, but EBV-positive cervical node(s) involvement
Tis	Carcinoma in situ
T1	Tumor confined to the nasopharynx, or extenion to oropharynx and/or nasal cavity without parapharyngeal involvement
T2	Tumor with extension to parapharyngeal space, and/or adjacent soft tissue involvement (medial pterygoid, lateral pterygoid, prevertebral muscles)
T3	Tumor with infiltration of bony structures at skull base, cervical vertebra, pterygoid structures, and/or paranasal sinuses
T4	Tumor with intracranial extension, involvement of cranial nerves, hypopharynx, orbit, parotid gland, and/or extensive soft tissue infiltration beyond the lateral surface of the lateral pterygoid muscle
Regional lymph nodes (N)	
NX	Regional nodes cannot be assessed
N0	No regional lymph node metastasis
N1	Unilateral metastasis in cervical lymph node(s) and/or unilateral or bilateral metastasis in retropharyngeal lymph node(s), 6 cm or smaller in greatest dimension, above the caudal border of cricoid cartilage
N2	Bilateral metastasis in cervical lymph node(s), 6 cm or smaller in greatest dimension, above the caudal border of cricoid cartilage
N3	Unilateral or bilateral metastasis in cervical lymph node(s), larger than 6 cm in greatest dimension, and/or extension below the caudal border of cricoid cartilage
Distant metastasis (M)	
cM0	No distant metastasis
cM1	Distant metastasis
pM1	Distant metastasis, microscopically confirmed

Head and Neck. Used with permission of the American College of Surgeons, Chicago, Illinois. The original and primary source for this information is the AJCC Cancer Staging Manual, Eighth Edition (2017) published by Springer International Publishing

Table 2.2 Prognostic stage groups

Stage	T	N	M
0	Tis	N0	M0
I	T1	N0	M0
II	T0–T1	N1	M0
	T2	N0–N1	M0
III	T0–T3	N2	M0
	T3	N1–N2	M0
IVA	T4	N0–N2	M0
	T Any	N3	M0
IVB	T Any	N Any	M1

2.1.3 Evidence Based Treatment Approaches

Stage T1N0M0 is recommended radiotherapy alone as the standard treatment. Concurrent chemoradiotherapy (CRT) has been the standard of care for non-metastatic advanced stage (stages T1, N1–3, M0 and T2–4, Any N, M0)

nasopharyngeal carcinoma, with adjuvant chemotherapy; induction chemotherapy followed by concurrent chemoradiotherapy has recently been considered an acceptable standard approach [1, 2].

RT alone was proved to be an effective treatment specifically for T1 disease in the MDACC series where RT alone succeeded a 5 year local control rates of 93%, 79%, 68%, and 53% for T1, T2, T3, and T4, respectively; defining poor prognostic factors for local control as T category, squamous histology, and cranial nerve deficits [3].

Concurrent chemoradiotherapy was encouraged with the phase III trial enrolling 230 stage II nasopharyngeal cancer patients for concurrent chemoradiotherapy with weekly cisplatin (30 mg/m^2) versus radiotherapy alone (Table 2.3) [4]. The concurrent arm demonstrated significantly improved overall survival of 94.5% at 5 years, in comparison to 85.8% for radiotherapy alone; along with improved distant metastasis free survival (94.8% vs. 83.9%) but no difference in locoregional relapse free survival (93.0% vs. 91.1%).

Intergroup 0099/RTOG 8817 phase 3 study concluded a significant disease free (69% vs. 24% at 5 years), and overall survival (78% vs. 47% at 5 years) benefit for concurrent cisplatin 100 mg/m^2 every 3 weeks and adjuvant 3 cycles chemotherapy of cisplatin 80 mg/m^2 and fluorouracil 1000 mg/m^2/day for stage III and IV nasopharyngeal cancer patients in comparison to RT alone (70 Gy, 35–39 fractions, 1.8–2.0 Gy/fraction/day, in both arms [5]. Concurrent chemoradiotherapy favored over radiotherapy alone at 5 years for disease free and overall survival in other trials as Taiwan, [6] Singapore, [7] China, [8] and Hong Kong [9, 10] randomized trials.

Though considered experimental, sequential therapy including induction chemotherapy followed by concurrent chemoradiotherapy has been in practical life for patients in case of high risk of distant metastasis of high nodal disease burden, supraclavicular disease, or in case of large T4 primary tumors, tumors compressing the critical organs at risk such as optic pathways, brainstem, temporal lobes increasing technical effort to deliver efficient and safe radiotherapy doses. Neoadjuvant/ Induction chemotherapy approach followed by concurrent chemoradiotherapy has not demonstrated overall survival benefit overall concomitant chemoradiotherapy yet, but has concluded that a progression free survival and/or distant metastasis free survival could be provided with acceptable toxicity (Table 2.4) [18]. Phase II randomized trial comparing concomitant radiotherapy with weekly cisplatin and induction chemotherapy with docetaxel and cisplatin followed by concomitant radiotherapy with weekly cisplatin demonstrated with similar quality of life scores that there was a trend 3 year progression-free survival trend to improve with sequential therapy (88% vs. 60%, $p = 0.12$) in addition to significant increase in overall survival (94% vs. 68%) [16]. Recent phase III trials comparing sequential regimens with concurrent chemoradiotherapy alone have been published from Asia [1, 2]. Sun et al. documented their open-label, phase 3, multicenter, randomized controlled trial at 10 institutions in China with the primary endpoint of failure-free survival for induction chemotherapy (3 cycles of -TPF- docetaxel, 60 mg/m^2 on day 1, intravenous cisplatin, 60 mg/m^2 on day 1, and continuous intravenous fluorouracil, 600 mg/m^2 per day from day 1 to 5, every 3 weeks) plus concurrent chemoradiotherapy

Table 2.3 Randomized prospective trials of concurrent chemoradiotherapy for locally advanced nasopharyngeal cases

				CRT	RT	
Study	#	Experimental arm	Standard arm	Disease free survival/overall survival		p
Intergroup 0099; Al-Sarraf et al. [5, 11]	150	70 Gy with cisplatin + 3 cycles of cisplatin/5FU	70 Gy	58%/67%	29%/37%	<0.001/0.005
Singapore; Wee et al. [7]	221	70 Gy with cisplatin + 3 cycles of cisplatin/5FU	70 Gy	72% (3 years)/80% (3 years)	53% (3 years)/65%	0.01/0.01
Taiwan; Lin et al. [6]	284	70–74 Gy with cisplatin	70–74 Gy	72%/72%	53%/53%	0.0012/0.0022
Hong Kong; Lee et al. [9]	348	66 Gy with cisplatin + 3 cycles of cisplatin/5FU	66 Gy	72%/78%	62%/54%	0.027/0.97
China; Zhang et al. [8]	115	70–74 Gy + 10 Gy boost with oxaliplatin	70–74 Gy + 10 Gy boost	96% (2 years)/100%	83% (2 years)/77%	0.02/0.01
Hong Kong; Chan et al. [10]	350	66 Gy + 10–20 Gy boost with cisplatin	66 Gy + 10–20 Gy boost	60%/70%	52%/78%	NS/0.065
China; Chen et al. [12]	506	60–66 Gy with cisplatin + 3 cycles of cisplatin/5FU	60–66 Gy with cisplatin	86% (2 years)/NA	84% (2 years)/ NA	0.13/NS

NS not significant, *CRT* chemoradiotherapy, *RT* radiotherapy

Table 2.4 Prospective randomized trials of neoadjuvant chemotherapy for locally advanced nasopharyngeal cases

Trials	n	Experimental arm	Standard arm	Experimental arm	Standard arm	p
				Disease free survival/overall survival		
International nasopharyngeal cancer study [13]	339	3 cycles of cisplatin + epirubicin + bleomycin, then 70 Gy	70 Gy	54% (2 years)/NA	40% (2 years)/NA	<0.001/ NS
China; Ma et al. [14]	456	2–3 cycles of cisplatin + bleomycin + 5FU, then 70 Gy	70 Gy	59%/63%	49%/56%	0.05/0.11
AOCOA; Chua et al. [15]	334	2–3 cycles of cisplatin + epirubicin, then 70 Gy	70 Gy	48% (3 years)/78% (3 years)	42% (3 years)/71% (3 years)	NS/NS
Hong Kong; Hui et al. [16]	65	2 cycles of docetaxel + cisplatin, then 70 Gy with cisplatin	70 Gy with cisplatin	59.5% (3 years)/94.1% (3 years)	88.2% (3 years)/67.7% (3 years)	0.12/0.012
China; Xu et al. [17]	338	2 cycles of cisplatin/5FU, then 70 Gy with cisplatin/5FU + 4 cycles of cisplatin/5FU	70 Gy with cisplatin/5FU + 4 cycles of cisplatin/5FU	82.5%/94.5% (3 years)	78.5%/95.9% (3 years)	0.16/0.54
China; Sun et al. [1]	477	3 cycles of docetaxel/cisplatin/5FU every 3 weeks, then ≥66 Gy IMRT with cisplatin every 3 weeks	≥66 Gy IMRT with cisplatin 100 mg/m^2 every 3 weeks	80% (3 years)/NA	72% (3 years)/NA	0.034/NA
China; Cao et al. [2]	476	2 cycles of cisplatin/5FU every 3 weeks, then ≥66 Gy with cisplatin every 3 weeks	≥66 Gy with cisplatin 80 mg/m^2 every 3 weeks	82% (3 years)/88.2% (3 years)	74.1% (3 years)/88.5% (3 years)	0.028/NS

NS not significant, *CRT* chemoradiotherapy, *RT* radiotherapy

(intensity-modulated radiotherapy with 3 cycles of 100 mg/m^2 cisplatin every 3 weeks) or concurrent chemoradiotherapy alone [1]. After a median follow-up of 45 months, 3-year failure-free survival was 80% in the sequential group and 72% in the concurrent chemoradiotherapy alone group (hazard ratio 0.68, $p = 0.034$); revealing most common grade 3 or 4 adverse events increased in sequential group as neutropenia (42% vs. 7%), leucopenia (41% vs. 41.17%), and stomatitis (41% vs. 35%). This Chinese trial in locoregionally advanced nasopharyngeal carcinoma showed that addition of TPF induction chemotherapy to concurrent chemoradiotherapy significantly improved failure-free survival with acceptable toxicity, awaiting long-term follow-up [1]. An other Chinese trial by Cao et al. published their phase III multicentre randomised controlled trial with the primary endpoint of disease-free survival (DFS) and distant metastasis-free survival (DMFS) for induction chemotherapy (2 cycles of -PF- intravenous cisplatin, 80 mg/m^2 on day 1, and continuous intravenous fluorouracil, 800 mg/m^2 per day from day 1 to 5, every 3 weeks) plus concurrent chemoradiotherapy (intensity-modulated or 3 dimensional conformal radiotherapy with 3 cycles of 80 mg/m^2 cisplatin every 3 weeks) or concurrent chemoradiotherapy alone [2]. The sequential arm with the 16.0% grade 3–4 neutropenia achieved higher 3-year DFS rate than the concurrent alone arm (82.0% vs. 74.1%, $P = 0.028$), while marginal statistical significance for 3-year DMFS rate (86.0% vs. 82.0%, $P = 0.056$), without any significant differences in OS or locoregional relapse-free survival (LRRFS) rates (OS: 88.2% vs. 88.5%, $P = 0.815$; LRRFS: 94.3% vs. 90.8%, $P = 0.430$). Induction arm was shown to improve tumor control, particularly at distant sites, in comparison to chemoradiotherapy alone without any early gain in OS [2].

2.1.4 Immobilization and Simulation

- Recommend the patient not to have any hair cut during the treatment weeks
- Position in supine with the neck extended and the head on headrest
- Wire surgical scars
- Use tongue depressors/displacers or jaw openers before thermoplastic mask if needed
- Use shoulder retractors for removing shoulders away to allow appropriate low-neck irradiation if required
- Use thermoplastic head and neck mask in possibly comfortable and reproducible position for the patient (Fig. 2.5)
- Check tightness of the mask for any space between the patient's skin and the mask, repeat this step for inter-fraction edema or weight loss to be proactive for adaptive approach
- Intravenous contrast is preferred during CT simulation to improve the visualization of the primary tumor and nodal disease as well as the parotids/submandibular glands to assist in contouring, if patient's renal functional status allows and if adequate measures for any possible anaphylactic reactions could be taken

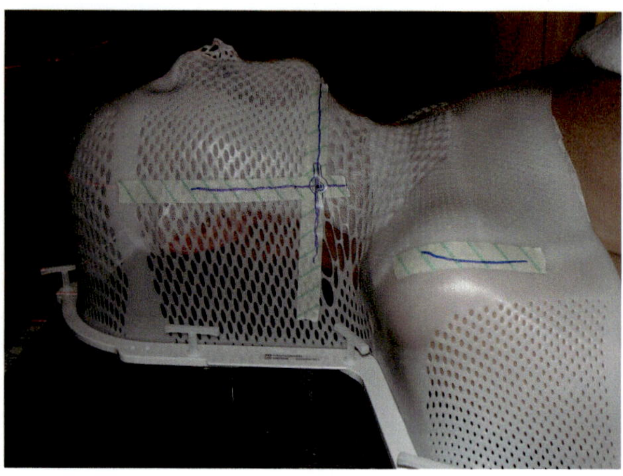

Fig. 2.5 Thermoplastic mask

- Generate CT topograms before the acquisition of the planning simulation scan to review and verify patient alignment and perform any relevant adjustments.
- Treatment planning CT is acquired using a slice-thickness of 1–3 mm covering cranium from top to the entire supra-clavicular region

2.1.5 Target Volume Delineation Guidelines

Case contouring was shown in Fig. 2.6.

Gross Tumor Volume (GTV): The gross disease at the primary disease site or any involved (>1 cm or with a necrotic center or PET positive) lymph nodes determined from physical/endoscopic examination, CT, MRI, PET-CT. The spreading pattern requires critical questioning for delineation [19, 20].

Check superiorly: skull base, foramen lacerum for VI nerve; foramen ovale; mandibular nerve in the parapharyngeal space; cavernous sinus for III, IV, ophthalmic division of V, and VI nerves.

Check anteriorly: nasal fossa or pterygopalatine fossa through sphenopalatine foramen; foramen rotundum to intracranial fossa; inferior orbital fissure into the orbital apex; superior orbital fissure to intracranium.

Check laterally: parapharyngeal space; medial or lateral pterygoid muscles (any trismus?); retrostyloid compartment related with the carotid space to cranial nerves IX, X, XI and XII; jugular foramen related with posterior cranial fossa and IX, X and XI cranial nerves.

Check inferiorly: submucosal plane into the oropharynx.

Check posteriorly: prevertebral muscles.

Clinical Target Volume (CTV):

Though the final tailoring of each case related with the treatment volumes should be based on full consideration of the individual factors and treatment facility abilities, target delineation should be consistent intra-departmentally based on

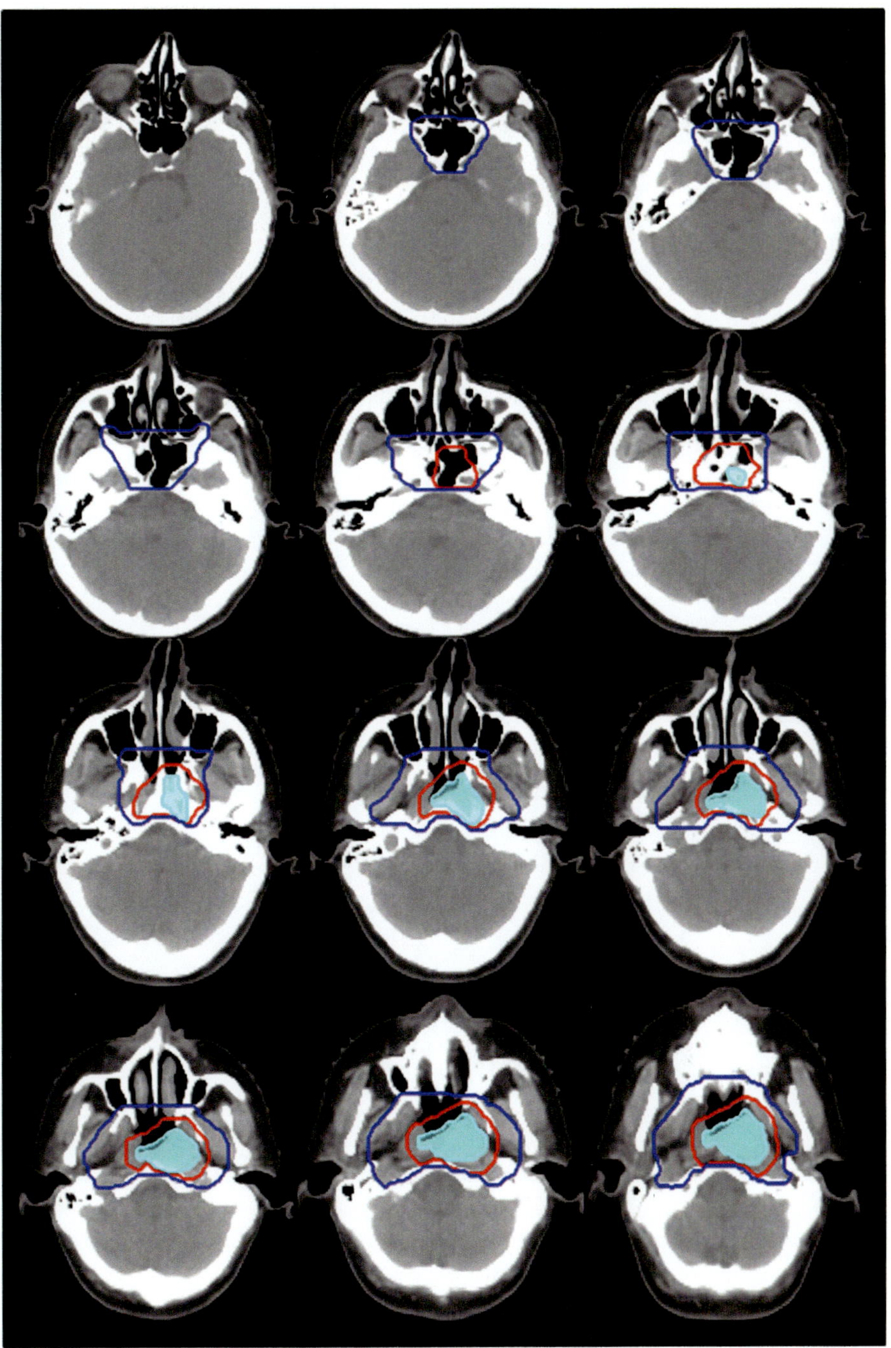

Fig. 2.6 Contouring the CTV1 (red), CTV2 (blue) and CTV3 (yellow)

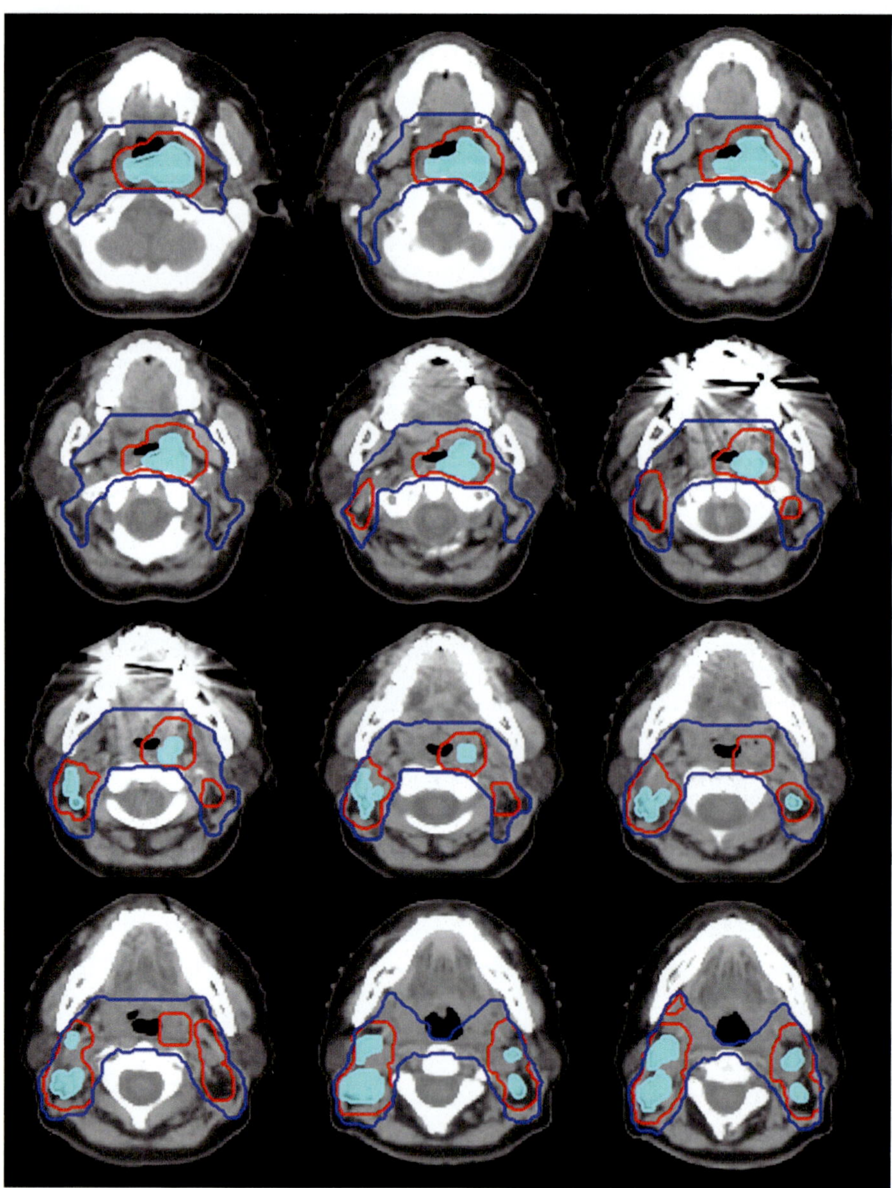

Fig. 2.6 (continued)

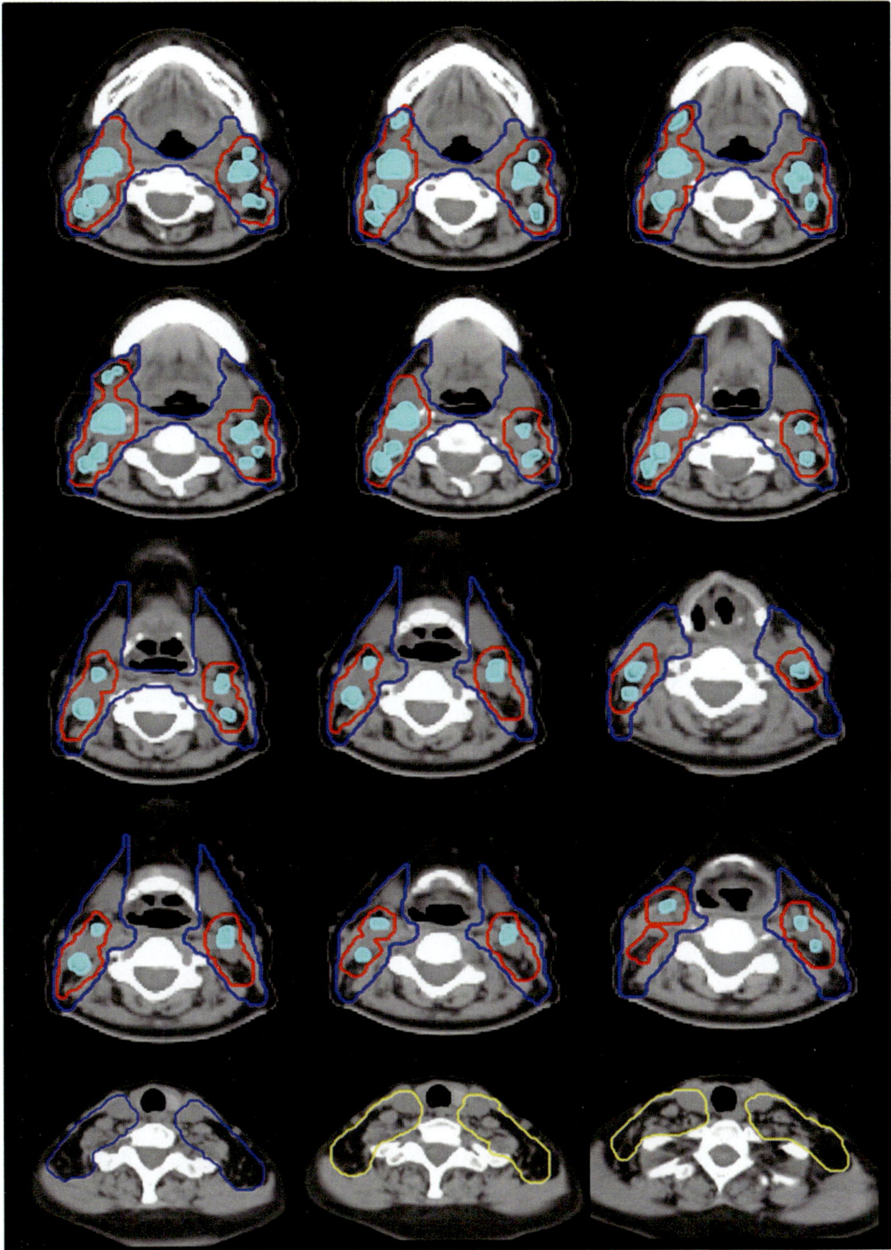

Fig. 2.6 (continued)

relevant literature; such as a recent international guideline for the delineation of the clinical target volumes (CTV) for nasopharyngeal carcinoma [21].

We aim to define overall 3 CTV treatment volumes based on risk definitions;

CTV 1:GTV-Primary and GTV-Nodal with a margin of 5 mm given circumferentially around the GTV which is as low as 0–1 mm adjacent to critical organs at risk such as chiasm, brain stem.

The entire nasopharynx aside from the tumor being in whether CTV1 or CTV2 is not a common consensus, most nasopharyngeal cancer endemic Asian sites recommend whole nasopharynx to be in CTV1 while most non-Asian centers cover the rest of nasopharynx in CTV2.

CTV 2, high risk for microscopic subclinical disease including potential routes of spread for primary and nodal tumor. CTV 2 covers entire nasopharynx, anterior one third (entire if involved) of the clivus, skull base including bilateral foramen ovale and rotundum, pterygoid fossa, bilateral upper deep jugular and parapharyngeal space, inferior sphenoid sinus (all if T3-T4), posterior third of the nasal cavity and maxillary sinuses covering pterygopalatine fossa, cavernous sinus if T3, T4, bulky disease involving the roof of the nasopharynx.

CTV 2 covers nodal target bilaterally if both neck is involved, CTV 2 covers ipsilaterally if contralateral neck is free of gross nodal involvement. If bilateral neck is involved, CTV 2 includes bilateral retropharyngeal, level 1b, 2–5. If lower neck is uninvolved, CTV 2 omits level 4 and 5b to be covered in CTV 3.

CTV 3, the lower risk subclinical disease mainly low anterior neck, and contralateral neck if free of gross nodal involvement.

Planning Target Volume (PTV): Additional margin given around the CTV's to compensate for the treatment set up and possible internal organ motion. If the institution has not performed a study to define the appropriate magnitude of PTV such as 3 mm, a minimum geometric expansion in all directions of 5 mm is recommended.

2.1.6   Treatment Planning

The patient with locally-advanced nasopharyngeal carcinoma presented here was treated with concurrent CRT (cisplatin 100 mg/m^2, every 21 days) utilizing SIB-VMAT technique with CTV1 = 70 Gy, CTV2 = 63 Gy, and CTV3 = 57 Gy in 33 fractions, respectively (Fig. 2.7).

The recommended normal tissue constraints are detailed in Table 2.5.

The recommended target volume doses are detailed in Table 2.6.

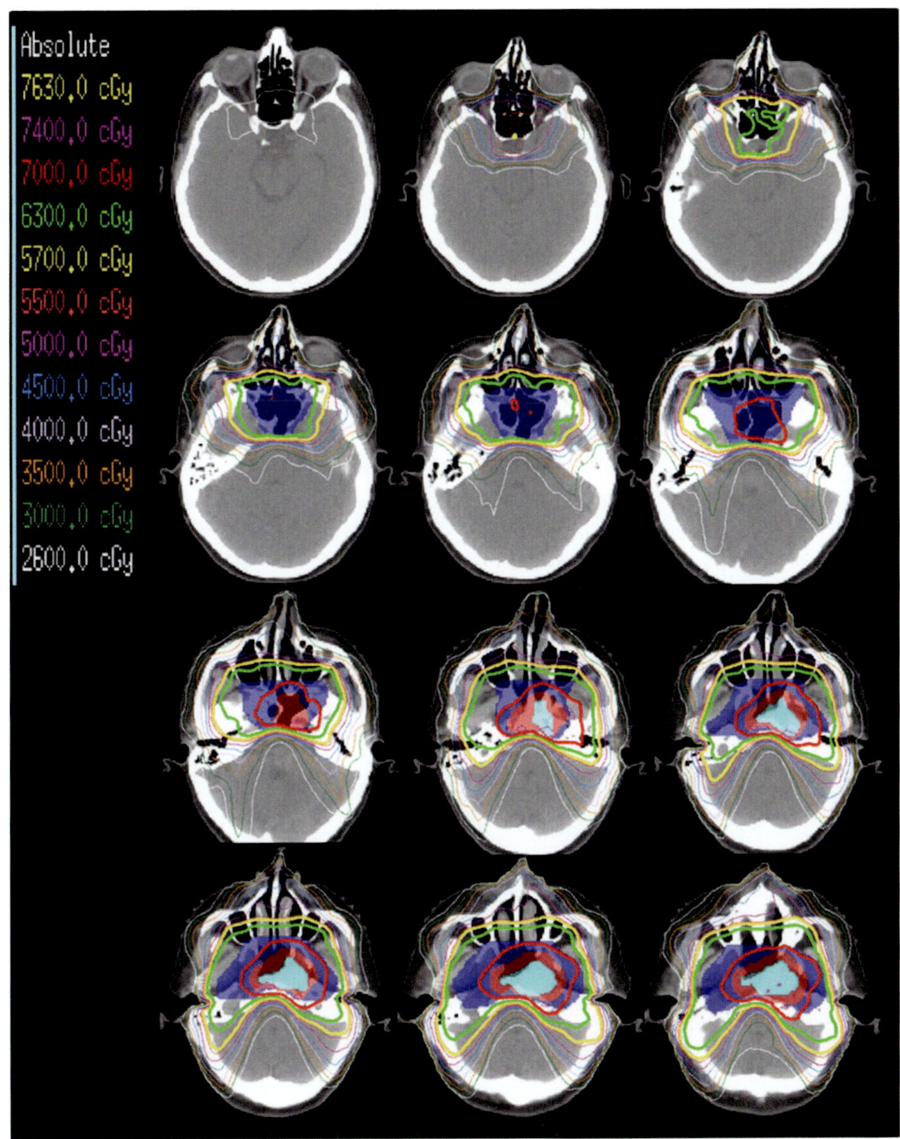

Fig. 2.7 Treatment plan for CTV70, CTV63 and CTV57

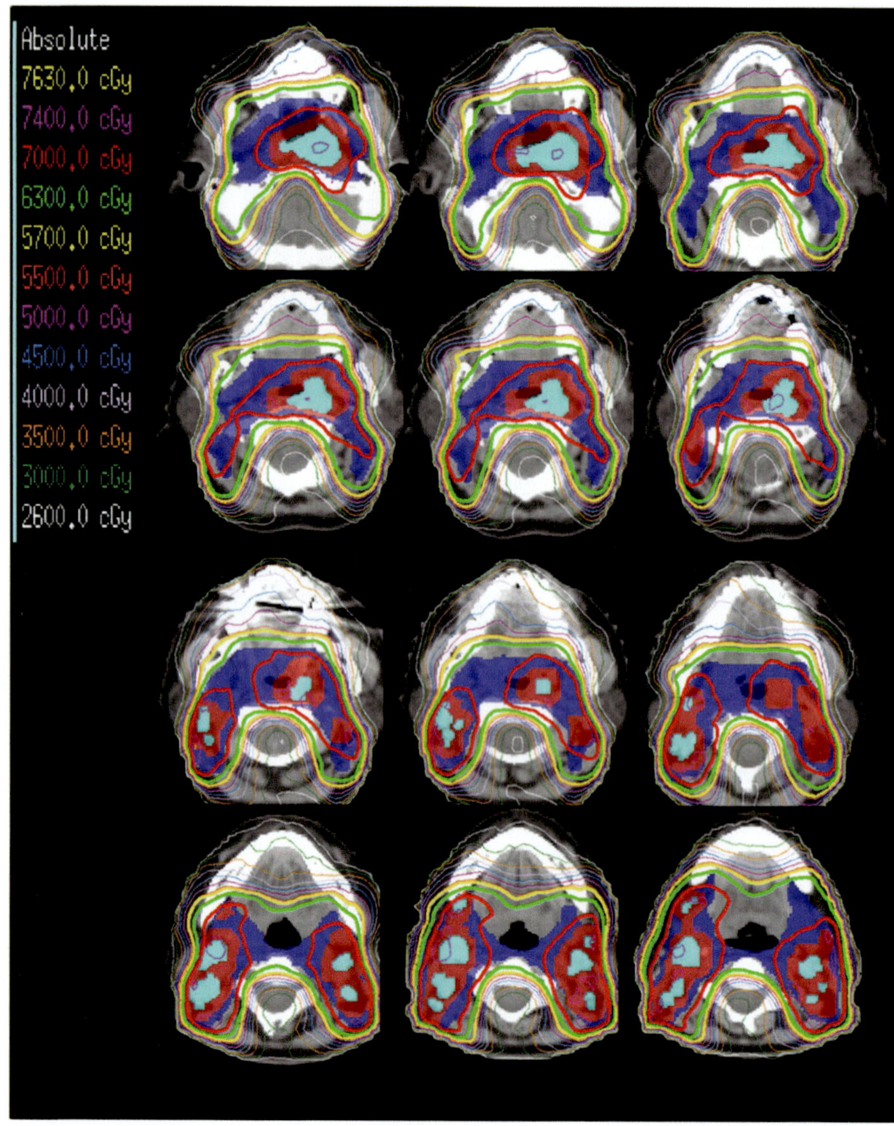

Fig. 2.7 (continued)

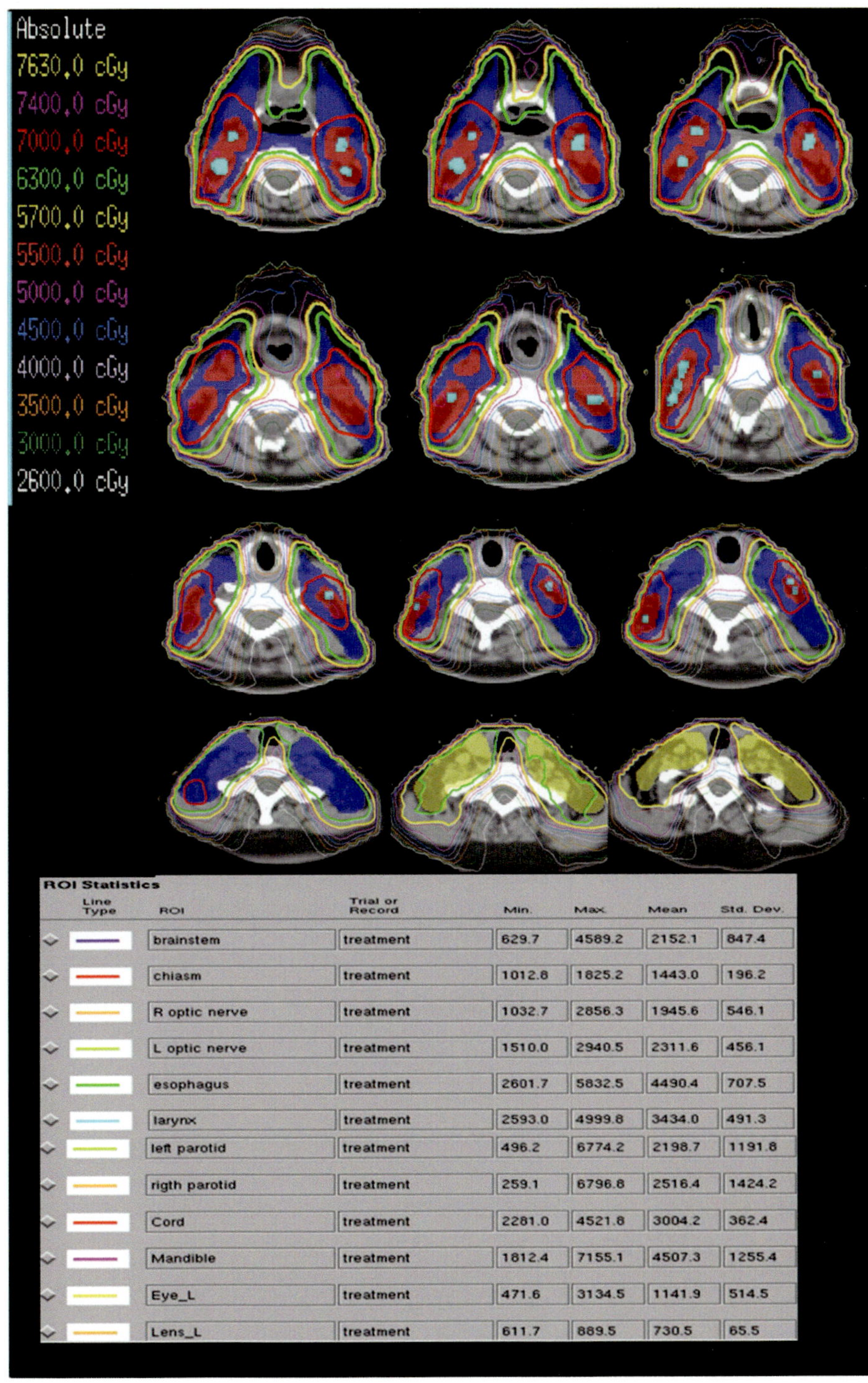

ROI Statistics

Line Type	ROI	Trial or Record	Min.	Max.	Mean	Std. Dev.
	brainstem	treatment	629.7	4589.2	2152.1	847.4
	chiasm	treatment	1012.6	1825.2	1443.0	196.2
	R optic nerve	treatment	1032.7	2856.3	1945.6	546.1
	L optic nerve	treatment	1510.0	2940.5	2311.6	456.1
	esophagus	treatment	2601.7	5832.5	4490.4	707.5
	larynx	treatment	2593.0	4999.8	3434.0	491.3
	left parotid	treatment	496.2	6774.2	2198.7	1191.8
	rigth parotid	treatment	259.1	6796.8	2516.4	1424.2
	Cord	treatment	2281.0	4521.8	3004.2	362.4
	Mandible	treatment	1812.4	7155.1	4507.3	1255.4
	Eye_L	treatment	471.6	3134.5	1141.9	514.5
	Lens_L	treatment	611.7	889.5	730.5	65.5

Fig. 2.7 (continued)

Table 2.5 Normal tissue constraints

Structure	Constraints
Brain	Dmax <54 Gy
Brainstem	Dmax <54 Gy (no more than 1% to exceed 60 Gy)
Spinal cord	Dmax <45 Gy (no more than 1% to exceed 50 Gy)
Optic nerves	Dmax <54 Gy
Chiasm	Dmax <54 Gy
Mandible (TM joint)	Dmax <70 Gy
Brachial plexus	Dmax <66 Gy
Oral cavity (excluding PTV's)	Mean dose <40 Gy
Submandibular/sublingual glands	As low as possible
Parotid glands	Mean dose <26 Gy At least 20 cc of the combined volume of both parotid glands <20 Gy At least 50% of one gland <30 Gy (in at least one gland)
Esophagus, postcricoid pharynx	Mean dose <45 Gy
Each cochlea	Dmax <35 Gy if possible, no more than 5% receives 55 Gy or more
Eyes	Dmax <50 Gy
Lens	Dmax <10 Gy, try to achieve <5 Gy (as low as possible)
Glottic larynx	Mean dose <36–45 Gy

Table 2.6 Target volume doses for nasopharyngeal cancer

TNM	CTV1 (70 Gy/33 fr)	CTV2 (59.4–63 Gy/33 fr)	CTV3 (54–57 Gy/33 fr)
T1–2 N0	GTVp + 1–5 mm	NA	Bilateral RP, Ipsilateral Ib, bilateral II–III–Va (lower neck- level IV and supraclavicular nodes can be omitted) [22]
T1–4 N1	GTVp + GTVn + 5 mm (1 mm)	Ipsilateral Ib–V, bilateral RP	Contralateral Ib, II–V
T1–4 N2	GTVp + GTVn + 5 mm (1 mm)	Ib–V, bilateral RPLN	Bilateral 4 and 5b if lower neck is uninvolved
T1–4 N3	GTVp + GTVn + 5 mm (1 mm)	Ib–V, bilateral RPLN	NA

2.1.7 Treatment Algorithm for Nasopharyngeal Cancer

Treatment Algorithm for nasopharyngeal cancer is summarized in Fig. 2.8.

2.1.8 Follow Up Algorithm for Nasopharyngeal Cancer

Follow-up Algorithm for nasopharyngeal cancer is summarized in Fig. 2.9.

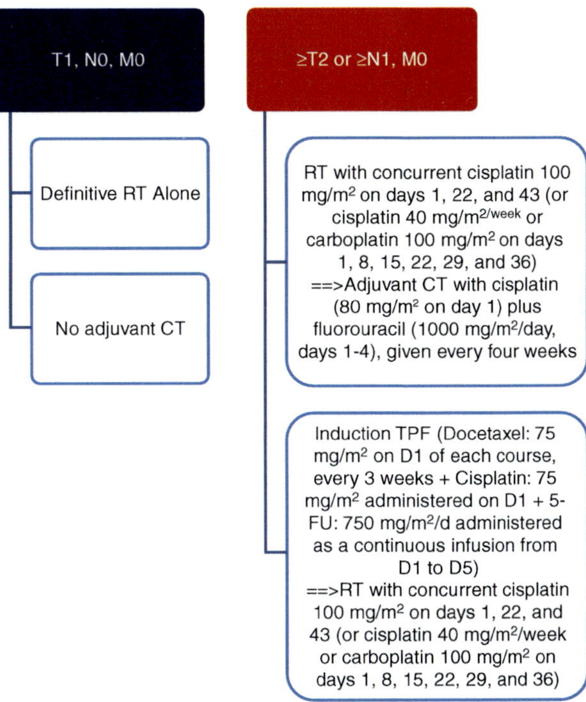

Fig. 2.8 Treatment Algorithm for nasopharyngeal cancer

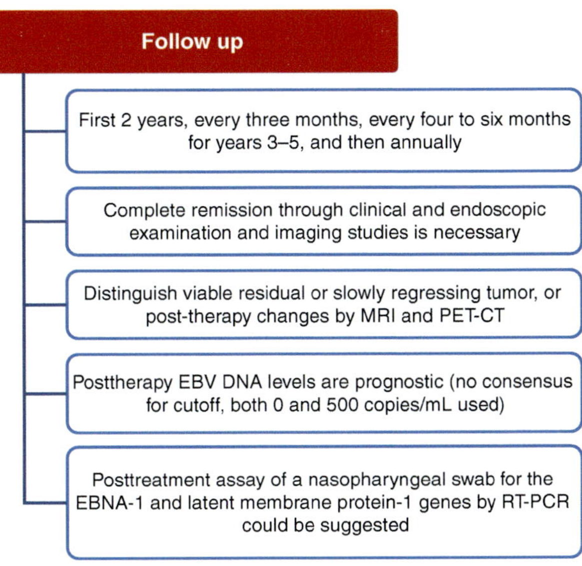

Fig. 2.9 Follow-up Algorithm for nasopharyngeal cancer

2.2 Oropharynx

Overview

Epidemiology

Tobacco and alcohol were historical major risk factors, while human papillomavirus (HPV) infection has become the current risk factor constituting approximately 70% of incidences, mainly in younger adults.

Pathological and Biological Features

Oropharyngeal subsites are soft palate, palatine tonsils, tonsillar pillars, base of tongue including lingual tonsils, posterior to circumvallate papillae, and pharyngeal wall. The most common locations are anterior tonsillar pillar and tonsil, as primary lymphatic drainage is to the retropharyngeal, level II and III nodes.

Oropharyngeal cancer is squamous cell (SCC) oriented in 95% of the cases defined as well-, moderately- or poorly-differentiated. HPV related SCC has a better prognosis. Others are adenocarcinoma, mucoepidermoid, adenoid cystic, melanoma, small cell carcinoma, non-Hodgkin's lymphoma.

Definitive Therapy

Early stage disease requires a single modality approach with surgery or radiotherapy, tailored individually per patient factors, leading to similar rates of local control and survival retrospectively. Bilateral neck needs elective treatment in almost all except for well lateralized tonsil primaries.

Locally advanced, without distant metastasis, stages III and IVA/B cancers need to be evaluated in a multidisciplinary approach to decide the initial modality to be surgery or not where radiotherapy and/or chemotherapy will also be on board; chemoradiotherapy with functional organ preservation approach or surgery and adjuvant chemoradiotherapy (for high-risk features: positive or close resection margins, nodal extracapsular extension, lymphovascular and perineural invasion).

Key Words: Oropharynx cancer, Radiotherapy

2.2.1 Case Presentation

Forty-five years old male who is an ex-smoker with 10 pack year history of smoking presented with a difficulty in swallowing with an obstruction feeling in his throat and 4 weeks old bilateral neck swelling which was prominent on the left. He denied any weight loss, trismus, odynophagia, otalgia, recent voice changes, hemoptysis, aspiration, cough, or dyspnea. He had no significant past medical history. The scope was introduced into the left nasal cavity. Nasopharyngeal mucosa and bilateral fossa of Rosenmuller were normal. As the scope was advanced, there was narrowed airway with a left sided oropharyngeal tumor localized in left vallecula. There were no lesions of the gingiva, buccal mucosa, floor of mouth, oral tongue by visualization. The scope was advanced further. There was no evidence of disease in the larynx, and hypopharynx. Vocal cords were mobile. In examination, base of tongue was soft in palpation. Cranial nerves II–XII are grossly intact without any facial numbness. Palate elevates symmetrically. Tongue protrudes normally. The bilateral neck was also palpable for positive nodes. The MRI revealed a left sided 14 × 17 × 19 mm lesion filling the vallecular behind the base of tongue, possibly originating from lingual tonsil (Figs. 2.9 and 2.10). The tumor was not invading the base of tongue and not invading the hypopharyngeal wall, but pressing on the epiglottis medially, touching lateral pharyngeal wall laterally. The lesion was bordered by lingual tonsil superiorly and hyoid inferiorly. Multiple ipsilateral neck nodal disease was mainly at level IIA, IIB, III, IV, VA, the largest localized at left level IIA measuring 40 × 25 mm without any extranodal extension. Contralateral right nodal disease was mainly at anterior and posterior jugular chain, the largest localized at left level IIA posterior to submandibular gland measuring 16 × 7 mm without any extranodal extension. A biopsy was performed from the prominent tumor confirming moderately differentiated squamous cell carcinoma, with p16 overexpression. He was staged as T3N2M0, advanced stage oropharyngeal cancer (Fig. 2.11).

2.2.2 Staging

As the AJCC seventh edition staging of oropharyngeal cancers reflected the behavior of tobacco-related squamous cell cancer but not HPV+ disease, it had hazard discrimination with loss of the ability to differentiating between stages. Therefore AJCC 8th edition has been revised according to two distinct systems depending on whether or not they overexpress p16 to separate HPV+ or HPV− disease (Tables 2.7, 2.8, 2.9, 2.10, 2.11, and 2.12).

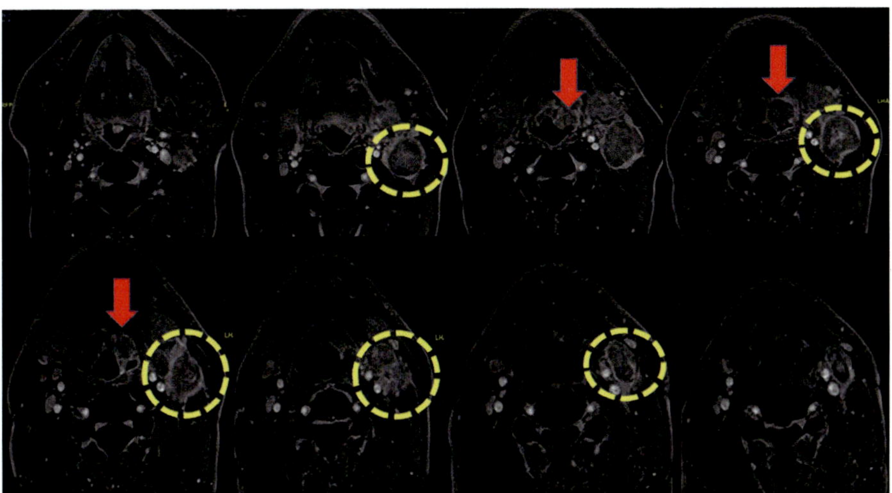

Fig. 2.10 Axial MRI images displaying left sided oropharyngeal tumor localized in left vallecula (red arrow) and large node on left neck (yellow circle)

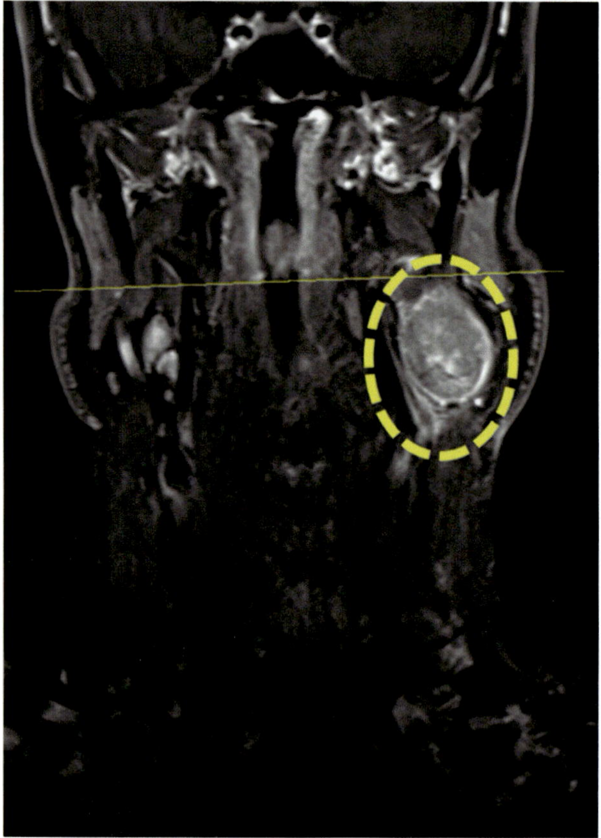

Fig. 2.11 Coronal MRI image displaying large node on left neck (yellow circle)

Table 2.7 TNM classification of HPV-mediated (p16+) oropharyngeal cancer

Primary tumor (T)	
T0	No primary tumor identified
T1	Tumor ≤2 cm in greatest dimension
T2	Tumor >2 cm but not more than 4 cm in greatest dimension
T3	Tumor >4 cm in greatest dimension or extension to lingual surface of the epiglottis
T4	Moderately advanced local disease
	Tumor invades the larynx, extrinsic muscle of the tongue, medial pterygoid, hard palate, or mandible or beyond[a]
Regional lymph nodes (N)	
Clinical N (cN)	
NX	Regional nodes cannot be assessed
N0	No regional lymph node metastasis
N1	One or more ipsilateral lymph nodes, none >6 cm
N2	Contralateral or bilateral lymph nodes, none >6 cm
N3	Lymph node(s) >6 cm

Table 2.7 (continued)

Pathological N (pN)	
NX	Regional nodes cannot be assessed
N0	No regional lymph node metastasis
N1	Metastasis in 4 or fewer lymph nodes
N2	Metastasis in more than 4 lymph nodes
Distant metastasis (M)	
cM0	No distant metastasis
cM1	Distant metastasis
pM1	Distant metastasis, microscopically confirmed

Head and Neck. Used with permission of the American College of Surgeons, Chicago, Illinois. The original and primary source for this information is the AJCC Cancer Staging Manual, Eighth Edition (2017) published by Springer International Publishing
[a]Mucosal extension to lingual surface of epiglottis from primary tumors of the base of the tongue and vallecula does not constitute invasion of the larynx

Table 2.8 Clinical prognostic groups for HPV-mediated (p16+) oropharyngeal cancer (cTNM)

Stage	T	N	M
I	T0–T2	N0	M0
	T0–T2	N1	M0
II	T0–T2	N2	M0
	T3	N0–N2	M0
III	T0–T3	N3	M0
	T4	N0–N3	M0
IV	T Any	N Any	M1

Table 2.9 Pathological prognostic groups for HPV-mediated (p16+) oropharyngeal cancer (pTNM)

Stage	T	N	M
I	T0–T2	N0	M0
	T0–T2	N1	M0
II	T0–T2	N2	M0
	T3–T4	N0	M0
	T3–T4	N1	M0
III	T3–T4	N2	M0
IV	T Any	N Any	M1

Table 2.10 TNM classification of non–HPV-mediated (p16) oropharyngeal cancer

Primary tumor (T)aa	
TX	Primary tumor cannot be assessed
Tis	Carcinoma in situ
T1	Tumor ≤2 cm in greatest dimension
T2	Tumor >2 cm but not more than 4 cm in greatest dimension
T3	Tumor >4 cm in greatest dimension or extension to lingual surface of the epiglottis

(continued)

Table 2.10 (continued)

T4	Moderately advanced or very advanced local disease Tumor invades the larynx, extrinsic muscle of the tongue, medial pterygoid, hard palate, or mandible or beyond[a]
T4a	Moderately advanced local disease Tumor invades the larynx, extrinsic muscle of the tongue, medial pterygoid, hard palate, or mandible[a]
T4b	Very advanced local disease Tumor invades lateral pterygoid muscle, pterygoid plates, lateral nasopharynx, or skull base or encases carotid artery

Regional lymph nodes (N)

Clinical N (cN)

NX	Regional lymph nodes cannot be assessed
N0	No regional lymph node metastasis
N1	Metastasis in a single ipsilateral lymph node ≤3 cm in greatest dimension and ENE (−)
N2	Metastasis in a single ipsilateral lymph node >3 cm but not more than 6 cm in greatest dimension and ENE (−); or metastases in multiple ipsilateral lymph nodes, none >6 cm in greatest dimension and ENE (−); or in bilateral or contralateral lymph nodes, none >6 cm in greatest dimension and ENE (−)
N2a	Metastasis in a single ipsilateral lymph node >3 cm but not more than 6 cm in greatest dimension and ENE (−)
N2b	Metastasis in multiple ipsilateral lymph nodes, none >6 cm in greatest dimension and ENE (−)
N2c	Metastasis in bilateral or contralateral lymph nodes, none >6 cm in greatest dimension and ENE (−)
N3	Metastasis in a lymph node >6 cm in greatest dimension and ENE (−); or metastasis in any node(s) with clinically overt ENE (+)
N3a	Metastasis in a lymph node >6 cm in greatest dimension and ENE (−)
N3b	Metastasis in any node(s) with clinically overt ENE (+)

Pathological N (pN)

NX	Regional lymph nodes cannot be assessed
N0	No regional lymph node metastasis
N1	Metastasis in a single ipsilateral lymph node ≤3 cm in greatest dimension and ENE (−)
N2	Metastasis in a single ipsilateral lymph node, 3 cm or smaller in greatest dimension and ENE (+); or a single ipsilateral node >3 cm but not more than 6 cm in greatest dimension and ENE (−); or metastases in multiple ipsilateral lymph nodes, none >6 cm in greatest dimension and ENE (−); or in bilateral or contralateral lymph nodes, none >6 cm in greatest dimension and ENE (−)
N2a	Metastasis in a single ipsilateral lymph node, 3 cm or smaller in greatest dimension and ENE (+); or a single ipsilateral node >3 cm but not more than 6 cm in greatest dimension and ENE (−)
N2b	Metastasis in multiple ipsilateral lymph nodes, none >6 cm in greatest dimension and ENE (−)
N2c	Metastasis in bilateral or contralateral lymph node(s), none >6 cm in greatest dimension and ENE (−)
N3	Metastasis in a lymph node >6 cm in greatest dimension and ENE (−); or in a single ipsilateral node >3 cm in greatest dimension and ENE (+); or multiple ipsilateral, contralateral, or bilateral nodes, any with ENE (+); or a single contralateral node of any size and ENE (+)

N3a	Metastasis in a lymph node >6 cm in greatest dimension and ENE (−)
N3b	Metastasis in a single ipsilateral node >3 cm in greatest dimension and ENE (+); or multiple ipsilateral, contralateral, or bilateral nodes, any with ENE (+); or a single contralateral node of any size and ENE (+)
Distant metastasis (M)	
cM0	No distant metastasis
cM1	Distant metastasis
pM1	Distant metastasis, microscopically confirmed

[a]Mucosal extension to lingual surface of epiglottis from primary tumors of the base of the tongue and vallecula does not constitute invasion of the larynx.

Table 2.11   Prognostic stage groups for non–HPV-mediated (p16−) oropharyngeal cancer

Stage	T	N	M
0	Tis	N0	M0
I	T1	N0	M0
II	T2	N0	M0
III	T3	N0	M0
	T1	N1	M0
	T2	N1	M0
	T3	N1	M0
IVA	T4a	N0	M0
	T4a	N1	M0
	T1	N2	M0
	T2	N2	M0
	T3	N2	M0
	T4a	N2	M0
IVB	T Any	N3	M0
	T4b	N Any	M0
IVC	T Any	N Any	M1

Table 2.12   Histologic grade

Histologic grade (G)	
GX	Grade cannot be assessed
G1	Well differentiated
G2	Moderately differentiated
G3	Poorly differentiated
G4	Undifferentiated

The tumor suppressor protein p16 overexpression [diffuse $\geq 75\%$ tumor expression, with at least moderate (+2/3) staining intensity] has been reliable inexpensive and widely available surrogate biomarker with immunohistochemistry which is easy to interpret, and an independent positive prognosticator for oropharyngeal cancer.

Changes for HPV Negative OPC Staging

T Classification: Unchanged except T0 removed.

N Classification: Unchanged with the exception of Extra Nodal Extension (ENE: Clinically evident as fixed, deep muscle or skin invasion) dividing N3 into N3a (lymph node >6 cm in dimension, no ENE) and N3b (any ENE+) M Classification: Unchanged.

Overall Stage: Unchanged except moving all ENE+ to N3b increased proportion of patients in stage IVb group Changes for HPV positive OPC Staging.

T Classification: Unchanged except removal of carcinoma in situ (Tis) and T4b (indistinguishable survival curves of T4a and T4b).

N Classification: ENE is not included in HPV positive tumors. Important difference is between clinical and pathologic staging as clinical staging is based on laterality and size of nodes whereas pathologic staging postoperatively is based on number of nodes (N1: 1–4 Nodes, N2: 5 or more nodes).

M Classification: Unchanged.

Overall Stage: Radical Change as stage IV is reserved for M1 disease.

NCCN Clinical Practice Guidelines in Oncology: Head and Neck Cancers. National Comprehensive Cancer Network. Available at http://www.nccn.org/professionals/physician_gls/pdf/head-and-neck.pdf. Version 2. 2017—May 8, 2017; Accessed 5 Feb 2018.

2.2.3 Evidence Based Treatment Approaches

Although there is no prospective randomized comparison between surgery or radiotherapy for stage T1-2N0–1 disease, preferred approach is single modality as primary surgery (transoral or open resection) or radiotherapy alone with similar rates of local control and survival [23–25].

Concurrent chemoradiotherapy is typically the main choice of treatment for locally advanced stages III and IVA/B cancers without distant metastases (Table 2.13) [26–33]. Multidisciplinary evaluation is important to define the resectability of primary and neck nodal disease to decide whether proceed with initial surgery for primary and neck with adjuvant radiotherapy for close resection margins, lymphovascular and perineural invasion, pT3–T4, N2 or N3, nodal disease levels IV–V or adjuvant chemoradiotherapy for positive surgical margins and/or nodal extracapsular invasion (Table 2.14) [34–37].

Neoadjuvant/Induction chemotherapy followed by radiotherapy ± concurrent chemotherapy is becoming a more acceptable approach to be considered in heavy nodal volume with an increased risk of distant metastases [27, 28, 38–41]. In case of ineligibility for concurrent adequate dose of cisplatin, cetuximab as a single agent alternative could be concurrently used with radiotherapy for locoregionally advanced head and neck cancer, however cetuximab did not improve progression-free or overall survival when given additionally to the standard chemoradiotherapy with cisplatin [42].

Table 2.13 Definitive concurrent radiation plus chemotherapy trials

Study	#	Radiotherapy schedule		Concomitant chemotherapy	DFS or PFS RT/CRT	OS RT/CRT
		Standard	Experimental			
GORTEC 94-01; Denis, Garaud et al. [26]	226	70 Gy; 2 Gy/fraction	70 Gy; 2 Gy/fraction	3 cycles of carboplatin +5FU	14.6%/26.6%	15.8/22.4
SAKK; Huguenin, Beer et al. [30]	224	74.4 Gy; 1.2 Gy/fraction twice daily	74.4 Gy; 1.2 Gy/fraction twice daily	2 cycles of Cisplatin	–/–	32%/46%
German 95–06; Budach, Stuschke et al. [31]	384	30 Gy; 2 Gy/fraction + 40.6 Gy; 1.4 Gy/fraction twice daily to a total of 70.6 Gy	14 Gy; 2 Gy/fraction + 63.6 Gy; 1.4 Gy/fraction twice daily to a total of 77.6 Gy	5FU + mitomycin	26.6%/29.3%	23.7%/28.6%
FNCLCC/ GORTEC; Bensadoun, Benezery et al. [32]	163	80.4 Gy; 1.2 Gy/fraction twice daily, 5 days per week	80.4 Gy; 1.2 Gy/fraction twice daily, 5 days per week	3 cycles of Cisplatin + 5FU	25.2%(2 years) /48.2%(2 years)	20.1%(2 years)/37.8% (2 years)
RTOG 0129; Ang, Zhang et al. [33]	743	70 Gy; 2 Gy/fraction	72 Gy; 42 fractions over 6 weeks	2–3 cycles of Cisplatin	–/–	59%/56%

Table 2.14 Postoperative concurrent radiation plus chemotherapy trials

Study		RTOG 9501; (Cooper, Pajak et al., Cooper, Zhang et al. [36, 37]	EORTC 22931; Bernier, Domenge et al. [34]
#		416	334
Median follow up, months		45.9 (120)	60
% Oropharyngeal cancer		43	30
Radiotherapy alone (RT)		60 Gy in 6 weeks	66 Gy in 6.5 weeks
Concurrent radiotherapy and chemotherapy (CRT)		60 Gy in 6 weeks plus cisplatin 100 mg/m^2 on days 1, 22, and 43	66 Gy in 6.5 weeks plus cisplatin 100 mg/m^2 on days 1, 22, and 43
Inclusion criteria	Positive resection margin	+ (6% of patients)	+ (13% of patients)
	Extracapsular extension	+ (49% of patients)	+ (41% of patients)
	≥2 nodes involved	+	−
	Perineural involvement	−	+
	Vascular tumor embolism	−	+
	Oral cavity or oropharyngeal tumor with involvement of level IV or V lymph nodes	−	+
Overall survival	RT	47% (27%)	40%
	CRT	56% (29%)	53%
Local regional recurrence	RT	33% (28.8%)	31%
	CRT	22% (22.3%)	18%
Disease free survival	RT	36% (19.1%)	36%
	CRT	47% (20.1%)	47%
Conclusion by Bernier, Cooper et al. [35]		Concurrent chemoradiotherapy increased local-regional control and disease-free survival of subgroup of patients with either microscopically involved resection margins and/or extracapsular spread	

HPV-positive oropharyngeal cancer (HPVOPC) is considered as a different entity from HPV-negative cancers, based on the response to treatments and survival [43]. Patients with HPVOPC commonly admit with a smaller primary and large cervical lymph nodes [44–46]. Oropharyngeal cancer has initially been suggested to be classified on the basis of four factors defining increased mortality risk as low (HPV+, ≤10packyear smoking or >10packyear and N0–N2a), intermediate (HPV+, >10packyear smoking and N2b–N3 or HPV−, ≤10packyear smoking, T2–3), or high risk (HPV−, ≤10packyear smoking, T4 or HPV−, >10packyear smoking) of death; [47, 48] now the staging system has completely been revised in AJCC 8th edition. As there are ongoing trials, current recommendation is treating regardless of the HPV status according to the stage (Table 2.15).

2.2.4 Target Volume Determination and Delineation Guidelines

Case contouring is given in Fig. 2.12.

Gross Tumor Volume (GTV): The gross disease at the primary disease site or any involved (>1 cm or with a necrotic center or PET positive) lymph nodes determined from physical/endoscopic examination, CT, MRI, PET-CT. Two major sites is covered below; base of tongue and tonsil:

Table 2.15 Ongoing phase 3 randomized trials in HPV-positive or HPV-negative oropharyngeal cancer patients

Trial	HPV status	Inclusion criteria	Exclusion criteria	Treatment
EORTC-1219	(−)	Oropharynx/larynx/hypopharynx primary tumor, stage III or IV (M0)	–	Accelerated 70 Gy in 6 weeks RT plus cisplatin vs. accelerated RT plus cisplatin plus nimorazole
RTOG-1016	(+)	T1–2,N2a–N3 or T3–4,any N	–	Accelerated 70 Gy IMRT plus high-dose cisplatin vs. accelerated IMRT plus cetuximab
TROG 12.01	(+)	Stage III (excluding T1–2 N1) or IV if ≤10 packyear smoking history. If >10 packyear smoking history, only N0–N2a	T4, N3 or M1	RT plus weekly cetuximab vs. RT plus weekly cisplatin
The Quarterback Trial	(+)	Oropharynx/unknown primary/nasopharynx, stage III or IV disease (M0)	Active smokers or smoking >20 packyear	Responders of 3 cycles of induction TPF randomized to 70 Gy RT plus weekly carboplatin vs RT (56 Gy) plus weekly carboplatin plus cetuximab
De-ESCALaTE	(+)	Stage III–IVa (T3N0–T4N0, and T1N1–T4N3) ≥N2b disease and smoking history	>10 packyear excluded	RT plus high-dose cisplatin vs RT plus cetuximab
ADEPT	(+)	Transoral resection (R0 margin) T1–4a, pN-positive with extracapsular spread	–	60 Gy IMRT in 6 weeks vs. IMRT plus cisplatin

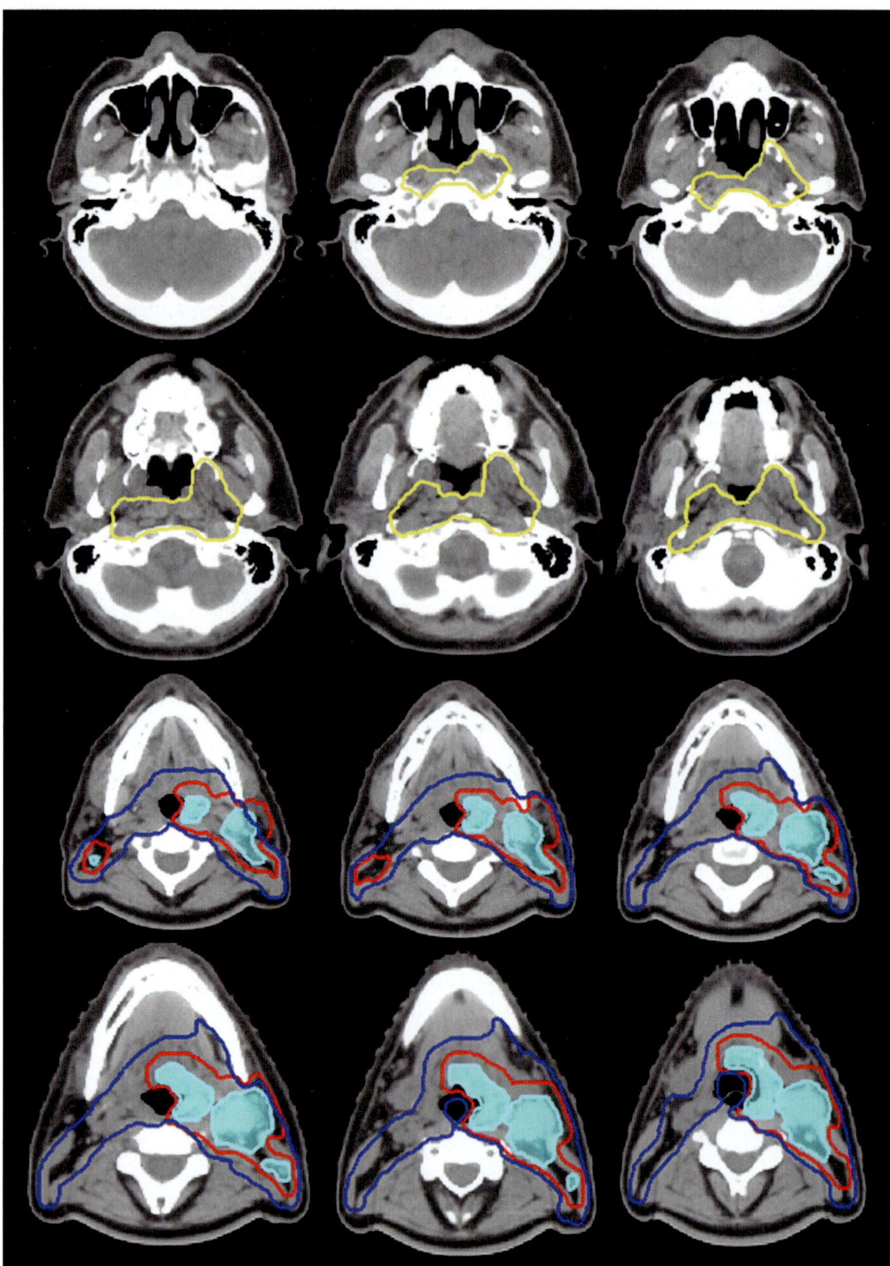

Fig. 2.12 Contouring the CTV1 (red), CTV2 (blue) and CTV3 (yellow)

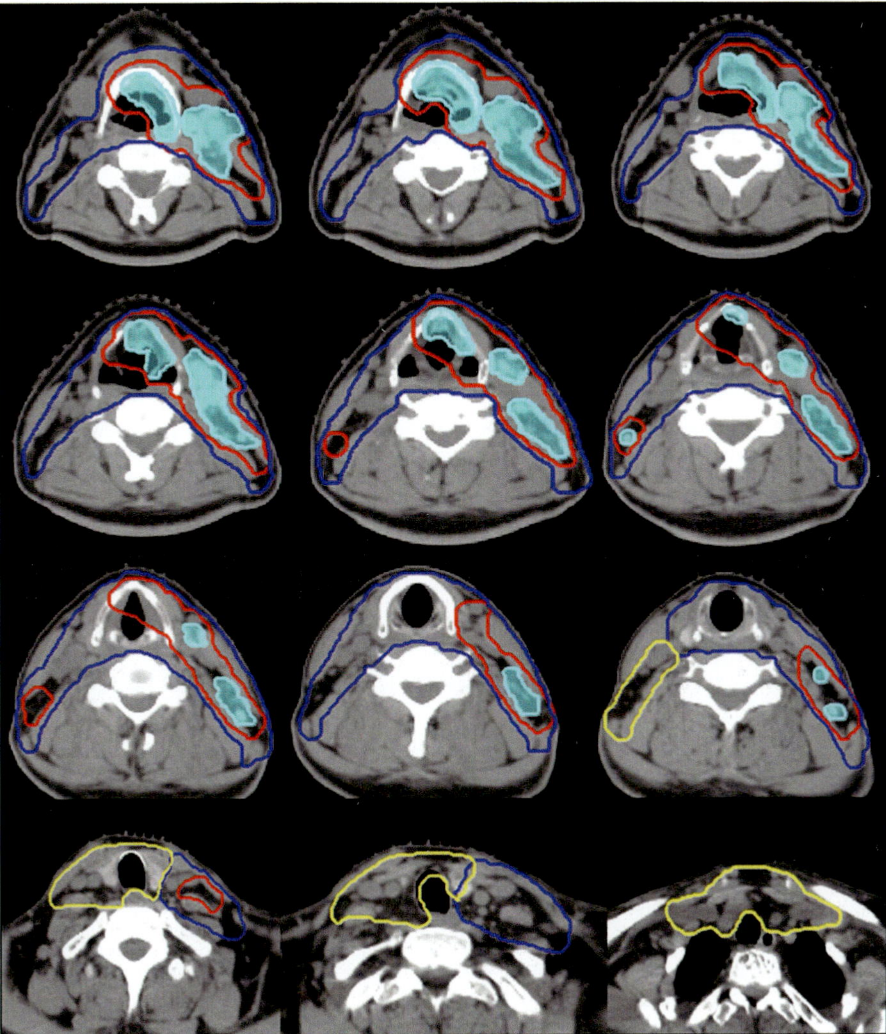

Fig. 2.12 (continued)

Check anteriorly: lingual surface of epiglottis, retromolar trigone, buccal mucosa, anterior tonsillar pillar, tonsillar fossa, oral tongue, mandible.

Check laterally: medial or lateral pterygoid muscles; retrostyloid compartment related with the carotid space to cranial nerves IX, X, XI and XII; jugular foramen related with posterior cranial fossa and IX, X and XI cranial nerves.

Check posteriorly: posterior tonsillar pillar, prevertebral fascia.

Check inferiorly: floor of the mouth, larynx, pyriform sinus, hypopharyngeal wall.

Check superiorly: soft palate, hard palate.

Clinical Target Volume (CTV): Though the final tailoring of each case related with the treatment volumes should be based on full consideration of the individual factors and treatment facility abilities, target delineation should be consistent intra-departmentally based on relevant literature; such as a recent international guideline for the delineation of the clinical target volumes (CTV) for oropharyngeal carcinoma [49].

2.2.4.1 Tonsil CTV1p

Expansion of GTV with 5–10 mm is recommended, while CTV1 of tonsil primary needs to be considered as a region/territory and a uniform expansion is not enough whereas a uniform expansion is suitable for a base of tongue primary.

Contours in air needs to be trimmed.

Anatomic landmarks which are necessary to be covered are maxillary tuberosity, minimal ($\approx$3 mm) ipsilateral base of tongue, minimal ($\approx$3 mm) ipsilateral glossopharyngeal sulcus, ipsilateral retromolar trigone, superior tip of hyoid inferiorly.

2.2.4.2 Tonsil CTV2

Anatomic landmarks which are necessary to be covered are ipsilateral soft and hard palate to midline, ipsilateral glossotonsillar sulcus, ipsilateral base of tongue, pterygoid plate (in CTV3 if N0), half of lateral pterygoid muscle (if trismus or radiological involvement, entire muscle), ipsilateral lateral pharyngeal wall at least to aryepiglottic fold inferiorly, ipsilateral parapharyngeal space, bilateral retrostyloid spaces if node positive.

Ipsilateral neck alone is sufficient for well-lateralized, small T1 tonsil primary without extension to soft palate or base of tongue, or node negative or low bulk N1.

CTV2 needs to cover levels IB–V if node positive; IA needs coverage if there is extension to oral tongue or oral cavity; IB–IV or IB–V is based on location of nodal disease; ipsilateral level IB is in CTV2 if involved nodes are closer or might be in CTV3 if involved nodes are farther away. Contralateral level IB is spared if node negative, or level II is not involved.

Retropharyngeal nodal coverage starts cranially at jugular foramen if node positive, at tip of atlas or transverse process of C1 if node negative, ends inferiorly at bottom of hyoid or bottom of C2.

2.2.4.3 Base of Tongue CTV1

A uniform expansion of GTV with 8–10 mm for base of tongue.

Contours in air is trimmed.

Entire vallecula is in CTV1 if there is extension to vallecula.

2.2.4.4 Base of Tongue CTV2

Include circumferential 1 cm of remaining base of tongue for well lateralized T1 tumors, include remaining base of tongue for >T1.

Other than base of tongue, include circumferential 8–10 mm margin to all sites.

Include ipsilateral glossotonsillar sulcus anteriorly and inferiorly, minimum 1–1.5 cm pre-epiglottic space caudal to GTV, ipsilateral posterior pharyngeal wall with at least 1 cm circumferentially over CTV1.

Pterygoid plates and soft palate are covered if tonsil is involved.

Cover levels IB–V in CTV2 if node positive (tailoring between IB–IV or IB–V based on nodal disease location), level V is not necessary to be involved in low neck CTV3.

Cover ipsilateral level IB in CTV2 if involved node is closer, in CTV3 if involved node is farther away.

Spare contralateral level IB if node negative, or level II is not involved.

Cover IA if oral tongue or oral cavity is invaded.

Cover retropharyngeal nodes from jugular foramen if node positive, from tip of atlas or transverse process of C1 if node negative to inferiorly to bottom of hyoid or bottom of C2.

Cover bilateral retrostyloid spaces in CTV2 if node positive, can omit if node negative.

Planning Target Volume (PTV): Additional margin given around the CTV's to compensate for the treatment set up and possible internal organ motion. If the institution has not performed a study to define the appropriate magnitude of PTV such as 3 mm, a minimum geometric expansion in all directions of 5 mm is recommended.

2.2.5 Treatment Planning

The patient with locally-advanced tonsillar carcinoma presented here was treated with concurrent CRT (cisplatin 100 mg/m^2, every 21 days) utilizing SIB-VMAT technique with CTV1 = 70 Gy, CTV2 = 63 Gy, and CTV3 = 57 Gy in 33 fractions, respectively (Tables 2.16, 2.17 and Fig. 2.13).

2.2.6 Treatment Algorithm for Oropharyngeal Cancer

Treatment Algorithm for orophrayngeal cancer is summarized in Figs. 2.8 and 2.14.

2.2.7 Follow-Up Algorithm for Oropharyngeal Cancer

Follow-up Algorithm for oropharyngeal cancer is summarized in Figs. 2.9 and 2.15.

Table 2.16 Target volume doses for tonsil

TNM	CTV1 (70 Gy/33 fr)	CTV2 (59.4–63 Gy/33 fr) might be individualized as ≈2 cm below the lowest positive node to continue with CTV for the rest	CTV3 (54–57 Gy/33 fr)
N0, small T1 without extension to soft palate or base of tongue, well-lateralized	GTVp +5 mm + tonsillar territory	Ipsilateral Ib, II (might use CTV3 dose)	Ipsilateral III, IV and Va (individualized)
T1–2 N0	GTVp +5 mm + tonsillar territory	Ipsilateral Ib, II–III (might use CTV3 dose)	Contralateral II-III-IV-Va (individualized) bilateral RP (bilateral IV and Vb if lower neck is uninvolved)
T1–4N1–N2b (single node N3)	GTVp + GTVn + 5 mm + tonsillar territory	Ipsilateral Ib (Ia if oral tongue involved), Ipsilateral II-III-IV-Va, Ipsilateral RP	Contralateral II-III-IV-Va, contralateral RP (bilateral IV and Vb if lower neck is uninvolved)
T1–4N2c-3	GTVp + 5 mm + tonsillar territory + GTVn	Bilateral Ib–V, RPLN	Bilateral IV and V if lower neck is uninvolved

Tonsillar territory: region including maxillary tuberosity, ipsilateral minimal base of tongue, ipsilateral glossopharyngeal sulcus, ipsilateral retromolar trigone, superior tip of hyoid

Table 2.17 Target volume doses for base of tongue

TNM	CTV1 (70 Gy/33 fr)	CTV2 (59.4–63 Gy/33 fr) might be individualized as ≈2 cm below the lowest positive node to continue with CTV for the rest	CTV3 (54–57 Gy/33 fr)
T1–2 N0	GTVp + 5 mm	NA	Bilateral II-III-IV, bilateral RP
T1–4N1–N2b (single node N3)	GTVp + GTVn + 5 mm	Ipsilateral Ib (Ia if oral tongue involved), Ipsilateral II-III-IV-Va, Ipsilateral RP	Contralateral II-III-IV-Va, contralateral RP (bilateral IV and Vb if lower neck is uninvolved)
T1–4N2c-3	GTVp + GTVn + 5 mm	Ib–Va, bilateral RPLN	Bilateral IV and Vb if lower neck is uninvolved

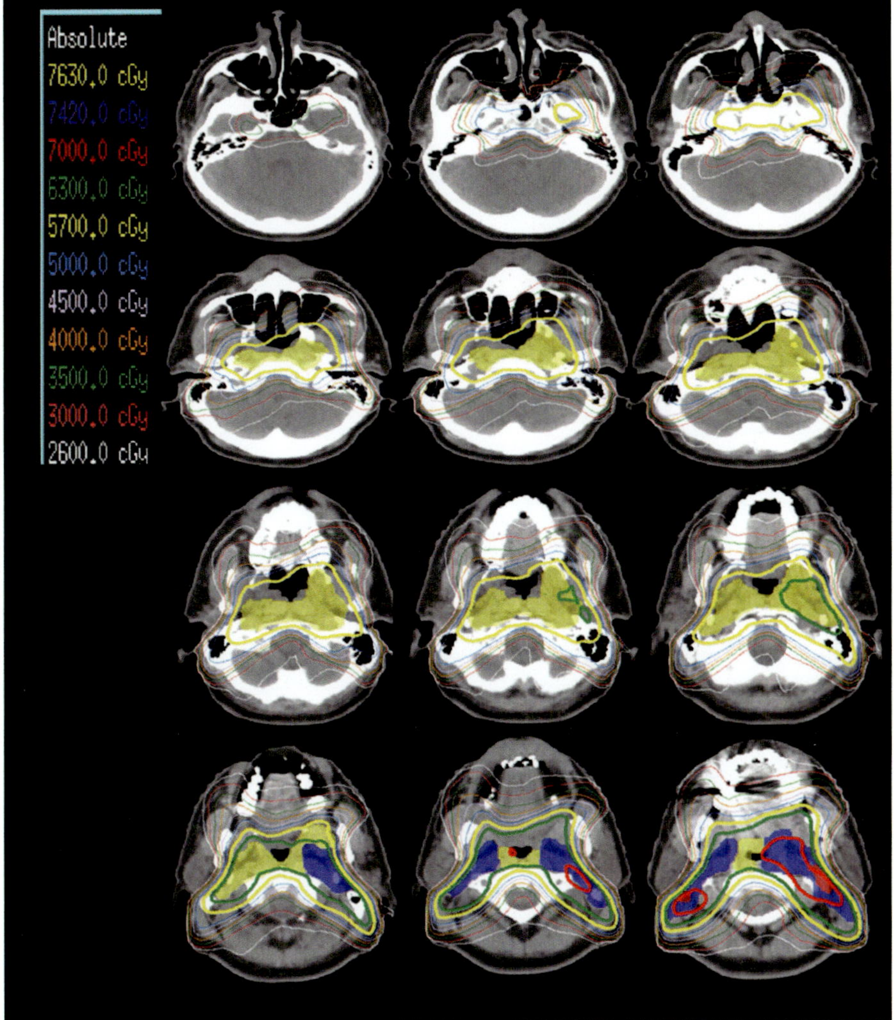

Fig. 2.13 Treatment plan

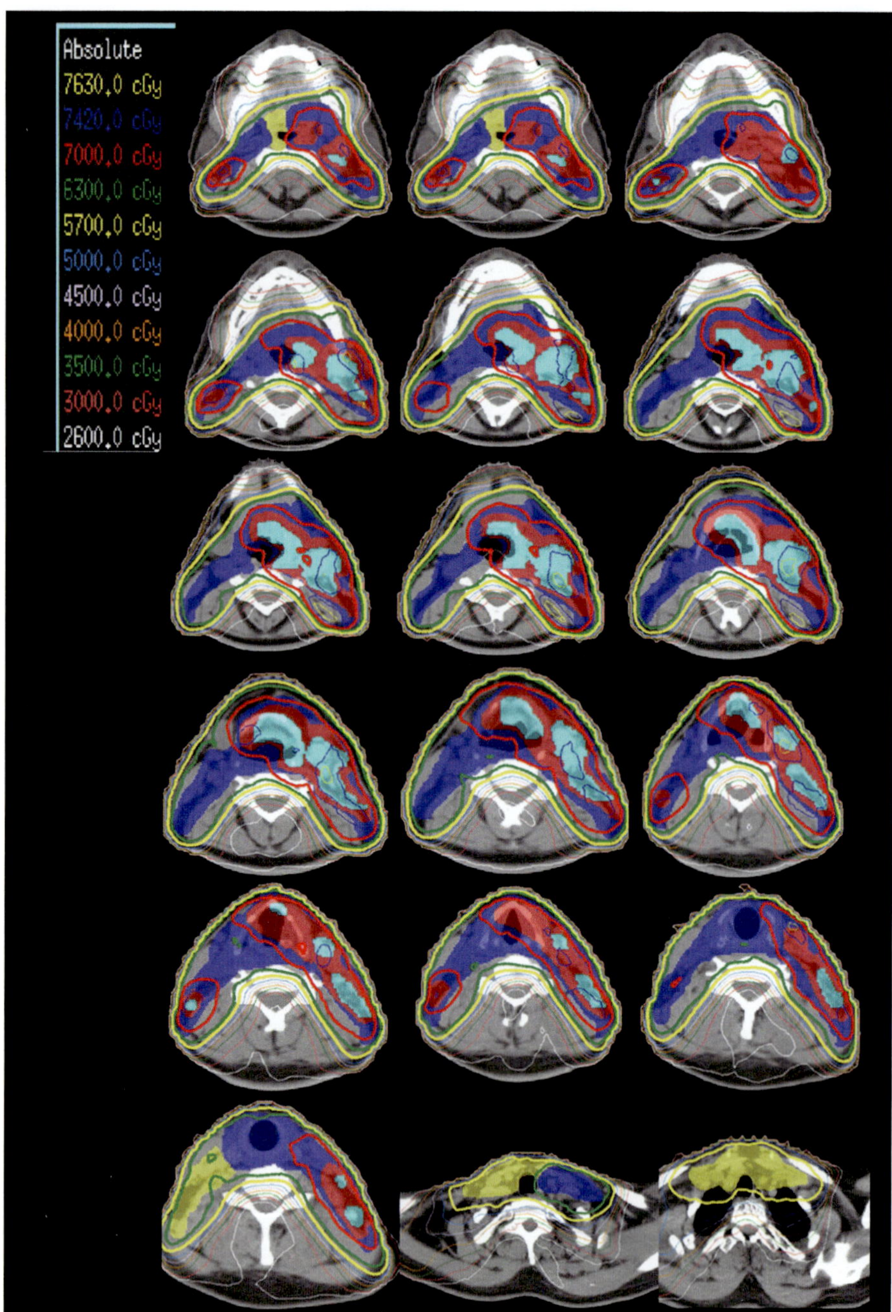

Fig. 2.13 (continued)

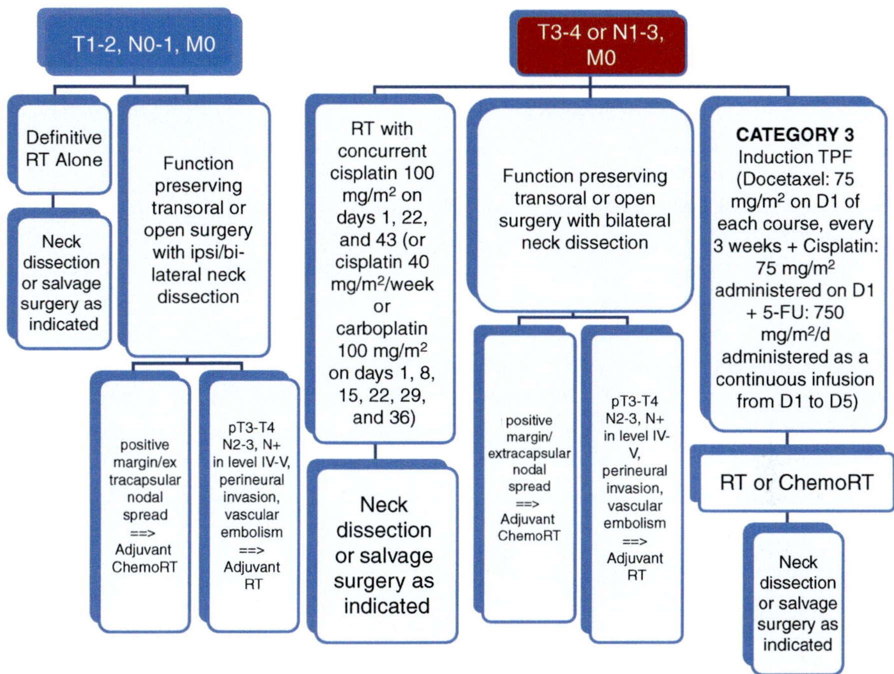

Fig. 2.14 Treatment Algorithm for oropharyngeal cancer

Fig. 2.15 Follow-up Algorithm for oropharyngeal cancer

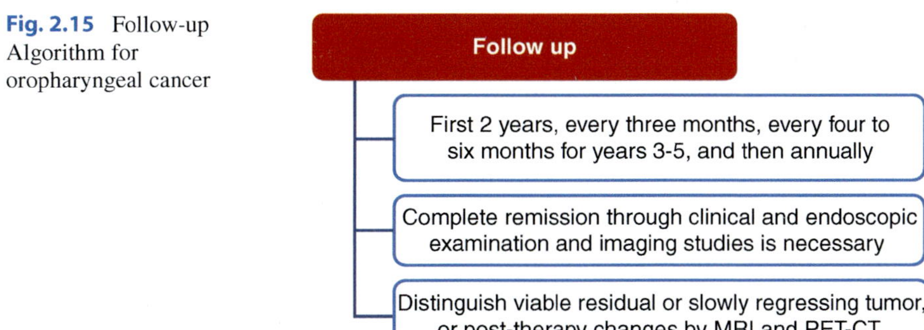

2.3 Larynx

Overview

Incidence, Etiology, and Epidemiology

Larynx cancer is the most common head and neck carcinoma.

Larynx is divided into three subsites as supraglottis, glottis (most common cancer site), and subglottis. The natural barriers for laryngeal cancer are thyroid and cricoid cartilages bearing two weak sites as anterior commissure, and laryngeal ventricle.

The major risk factor is tobacco (packet per day x time of exposure in years), as alcohol is the second.

Pathological Features

>95% are squamous cell carcinoma.

Definitive Therapy

Admission and expected functional outcome, patient preference, age, tumor localization and extension, positive nodal disease and burden are on board for management. The goal with any selected single/multiple modality is to achieve maximal laryngeal preservation if possible without any predicted decrease in locoregional control and overall survival; radiotherapy or conservative surgery are similarly efficient in early stage disease, induction chemotherapy followed by radiotherapy or concurrent chemoradiotherapy are equally efficient for organ preservation, as well as surgery and postoperative radiotherapy (close or positive margins, multiple lymph node involvement, and/or extracapsular extension) ± chemotherapy in locoregionally advanced disease.

Key Words: Larynx cancer, Radiotherapy

2.3.1 Case Presentation

Fifty-eight years old female, admitted with a difficulty in swallowing and hoarseness accompanied by no major neck mass as well as no dyspnea, aspiration, pain, odynophagia, otalgia, dysphagia, hemoptysis, or weight loss. Her medical history is significant for 60 pack year history of smoking, and diabetes.

Her physical exam revealed small bilateral mobile non conglomerated subcentimeter nodes. The scope was introduced into the left nasal cavity. Nasopharyngeal mucosa was normal with well-defined bilateral Rosenmuller fossa, posterior pharyngeal/oropharyngeal wall, soft palate, tonsils, vallecula or base of tongue. The airway was narrow due to a supraglottic lesion measuring approximately 30 mm initiating at left aryepiglottic fold, extending to left vocal cord inferiorly while invading bilateral arytenoid cartilage. The vocal cords were moving normally.

His PET-CT, CT and MRI scans defined the supraglottic lesion measuring 30 × 25 mm extending from left aryepiglottic fold, to left vocal cord invading bilateral arytenoid cartilage and paralaryngeal blurred fatty planes. The inner part of the thyroid cartilage on left seemed minimally invaded (Figs. 2.16 and 2.17).

Bilateral neck nodal metastases were present in level 1B (measuring 6 mm on right, 8 mm on left) and level 2 (measuring 8 mm on right, 7 mm on left) Neck ultrasound guided bilateral level 2 nodal biopsy with fine needle aspiration revealed squamous cell cancer, as well as the surgical biopsy of supraglottic tumor as moderately differentiated invasive squamous carcinoma. She was staged as T3N2M0 (stage IVA) supraglottic laryngeal squamous cell cancer.

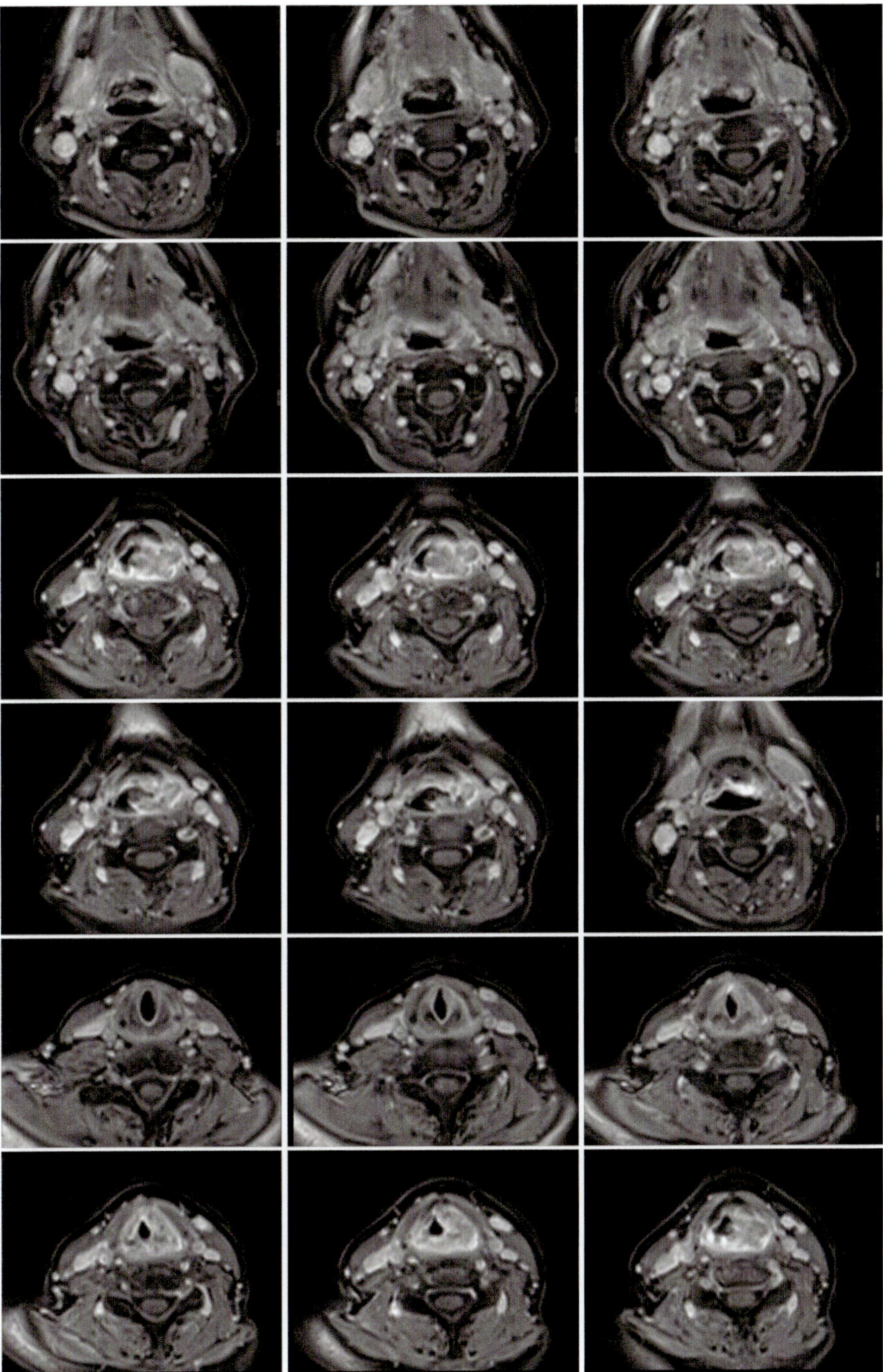

Fig. 2.16 Magnetic resonance imaging of the patient

2.3.2 Staging

American Joint Committee on Cancer staging for laryngeal carcinoma (AJCC 8th edition) was given Table 2.18. Only N staging was revised in new edition. N staging was given previously in Sect. 2.2.2 (Staging).

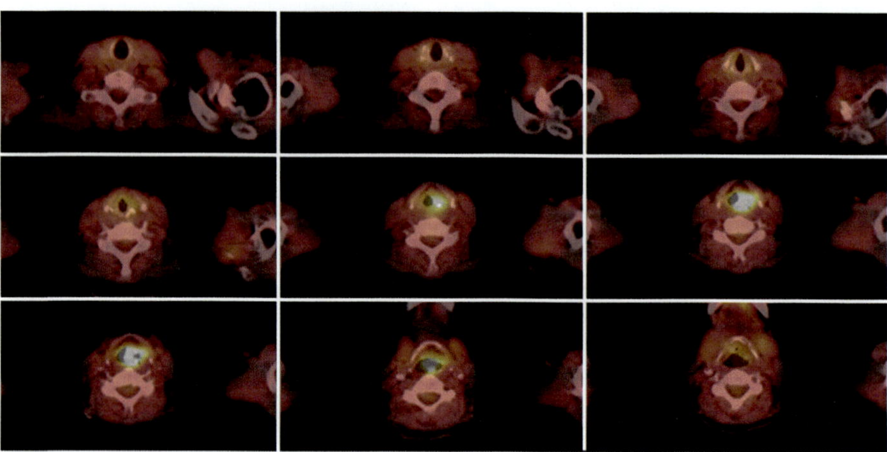

Fig. 2.17 Positron emission tomography imaging of the patient

Table 2.18 American Joint Committee on Cancer staging for laryngeal carcinoma (AJCC 8th edition)

Primary tumor (T)	
Tis	Carcinoma in situ
Supraglottis	
T1	Tumor limited to one subsite of supraglottis with normal vocal cord mobility
T2	Tumor invades mucosa of more than one adjacent subsite of supraglottis or glottis or region outside the supraglottis (e.g., mucosa of base of tongue, vallecula, medial wall of pyriform sinus) without fixation of the larynx
T3	Tumor limited to larynx with vocal cord fixation and/or invades any of the following: Postcricoid area, preepiglottic space, paraglottic space, and/or inner cortex of thyroid cartilage
T4a	Moderately advanced local disease: Tumor invades through the thyroid cartilage and/or invades tissues beyond the larynx (e.g., trachea, soft tissues of neck including deep extrinsic muscle of the tongue, strap muscles, thyroid, or esophagus)
T4b	Very advanced local disease: Tumor invades prevertebral space, encases carotid artery, or invades mediastinal structures
Glottis	
T1	Tumor limited to the vocal cord(s) (may involve anterior or posterior commissure) with normal mobility
T1a	Tumor limited to one vocal cord
T1b	Tumor involves both vocal cords

(continued)

Table 2.18 (continued)

T2	Tumor extends to supraglottis and/or subglottis, and/or with impaired vocal cord mobility
T3	Tumor limited to the larynx with vocal cord fixation and/or invasion of paraglottic space, and/or inner cortex of the thyroid cartilage
T4a	Moderately advanced local disease: Tumor invades through the outer cortex of the thyroid cartilage and/or invades tissues beyond the larynx (e.g., trachea, soft tissues of neck including deep extrinsic muscle of the tongue, strap muscles, thyroid, or esophagus)
T4b	Very advanced local disease: Tumor invades prevertebral space, encases carotid artery, or invades mediastinal structures
Subglottis	
T1	Tumor limited to the subglottis
T2	Tumor extends to vocal cord(s) with normal or impaired mobility
T3	Tumor limited to larynx with vocal cord fixation
T4a	Moderately advanced local disease: Tumor invades cricoid or thyroid cartilage and/or invades tissues beyond the larynx (e.g., trachea, soft tissues of neck including deep extrinsic muscles of the tongue, strap muscles, thyroid, or esophagus)
T4b	Very advanced local disease: Tumor invades prevertebral space, encases carotid artery, or invades mediastinal structures
Distant metastasis (M)	
M0	No distant metasttasis
M1	Distant metastasis
Stage groups	
Stage 0	Tis N0 M0
Stage I	T1 N0 M0
Stage II	T2 N0 M0
Stage III	T3 N0 M0
	T1 N1 M0
	T2 N1 M0
	T3 N1 M0
Stage IVA	T4a N0 M0
	T4a N1 M0
	T1 N2 M0
	T2 N2 M0
	T3 N2 M0
	T4a N2 M0
Stage IVB	T4b Any N M0
	Any T N3 M0
Stage IVC	Any T Any N M1

Used with permission of the American College of Surgeons, Chicago, Illinois. The original and primary source for this information is the AJCC Cancer Staging Manual, Eighth Edition (2017) published by Springer International Publishing

2.3.3 Evidence Based Treatment Approaches

The multidisciplinary effort is mainly on preserving functional larynx, if possible, without any detrimental decrease in local control and overall survival rates in any stage of laryngeal carcinoma.

2.3.3.1 Glottic/Supraglottic Larynx

Surgery with transoral laser excision is generally the first treatment option for carcinoma in situ, while RT is a good alternative. Larynx preservation with radiotherapy is recommended for T1–2N0M0 and selected T3N0M0 cases, with salvage surgery for any incomplete response, as definitive treatment with partial laryngectomy or endoscopic/open surgery is a good alternative to larynx preservation. Adjuvant radiotherapy ± chemotherapy is based on postoperative pathology. If total laryngectomy is indicated for T3N0–1M0 disease for definitive treatment, concurrent chemoradiotherapy or induction chemotherapy and consolidative radiotherapy are encouraged as the preferred option, while laryngectomy in N0 or laryngectomy and ipsilateral/bilateral neck dissection in N1. Salvage surgery is always on board if disease persists in primary or neck. Postoperative adverse features such as positive extracapsular extension or positive margins, adjuvant concurrent chemoradiotherapy is indicated, while radiotherapy alone for ≥2 nodes involved, perineural involvement, and vascular tumor embolism. If induction chemotherapy is the first step, definitive radiotherapy alone is recommended for complete responders, radiotherapy ± concurrent chemotherapy for incomplete responders. Incomplete response after definitive radiotherapy requires surgical salvage. Discussion with T4a should include laryngectomy and unilateral/bilateral lymph node dissection, on the other hand, selected T4a patients refusing surgery need to be treated with concurrent chemoradiotherapy or induction chemotherapy followed by radiotherapy/chemoradiotherapy.

2.3.3.2 Subglottic Larynx

Subglottic tumor alone which is very rare if not transglottic, mostly presenting with advanced T3–4N+ disease, requires definitive radiotherapy, chemoradiotherapy, or total laryngectomy ± adjuvant radiotherapy/chemoradiotherapy. Salvage surgery is inevitable if response is not complete following evaluation after first option radiotherapy/chemoradiotherapy.

T1 and T2 glottic/supraglottic tumors can be recommended transoral laser excision or RT are options, and, RT is generally the first choice of treatment with surgery being reserved for RT failures due to the fact that voice quality deteriorates with increasing resection; local control rates following RT at 5 years are 85–95% for T1 and 60–89% for T2 glottic tumors and supraglottic 100% for T1 and 86% for T2 supraglottic tumors [50, 51]. Increasing treatment duration with less than 2 Gy per fraction decreases local control, therefore >2 Gy/fraction/day is general recommendation; such as the prospective randomized study by Yamazaki et al. emphasized that 2.25 Gy/fr (n = 91) versus 2 Gy/fr (n = 89) significantly increased local control rates (94% vs. 77%; p = 0.004) [52]. *Nodal radiotherapy is not recommended as nodal metastases is extremely rare for early stage glottis T1 (0%), T2a (3%) and T2b (8%); [53] whereas recurrences in primary should indicate considering nodal metastases up to 20–25% which might trigger distant metastases* [54].

In case of local-regionally advanced laryngeal (T1–2N+ disease or T3) carcinoma, total laryngectomy or induction chemotherapy followed by surgery or radiotherapy/chemoradiotherapy, or concurrent chemoradiotherapy are treatment options. Two benchmark studies cleared the path for larynx preservation standard approach as induction chemotherapy followed by radiotherapy or upfront concurrent chemoradiotherapy for locally advanced laryngeal carcinoma (Table 2.19) [55–57].

Larynx preservation era initiated with Veterans Affairs Laryngeal Cancer Study in 1991 leading to a shift in advanced-stage laryngeal cancer primary treatment with non-surgical approach reserving total laryngectomy for salvage, randomizing 332 stage III or IV laryngeal cancer patients into induction chemotherapy with cisplatin and fluorouracil followed by RT or surgery followed by RT groups; [55] larynx preservation was 64% in the induction chemotherapy arm with fewer local failures in the surgery group ($P = 0.0005$) and fewer distant metastases in the chemotherapy group ($P = 0.016$) [55]. RTOG 91-11 study randomized 547 patients with stage III or IV laryngeal cancer into three arms of induction chemotherapy (cisplatin and fluorouracil) followed by radiotherapy, radiotherapy given concurrently with cisplatin, and radiotherapy alone in order to define appropriate timing of chemotherapy (induction vs. concurrent), [56, 57] where both chemotherapy arms were shown to increase disease-free survival in comparison to radiotherapy alone. Larynx preservation with an intact larynx at 2 years was significantly higher with 88% in the concurrent schema versus 75% ($P = 0.005$) in induction and 70% in radiotherapy alone arms ($P < 0.001$); locoregional control rate was also similarly higher in the concurrent chemoradiotherapy arm than the chemotherapy and RT alone group (concurrent, 78% vs. induction, 61% vs. radiotherapy alone, 56%) [56, 57].

Three-dimensional conformal radiotherapy is a viable technique for early stage laryngeal carcinomas, while carotid sparing intensity modulated radiotherapy is also appealing [58–60].

Intensity modulated radiotherapy based techniques are preferred modalities for locally advanced laryngeal carcinoma patients due to better organ at risk sparing abilities [61, 62].

2.3.4 Target Volume Determination and Delineation Guidelines

Case contouring was shown in Fig. 2.18.

If there is induction chemotherapy, defining pre-chemotherapy target volumes carry importance to allow coverage of the regressed GTV to be delineated at least in CTV2 with co-registration of pre- and post-chemotherapy images.

Table 2.19 Randomized larynx preservation trials

Studies	#	Treatment arms			Overall survival	Larynx preservation
VA, Wolf et al. [55]	332	Surgery + radiotherapy	Induction chemotherapy + radiotherapy		68% (2 years) 68% (2 years)	– 64% (2 years)
RTOG-91-11, Forastiere et al. [56, 57]	547	Induction chemotherapy + radiotherapy	Concurrent chemoradiotherapy	Radiotherapy	38.5% (10 years) 27.5% (10 years) 31.5% (10 years)	67.5% (10 years) 81.7% (10 years) 63.8% (10 years)
EORTC 24891, Lefebvre et al. [64]	202	Surgery + Radiotherapy	Induction chemotherapy + radiotherapy		32.6% (5 years) 13.8% (10 years) 38% (5 years) 13.1% (10 years)	– – 21.9 (5 years) 8.7% (10 years)
GETTEC, Richard et al. [65]	68	S + RT	Induction chemotherapy + radiotherapy		84% (2 years) 69% (2 years)	– 42% (2 years)
GORTEC 2000–01, Janoray et al. [66, 67]	213	PF Induction chemotherapy + radiotherapy	TPF induction chemotherapy + radiotherapy		60% (3 years) 60% (3-years)	57.5% (3 years) 70.3% (3-years)

TAX 324, Posner et al. (subgroup) [68]	166	PF Induction chemotherapy + chemoradiotherapy	TPF Induction chemotherapy + chemoradiotherapy		40% (3-years) 57% (3 years)	32% (3-years) 52% (3 years)
EORTC 24954, Lefebvre et al. [69]	450	Sequential PF Induction chemotherapy + radiotherapy	Alternating PF Induction chemotherapy + radiotherapy		62.2% (3 years) 48.5% (5 years) 64.8% (3 years) 51.9% (5 years)	39.5% (3 years) 30.5% (5 years) 45.4% (3 years) 36.2% (5 years)
TREMPLIN [70]	153	TPF induction chemotherapy + chemoradiotherapy (Platin based)	TPF induction chemotherapy + chemoradiotherapy (Cetixumab)		92% (18 months) 89% (18 months)	87% (18 months) 82% (18 months)

Abbreviations: *TPF* docetaxel, cisplatin, fluorouracil

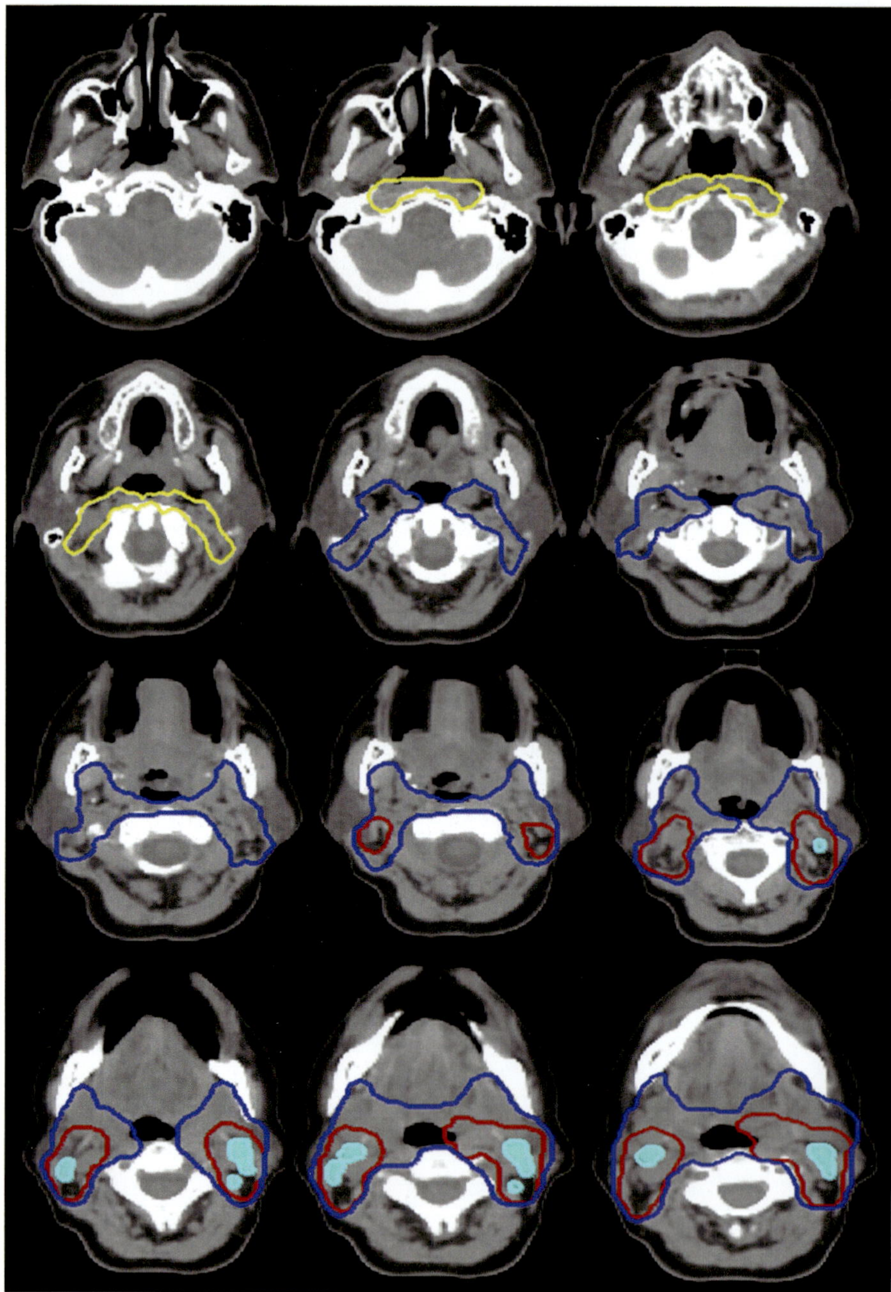

Fig. 2.18 Contouring the CTV1 (red), CTV2 (blue) and CTV3 (yellow)

Fig. 2.18 (continued)

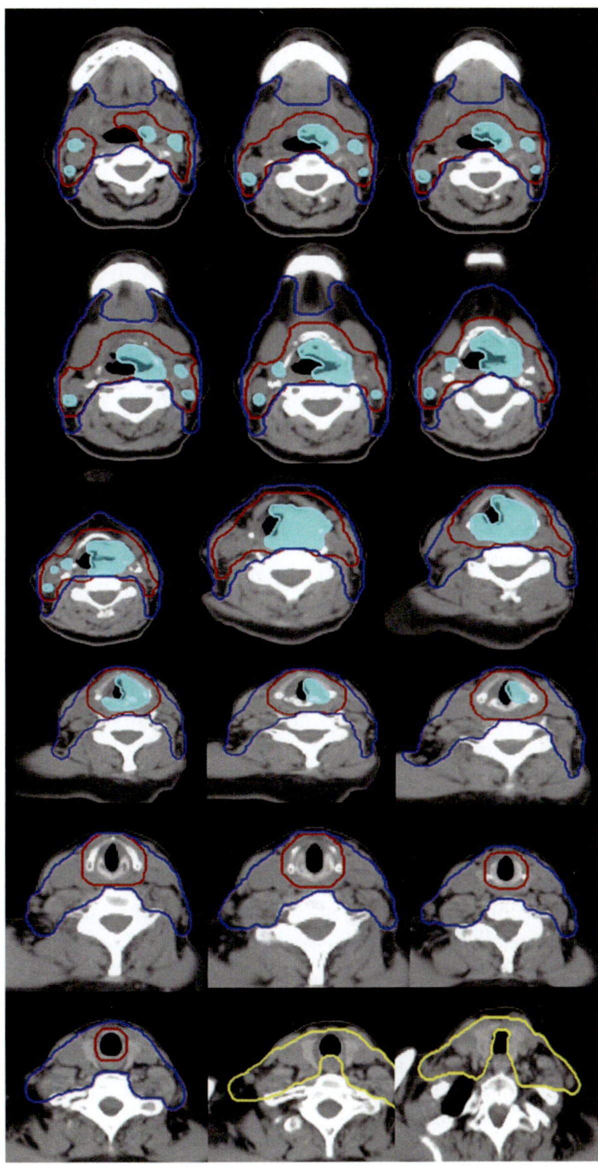

Gross Tumor Volume (GTV): The gross disease at the primary disease site or any involved (>1 cm or with a necrotic center or PET positive) lymph nodes determined from physical/endoscopic examination, CT, MRI, PET-CT.

Clinical Target Volume (CTV): Though the final tailoring of each case related with the treatment volumes should be based on full consideration of the individual factors and treatment facility abilities, target delineation should be consistent intra-departmentally based on relevant literature; such as a recent international guideline for the delineation of the clinical target volumes (CTV) for laryngeal carcinoma primary and nodal disease [49, 63].

CTV for T1–2N0 glottic cancer requires the entire larynx as an anatomic landmark to be covered, from top of thyroid notch to the bottom of the thyroid cartilage.

Risk definition implies three CTV for definitive radiotherapy in locally advanced laryngeal tumors.

CTV1: A uniform expansion of GTV with 5–8 mm at all directions, but may be reduced to as low as 1 mm in close proximity of critical structures.

CTV2: A uniform expansion of CTV1 with at least 10 mm at all directions, to cover potential microscopic mucosal and submucosal routes of disease spread.

CTV2 needs to cover levels II–IV if node positive; IB needs coverage if level 2 is positive.

Level 5 is covered if level II–IV are heavily involved. If bulky nodal volume present, tailoring retropharyngeal node coverage due to retrograde lymphatic flow might be an option which is not necessary in routine. Level VI requires to be covered in presence of subglottic extension or subglottic lesions.

CTV3: cover levels II–IV of the uninvolved neck.

Planning Target Volume (PTV): Additional margin given around the CTV's to compensate for the treatment set up and possible internal organ motion. If the institution has not performed a study to define the appropriate magnitude of PTV such as 3 mm, a minimum geometric expansion in all directions of 5 mm is recommended.

2.3.5 Treatment Planning

The patient with locally-advanced laryngeal carcinoma presented here was treated with concurrent CRT (cisplatin 100 mg/m^2, every 21 days) utilizing SIB-VMAT technique with CTV1 = 70 Gy, CTV2 = 63 Gy, and CTV3 = 57 Gy in 35 fractions, respectively (Fig. 2.19).

Guidelines for Target Volume Doses (Table 2.20).
Guidelines for Normal Tissue Constraints
As given in Table 2.5.

2.3.6 Treatment Algorithm for Larynx Cancer

Treatment Algorithm for larynx cancer is summarized in Figs. 2.20, 2.21, and 2.22.

2.3.7 Follow-Up Algorithm for Larynx Cancer

Please see Sect. 2.2.7.

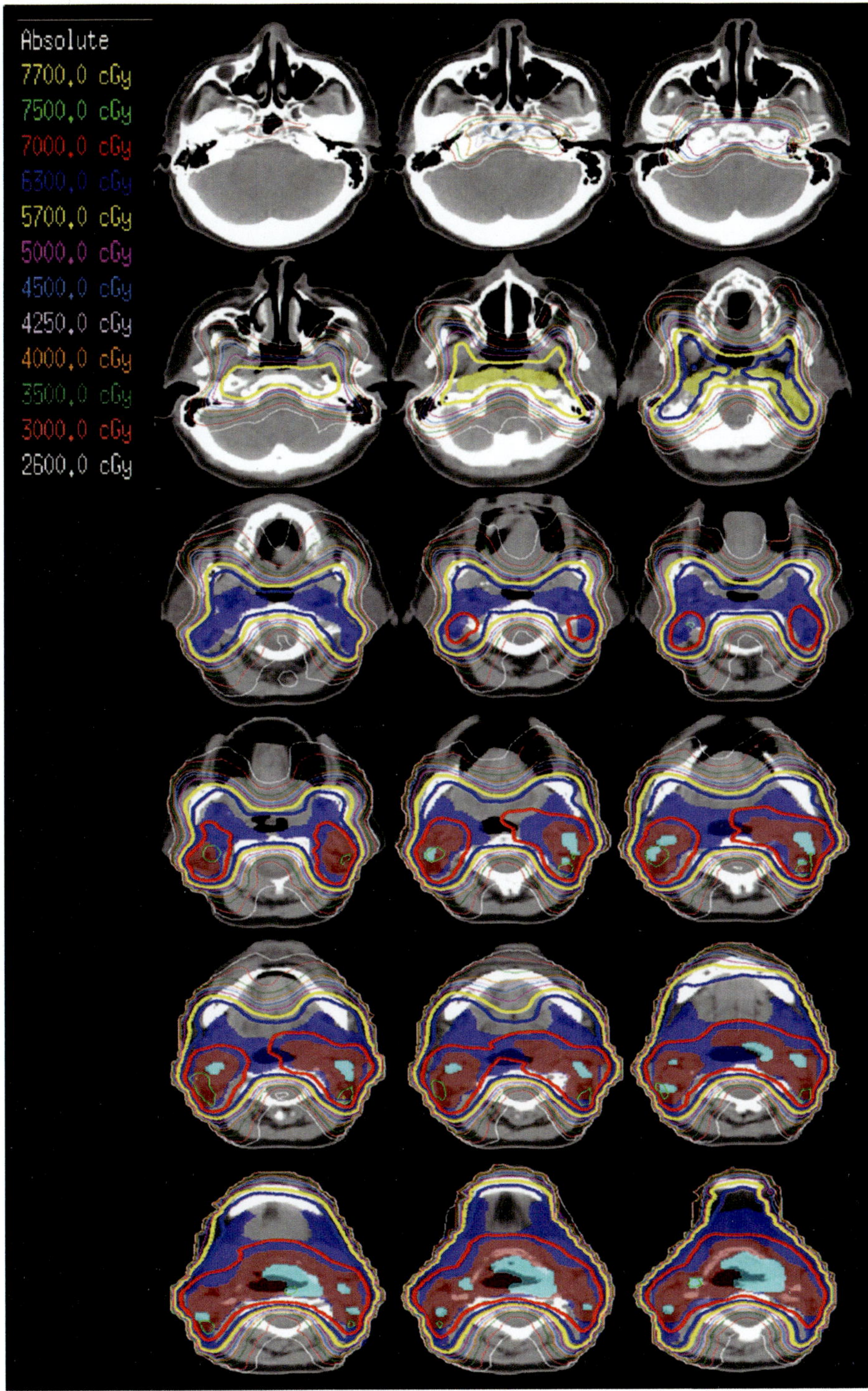

Fig. 2.19 Treatment plan

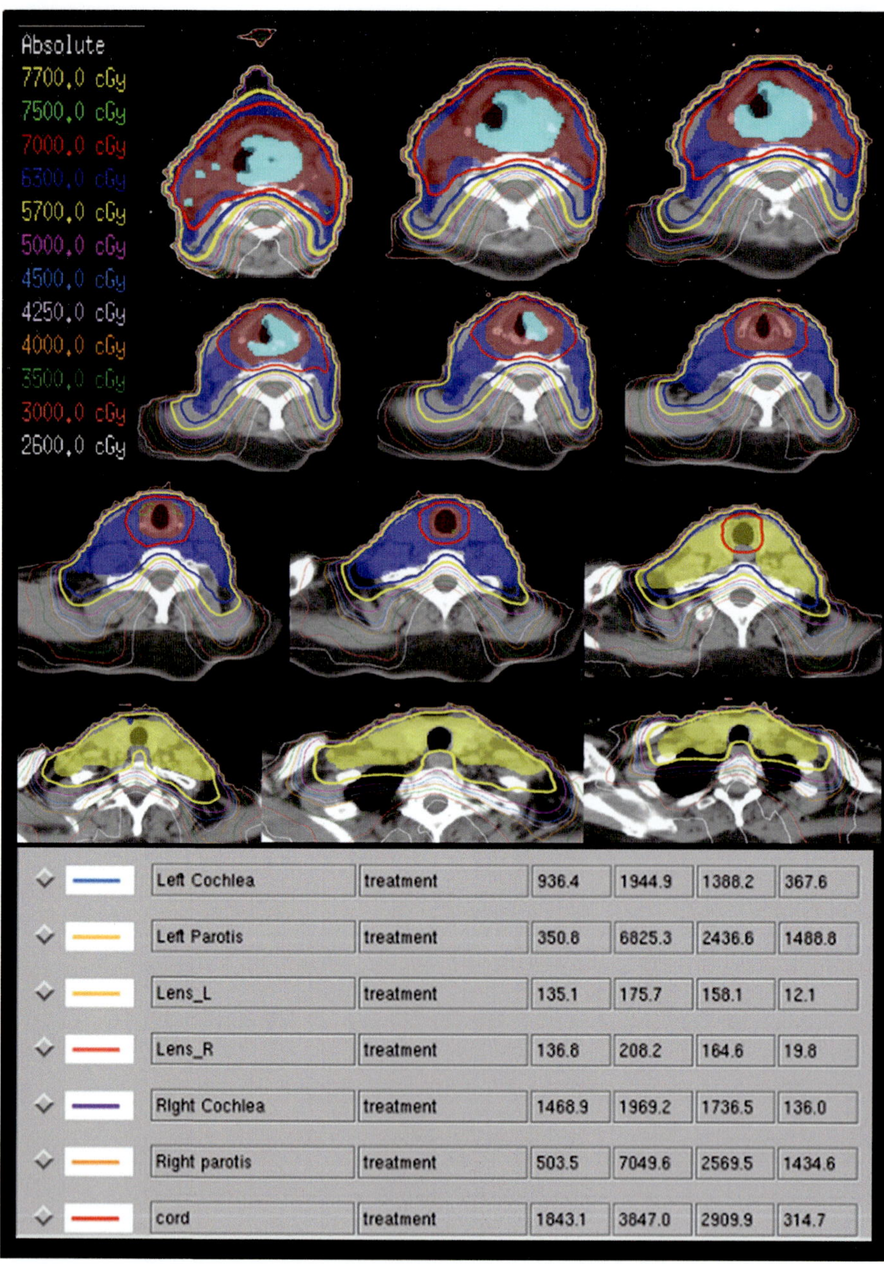

—	Left Cochlea	treatment	936.4	1944.9	1388.2	367.6
—	Left Parotis	treatment	350.8	6825.3	2436.6	1488.8
—	Lens_L	treatment	135.1	175.7	158.1	12.1
—	Lens_R	treatment	136.8	208.2	164.6	19.8
—	Right Cochlea	treatment	1468.9	1969.2	1736.5	136.0
—	Right parotis	treatment	503.5	7049.6	2569.5	1434.6
—	cord	treatment	1843.1	3847.0	2909.9	314.7

Fig. 2.19 (continued)

Table 2.20   Target volume doses for laryngeal cancer

TNM	CTV1 (70 Gy/33–35 fr) (T1–2N0, 65.25 Gy/2.25 fr)	CTV2 (59.4–63 Gy/33–35 fr) might be individualized as ≈2 cm below the lowest positive node to continue with CTV for the rest	CTV3 (54–57 Gy/33–35 fr)
T1–2 N0	GTVp + 5 mm + entire remaining larynx	NA	NA
T1–4N1–N3	GTVp + GTVn + 5 mm	Ipsilateral Ib (if level 2b involved), Ipsilateral II-III-IV	Contralateral II–III–IV

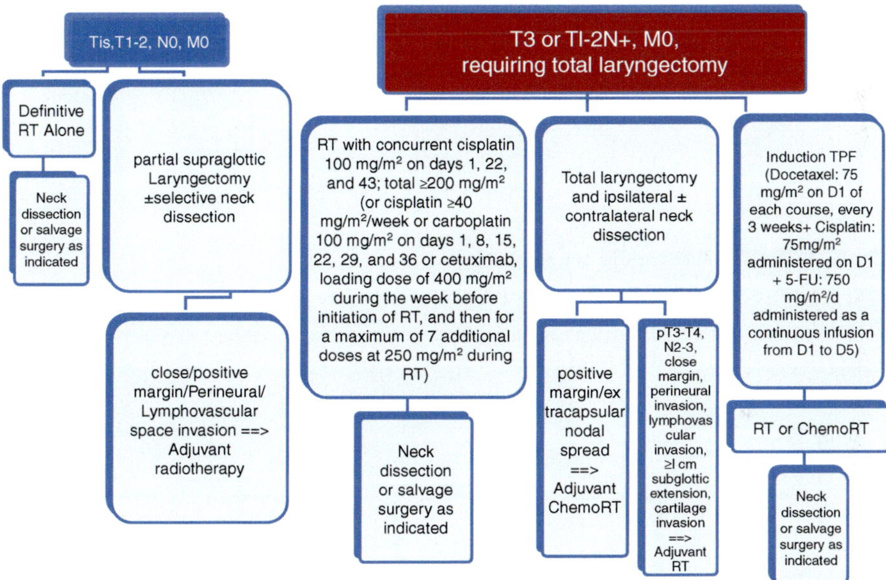

Fig. 2.20   Treatment Algorithm for supraglottic larynx cancer

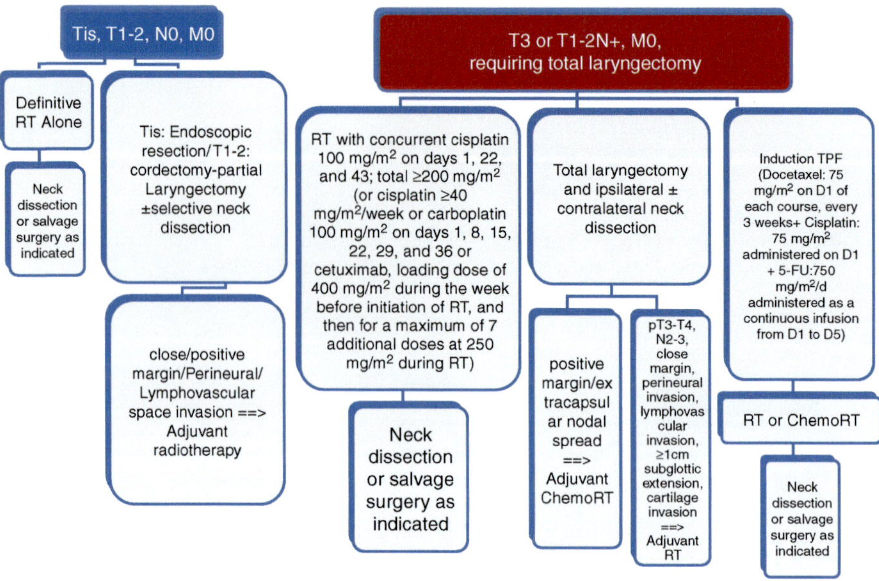

Fig. 2.21 Treatment Algorithm for glottis larynx cancer

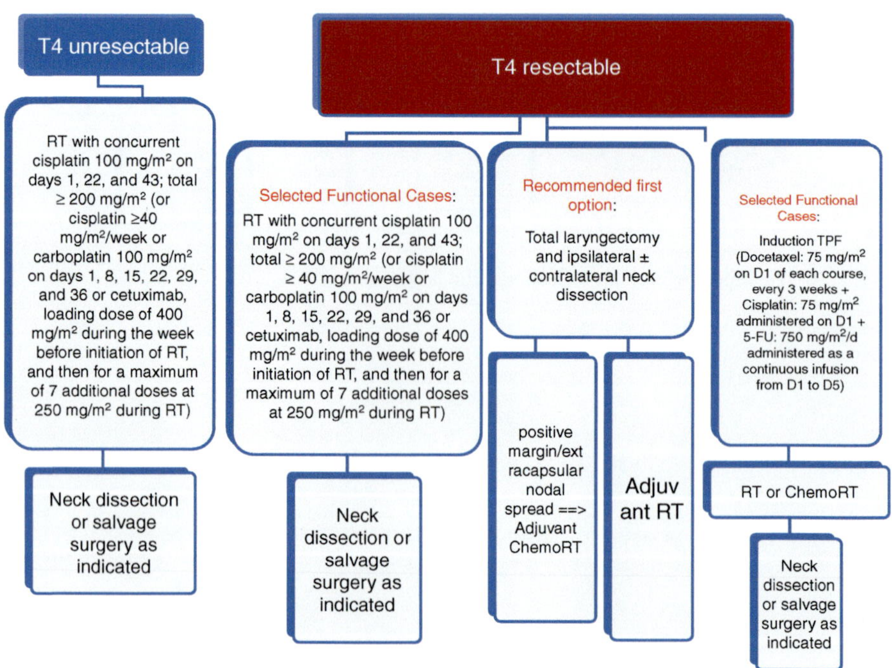

Fig. 2.22 Treatment Algorithm for T4 larynx cancer

References

1. Sun Y, Li WF, Chen NY, Zhang N, Hu GQ, Xie FY, Sun Y, Chen XZ, Li JG, Zhu XD, et al. Induction chemotherapy plus concurrent chemoradiotherapy versus concurrent chemoradiotherapy alone in locoregionally advanced nasopharyngeal carcinoma: a phase 3, multicentre, randomised controlled trial. Lancet Oncol. 2016;17(11):1509–20.
2. Cao SM, Yang Q, Guo L, Mai HQ, Mo HY, Cao KJ, Qian CN, Zhao C, Xiang YQ, Zhang XP, et al. Neoadjuvant chemotherapy followed by concurrent chemoradiotherapy versus concurrent chemoradiotherapy alone in locoregionally advanced nasopharyngeal carcinoma: a phase III multicentre randomised controlled trial. Eur J Cancer. 2017;75:14–23.
3. Sanguineti G, Geara FB, Garden AS, Tucker SL, Ang KK, Morrison WH, Peters LJ. Carcinoma of the nasopharynx treated by radiotherapy alone: determinants of local and regional control. Int J Radiat Oncol Biol Phys. 1997;37(5):985–96.
4. Chen QY, Wen YF, Guo L, Liu H, Huang PY, Mo HY, Li NW, Xiang YQ, Luo DH, Qiu F, et al. Concurrent chemoradiotherapy vs radiotherapy alone in stage II nasopharyngeal carcinoma: phase III randomized trial. J Natl Cancer Inst. 2011;103(23):1761–70.
5. Al-Sarraf M, LeBlanc M, Giri PG, Fu KK, Cooper J, Vuong T, Forastiere AA, Adams G, Sakr WA, Schuller DE, et al. Chemoradiotherapy versus radiotherapy in patients with advanced nasopharyngeal cancer: phase III randomized intergroup study 0099. J Clin Oncol. 1998;16(4):1310–7.
6. Lin JC, Jan JS, Hsu CY, Liang WM, Jiang RS, Wang WY. Phase III study of concurrent chemoradiotherapy versus radiotherapy alone for advanced nasopharyngeal carcinoma: positive effect on overall and progression-free survival. J Clin Oncol. 2003;21(4):631–7.
7. Wee J, Tan EH, Tai BC, Wong HB, Leong SS, Tan T, Chua ET, Yang E, Lee KM, Fong KW, et al. Randomized trial of radiotherapy versus concurrent chemoradiotherapy followed by adjuvant chemotherapy in patients with American joint committee on cancer/international union against cancer stage III and IV nasopharyngeal cancer of the endemic variety. J Clin Oncol. 2005;23(27):6730–8.
8. Zhang L, Zhao C, Peng PJ, Lu LX, Huang PY, Han F, Wu SX. Phase III study comparing standard radiotherapy with or without weekly oxaliplatin in treatment of locoregionally advanced nasopharyngeal carcinoma: preliminary results. J Clin Oncol. 2005;23(33):8461–8.
9. Lee AW, Tung SY, Chua DT, Ngan RK, Chappell R, Tung R, Siu L, Ng WT, Sze WK, Au GK, et al. Randomized trial of radiotherapy plus concurrent-adjuvant chemotherapy vs radiotherapy alone for regionally advanced nasopharyngeal carcinoma. J Natl Cancer Inst. 2010;102(15):1188–98.
10. Chan AT, Leung SF, Ngan RK, Teo PM, Lau WH, Kwan WH, Hui EP, Yiu HY, Yeo W, Cheung FY, et al. Overall survival after concurrent cisplatin-radiotherapy compared with radiotherapy alone in locoregionally advanced nasopharyngeal carcinoma. J Natl Cancer Inst. 2005;97(7):536–9.
11. Al-Sarraf M, LeBlanc M, Giri PG, Fu KK, Cooper J, Vuong T, Forastiere AA, Adams G, Sakr WA, Schuller DE, et al. Superiority of 5-year survival with chemoradiotherapy vs. radiotherapy in patients with locally advanced nasopharyngeal cancer. Intergroup 0099 phase III study. Final report. Proc Am Soc Clin Oncol. 2001;20:2279.
12. Chen L, Hu CS, Chen XZ, Hu GQ, Cheng ZB, Sun Y, Li WX, Chen YY, Xie FY, Liang SB, et al. Concurrent chemoradiotherapy plus adjuvant chemotherapy versus concurrent chemoradiotherapy alone in patients with locoregionally advanced nasopharyngeal carcinoma: a phase 3 multicentre randomised controlled trial. Lancet Oncol. 2012;13(2):163–71.
13. International Nasopharynx Cancer Study Group, VUMCA I Trial. Preliminary results of a randomized trial comparing neoadjuvant chemotherapy (cisplatin, epirubicin, bleomycin) plus radiotherapy vs. radiotherapy alone in stage IV(> or = N2, M0) undifferentiated nasopharyngeal carcinoma: a positive effect on progression-free survival. Int J Radiat Oncol Biol Phys. 1996;35(3):463–9.

14. Ma J, Mai HQ, Hong MH, Min HQ, Mao ZD, Cui NJ, Lu TX, Mo HY. Results of a prospective randomized trial comparing neoadjuvant chemotherapy plus radiotherapy with radiotherapy alone in patients with locoregionally advanced nasopharyngeal carcinoma. J Clin Oncol. 2001;19(5):1350–7.

15. Chua DT, Sham JS, Choy D, Lorvidhaya V, Sumitsawan Y, Thongprasert S, Vootiprux V, Cheirsilpa A, Azhar T, Reksodiputro AH. Preliminary report of the Asian-Oceanian clinical oncology association randomized trial comparing cisplatin and epirubicin followed by radiotherapy versus radiotherapy alone in the treatment of patients with locoregionally advanced nasopharyngeal carcinoma. Asian-Oceanian clinical oncology association nasopharynx cancer study group. Cancer. 1998;83(11):2270–83.

16. Hui EP, Ma BB, Leung SF, King AD, Mo F, Kam MK, Yu BK, Chiu SK, Kwan WH, Ho R, et al. Randomized phase II trial of concurrent cisplatin-radiotherapy with or without neoadjuvant docetaxel and cisplatin in advanced nasopharyngeal carcinoma. J Clin Oncol. 2009;27(2):242–9.

17. Xu T, Hu C, Zhu G, He X, Wu Y, Ying H. Preliminary results of a phase III randomized study comparing chemotherapy neoadjuvantly or concurrently with radiotherapy for locoregionally advanced nasopharyngeal carcinoma. Med Oncol. 2012;29(1):272–8.

18. OuYang PY, Xie C, Mao YP, Zhang Y, Liang XX, Su Z, Liu Q, Xie FY. Significant efficacies of neoadjuvant and adjuvant chemotherapy for nasopharyngeal carcinoma by meta-analysis of published literature-based randomized, controlled trials. Ann Oncol. 2013;24(8):2136–46.

19. Li WF, Sun Y, Chen M, Tang LL, Liu LZ, Mao YP, Chen L, Zhou GQ, Li L, Ma J. Locoregional extension patterns of nasopharyngeal carcinoma and suggestions for clinical target volume delineation. Chin J Cancer. 2012;31(12):579–87.

20. Dubrulle F, Souillard R, Hermans R. Extension patterns of nasopharyngeal carcinoma. Eur Radiol. 2007;17(10):2622–30.

21. Lee AW, Ng WT, Pan JJ, Poh SS, Ahn YC, AlHussain H, Corry J, Grau C, Gregoire V, Harrington KJ, et al. International guideline for the delineation of the clinical target volumes (CTV) for nasopharyngeal carcinoma. Radiother Oncol. 2018;126(1):25–36.

22. Li JG, Yuan X, Zhang LL, Tang YQ, Liu L, Chen XD, Gong XC, Wan GF, Liao YL, Ye JM, et al. A randomized clinical trial comparing prophylactic upper versus whole-neck irradiation in the treatment of patients with node-negative nasopharyngeal carcinoma. Cancer. 2013;119(17):3170–6.

23. Adelstein DJ, Ridge JA, Brizel DM, Holsinger FC, Haughey BH, O'Sullivan B, Genden EM, Beitler JJ, Weinstein GS, Quon H, et al. Transoral resection of pharyngeal cancer: summary of a National Cancer Institute Head and Neck Cancer Steering Committee Clinical Trials Planning Meeting, November 6-7, 2011, Arlington, Virginia. *Head Neck*. 2012;34(12):1681–703.

24. Li RJ, Richmon JD. Transoral endoscopic surgery: new surgical techniques for oropharyngeal cancer. Otolaryngol Clin N Am. 2012;45(4):823–44.

25. Selek U, Garden AS, Morrison WH, El-Naggar AK, Rosenthal DI, Ang KK. Radiation therapy for early-stage carcinoma of the oropharynx. Int J Radiat Oncol Biol Phys. 2004;59(3):743–51.

26. Denis F, Garaud P, Bardet E, Alfonsi M, Sire C, Germain T, Bergerot P, Rhein B, Tortochaux J, Calais G. Final results of the 94-01 French Head and Neck Oncology and Radiotherapy Group randomized trial comparing radiotherapy alone with concomitant radiochemotherapy in advanced-stage oropharynx carcinoma. J Clin Oncol. 2004;22(1):69–76.

27. Hitt R, Grau JJ, Lopez-Pousa A, Berrocal A, Garcia-Giron C, Irigoyen A, Sastre J, Martinez-Trufero J, Brandariz Castelo JA, Verger E, et al. A randomized phase III trial comparing induction chemotherapy followed by chemoradiotherapy versus chemoradiotherapy alone as treatment of unresectable head and neck cancer. Ann Oncol. 2014;25(1):216–25.

28. Pignon JP, Bourhis J, Domenge C, Designe L. Chemotherapy added to locoregional treatment for head and neck squamous-cell carcinoma: three meta-analyses of updated individual data. MACH-NC collaborative group. Meta-analysis of chemotherapy on head and neck cancer. Lancet. 2000;355(9208):949–55.

29. Pignon JP, le Maitre A, Maillard E, Bourhis J. Meta-analysis of chemotherapy in head and neck cancer (MACH-NC): an update on 93 randomised trials and 17,346 patients. Radiother Oncol. 2009;92(1):4–14.
30. Huguenin P, Beer KT, Allal A, Rufibach K, Friedli C, Davis JB, Pestalozzi B, Schmid S, Thoni A, Ozsahin M, et al. Concomitant cisplatin significantly improves locoregional control in advanced head and neck cancers treated with hyperfractionated radiotherapy. J Clin Oncol. 2004;22(23):4665–73.
31. Budach V, Stuschke M, Budach W, Baumann M, Geismar D, Grabenbauer G, Lammert I, Jahnke K, Stueben G, Herrmann T, et al. Hyperfractionated accelerated chemoradiation with concurrent fluorouracil-mitomycin is more effective than dose-escalated hyperfractionated accelerated radiation therapy alone in locally advanced head and neck cancer: final results of the radiotherapy cooperative clinical trials group of the German Cancer society 95-06 prospective randomized trial. J Clin Oncol. 2005;23(6):1125–35.
32. Bensadoun RJ, Benezery K, Dassonville O, Magne N, Poissonnet G, Ramaioli A, Lemanski C, Bourdin S, Tortochaux J, Peyrade F, et al. French multicenter phase III randomized study testing concurrent twice-a-day radiotherapy and cisplatin/5-fluorouracil chemotherapy (BiRCF) in unresectable pharyngeal carcinoma: results at 2 years (FNCLCC-GORTEC). Int J Radiat Oncol Biol Phys. 2006;64(4):983–94.
33. Ang K, Zhang Q, Wheeler RH, Rosenthal DI, Nguyen-Tan F, Kim H, Lu C, Axelrod RS, Silverman CI, Weber RS. A phase III trial (RTOG 0129) of two radiation-cisplatin regimens for head and neck carcinomas (HNC): impact of radiation and cisplatin intensity on outcome. J Clin Oncol. 2010;28(15s):5507.
34. Bernier J, Domenge C, Ozsahin M, Matuszewska K, Lefebvre JL, Greiner RH, Giralt J, Maingon P, Rolland F, Bolla M, et al. Postoperative irradiation with or without concomitant chemotherapy for locally advanced head and neck cancer. N Engl J Med. 2004;350(19):1945–52.
35. Bernier J, Cooper JS, Pajak TF, van Glabbeke M, Bourhis J, Forastiere A, Ozsahin EM, Jacobs JR, Jassem J, Ang KK, et al. Defining risk levels in locally advanced head and neck cancers: a comparative analysis of concurrent postoperative radiation plus chemotherapy trials of the EORTC (#22931) and RTOG (# 9501). *Head Neck.* 2005;27(10):843–50.
36. Cooper JS, Pajak TF, Forastiere AA, Jacobs J, Campbell BH, Saxman SB, Kish JA, Kim HE, Cmelak AJ, Rotman M, et al. Postoperative concurrent radiotherapy and chemotherapy for high-risk squamous-cell carcinoma of the head and neck. N Engl J Med. 2004;350(19):1937–44.
37. Cooper JS, Zhang Q, Pajak TF, Forastiere AA, Jacobs J, Saxman SB, Kish JA, Kim HE, Cmelak AJ, Rotman M, et al. Long-term follow-up of the RTOG 9501/intergroup phase III trial: postoperative concurrent radiation therapy and chemotherapy in high-risk squamous cell carcinoma of the head and neck. Int J Radiat Oncol Biol Phys. 2012;84(5):1198–205.
38. Ko EC, Genden EM, Misiukiewicz K, Som PM, Kostakoglu L, Chen CT, Packer S, Kao J. Toxicity profile and clinical outcomes in locally advanced head and neck cancer patients treated with induction chemotherapy prior to concurrent chemoradiation. Oncol Rep. 2012;27(2):467–74.
39. Vokes EE, Stenson K, Rosen FR, Kies MS, Rademaker AW, Witt ME, Brockstein BE, List MA, Fung BB, Portugal L, et al. Weekly carboplatin and paclitaxel followed by concomitant paclitaxel, fluorouracil, and hydroxyurea chemoradiotherapy: curative and organ-preserving therapy for advanced head and neck cancer. J Clin Oncol. 2003;21(2):320–6.
40. Posner MR, Hershock DM, Blajman CR, Mickiewicz E, Winquist E, Gorbounova V, Tjulandin S, Shin DM, Cullen K, Ervin TJ, et al. Cisplatin and fluorouracil alone or with docetaxel in head and neck cancer. N Engl J Med. 2007;357(17):1705–15.
41. Cohen EEW, Karrison T, Kocherginsky M, Huang CH, Agulnik M, Mittal BB, Yunus F, Samant S, Brockstein B, Raez LE, et al. DeCIDE: a phase III randomized trial of docetaxel (D), cisplatin (P), 5-fluorouracil (F) (TPF) induction chemotherapy (IC) in patients with N2/N3 locally advanced squamous cell carcinoma of the head and neck (SCCHN). J Clin Oncol. 2012;30(15s):5500.
42. Ang K, Zhang Q, Rosenthal DI, Nguyen-Tan F, Wheeler RH, Sherman EJ, Weber RS, Galvin JM, Schwartz DL, El-Naggar AK, et al. A randomized phase III trial (RTOG 0522) of

concurrent accelerated radiation plus cisplatin with or without cetuximab for stage III-IV head and neck squamous cell carcinomas (HNC). J Clin Oncol. 2011;29(15s):5500.

43. Urban D, Corry J, Rischin D. What is the best treatment for patients with human papillomavirus-positive and -negative oropharyngeal cancer? Cancer. 2014;120(10):1462–70.

44. Hafkamp HC, Manni JJ, Haesevoets A, Voogd AC, Schepers M, Bot FJ, Hopman AH, Ramaekers FC, Speel EJ. Marked differences in survival rate between smokers and nonsmokers with HPV 16-associated tonsillar carcinomas. Int J Cancer. 2008;122(12):2656–64.

45. Goldenberg D, Begum S, Westra WH, Khan Z, Sciubba J, Pai SI, Califano JA, Tufano RP, Koch WM. Cystic lymph node metastasis in patients with head and neck cancer: an HPV-associated phenomenon. *Head Neck*. 2008;30(7):898–903.

46. Huang SH, O'Sullivan B, Xu W, Zhao H, Chen DD, Ringash J, Hope A, Razak A, Gilbert R, Irish J, et al. Temporal nodal regression and regional control after primary radiation therapy for N2-N3 head-and-neck cancer stratified by HPV status. Int J Radiat Oncol Biol Phys. 2013;87(5):1078–85.

47. Ang KK, Harris J, Wheeler R, Weber R, Rosenthal DI, Nguyen-Tan PF, Westra WH, Chung CH, Jordan RC, Lu C, et al. Human papillomavirus and survival of patients with oropharyngeal cancer. N Engl J Med. 2010;363(1):24–35.

48. O'Sullivan B, Huang SH, Siu LL, Waldron J, Zhao H, Perez-Ordonez B, Weinreb I, Kim J, Ringash J, Bayley A, et al. Deintensification candidate subgroups in human papillomavirus-related oropharyngeal cancer according to minimal risk of distant metastasis. J Clin Oncol. 2013;31(5):543–50.

49. Gregoire V, Evans M, Le QT, Bourhis J, Budach V, Chen A, Eisbruch A, Feng M, Giralt J, Gupta T, et al. Delineation of the primary tumour clinical target volumes (CTV-P) in laryngeal, hypopharyngeal, oropharyngeal and oral cavity squamous cell carcinoma: AIRO, CACA, DAHANCA, EORTC, GEORCC, GORTEC, HKNPCSG, HNCIG, IAG-KHT, LPRHHT, NCIC CTG, NCRI, NRG Oncology, PHNS, SBRT, SOMERA, SRO, SSHNO, TROG consensus guidelines. Radiother Oncol. 2018;126(1):3–24.

50. Tomeh C, Holsinger FC. Laryngeal cancer. *Curr Opin Otolaryngol Head Neck Surg*. 2014;22(2):147–53.

51. Hinerman RW, Mendenhall WM, Amdur RJ, Stringer SP, Villaret DB, Robbins KT. Carcinoma of the supraglottic larynx: treatment results with radiotherapy alone or with planned neck dissection. *Head Neck*. 2002;24(5):456–67.

52. Yamazaki H, Nishiyama K, Tanaka E, Koizumi M, Chatani M. Radiotherapy for early glottic carcinoma (T1N0M0): results of prospective randomized study of radiation fraction size and overall treatment time. Int J Radiat Oncol Biol Phys. 2006;64(1):77–82.

53. Mendenhall WM, Amdur RJ, Morris CG, Hinerman RW. T1-T2N0 squamous cell carcinoma of the glottic larynx treated with radiation therapy. J Clin Oncol. 2001;19(20):4029–36.

54. Mendenhall WM, Werning JW, Hinerman RW, Amdur RJ, Villaret DB. Management of T1-T2 glottic carcinomas. Cancer. 2004;100(9):1786–92.

55. Wolf GT, Fisher SG, Hong WK, Hillman R, Spaulding M, Laramore GE, Endicott JW, McClatchey K, Henderson WG. Induction chemotherapy plus radiation compared with surgery plus radiation in patients with advanced laryngeal cancer. N Engl J Med. 1991;324(24):1685–90.

56. Forastiere AA, Goepfert H, Maor M, Pajak TF, Weber R, Morrison W, Glisson B, Trotti A, Ridge JA, Chao C, et al. Concurrent chemotherapy and radiotherapy for organ preservation in advanced laryngeal cancer. N Engl J Med. 2003;349(22):2091–8.

57. Forastiere AA, Zhang Q, Weber RS, Maor MH, Goepfert H, Pajak TF, Morrison W, Glisson B, Trotti A, Ridge JA, et al. Long-term results of RTOG 91-11: a comparison of three nonsurgical treatment strategies to preserve the larynx in patients with locally advanced larynx cancer. J Clin Oncol. 2013;31(7):845–52.

58. Chakraborty S, Muttath G. Carotid sparing intensity-modulated radiotherapy in early glottic cancers: a case of Maslow's hammer? J Cancer Res Ther. 2015;11(2):495–6.

59. Chatterjee S, Guha S, Prasath S, Mallick I, Achari R. Carotid sparing hypofractionated tomotherapy in early glottic cancers: refining image guided IMRT to improve morbidity. J Cancer Res Ther. 2013;9(3):452–5.

60. Zumsteg ZS, Riaz N, Jaffery S, Hu M, Gelblum D, Zhou Y, Mychalczak B, Zelefsky MJ, Wolden S, Rao S, et al. Carotid sparing intensity-modulated radiation therapy achieves comparable locoregional control to conventional radiotherapy in T1-2N0 laryngeal carcinoma. Oral Oncol. 2015;51(7):716–23.
61. Loimu V, Collan J, Vaalavirta L, Back L, Kapanen M, Makitie A, Tenhunen M, Saarilahti K. Patterns of relapse following definitive treatment of head and neck squamous cell cancer by intensity modulated radiotherapy and weekly cisplatin. Radiother Oncol. 2011;98(1):34–7.
62. Skinner WK, Muse ED, Yaparpalvi R, Guha C, Garg MK, Kalnicki S. Obtaining normal tissue constraints using intensity modulated radiotherapy (IMRT) in patients with oral cavity, oropharyngeal, and laryngeal carcinoma. Med Dosim. 2009;34(4):279–84.
63. Gregoire V, Ang K, Budach W, Grau C, Hamoir M, Langendijk JA, Lee A, Le QT, Maingon P, Nutting C, et al. Delineation of the neck node levels for head and neck tumors: a 2013 update. DAHANCA, EORTC, HKNPCSG, NCIC CTG, NCRI, RTOG, TROG consensus guidelines. Radiother Oncol. 2014;110(1):172–81.
64. Lefebvre JL, Andry G, Chevalier D, Luboinski B, Collette L, Traissac L, de Raucourt D, Langendijk JA. Laryngeal preservation with induction chemotherapy for hypopharyngeal squamous cell carcinoma: 10-year results of EORTC trial 24891. Ann Oncol. 2012;23(10):2708–14.
65. Richard JM, Sancho-Garnier H, Pessey JJ, Luboinski B, Lefebvre JL, Dehesdin D, Stromboni-Luboinski M, Hill C. Randomized trial of induction chemotherapy in larynx carcinoma. Oral Oncol. 1998;34(3):224–8.
66. Janoray G, Pointreau Y, Garaud P, Chapet S, Alfonsi M, Sire C, Jadaud E, Calais G: Long-term results of a multicenter randomized phase III trial of induction chemotherapy with cisplatin, 5-fluorouracil, +/− docetaxel for larynx preservation. J Natl Cancer Inst 2016;108(4). https://doi.org/10.1093/jnci/djv368.
67. Pointreau Y, Garaud P, Chapet S, Sire C, Tuchais C, Tortochaux J, Faivre S, Guerrif S, Alfonsi M, Calais G. Randomized trial of induction chemotherapy with cisplatin and 5-fluorouracil with or without docetaxel for larynx preservation. J Natl Cancer Inst. 2009;101(7):498–506.
68. Posner MR, Norris CM, Wirth LJ, Shin DM, Cullen KJ, Winquist EW, Blajman CR, Mickiewicz EA, Frenette GP, Plinar LF, et al. Sequential therapy for the locally advanced larynx and hypopharynx cancer subgroup in TAX 324: survival, surgery, and organ preservation. Ann Oncol. 2009;20(5):921–7.
69. Lefebvre JL, Rolland F, Tesselaar M, Bardet E, Leemans CR, Geoffrois L, Hupperets P, Barzan L, de Raucourt D, Chevalier D, et al. Phase 3 randomized trial on larynx preservation comparing sequential vs alternating chemotherapy and radiotherapy. J Natl Cancer Inst. 2009;101(3):142–52.
70. Lefebvre JL, Pointreau Y, Rolland F, Alfonsi M, Baudoux A, Sire C, de Raucourt D, Malard O, Degardin M, Tuchais C, et al. Induction chemotherapy followed by either chemoradiotherapy or bioradiotherapy for larynx preservation: the TREMPLIN randomized phase II study. J Clin Oncol. 2013;31(7):853–9.

Lung Cancer

3

Ugur Selek, Duygu Sezen, and Yasemin Bolukbasi

3.1 Non-small Cell Lung Cancer

Overview

Epidemiology: Non small-cell lung cancer (NSCLC) is most common non-cutaneous cancer in the world which is again the most common cause of cancer related death worldwide. Smoking (active/passive) is related with more than 90% of cases, which requires low-dose CT screening with strong smoking history [1].

Pathological and Biological Features: Adenocarcinoma (40%), squamous cell carcinoma (25%) and large cell carcinoma (10%) constitute the main pathological subtypes.

TTF-1 is only positive in adenocarcinomas of primary lung and thyroid, while napsin positivity is distinguishing as being 80% positive in lung and 10% in thyroid.

U. Selek (✉) · Y. Bolukbasi
Department of Radiation Oncology, School of Medicine, Koç University, Istanbul, Turkey

Department of Radiation Oncology, The University of Texas MD Anderson Cancer Center, Houston, TX, USA

D. Sezen
Department of Radiation Oncology, School of Medicine, Koç University, Istanbul, Turkey

© Springer Nature Switzerland AG 2019
G. Ozyigit, U. Selek (eds.), *Radiation Oncology*,
https://doi.org/10.1007/978-3-319-97145-2_3

Former "bronchoalveolar carcinoma" is currently documented as "Adenocarcinoma in situ (AIS) or minimally invasive adenocarcinoma (MIS)" with weak association with smoking.

Subtype analysis of NSCLC for all patients whose tumor contains an element of adenocarcinoma requires determination of presence or absence of a driver mutation as epidermal growth factor receptors (EGFR), anaplastic lymphoma kinase (ALK), and c-ROS oncogene 1 (ROS1) mutations for not only being identifiable but their targeted treatment resulting in responses better than that with standard chemotherapy [2, 3].

Immunotherapy has recently been an effective option for those with a high level of programmed death ligand 1 (PD-L1) expression (membranous PD-L1 expression on at least 50 percent of tumor cells), regardless of the staining intensity [4].

Prognostic factors include stage, weight loss (>10% body weight over 6 months), performance status, pleural effusion [5, 6].

Definitive Therapy: Despite locally advanced (stage III) and disseminated (stage IV) disease, early stage I-II disease is often curable with aggressive definitive therapy. Eligible patients having adequate function pulmonary volume without serious medical comorbidity are surgical lobectomy candidates for patients with stage I or II NSCLC rather than radiation therapy; while stereotactic body radiation therapy (SBRT)/stereotactic ablative radiotherapy (SABR) is a viable alternative with growing evidence as definitive treatment in selected stage I patients. For patients with larger primary tumors who are not surgical candidates, standard-fractionation radiation therapy is applicable. Adjuvant chemotherapy is recommended after complete resection of stage IB NSCLC with high-risk features & stage II NSCLC with a cisplatin-based doublet. Postoperative radiotherapy is indicated for patients with positive surgical resection margins for stage I-II NSCLC.

Keywords: Non-small cell lung cancer, Radiotherapy

3.1.1 Case Presentation

60 years old male with 40 packet year smoking history and no significant past medical history admitted with dyspnea and hiccups. He had no dysphagia, odynophagia, or swallowing, and chewing problems. His physical exam was normal in general except right sided rhonchus in pulmonary auscultation. As he has been a heavy smoker, a chest CT was ordered revealing right hilar parenchymal tumor encasing the main bronchus with multiple stations of mediastinal nodal disease (starting at right level 2 upper mediastinum and continuing to level 10 & 11 ipsilaterally in addition to contralateral small nodes). PET CT (Fig. 3.1) confirmed the CT findings as major tumor bulk on right mediastinum and hilum, but low SUV on left sided

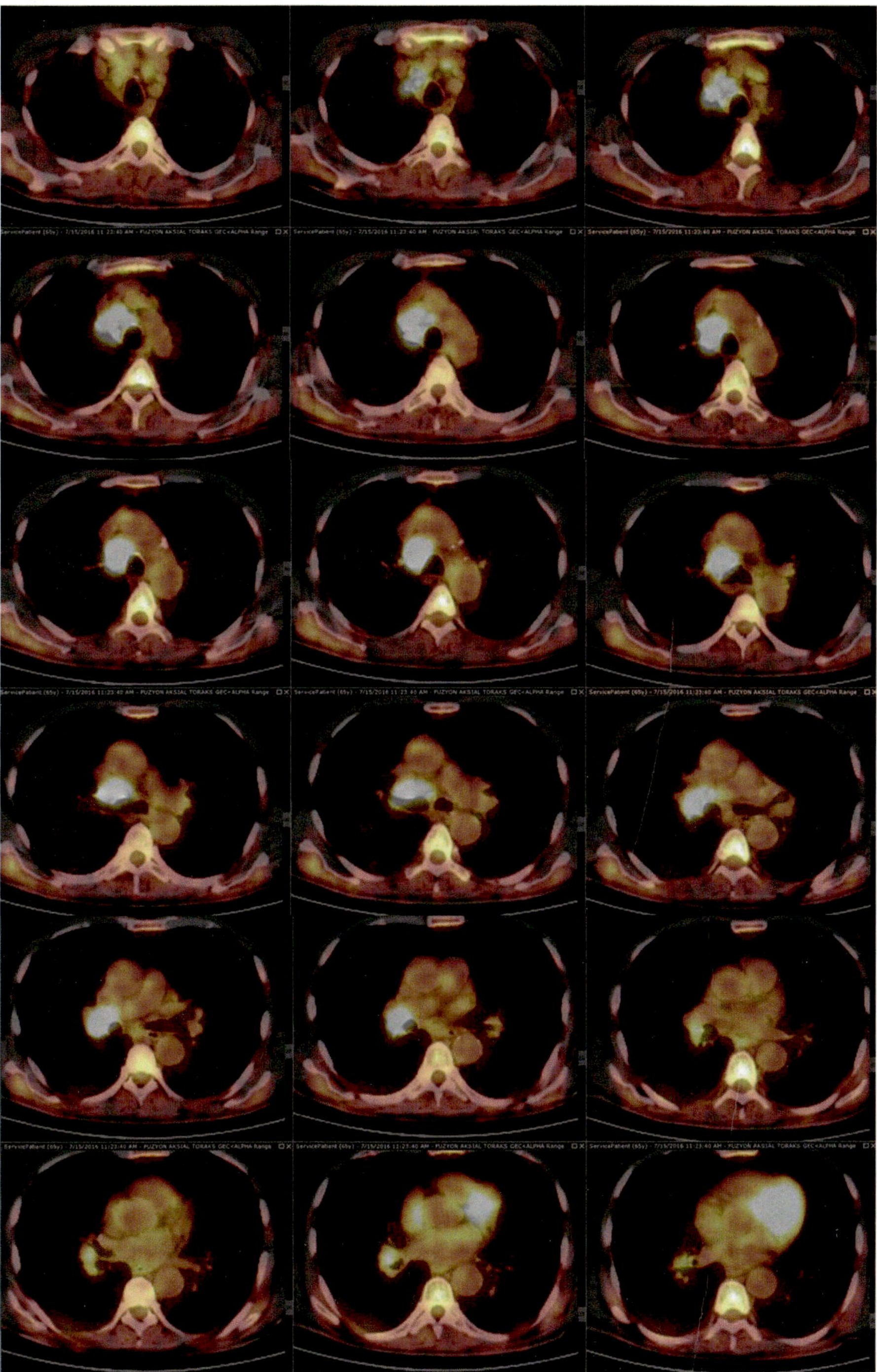

Fig. 3.1 Axial PET-CT fusion images defining multiple stations of mediastinal disease

small nodes. Endobronchial ultrasound guided biopsies revelaed squamous cell carcinoma both in primary and multiple stations. He was staged as T2N3M0, locoregionally advanced non-small cell lung cancer.

3.1.2 Staging

Systemic physical examination is important depending on the high incidence of metastases.

Routine complete blood count as well as biochemistry including blood urea/creatinine, liver function tests etc.

Eligibility criteria for definitive concurrent chemoradiotherapy is generally considered as;

KPS $\geq$ 70, FEV-1 > 1 L, FVC $\geq$ 45%, Absolute neutrophil > 1500/μL, Trombosite > 100,000/μL, Serum creatinine < 1.5× normal.

Pathological examination is required by less likely using sputum, but mostly fine needle aspiration, endobronchial or CT-guided biopsy, or mediastinoscopy guided biopsy.

Radiological imaging includes CT of chest and abdomen, MRI brain, preferably PET/CT, radionuclide bone scan.

Smoking cessation is important.

At diagnosis, three groups reflecting the extent of the NSCLC and the treatment approach are detailed:

Surgically resectable disease (mainly stage I, stage II, and selected stage III tumors): the best prognostic cohort, eligible for curative surgery or eligible for curative radiotherapy with resectable but medical contraindicated to surgery. Resected stage II or stage IIIA NSCLC might benefit postoperative cisplatin-based combination chemotherapy.

Locally (T3–T4) and/or regionally (N2–N3) advanced disease: Require combined modalities. If unresectable or N2–N3, radiotherapy with chemotherapy is recommended. If resectable for selected T3 or N2, either preoperative or postoperative chemotherapy or chemoradiotherapy.

Distant metastatic disease: radiotherapy or platinum-based chemotherapy for palliation of symptoms of the primary tumor. Selected oligometastatic disease might be recommended definitive treatment based on response [7].

> **The Revised International System for Staging Lung Cancer**
> The Revised International System for Staging Lung Cancer was adopted in 2010 by the AJCC and the Union Internationale Contre le Cancer [8, 9]. The 8th Edition of TNM in Lung Cancer (Table 3.1), has recently been changed to be the standard of non-small cell lung cancer staging since January 1st, 2018; issued by the IASLC (International Association for the Study of Lung Cancer) and replaces the TNM 7th edition [10–13].

Table 3.1 The 8th edition of TNM in lung cancer

T: Primary tumor	
Tx	Primary tumor cannot be assessed or tumor proven by presence of malignant cells in sputum or bronchial washings but not visualized by imaging or bronchoscopy
T0	No evidence of primary tumor
Tis	Carcinoma in situ
T1	Tumor ≤3 cm in greatest dimension surrounded by lung or visceral pleura without bronchoscopic evidence of invasion more proximal than the lobar bronchus (i.e., not in the main bronchus)
T1a(mi)	**Minimally invasive adenocarcinoma**
T1a	**Tumor ≤ 1 cm in greatest dimension**
T1b	**Tumor > 1 cm but ≤ 2 cm in greatest dimension**
T1c	**Tumor > 2 cm but ≤ 3 cm in greatest dimension**
T2	Tumor >3 cm **but ≤ 5 cm** or tumor with any of the following features: • **Involves main bronchus regardless of distance from the carina but without involvement of the carina** • Invades visceral pleura • **Associated with atelectasis or obstructive pneumonitis that extends to the hilar region, involving part or all of the lung**
T2a	**Tumor > 3 cm but ≤ 4 cm in greatest dimension**
T2b	**Tumor > 4 cm but ≤ 5 cm in greatest dimension**
T3	**Tumor > 5 cm but ≤ 7 cm in greatest dimension** or associated with separate tumor nodule(s) in the same lobe as the primary tumor or directly invades any of the following structures: chest wall (including the parietal pleura and superior sulcus tumors), phrenic nerve, parietal pericardium
T4	**Tumor > 7 cm in greatest dimension** or associated with separate tumor nodule(s) in a different ipsilateral lobe than that of the primary tumor or invades any of the following structures: **diaphragm**, mediastinum, heart, great vessels, trachea, recurrent laryngeal nerve, esophagus, vertebral body, and carina
N: Regional lymph node involvement	
Nx	Regional lymph nodes cannot be assessed
N0	No regional lymph node metastasis
N1	Metastasis in ipsilateral peribronchial and/or ipsilateral hilar lymph nodes and intrapulmonary nodes, including involvement by direct extension
N2	Metastasis in ipsilateral mediastinal and/or subcarinal lymph node(s)
N3	Metastasis in contralateral mediastinal, contralateral hilar, ipsilateral or contralateral scalene, or supraclavicular lymph node(s)
M: Distant metastasis	
M0	No distant metastasis
M1	Distant metastasis present
M1a	Separate tumor nodule(s) in a contralateral lobe; tumor with pleural or pericardial nodule(s) or malignant pleural or pericardial effusion
M1b	**Single extrathoracic metastasis**
M1c	**Multiple extrathoracic metastases in one or more organs**

(continued)

Table 3.1 (continued)

Stage groupings				
Occult carcinoma	TX		N0	M0
Stage 0	Tis		N0	M0
Stage IA1	**T1a(mi)**		**N0**	**M0**
	T1a		**N0**	**M0**
Stage IA2	**T1b**		**N0**	**M0**
Stage IA3	**T1c**		**N0**	**M0**
Stage IB	T2a		N0	M0
Stage IIA	T2b		N0	M0
Stage IIB	**T1a to c**		**N1**	**M0**
	T2a		**N1**	**M0**
	T2b		N1	M0
	T3		N0	M0
Stage IIIA	**T1a to c**		**N2**	**M0**
	T2a to b		N2	M0
	T3		N1	M0
	T4		N0	M0
	T4		N1	M0
Stage IIIB	**T1a to c**		**N3**	**M0**
	T2a to b		N3	M0
	T3		**N2**	**M0**
	T4		N2	M0
Stage IIIC	**T3**		**N3**	**M0**
	T4		**N3**	**M0**
Stage IVA	**Any T**		**Any N**	**M1a**
	Any T		**Any N**	**M1b**
Stage IVB	**Any T**		**Any N**	**M1c**

> **Changes in T Stage Are as Follows [14]**
>
> T1 into T1a ($\leq$1 cm), T1b (>1 to $\leq$2 cm), and T1c (>2 to $\leq$3 cm);
>
> T2 into T2a (>3 to $\leq$4 cm) and T2b (>4 to $\leq$5 cm); involvement of main bronchus regardless of distance from carina; partial and total atelectasis/pneumonitis;
>
> T3 as greater than 5 to less than or equal to 7 cm;
>
> T4 as greater than 7 cm; diaphragm invasion;
>
> Mediastinal pleura invasion is not a T descriptor anymore.

3.1.3 Evidence Based Treatment Approaches

Stages I and II NSCLC: Lobectomy with systematic lymph node dissection over pneumonectomy is the recommended treatment modality for patients with stages I and II NSCLC [15–17]. SBRT/SABR is a viable alternative with growing evidence as definitive treatment in selected stage I patients [18–25].

As accurate mediastinal nodal staging is crucial for SABR eligibility of stage I & II NSCLC patients, PET/CT started to be replacing the need for mediastinoscopy in recent years. [26, 27]. Senthi et al. retrospectively evaluated their series of 676 medically inoperable PET staged early stage NSCLC patients, treated with SABR (54–60 Gy, three to eight once-daily fractions) between April 2003 and Dec 2011 [18], and documented an actuarial two-year regional recurrence rates of 7.8% while local and distant recurrence rates were 4.9% and 14.7%, respectively. Initially, patients bearing early stage NSCLC with high surgical risk and medical inoperability were the target population for SABR and were compared with surgical series [28–33]. Phase II RTOG 0236 trial prescribing SABR in stage I medically inoperable NSCLC patients enrolled a poor functional status cohort with a baseline hypoxemia and/or hypercapnia, a baseline FEV1 < 40% predicted, baseline severely reduced diffusion capacity, post-operative predicted FEV1 < 30% predicted, etc. [21] and Timmerman et al. reported encouraging median survival of 48 months win comparison to 13 months for an untreated T1 N0 M0 patient [23]. Onishi et al. retrospectively analyzed multiinstitutional data from 14 Japanese centers revealing 87 Stage I medically operable NSCLC patients who refused surgery [24], and stated cumulative local control rates of 92% for T1 and 73% for T2 at 5 years in addition to 72% and 62% overall survival for Stage IA and IB respectively at five years with a median follow-up of 55 months. Lagerward et al. presented outcomes of 177 potentially operable patients treated with SABR from their institutional prospective database and documented an exciting median overall survival of 61.5 months with 94.7% and 84.7% survival rates at 1 and 3 years respectively [34]. The Japan Clinical Oncology Group (JCOG) documented the SABR outcome of operable peripheral stage IA NSCLC patients in phase II JCOG 0403 trial with 76% overall survival and 69% locally progression-free survival rates at 3 years [35]. Retrospective series including clinical stage I NSCLC patients treated with surgery or SABR were studied by matched-pair analysis and propensity score comparisons [36–38]; defining SABR as a comparable definitive treatment choice with definitive surgery in early stage NSCLC patients matched for selection factors to reduce the bias due to confounding variables [36–38]. Solda et al. recently reported about 3771 patients treated with SABR for NSCLC recognized comparable survival outcome to surgery (2 year survival with SABR 70% versus 68% with surgery) regardless of co-morbidity [38]. Meta-analysis by Zheng et al. (4850 SABR and 7071 surgery) underlined no significant OS and disease free survival difference in stage I NSCLC between SABR and surgery [39]. Prospective phase III studies for operable early stage NSCLC patients comparing SABR versus surgery (optimal lobectomy with mediastinal dissection) were Dutch multicenter study (ROSEL) and international cooperative clinical trial (STARS) with very close inclusion criteria. Chang et al. combined two datasets and documented the first findings of two randomized phase III trials comparing the current standard of care of surgery and SABR for operable stage I NSCLC patients [40]. Despite fairly small—58 patients—sample size and limited follow up time, non-invasive SABR appeared to be non-inferior to lobectomy, perhaps better, with 95% (only one death) estimated overall survival at 3 years versus 79% (six deaths) with surgery; in addition to better recurrence-free survival at 3 years (SABR, 86% vs. Surgery, 80%) [40]; with better tolerance and no high-grade toxicity in this

SABR cohort [40, 41]. There are continuing prospective efforts in stage I peripheral NSCLC patients such as United Kingdom SABRT TH study (NCT02629458) to compare SABR with lobectomy or sublobar resection in patients considered having higher surgical risk of complications; RTOG3502/POSTLIV study (NCT01753414) to compare radical resection versus SABR; and University of Texas Southwestern STABLE-MATES study (NCT02468024) to compare sublobar resection with SABR; Veterans Affairs VALOR study in both peripheral and central stage I NSCLC patients to compare lobectomy or segmentectomy with SABR [42]. A recent meta-analysis on survival outcome after SBRT and Surgery for early stage NSCLC, Yu et al. found more favorable outcomes with stage I NSCLC treated with SBRT where the surgery had no obvious advantages in this meta-analysis [43]. In contrary, another recent meta-analysis by Li et al. comparing SABR versus surgery for patients with T1-3 N0 M0 NSCLC concluded that surgery, both lobectomy and sublobectomy, might be superior to SBRT/SABR with regard to survival [44]. Videtic et al. has just released the executive Summary of The American Society for Radiation Oncology (ASTRO) Evidence-Based Guideline on SBRT for early-stage NSCLC [25]; and concluded that SBRT has gained an significant role in particularly treating medically inoperable early-stage NSCLC patients with limited other treatment options (Figs. 3.2 and 3.3) [25].

Stage III NSCLC covers a very mixed group of patients due to extent and localization of primary and nodal disease, leading into a controversial management strategies, where common consensus guidelines are generally followed such as American Society for Radiation Oncology (ASTRO) and American Society of Clinical Oncology (ASCO) [45–47]. Mediastinal lymph nodes which are enlarged on CT or metabolically active on PET-CT requires pathologic confirmation of tumor involvement who are otherwise potentially resectable. If mediastinal lymph nodes are negative, then lobectomy with systematic lymph node dissection, similar to stage I and stage II disease, is next step; if pathologically involved by tumor, definitive chemoradiation, as well as bi- or tri-modality therapy for selected cases, is recommended. Preoperative pathologic evaluation of mediastinal lymph nodes for a peripheral T1a primary lesion, in case of no suspicious CT and/or PET-CT guided N1 or N2-3 lymph node involvement, is controversial. For potentially resectable central T2, T3, and T4 tumors, invasive mediastinal staging is indicated if there is enlarged hilar lymph nodes by CT and/or clinical N1 involvement by PET, even without prominent mediastinal nodal involvement [48, 49].

T3 N1 M0 NSCLC (stage IIIA): Patients are triaged with initial invasive mediastinal staging with systematic lymph node dissection followed by lobectomy, and finally consulted for adjuvant chemotherapy for those with completely resected disease. If surgery with clear margins is not technically possible, concurrent chemoradiotherapy is recommended.

T4 lesions were identified as unresectable and classified as stage IIIB, while resectable T4N0-1 lesions are rare, therefore the initial recommendation is definitive chemoradiotherapy.

Mediastinal nodal involvement in the final pathology is not surprising in approximately 20% of surgically treated cases based on careful preoperative evaluation (endobronchial ultrasound -EBUS and/or mediastinoscopy). In postoperative mediastinal nodal involvement, adjuvant chemotherapy with platinum-based doublet regimens and mostly adjuvant postoperative radiotherapy sequentially after chemotherapy are recommended [50]. Targeted therapy for those with or without driver mutations, the use of adjuvant targeted therapy including cetuximab, erlotinib, and crizotinib is not indicated.

Postoperative radiotherapy (PORT): indicated in positive surgical margins or pathologically N2 disease without much controversy [50–52]. Positive surgical margins increases local recurrences leading to decreased survival, so the general

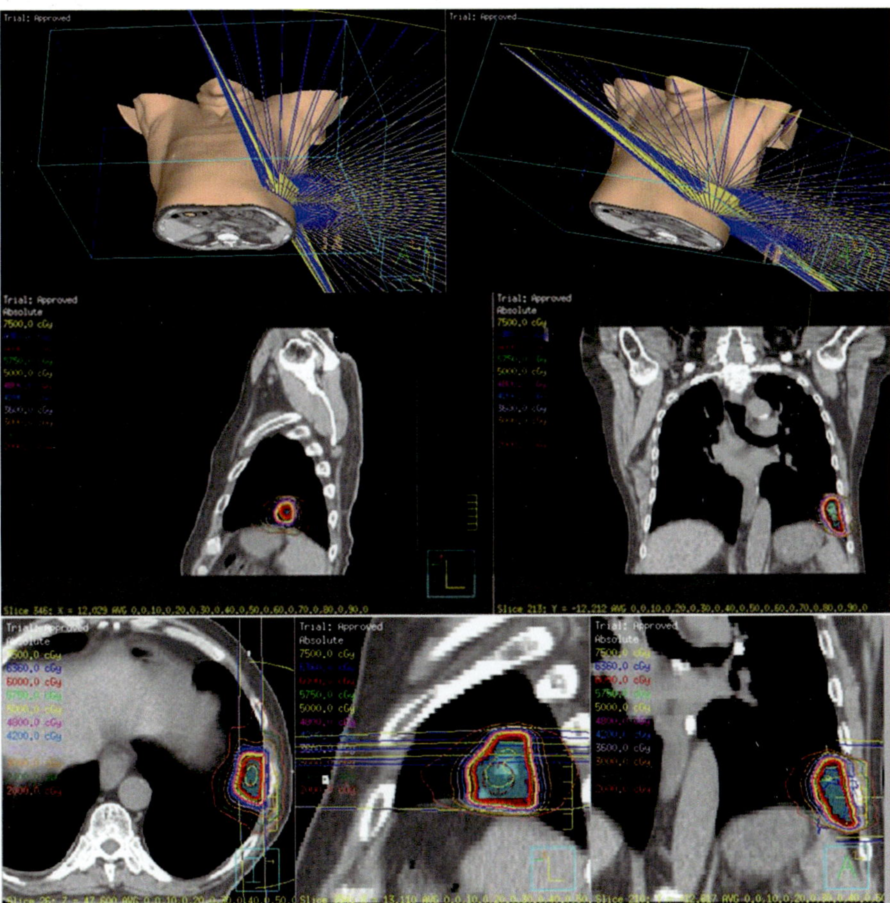

Fig. 3.2 Stereotactic ablative radiotherapy for an early stage NSCLC in four fractions, iGTV 60Gy and PTV 50 Gy in four fractions

Plan Summary Sheet

Beam Setup

Beam	Machine	Energy	Modality	Prescription	Isocenter	SSD (cm) Start /Avg	MU Per Fraction
0–178	AHITruebeam	6 MV	Photons	50Gy in 4 Fr	CT ISO	89.02 / 94.11	**818**
178–0	AHITruebeam	6 MV	Photons	50Gy in 4 Fr	CT ISO	91.85 / 94.11	**717**
A0–178	AHITruebeam	6 MV	Photons	50Gy in 4 Fr	CT ISO	89.02 / 94.11	**818**
A178–0	AHITruebeam	6 MV	Photons	50Gy in 4 Fr	CT ISO	91.85 / 94.11	**717**

Beam	Collimators (cm) (Control Pt 1) X1	X2	Y2	Y1	Gantry Start / Stop	Couch	Coll	Block	Wedge	Bolus	Comp
0–178	2.3	2.7	3.5	3.0	0 / 178	0	12	MLC	None	No	No
178–0	2.1	2.9	4.0	2.5	178 / 0	0	348	MLC	None	No	No
A0–178	2.3	2.7	3.5	3.0	0 / 178	0	12	MLC	None	No	No
A178–0	2.1	2.9	4.0	2.5	178 / 0	0	348	MLC	None	No	No

Prescriptions

50Gy in 4 Fr

Prescribe 1250 cGy per fraction to 80% of "PTV 50 Gy in 4 fr" mean dose for 4 fractions.
Actual "PTV 50 Gy in 4 fr" mean dose from all prescriptions/beams is 6247.76 cGY.
4 beams are assigned to this prescription.

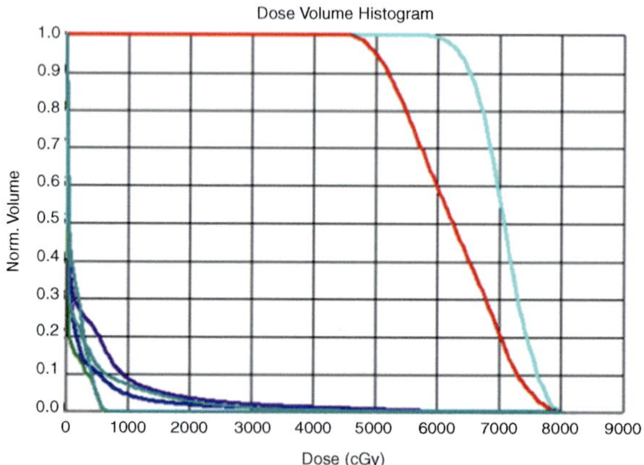

Dose Volume Histogram

ROI Statistics

Line Type	ROI	Trial or Record	Min.	Max.	Mean	Std. Dev.
	iGTV 60 Gy in 4fr	Approved	5618.6	8010.6	7069.8	420.5
	PTV 50 Gy in 4 fr	Approved	4305.2	8010.6	6247.8	792.8
	Cord1	Approved	0.2	625.6	72.1	150.6
	L Lung	Approved	0.7	7501.8	319.9	755.5
	Total Lung	Approved	0.7	7501.8	185.8	549.4
	Heart	Approved	9.4	687.4	138.1	161.9
	Chest wall	Approved	--	7960.5	231.0	627.8

Fig. 3.2 (continued)

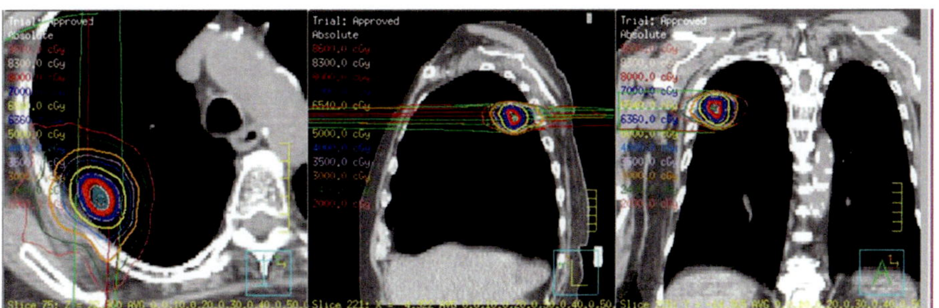

Plan Summary Sheet

Beam Setup

Beam	Machine	Energy	Modality	Prescription	Isocenter	SSD (cm) Start / (cm)	MU Per Fraction
182–0	AHITruebeam	6 MV	Photons	80Gy in 10 fr	iso	92.73 / 88.22	**1087**
0–182	AHITruebeam	6 MV	Photons	80Gy in 10 fr	iso	85.78 / 88.22	**1044**

Beam	Collimators (cm) (Control Pt 1) X1	X2	Y2	Y1	Gantry Start / Stop	Couch	Coll	Block	Wedge	Bolus	Comp
182–0	2.5	1.4	1.5	2.2	182 / 0	0	352	MLC	None	No	No
0–182	2.4	2.3	1.5	2.2	0 / 182	0	352	MLC	None	No	No

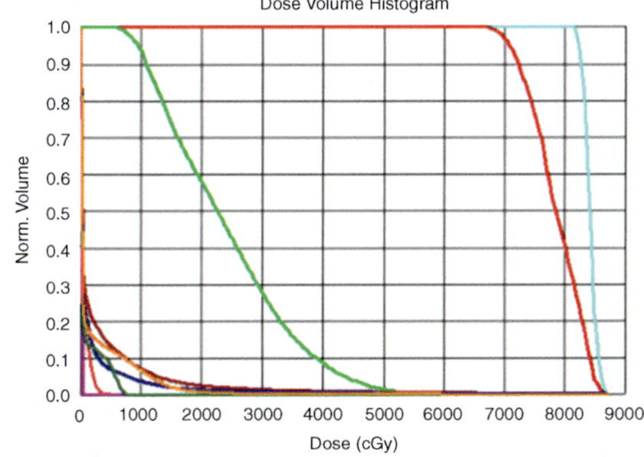

ROI Statistics

Line Type	ROI	Trial or Record	Min.	Max.	Mean	Std. Dev.
	PTV70Gy in 10 fr	Approved	6439.5	8700.1	7835.9	446.4
	costa	Approved	513.1	5942.4	2364.8	1067.3
	Lung_R1	Approved	0.0	8700.1	243.8	707.2
	Lung_L1	Approved	0.8	525.2	42.7	71.4
	heart	Approved	1.0	10.9	3.1	1.7
	Total Lung	Approved	0.0	8700.1	146.1	519.3
	Cord1	Approved	1.2	786.4	80.7	177.1
	Chest Wall	Approved	--	5969.9	187.7	409.2

Fig. 3.3 Stereotactic ablative radiotherapy for an early stage NSCLC in ten fractions, iGTV 80Gy and PTV 70 Gy in ten fractions

consensus is to recommend postoperative radiotherapy [53–55]. The unresolved controversy is related with close surgical margins and about the definition of adequate margins [56–58]. Therefore, clinical insight from surgeon is very important during evaluating the indication [59]. PORT seems to improve locoregional outcome specifically in N2 disease independent from chemotherapy effect, and N1 disease when no chemotherapy administered [52, 60–64]. PORT in N2 disease is being explored in phase 3 "The Lung Adjuvant Radiotherapy (LungART)" trial to provide prospective information [65–67].

Retrospective analysis of ANITA study, evaluating the adjuvant vinorelbine prospectively on 840 IB-IIIA patients, underlined the effectivity of PORT in N2 disease [52], and SEER data analysis involving more than 7000 patients confirmed the survival advantage of PORT in N2 patients [68]. The detrimental effect of PORT on survival documented by 1998 PORT metaanalysis, updated in 2013 including nine studies, is important to understand that the poor technology in older series and lack of conformal sparing the organs at risk can result in decrease outcome [69–71]. Modern radiotherapy techniques, focusing on critical threshold doses of organs at risk, might provide better outcome such as the meta-analysis defining the potential of 10% local control benefit by PORT in stage IIIA-N2 might turn into 13% survival benefit at 5 years [72]; as well as the survival benefit of PORT noted in 2015 "The National Cancer Data Base" analysis of PORT for N2 disease [73, 74]. Matsuguma et al. published that PORT is more effective in involvement of multiple N2 stations [75], besides another Japan series noted that inadequate nodal dissection which is less than 10 and/or 4 or more nodal involvement are poor prognostic factors on survival [76]. SEER data pointed out that survival benefit of PORT was more prominent in group with N2 disease having a ratio of positive nodes/dissected nodes ≥ 50% [77]. MD Anderson Cancer Center analysis on 1402 patients between 1998 & 2009, staged I-III (N0-N1) who did not receive PORT, revealed that recurrence was evident in 9% which decreased survival [78]; multivariate factors increasing local recurrence independently were surgical procedure (wedge + segmentectomy × lobectomy + bilobectomy + pneumonectomy), tumor size larger than 2.7 cm and visceral pleural invasion; multivariate factors increasing regional recurrence independently were N1, visceral pleural invasion (VPI), and lymphovascular invasion (LVI) [78]. Hui et all documented that PORT is more helpful in patients staged IIIA-N2 NSCLC if 3 or more factors are present among smoking index (daily cigarettes × years of smoking) ≤ 400, cN2, pT3, squamous cell cancer histology, and ≥ 4 positive nodes [79]. Therefore, there is common ground to recommend PORT in very close/positive surgical margins and/or pathologic N2 disease, and routine PORT is not recommended for N1 disease, while multidisciplinary tailoring is recommended for N1 disease based on number of nodes involved, LVI, VPI, and extracapsular extension [59, 78].

Stage III NSCLC with mediastinal involvement (N2, N3): require a multidisciplinary institutional approach including input from medical oncology, radiation oncology, and thoracic surgery, which has not been clearly defined. Crucial factors prompting the decision are the patient's overall performance status, preferences of the patients' and medical team, as well as the probability of R0 complete resection based on the extension of the primary and nodal disease. Concurrent chemoradiotherapy is the first treatment choice in most patients with clinically evident N2 disease, delivering full-dose radiation therapy with platinum-based chemotherapy; as induction/neoadjuvant chemotherapy or chemoradiotherapy followed by surgery might be also applicable decisions in a tailored group of patients [80–82]. Randomized prospective phase III (Intergroup 0139, EORTC 08941 and ESPATUE) trials have not showed any survival advantage for consolidative surgery following either neoadjuvant concurrent chemoradiotherapy or induction chemotherapy followed by radiotherapy [83–88]; while Intergroup 0139 defined a significant increase in the primary tumor control and an improvement in five-year progression-free survival (22% versus 11%).

N3 disease dictates concurrent chemoradiotherapy as the standard of care [89]. Concurrent chemoradiotherapy in highly selected medically fit septuagenarians with stage III might also be as effective as younger patients to improve survival outcomes, with a relatively acceptable toxicity profile [90]. Sequential chemoradiotherapy or radiotherapy alone are viable treatment preferences for any ineligible candidate for concurrent chemoradiotherapy.

Stage III NSCLC who completed concurrent chemoradiotherapy without any progression can be recommended immunotherapy with PD-L1 antibody durvalumab, where a phase III trial recently documented that, relative to placebo, durvalumab after at least two cycles of platinum-based chemoradiotherapy increased the median progression free survival (16.8 versus 5.6 months; HR for disease progression or death 0.52), and median time to death or distant metastasis (23.2 versus 14.6 months) [91].

3.1.4 Radiotherapy Planning

Lung function guided radiotherapy selection is given below in Table 3.2 [92]. Stage guided treatment selection is summarized in Table 3.3.

3.1.4.1 Immobilization and Simulation
Intravenous contrast is preferred during CT simulation to improve the visualization of the primary tumor and nodal disease, if patient's renal functional status allows and if adequate measures for any possible anaphylactic reactions could be taken.

Generate CT topograms before the acquisition of the planning simulation scan to review and verify patient alignment and perform any relevant adjustments.

Planning CT is acquired using a slice-thickness of 1–3 mm covering from above the supraclavicular field to below diaphragm.

Table 3.2 Lung function guided radiotherapy selection

Class 0	Class I	Class II	Class III	Class IV
FEV1 ≥ 80% predicted	FEV1 ≥ 65 to 79% predicted	FEV1 ≥ 55 to 64% predicted	FEV1 ≥ 45 to 54% predicted	FEV1 < 45% predicted
DLCO ≥75% predicted	DLCO ≥65 to 74% predicted	DLCO ≥55 to 64% predicted	DLCO 45 to 54% predicted	DLCO <45% predicted
VO$_2$ max >25 mL/kg/min	VO$_2$ max 22 to 25 mL/kg/min	VO$_2$ max 18 to 21 mL/kg/min	VO$_2$ max 15 to 17 mL/kg/min	VO$_2$ max <15 mL/kg/min
Able to tolerate even pneumonectomy		Average risk for any surgical intervention	Average risk for any surgical intervention	Very high risk/ medically inoperable
				if LVEF ≤50%, more vulnerable
Definitive RT or SABR based on clinical requirement		Assessment of regional lung parenchymal function		
		Predicted post-RT FEV1 > 30% and DLCO >35%	Predicted post-RT FEV1 < 30% and DLCO <35% Palliative RT or SABR	
		Definitive RT or SABR	Strongly consider mean lung dose <8 Gy & and V20 < 10%	

SABR stereotactic ablative body radiotherapy, *RT* radiotherapy

Table 3.3 Stage guided treatment selection

Stage 1&2		Stage 3A			Stage 3A		Stage 3B	
T1N0 T2N0		T3N1 N2			T3N1 N2		T4 N3	
Operable	Inoperable	Eligible for surgery/single station N2			Inoperable/multiple station N2		Inoperable	
Surgery	SABR/RT	Surgery + Adjuvant CT	Induction CT	Induction CRT	Eligible	Ineligible	Eligible	Ineligible
		±Postop RT	+ Surgery	+ Surgery	CRT	Induction CT + RT	CRT	Induction CT + RT
			±Postop RT					

Postoperative adjuvant RT: gross residual disease, close or positive microscopic surgical margins/ any positive N2 node/any T4 disease excluding malignant pleural effusion and separate nodules in the same lobes/positive multiple hilar nodes with extracapsular involvement

3.1.4.2 Utilization of Motion Awareness and Management

Target motion in correlation with respiratory cycle is a major challenge for ideal delivery of radiotherapy. The conventional approaches is to both plan and deliver radiotherapy in normal breathing pattern without any respiratory management, but to prescribe dose to a larger estimated volume with additional margin to compensate the unknown motion under treatment. The lung tumor motion and methods to cope with it have long been studied in order to consider this change in lung cancer treatment planning [93–95]. The American Association of Physicists in Medicine (AAPM) Task Group 76 guidelines summarized the adequate methods to account this obscure motion by different methods as motion encompassing (slow CT scanning; combination of inhale and exhale breath-hold CT; 4Dimensional-CT/respiration-correlated CT); respiratory gating (internal fiducial markers or external markers to signal respiration); breath hold (self or device controlled with or without respiratory monitoring); abdominal compression for shallow breathing; and real time tracking [96]. The most well accepted and user friendly method seems to be 4D-CT during normal breathing to obtain an average internal target volume (ITV) model to cover and compensate respiration-related tumor motion [95, 97–99]. The ITV approach provides individualization in prescription by designing patient and motion specific margins of incorporating the extent of tumor motion.

As the motion could be managed with 4DCT and ITV utilization, dose calculation was another concern in IMRT due to the fact that motion information and change in density based on movement was not included in calculation in conventional setting and especially breathing-related intra-fraction organ motion was an issue. However, the plans after 4DCT simulation are generally reconstructed on an average intensity projection dataset and dose calculations are performed with treatment planning software including modern dose algorithms based on heterogeneity correction such as Monte Carlo, collapsed-cone, convolution/superposition, anisotropic analytical algorithm, and Acuros® XB [100–104]. Additionally, Bortfeld et al. has shown that the effect of organ motion in IMRT does not cause systematic errors in dose delivery and is averaging the dose distribution without motion over the path of the tumor motion and this is actually not different from conventional beams [105]. The vital component in planning is 4D-CT simulation, which should be used if available; if it is not available, other alternative options to produce an average image of the tumor at all respiratory phases such as spiral CT or slow CT scanning need to be considered. Based on the complex extent of dose shaping and conformity requirement in IMRT than 3DCRT, it ought to be expressed that motion awareness and 4D planning support to identify the margins of the runaway target are more critical for IMRT than for conventional 3D-CRT. Therefore, the planned IMRT doses with motion awareness including 4DCT dataset and current heterogeneity correction algorithms most definitely represent the doses delivered.

3.1.4.3 Target Volume Delineation Guidelines

Although elective nodal irradiation is not recommended, surgical lymph node levels are important to evaluate per case; International Association for the Study of Lung Cancer has published lymph node contouring atlas revealing levels 1–9 corresponding to N2 nodes, and levels 10–14 to N1 nodes [106].

Volume Definition (Contouring for Involved Field Irradiation)
GTV: Contoured based on CT image.

Internal GTV (iGTV): contouring the GTV based on 4D CT (Respiratory data sets are "binned" by phase: 0–100% at 10% interval): Define the GTV contour using the maximum intensity projection (MIP) and modify based on visual verification of contours in individual respiratory phases. Pulmonary extent is contoured on lung windows (−600/1600 HU), spiculated part of lesion is recommended to be considered as GTV. PET-CT scan is used to differentiate between atelectasis and tumor in parenchyma. Mediastinal extent and lymph nodes (>1 cm in the shortest dimension on CT and PET-CT positive nones) are contoured on mediastinal windows (+20/400 HU).

If neoadjuvant chemotherapy received: GTV include post-chemotherapy lung extent in addition to pre-chemotherapy positive nodal stations, as well as ipsilateral hilum if positive mediastinal nodal disease initially; if complete response post-chemotherapy, pre-chemotherapy positive nodal station and positive lung parenchymal involvement is defined as CTV to receive at least 50 Gy.

CTV = Internal Target Volume (ITV); ITV is determined to be the iGTV plus a margin that accounts for microscopic disease, therefore:

ITV = iGTV plus 8 mm margin for all histologies [107].

Should not extend beyond anatomic boundaries (chest wall, vertebral body, vessels, mediastinal wall etc.) except evidence of invasion.

No elective node in theory, however lobe-specific extent of systematic lymph node dissection algorithm might be followed for CTV2 (the right mid lobe or right lower lobe, or left lingular, left lower lobe lesion require subcarinal nodal station; and left upper lobe lesion requires aorticopulmonary window nodal station if positive mediastinal nodal disease) [108].

PTV: Definitive treatment is recommended to use ITV generally or respiratory gating (end of expiration) very selectively [109].

ITV: iGTV +8 mm margin accounts for respiratory motion, but not patient motion on table, therefore image guidance is the determining factor for PTV margin.

PTV_SABR for early stage disease = iGTV +5 mm.

PTV=ITV + 5 mm-1 cm margin (if once-weekly port films).

PTV=ITV + 5 mm (if daily orthogonal kV).

PTV=ITV + 3 mm (if daily orthogonal kV daily and CBCT daily or 2–3 times/week).

> **Postoperative Volume Definition (Contouring)**
> **GTV**: gross/microscopic positive margins or gross residual disease as indicated by CT, PET, operative note, and pathological report.
>
> **CTV**: iGTV+ 8 mm plus the surgical stump + positive mediastinal nodal stations (N2) as identified pathologically or radiologically + Ipsilateral hilum (N1) + if there is no mediastinal nodal dissection or adequate mapping, ipsilateral hilar (N1) and ipsilateral mediastinal nodes (N2) + high-risk areas due to surgeon input.
>
> **PTV**: As defined.

3.1.4.4 Case Contouring

The patient with locally-advanced T2N3M0 squamous cell carcinoma treated with concurrent CRT (cisplatin & etoposide) utilizing image guided simultaneous integrated volumetric modulated arc treatment (SIB-VMAT) technique with iGTV = 66Gy (2.2Gy/fraction), CTV = 60Gy (2Gy/fraction), in 30 fractions and 6 weeks (Figs. 3.4 and 3.5).

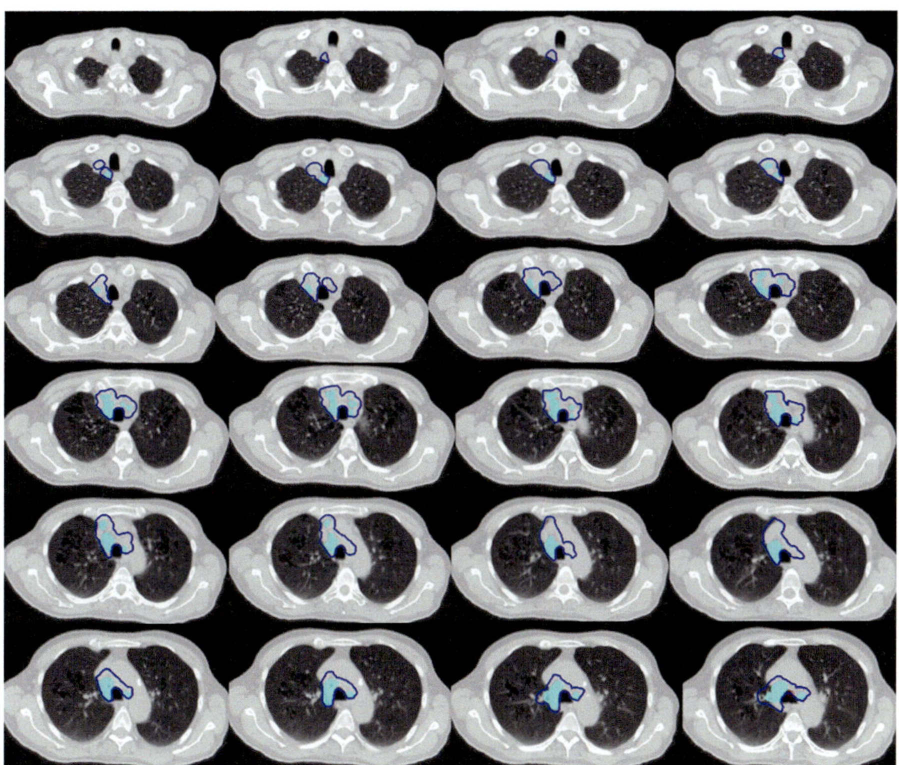

Fig. 3.4 Contouring for T2N3M0 NSCLC, iGTV 66Gy (skyblue), and CTV 60Gy (blue)

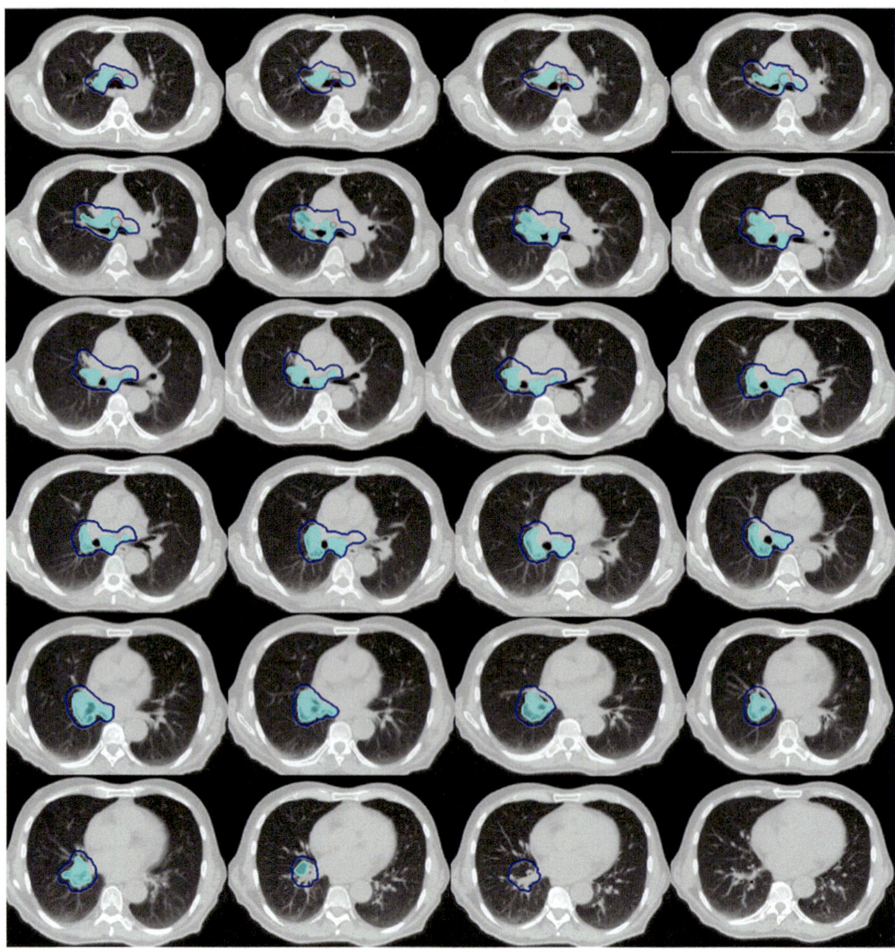

Fig. 3.4 (continued)

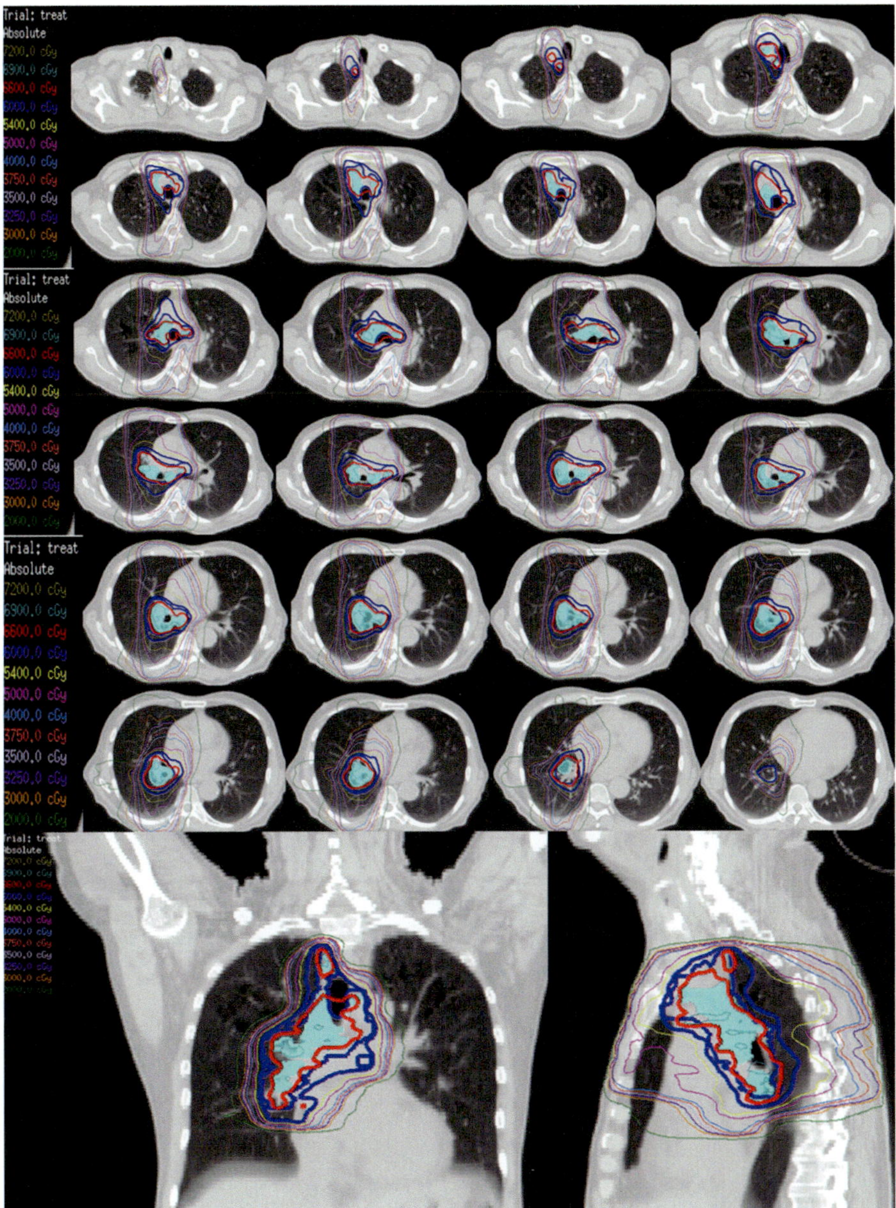

Fig. 3.5 Treatment plan for T2N3M0 NSCLC, iGTV 66Gy, and CTV 60Gy

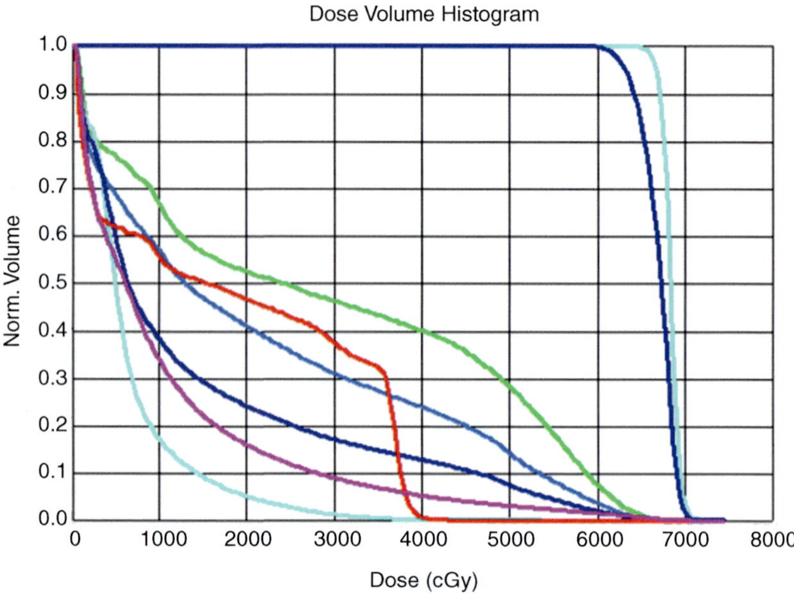

ROI Statistics

Line Type	ROI	Trial or Record	Min.	Max.	Mean	Std. Dev.
—	iGTV 66 Gy in 30 fr	treat	5996.6	7182.8	6829.8	98.4
—	esophagus	treat	63.0	6750.7	2827.7	2283.0
—	CTV 60 Gy in 30 fr	treat	4861.2	7252.5	6686.3	197.9
—	lung l	treat	33.8	5348.7	660.6	618.3
—	lung r	treat	23.5	7424.5	2098.9	2020.4
—	t lung	treat	23.5	7424.5	1424.3	1691.7
—	cord	treat	38.6	4294.1	1829.7	1580.4
—	Heart	treat	50.1	7056.6	1067.4	1323.8

Fig. 3.5 (continued)

3.1.4.5 Treatment Planning

Prescription Dose

Stereotactic Ablative Radiotherapy
60 Gy in 3 fractions, 50 Gy in 4 fractions or 70 Gy in 10 fractions, depending on tumor location/size, using computed tomography-based heterogeneity corrections and a convolution superposition calculation algorithm [110, 111].

Locoregionally Advanced
The results of phase III comparison of 60 Gy versus 74 Gy conformal chemoradiotherapy with or without cetuximab for stage III NSCLC in RTOG 0617 demonstrated 60 Gy is superior to 74 Gy in terms of overall survival and local-regional control, and "RTOG standard dose" is documented to be minimum 60 Gy, while a moderate dose escalation is encouraged between 60–70 Gy for locoregionally advanced NSCLC [112]. Based on our 4DCT and IMRT approach with strict OAR criteria, high dose radiotherapy seems a feasible and appropriate practice.
Radiotherapy with concurrent chemotherapy:

- 66 Gy (2.2 Gy/fraction/day) simultaneous integrated radiation boost to iGTV while prescribing 60 Gy (2 Gy/fraction/day) to the PTV in 30 fractions
- 60–66 Gy (2 Gy/fraction/day) to the PTV in 30 fractions

Radiotherapy alone after sequential chemotherapy or consolidation/ Palliation with radiotherapy alone:

- 45 Gy (3 Gy/fraction/day) to the PTV in 15 fractions
- 52.5 Gy (3.5 Gy/fraction/day) simultaneous integrated radiation boost to iGTV while prescribing 45 Gy (3 Gy/fraction/day) to the PTV in 15 fractions
- 60 Gy (3 Gy/fraction/day) to the PTV in 20 fractions for selected small volume disease which is not involving critical organs at risk
- 30 Gy (3 Gy/fraction/day) to the PTV in 10 fractions if life expectancy <6 months with poor KPS and/or with multiple visceral/brain metastasis

Postoperative Dose
Negative margins: 50 Gy (2 Gy/fraction/day) in 25 fractions.
Positive ECE: 54 Gy (2 Gy/fraction/day) in 27 fractions.
Microscopic positive margin: 60 Gy (2 Gy/fraction/day) in 30 fractions.
Gross residual disease: 66–70 Gy (2 Gy/fraction/day) in 33–35 frs.

Concurrent chemotherapy could be used in case of gross disease in postop setting.

Tailoring could be made such as simultaneous integrated boost to gross disease with 70 Gy (2Gy/fraction/day) while prescribing 63 Gy (1.8 Gy/fraction/day) to the remaining bed.

The recommended organs at risk doses are detailed in Tables 3.4 and 3.5 for SABR prescribed in 4 and 10 fractions.

Table 3.4 Normal tissue constraints for SABR [110, 111]

Organ at risk	50 Gy in 4 fractions	70 Gy in 10 fractions
Total lung	Mean dose ≤6 Gy, V5 ≤ 30%, V10 ≤ 17%, V20 ≤ 12%, V30 ≤ 7%	Mean dose ≤9 Gy, V40 ≤ 7%
Ipsilateral lung	Mean dose ≤10 Gy, V10 ≤ 35%, V20 ≤ 25%, V30 ≤ 15%	
Trachea	V35 ≤ 1 cc	V40 ≤ 1 cc, Dmax ≤60Gy
Bronchial tree	V35 ≤ 1 cc, Dmax ≤38Gy	V50 ≤ 1 cc, Dmax ≤60Gy
Hilar major vessels	V40 ≤ 1 cc, Dmax ≤56Gy	V50 ≤ 1 cc, Dmax ≤75Gy
Other Chest Great Vessels	V40 ≤ 1 cc, Dmax ≤56Gy	V50 ≤ 1 cc, Dmax ≤75Gy
Esophagus	V30 ≤ 1 cc, Dmax ≤35Gy	V40 ≤ 1 cc, Dmax ≤50Gy
Heart/Pericardium	V40 ≤ 1 cc, V20 ≤ 5 cc, Dmax ≤45Gy	V45 ≤ 1 cc, Dmax ≤60Gy
Spinal Cord	V20 ≤ 1 cc, Dmax ≤25Gy	V35 ≤ 1 cc, Dmax ≤40Gy
Chestwall	V30 ≤ 30 cc	V50 ≤ 60 cc, V40 ≤ 120 cc, V30 ≤ 250 cc, Dmax ≤82Gy
Skin	V30 ≤ 50 cc	V50 ≤ 60 cc, V40 ≤ 120 cc, V30 ≤ 250 cc, Dmax ≤82Gy
Brachial plexus	Dmax <35Gy, 0.2 cc less than 30 Gy	Dmax <55 Gy, 0.2 cc less than 50 Gy

Table 3.5 Normal tissue constraints for fractionated radiotherapy

Organ	RT alone	Chemo and RT	Chemo and RT before surgery
Spinal cord	D_{max} < 45 Gy D_{max} < 32 Gy (BID)	D_{max} < 45 Gy D_{max} < 32 Gy (BID)	D_{max} < 45 Gy D_{max} < 32 Gy (BID)
Lung	MLD ≤ 20 Gy V_{20} ≤ 40%	MLD ≤ 20 Gy V_{20} ≤ 35% V_{10} ≤ 45% V_{5} ≤ 65%	MLD ≤ 20 Gy V_{20} ≤ 20% V_{10} ≤ 40% V_{5} ≤ 55%
	[113] If possible: Ipsilateral V20 ≤ 52%; V30 ≤ 39%; MLD ≤ 22 Gy [114] *Grade 3 Pneumonia <2% if* V20 ≤ %25 V5 ≤ %60 V10 ≤ %42 V25 ≤ %20 V35 ≤ %15 V50 ≤ %10 [114] *Grade 3 Pneumonia increases in every 10% addition to limits:* V20 ≤ %25 → < %2 V20 ≤ %35 → %16 V20 ≤ %45 → %25 V20 ≤ %55 → %36		

Table 3.5 (continued)

Organ	RT alone	Chemo and RT	Chemo and RT before surgery
Heart	$V_{30} \leq 45\%$ Mean Dose <26 Gy		
Liver	$V_{30} \leq 40\%$ Mean Dose <30 Gy		
Esophagus	$D_{max} \leq 80$ Gy $V_{70} < 20\%$ $V_{50} < 40\%$ Mean Dose <34 Gy		
Brachial plexus	$D_{max} \leq 66$ Gy		

3.2 Small Cell Lung Cancer

Abstract

Epidemiology Small cell lung cancer (SCLC) accounts for 15–20% of lung cancer cases with decreasing incidence. Extensive stage disease constitutes almost 2/3 of patients at admission, while the remainder present with limited stage disease. In more 95% of cases, tobacco exposure is the main etiological factor. SCLC has a classic radiographic presentation with bulky hilar and mediastinal lymph node involvement.

Pathological and Biological Features SCLC is characterized by small cells with scant cytoplasm and nuclear features of fine, dispersed chromatin without distinct nucleoli. SCLC might be associated with paraneoplastic syndromes such as SIADH, ACTH production syndrome, and Eaton–Lambert syndrome. The vast majority of SCLCs express at least one neuroendocrine marker. Most important prognostic factors are stage and performance status.

Definitive Therapy SCLC was documented as highly sensitive to cytotoxic chemotherapy. Standard treatment for limited stage is systemic therapy and concurrent radiotherapy, however if very early staged small cell lung cancer as clinical T1-2N0M0 is evaluated, for N0 cases, mediastinal staging followed by lobectomy and mediastinal nodal dissection is not inappropriate to be recommended. For extensive stage patients, treatment starts with cisplatin/carboplatin based chemotherapy and thoracic ± metastatic site radiotherapy for selected patients. The median overall survival (OS) for patients with limited SCLC is median 20 months, metastatic SCLC receiving standard chemotherapy in range of 9–11 months over the past 20+ years, even in the most recent large randomized clinical trials. Prophylactic cranial radiotherapy (PCI) is recommended for all stages, as brain metastases incidence is 10–15% at presentation and 50–80% at 2-year after chemo-RT.

Keywords: Small cell lung cancer, Radiotherapy

3.2.1 Case Presentation

54 years old female with 50 packet year smoking history and no significant past medical history admitted with coughing and blood in sputum. Her physical exam was normal in general except right sided decreased breathing sounds and rhonchus in pulmonary auscultation. A chest CT was ordered revealing right hilar small tumor with conglomerated multiple stations of mediastinal nodal disease filling and expanding anterior mediastinum in addition to bilateral supraclavicular disease. PET CT confirmed the CT findings without distant metastases (Fig. 3.6). Endobronchial ultrasound guided biopsies revealed small cell carcinoma both in primary and mediastinum, as well as fine needle aspiration of CT guided biopsy confirmed contralateral supraclavicular nodes involvement. Her cranial MRI was normal without metastases. She was staged as limited stage small cell lung cancer.

3.2.2 Staging

Two staging systems are commonly used. The Veterans' Administration Lung Study Group (VALSG) presented a two-stage classification system in the 1950s [115]. Basically, this system categorizes SCLC as limited-stage (LS), in which the disease is limited to an area within the thorax that can be covered within a radiation port, and extensive-stage (ES), in which disease cannot be encompassed in a radiation field such as having malignant pleural or pericardial effusions or metastases consistent with hematogenous spread. The International Association for the Study of Lung Cancer (IASLC) also projected that the TNM lung cancer staging system be used in place of the VALSG system. Although the TNM system is in more details and could predict more precise the situation of the disease, the VALSG system is very practical staging system and widely used clinically.

Limited Stage (LS): disease fitting into a single radiation port, typically confined to one hemithorax and regional nodes.

Extensive Stage (ES): may include malignant pleural or pericardial effusions or metastases consistent with hematogenous spread.

3.2.3 Evidence Based Treatment Recommendation

For Limited stage disease, concurrent cisplatin and etoposide (4 cycles every 3 weeks) with early thoracic radiotherapy during cycle 1 or 2 (45 Gy for 1.5 Gy b.i.d. or 60–70 Gy for 1.8-2Gy QD). For <5% of patients with cT1-2N0 disease with negative mediastinoscopy (or endoscopic biopsy), lobectomy and mediastinal node dissection/sampling may be performed initially [116, 117]. If pN0, chemotherapy alone; if pN+, concurrent chemoradiation as above. Prophylactic cranial radiotherapy is recommended in all patients after completion of other treatments (25 Gy in 10 fractions).

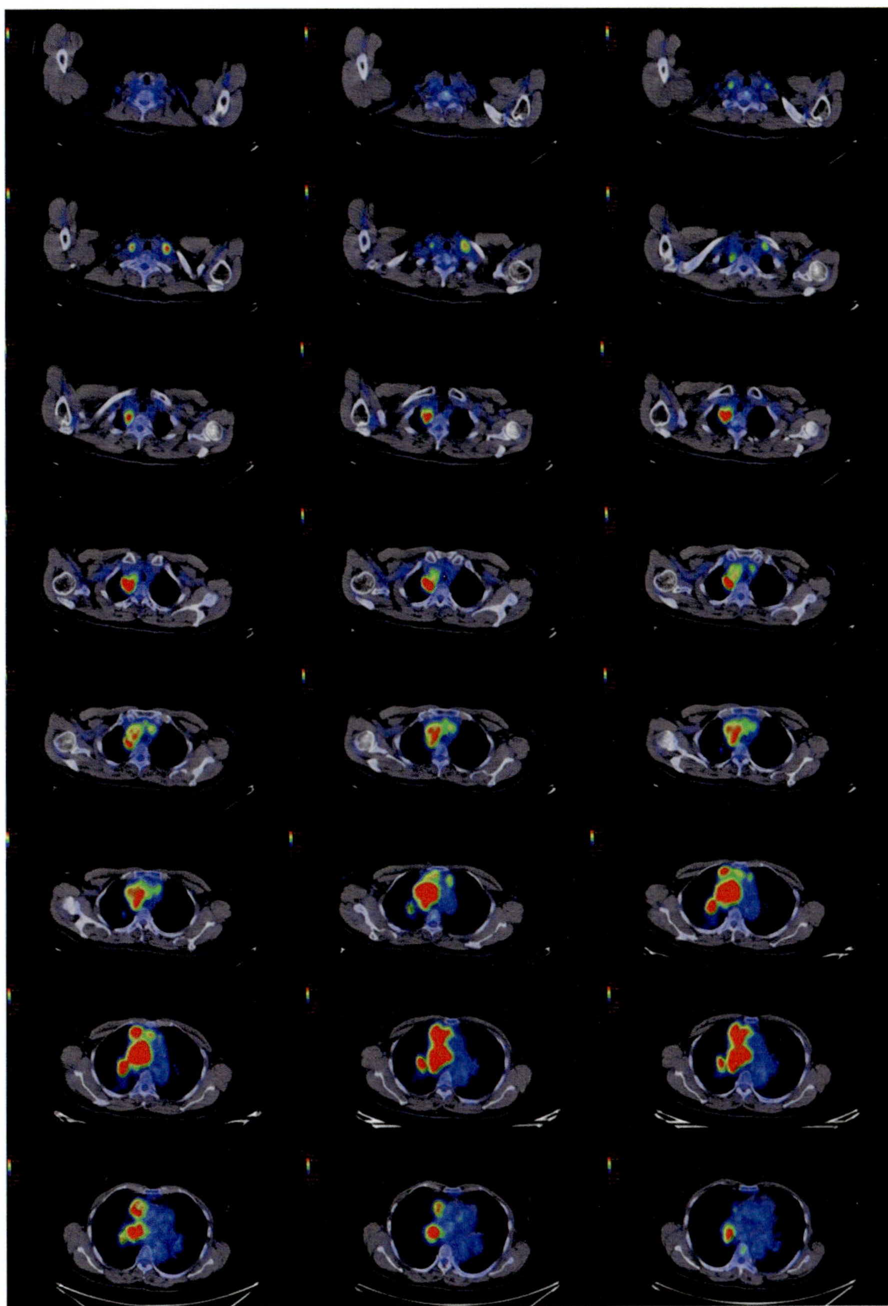

Fig. 3.6 Axial PET-CT fusion images defining multiple stations of mediastinal disease

Table 3.6 Stage guided treatment selection

		Limited stage	Extensive stage	
Clinical T1-2 N0 M0 (~5%) Pathological Mediastinal staging → If N+ continue with chemoradiotherapy; If N0, continue with lobectomy and mediastinal nodal dissection. Then with final pathology: If pN0 → systemic chemotherapy If pN1 → systemic chemotherapy ± involved field radiotherapy (sequential or concurrent) If pN2 → systemic chemotherapy + involved field concurrent radiotherapy		T3-4 or N + M0 Definitive Chemotherapy + Concurrent radiotherapy With first or second cycle	Definitive Chemotherapy	Definitive Chemotherapy
+ PCI		+ PCI	Good Response: Consolidation RT ± Chemo ± PCI	Poor Response: Palliative Chemotherapy ± ± Best Supportive care

For extensive disease, initial step is combination platinum-based chemotherapy. For patients with PR or CR to chemotherapy, prophylactic cranial RT (25 Gy in 10 fractions), consolidative thoracic/metastatic radiotherapy to primary and metastatic sites. If brain metastases present, whole brain radiotherapy (WBRT, 30–37.5 Gy in 10–15 fractions) is recommended.

Stage guided treatment selection is summarized in Table 3.6.

3.2.3.1 Limited Stage SCLC

Approximately 30% of patients with SCLC present with early stage disease. The clinical presentation without clinical or pathologic evidence of mediastinal lymph node involvement is rare and N0 SCLC usually undergo surgical resection [116, 117]. There are no prospective studies evaluating the value of adjuvant chemotherapy for operated patients. The retrospective analyses of National Cancer Database including 1574 cases between 2003 and 2011, demonstrated that overall survival (OS) was improved with adjuvant chemotherapy with or without adjuvant radiation [118]. Also furthermore, platinum-based neoadjuvant or adjuvant therapy was shown to provide superior OS for surgically staged patients in a retrospective review from Johns Hopkins University compared to patients receiving non-platinum regimens [119]. Often, LS-SCLCs have mediastinal lymph node involvement at the time of diagnosis and the standard treatment for these cancers is concurrent chemotherapy and radiation [117]. In 1992, meta-analysis by Pignon consists 13 trials and 2140 patients with LS-SCLC treated with chemo ± thoracic radiotherapy with a median follow-up of 43 months [120–122]. Thoracic radiotherapy improved 3-year overall survival by 5.4% vs. chemotherapy alone (14.3 vs. 8.9%). The optimal timing of radiation for LS-SCLC remains controversial. Metaanalyses of randomized controlled trials, assessing LS-SCLC patients receiving chemo and early vs. late timing of thoracic radiotherapy revealed an improved survival for early concurrent combination of radiotherapy with platinum-based chemotherapy [123, 124]. In addition to this finding, the amount of time from start to completion of thoracic radiotherapy in LD-SCLC may also effect overall survival. The completion of therapy in less than 30 days was associated with an improved 5-year survival rate (relative risk, 0.62; 95% confidence interval, 0.49–0.80; P = 0.0003) [123].

Turrisi et al. randomized 417 patients to receive a total of 45 Gy radiotherapy, either once-daily (1.8 Gy in 25 fractions) or twice-daily (1.5 Gy in 30 fractions) with concurrent cisplatin and etoposide [125]; the median survival improved from 19 months by once-daily to 23 months by twice-daily radiotherapy, after a median follow up of almost 8 years, and though twice daily radiotherapy decreased local failure (36 vs. 52%), also increased grade 3 esophagitis (27 vs. 11%). Despite this benefit, the widely clinical implementation of twice daily radiotherapy was limited due to scheduling/accommodation problems and significant acute side effects. The dose escalation interest from once daily 45 Gy radiotherapy in 25 fractions to a 60–70 Gy of once-daily radiation schema with concurrent chemotherapy has been evaluated in randomized trials [126–128]. The ideal timing to initiate radiotherapy with the concurrent chemotherapy is within the first two cycles of chemotherapy [124, 129, 130]. Komaki et al. reported RTOG 0239 phase II trial using accelerated high-dose thoracic radiotherapy (61.2 Gy in 5 weeks with large field to 28.8 Gy/1.8 Gy QD, then 14.4 Gy/1.8 Gy b.i.d. in the evening) concurrent with etoposide/cisplatin [131]; revealing two-year overall survival of 37% and local control of 80%, aside from 18% acute severe esophagitis. CALGB 30610/RTOG 0538 ongoing trial has planned to compare standard fractionation (70 Gy/2 Gy daily) versus Turrisi regimen (45 Gy/1.5 Gy BID) versus RTOG 0239 dose escalation (61.2 Gy in 5 weeks) schemas, and has been revised with closure of accelerated high-dose thoracic radiotherapy arm at interim analysis after the publication of RTOG 0239.

Recently reported CONVERT trial by Faivre-Finn et al., with 45 months of median follow up, randomized 547 patients to 45 Gy (1.5 Gy BID over 15 weekdays, 3 weeks) vs. 66 Gy (2 Gy daily QD over 33 weekdays, 6.5 weeks), each with 4 to 6 cycles of concurrent cisplatin/etoposide, followed by PCI as indicated, in order to demonstrate superiority of the once-daily regimen [132]. After a median follow up of 45 months, no statistically significant difference was acknowledged in overall survival at 2 years (BID 56% × QD 51%) and median survival (BID 30 months × QD 25 months, hazard radio for death for QD regimen was 1.18,

P = 0.14) The rate of grade 2 esophagitis, grade 3/4 esophagitis and grade 3/4 pneumonitis were 55% × 63%, 19% × 19%, 2.2% × 2.5%, respectively and found to be similar in both arms [132]. Due to the failure of CONVERT to define QD reqimen superior and lack of sufficient power to validate equivalence of the BID to QD regimens, BID 45 Gy is yet the gold standard, while QD 60–70 Gy is appealing easier in many practices be applicable in LS-SCLC. Hopefully, emerging evidence will be provided by ongoing CALGB 30610/RTOG 0538 study (NCT00632853; 45 Gy BID × 70 Gy QD).

3.2.3.2 Extensive Stage SCLC

Extensive stage SCLC is mostly not curable, therefore, except selected patients for definitive treatment approach, the general management is to increase quality of life as well as prolong disease free survival as much as possible. The first step is systemic therapy including platinum (cisplatin or carboplatin) combined with etoposide. As the first site progressing after initial chemotherapy is frequently the primary thoracic disease, the role of consolidative thoracic radiotherapy following chemotherapy was evaluated in ES-SCLC, principally in manageable extrathoracic disease burden [133–136]. Jeremic et al. randomized 109 patients already received three cycles of standard cisplatin/etoposide (PE) with complete or a partial response to either thoracic radiotherapy (54 Gy in BID 36 fractions over 18 week days, n = 55) in combination with chemotherapy followed by two cycles of PE or an additional four cycles of PE (n = 54) [136]; and documented significantly better survival rates with thoracic radiotherapy than those chemotherapy alone (median survival, 17 × 11 months; 5-year survival rate, 9.1% vs. 3.7%, respectively; P = 0.041). The phase 3 randomised controlled CREST Trial/NTR1527 enrolled 498 patients with ES-SCLC to receive thoracic radiotherapy of 30 Gy in 10 fractions or not after chemotherapy, while all patients were prescribed prophylactic radiotherapy (PCI) [133]; and Slotman et al. documented a significant survival advantage at 2 years with the use of thoracic radiotherapy (3% versus 13%, P = 0.004). The meta-analysis of the Jeremic trial and the CREST trials with a total of 604 patients (302 thoracic radiotherapy; 302 non-thoracic radiotherapy) underlined the consolidative thoracic radiotherapy to overall provide 20% improvement in overall survival and 25% improvement in progression-free survival [137]. Therefore, ES-SCLC patients with a partial/complete response to chemotherapy, are candidates to be evaluated for consolidative thoracic radiotherapy. Likewise, consolidative radiotherapy to multiple sites of metastasis with complete or partial response to chemotherapy has been evaluated in phase II RTOG 0937 trial enrolling 97 patients who all received PCI to consolidative radiotherapy to the thorax and up to four extracranial metastases or not [138]. Gore et al. documented that the overall survival at 1 year was not different between the groups (60.1% for PCI and 50.8% for PCI+ consolidation radiotherapy-PCI + cRT, p = 0.21), but time to progression favored consolidation radiotherapy as 3- and 12-month rates of progression were 53.3% versus 14.5% and 79.6% versus 75% for PCI versus PCI + cRT, respectively; with being more efficient in a subgroup having 1 metastasis compared to 2–4 metastases, as well as in partial response as opposed to a complete response after chemotherapy [138]. This indicates the requirement of individualization until future studies delineating the pathway for consolidative radiotherapy to metastatic sites in ES-SCLC.

3.2.3.3 PCI for Limited Stage

In case of a complete response, partial response or stable disease following chemoradiotherapy, subsequent prophylactic cranial irradiation (PCI) is commonly recommended. The meta-analysis analyzing seven trials involving 987 limited and extensive stage patients by Auperin et al. concluded that PCI in patients with a complete response after induction chemotherapy provided an improvement in 3-year overall survival of approximately 5.4% (15.3% in no PCI vs. 20.7% in PCI arm), as well as a reduction of the 3-year incidence of brain metastases (59 in no PCI vs. 33% in PCI arm) [139]. RTOG 0212/Intergroup trial by Le Pechoux et al. questioned the optimal dose for PCI in their cohort of 720 LS-SCLC patients having complete response to chemoradiotherapy by randomizing to standard dose (25 Gy/2.5 Gy QD) or to a higher dose (36 Gy/2 Gy QD or 36 Gy/1.5 Gy b.i.d.) of PCI [140]; and concluded that incidence of brains metastases were similar at 2 years, with a decreasing overall survival with higher dose at 2 years (37 vs. 42%). Consequently, 25 Gy is considered standard of care, aside from the discussion on the decline in both short-term quality of life and long-term cognitive functioning with PCI. Phase II multi-institutional RTOG 0933 trial is one of the studies exploring preservation of memory with conformal avoidance of the hippocampal neural stem-cell compartment during whole-brain radiotherapy [141].

3.2.3.4 PCI for Extensive Stage (ES-SCLC)

PCI is also often recommended in patients with ES-SCLC, based on EORTC 22993 trial in support of PCI in ES-SCLC, randomizing 286 patients with a response to 4–6 cycles of chemotherapy to PCI versus observation [142]. Slotman et al. revealed the decrement in risk of symptomatic brain metastases (HR 0.27, P < 0.001) and the increment in median overall survival (6.7 vs. 5.4 months, P = 0.003) with PCI [142]. The most criticized limitation of the study was the lack of proper brain imaging for staging or follow-up unless patients were symptomatic (only 29% with brain imaging). Recently, a multi-institutional Japanese trial by Takahashi et al. evaluated the same question of PCI in MR staging and follow up era, randomizing 224 patients with ES-SCLC, and concluded in the interim analysis that PCI has reduced the incidence of brain metastases but has not provided an improvement in survival (median overall survival of 11.6 months with PCI vs. 13.7 months with observation, HR 1.27, p = 0.094) [143]. This Japanese trial investigating PCI for patients with ES-SCLC was stopped early due to this interim analysis failing to confirm a survival benefit which might motivate the additional trials to rethink the role of PCI in ES-SCLC.

3.2.4 Radiotherapy Planning

3.2.4.1 Volume Definition (Contouring for Involved Field Irradiation)

Volume Definition (Contouring): Involved Field Irradiation as Defined in NSCLC
Allowing 1 or 2 cycles of chemotherapy before concurrent chemotherapy is acceptable if the volume is too large to start with concurrent chemoradiotherapy. Though traditional mediastinal fields covered ipsilateral hilum and bilateral mediastinum from thoracic inlet to subcarinal region, current practice is using involved field radiotherapy as in NSCLC. This approach is supported by Van Loon et al. with PET-based selective nodal irradiation for LD-SCLC resulting in a low rate of isolated nodal failures (3%), and with a low percentage of acute esophagitis [144]; as well as the retrospective data by Shirvani et al. confirming only 2% isolated nodal failure with same strategy [145].

3.2.4.2 Prescription Dose

Definitive thoracic radiotherapy with concurrent chemotherapy was prescribed with three options previously as compared in RTOG 0538, high-dose conventional radiotherapy of 70 Gy (2 Gy once daily over 7 weeks), or 61.2 Gy (1.8 Gy once daily for 16 days followed by 1.8 Gy twice daily for 9 days), or hyperfractionated 45 Gy (1.5 Gy twice daily over 3 weeks) in patients with limited-stage small cell lung cancer. Based on the results of RTOG 0239 [131], an interim analysis closed the arm 61.2 Gy based upon a comparison of treatment-related toxicity. Therefore the possible options for prescription are:

- 45 Gy (1.5 Gy/fraction BID) to PTV in 30 fractions in 15 week days
- 54 Gy (1.8 Gy/fraction BID) simultaneous integrated radiation boost to iGTV while prescribing 45 Gy (1.5 Gy/fraction BID) to the PTV in 30 fractions in 15 week days
- 70 Gy (2 Gy/fraction/day) to PTV in 35 fractions in 35 week days

Evaluating patients for response and regression with cone beam CT after 1st week which might require plan adaptation as there is no cut off for any modification: mostly subjective per physician disposal based on V20 at first plan and response.

Radiotherapy for Consolidation in extensive stage patients following chemotherapy

- 30 Gy–45 Gy (3 Gy/fraction/day, in 10–15 fractions) to the PTV
- Or for a more definitive dose consider 52.5 Gy (3.5 Gy/fraction/day) simultaneous integrated radiation boost to iGTV while prescribing 45 Gy (3 Gy/fraction/day) to the PTV in 15 fractions

3.2.4.3 Case Contouring

The patient with limited stage small cell carcinoma treated with concurrent CRT utilizing image guided simultaneous integrated volumetric modulated arc treatment (SIB-VMAT) technique with iGTV = 54Gy (1.8Gy/fraction), CTV = 45Gy (1.5Gy/fraction), in 30 fractions, twice per day, and 3 weeks (Figs. 3.7 and 3.8).

Normal Tissue Constraints for fractionated radiotherapy is summarized in Table 3.7.

3.2.5   Follow-Up Recommendations

Follow up for algorithm for NSCLC & SCLC is shown in Fig. 3.9.

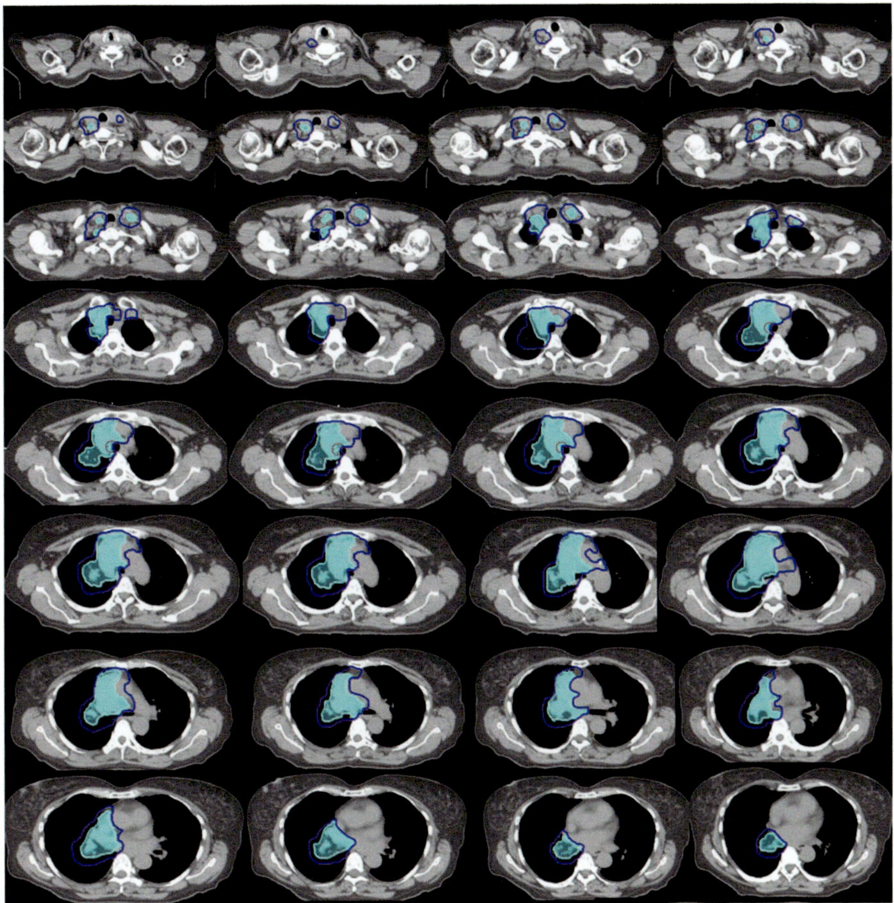

Fig. 3.7 Contouring for iGTV 54Gy (skyblue), and CTV 45Gy (blue)

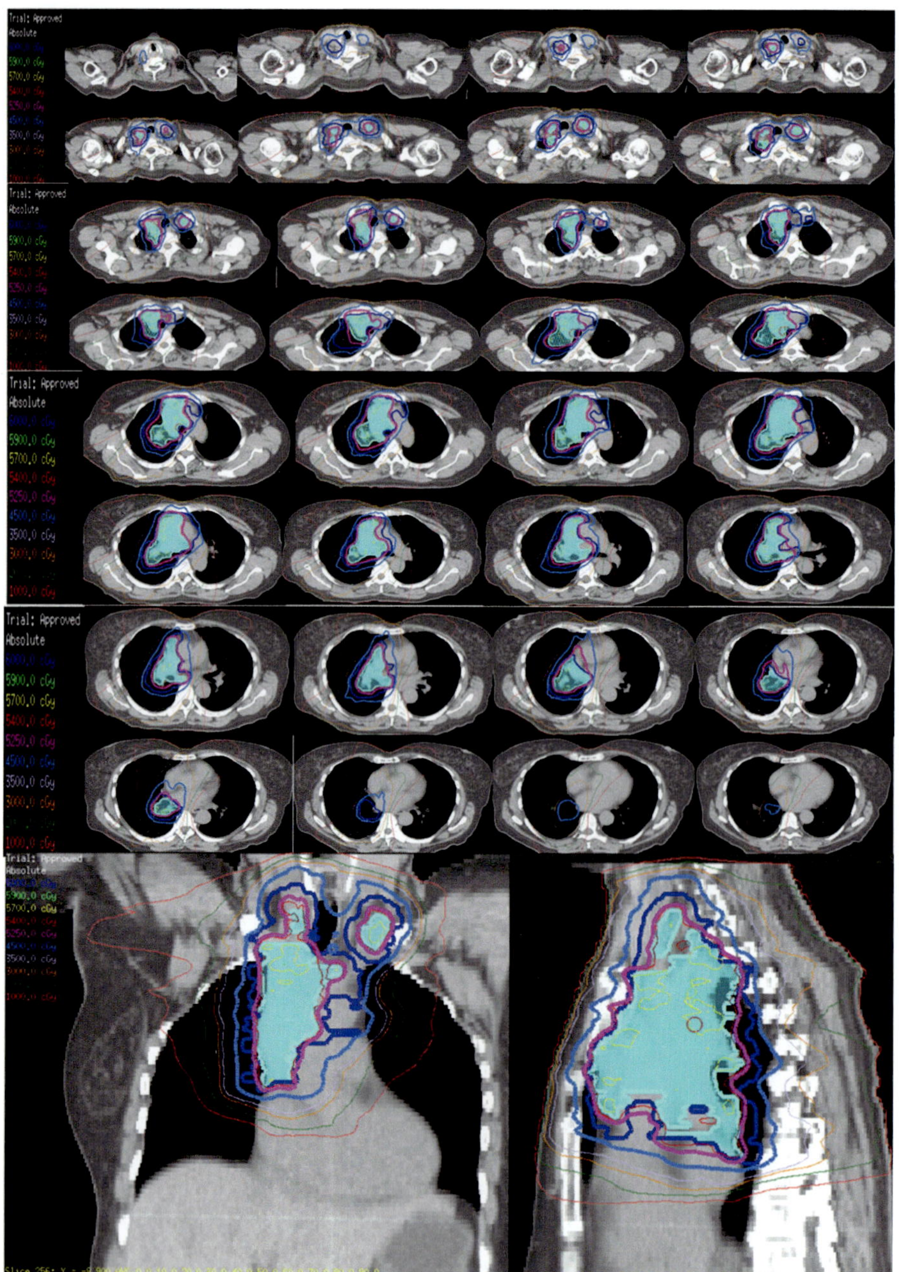

Fig. 3.8 Treatment plan for limited stage small cell lung cancer, iGTV 54Gy, and CTV 45Gy

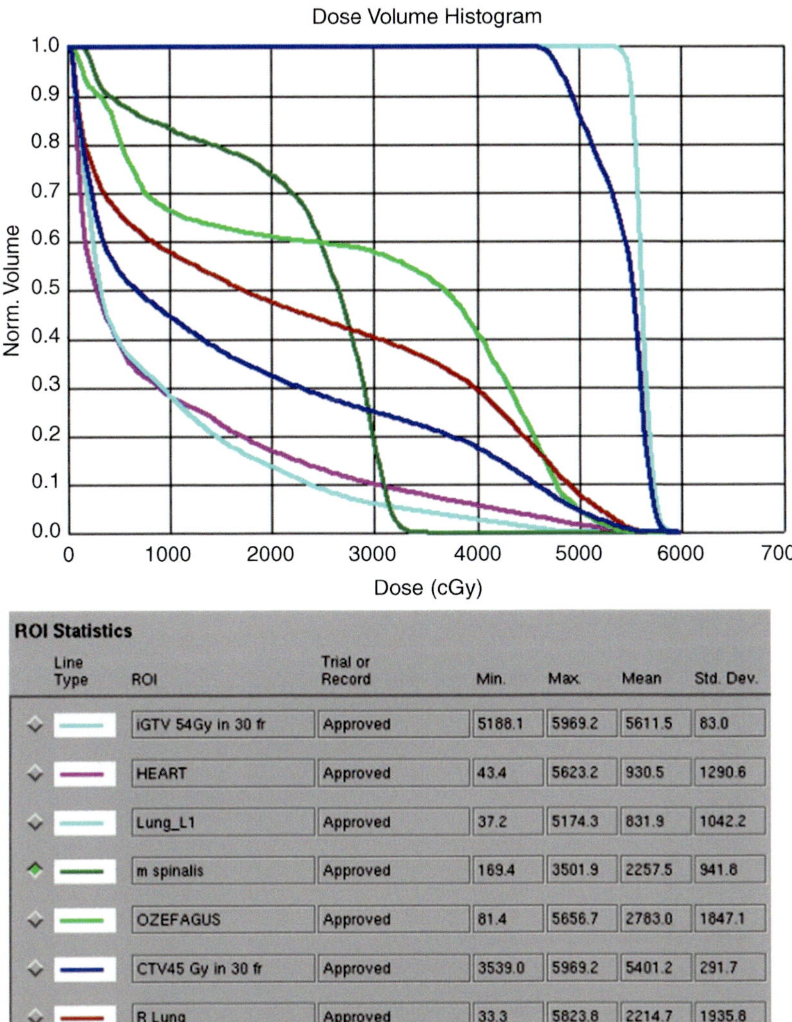

Line Type	ROI	Trial or Record	Min.	Max.	Mean	Std. Dev.
	iGTV 54Gy in 30 fr	Approved	5188.1	5969.2	5611.5	83.0
	HEART	Approved	43.4	5623.2	930.5	1290.6
	Lung_L1	Approved	37.2	5174.3	831.9	1042.2
	m spinalis	Approved	169.4	3501.9	2257.5	941.8
	OZEFAGUS	Approved	81.4	5656.7	2783.0	1847.1
	CTV45 Gy in 30 fr	Approved	3539.0	5969.2	5401.2	291.7
	R Lung	Approved	33.3	5823.8	2214.7	1935.8
	Total Lung	Approved	33.3	5823.8	1595.8	1740.4

Fig. 3.8   (continued)

Table 3.7 Normal tissue constraints for fractionated radiotherapy

Organ	RT alone	Chemo and RT	Chemo and RT before surgery
Spinal cord	$D_{max} < 45$ Gy $D_{max} < 32$ Gy (BID)	$D_{max} < 45$ Gy $D_{max} < 32$ Gy (BID)	$D_{max} < 45$ Gy $D_{max} < 32$ Gy (BID)
Lung	$MLD \leq 20$ Gy $V_{20} \leq 40\%$	$MLD \leq 20$ Gy $V_{20} \leq 35\%$ $V_{10} \leq 45\%$ $V_5 \leq 65\%$	$MLD \leq 20$ Gy $V_{20} \leq 20\%$ $V_{10} \leq 40\%$ $V_5 \leq 55\%$
	[113] If possible: Ipsilateral V20 $\leq$ 52%; V30 $\leq$ 39%; MLD $\leq$ 22 Gy [114] *Grade 3 Pneumonia <2% if* V20 $\leq$ %25 V5 $\leq$ %60 V10 $\leq$ %42 V25 $\leq$ %20 V35 $\leq$ %15 V50 $\leq$ %10 [114] *Grade 3 Pneumonia increases in every 10% addition to limits:* V20 $\leq$ %25 → <%2 V20 $\leq$ %35 → %16 V20 $\leq$ %45 → %25 V20 $\leq$ %55 → %36		
Heart	$V_{30} \leq 45\%$ Mean Dose <26 Gy		
Liver	$V_{30} \leq 40\%$ Mean Dose <30 Gy		
Esophagus	$D_{max} \leq 80$ Gy $V_{70} < 20\%$ $V_{50} < 40\%$ Mean Dose <34 Gy		
Brachial plexus	$D_{max} \leq 66$ Gy		

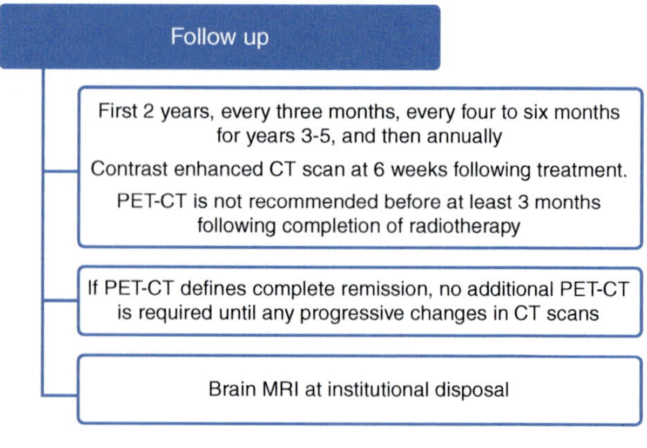

Fig. 3.9 Follow up for algorithm for NSCLC and SCLC

References

1. Aberle DR, Adams AM, Berg CD, Black WC, Clapp JD, Fagerstrom RM, Gareen IF, Gatsonis C, Marcus PM, Sicks JD. Reduced lung-cancer mortality with low-dose computed tomographic screening. N Engl J Med. 2011;365(5):395–409.
2. Sholl LM. Biomarkers in lung adenocarcinoma: a decade of progress. Arch Pathol Lab Med. 2015;139(4):469–80.
3. Lindeman NI, Cagle PT, Beasley MB, Chitale DA, Dacic S, Giaccone G, Jenkins RB, Kwiatkowski DJ, Saldivar JS, Squire J, et al. Molecular testing guideline for selection of lung cancer patients for EGFR and ALK tyrosine kinase inhibitors: guideline from the College of American Pathologists, International Association for the Study of Lung Cancer, and Association for Molecular Pathology. J Thorac Oncol. 2013;8(7):823–59.
4. Herbst RS, Baas P, Kim DW, Felip E, Perez-Gracia JL, Han JY, Molina J, Kim JH, Arvis CD, Ahn MJ, et al. Pembrolizumab versus docetaxel for previously treated, PD-L1-positive, advanced non-small-cell lung cancer (KEYNOTE-010): a randomised controlled trial. Lancet. 2016;387(10027):1540–50.
5. Topkan E, Parlak C, Selek U. Impact of weight change during the course of concurrent chemoradiation therapy on outcomes in stage IIIB non-small cell lung cancer patients: retrospective analysis of 425 patients. Int J Radiat Oncol Biol Phys. 2013;87(4):697–704.
6. Stinchcombe TE, Hodgson L, Herndon JE 2nd, Kelley MJ, Cicchetti MG, Ramnath N, Niell HB, Atkins JN, Akerley W, Green MR, et al. Treatment outcomes of different prognostic groups of patients on cancer and leukemia group B trial 39801: induction chemotherapy followed by chemoradiotherapy compared with chemoradiotherapy alone for unresectable stage III non-small cell lung cancer. J Thorac Oncol. 2009;4(9):1117–25.
7. Albain KS, Crowley JJ, LeBlanc M, Livingston RB. Survival determinants in extensive-stage non-small-cell lung cancer: the Southwest Oncology Group experience. J Clin Oncol. 1991;9(9):1618–26.
8. Mountain CF. Revisions in the international system for staging lung cancer. Chest. 1997;111(6):1710–7.
9. Edge SB, Compton CC. The American Joint Committee on Cancer: the 7th edition of the AJCC cancer staging manual and the future of TNM. Ann Surg Oncol. 2010;17(6):1471–4.
10. Detterbeck FC. The eighth edition TNM stage classification for lung cancer: what does it mean on main street? J Thorac Cardiovasc Surg. 2018;155(1):356–9.
11. Goldstraw P, Chansky K, Crowley J, Rami-Porta R, Asamura H, Eberhardt WE, Nicholson AG, Groome P, Mitchell A, Bolejack V. The IASLC lung cancer staging project: proposals for revision of the TNM stage groupings in the forthcoming (eighth) edition of the TNM classification for lung cancer. J Thorac Oncol. 2016;11(1):39–51.
12. Carter BW, Lichtenberger JP 3rd, Benveniste MK, de Groot PM, Wu CC, Erasmus JJ, Truong MT. Revisions to the TNM staging of lung cancer: rationale, significance, and clinical application. Radiographics. 2018;38(2):374–91.
13. AJCC (American Joint Committee on Cancer). Cancer staging manual. 8th ed. Chicago: Springer; 2017.
14. Rami-Porta R, Bolejack V, Crowley J, Ball D, Kim J, Lyons G, Rice T, Suzuki K, Thomas CF Jr, Travis WD, et al. The IASLC lung cancer staging project: proposals for the revisions of the T descriptors in the forthcoming eighth edition of the TNM classification for lung cancer. J Thorac Oncol. 2015;10(7):990–1003.
15. Ginsberg RJ, Rubinstein LV. Randomized trial of lobectomy versus limited resection for T1 N0 non-small cell lung cancer. Lung Cancer Study Group. Ann Thorac Surg. 1995;60(3):615–22. Discussion 622–613.
16. Manser R, Wright G, Hart D, Byrnes G, Campbell DA. Surgery for early stage non-small cell lung cancer. Cochrane Database Syst Rev. 2005;1:CD004699.

17. Lardinois D, De Leyn P, Van Schil P, Porta RR, Waller D, Passlick B, Zielinski M, Lerut T, Weder W. ESTS guidelines for intraoperative lymph node staging in non-small cell lung cancer. Eur J Cardiothorac Surg. 2006;30(5):787–92.
18. Senthi S, Lagerwaard FJ, Haasbeek CJ, Slotman BJ, Senan S. Patterns of disease recurrence after stereotactic ablative radiotherapy for early stage non-small-cell lung cancer: a retrospective analysis. Lancet Oncol. 2012;13(8):802–9.
19. Verstegen NE, Lagerwaard FJ, Haasbeek CJ, Slotman BJ, Senan S. Outcomes of stereotactic ablative radiotherapy following a clinical diagnosis of stage I NSCLC: comparison with a contemporaneous cohort with pathologically proven disease. Radiother Oncol. 2011;101(2):250–4.
20. Inoue T, Shimizu S, Onimaru R, Takeda A, Onishi H, Nagata Y, Kimura T, Karasawa K, Arimoto T, Hareyama M, et al. Clinical outcomes of stereotactic body radiotherapy for small lung lesions clinically diagnosed as primary lung cancer on radiologic examination. Int J Radiat Oncol Biol Phys. 2009;75(3):683–7.
21. Timmerman RD, Hu C, Michalski J, Straube W, Galvin J, Johnstone D, Bradley J, Barriger R, Bezjak A, Videtic GM, et al. Long-term results of RTOG 0236: a phase II trial of stereotactic body radiation therapy (SBRT) in the treatment of patients with medically inoperable stage I non-small cell lung cancer. Int J Radiat Oncol Biol Phys. 2014;90(Suppl 1):S30.
22. Chi A, Liao Z, Nguyen NP, Xu J, Stea B, Komaki R. Systemic review of the patterns of failure following stereotactic body radiation therapy in early-stage non-small-cell lung cancer: clinical implications. Radiother Oncol. 2010;94(1):1–11.
23. Raz DJ, Zell JA, Ou SH, Gandara DR, Anton-Culver H, Jablons DM. Natural history of stage I non-small cell lung cancer: implications for early detection. Chest. 2007;132(1):193–9.
24. Onishi H, Shirato H, Nagata Y, Hiraoka M, Fujino M, Gomi K, Karasawa K, Hayakawa K, Niibe Y, Takai Y, et al. Stereotactic body radiotherapy (SBRT) for operable stage I non-small-cell lung cancer: can SBRT be comparable to surgery? Int J Radiat Oncol Biol Phys. 2011;81(5):1352–8.
25. Videtic GMM, Donington J, Giuliani M, Heinzerling J, Karas TZ, Kelsey CR, Lally BE, Latzka K, Lo SS, Moghanaki D, et al. Stereotactic body radiation therapy for early-stage non-small cell lung cancer: executive summary of an ASTRO evidence-based guideline. Pract Radiat Oncol. 2017;7(5):295–301.
26. Rwigema JC, Lee P. Is staging mediastinoscopy necessary before stereotactic body radiotherapy for inoperable early stage lung cancer? J Thorac Dis. 2015;7(12):E612–4.
27. Rwigema JC, Chen AM, Wang PC, Lee JM, Garon E, Lee P. Incidental mediastinal dose does not explain low mediastinal node recurrence rates in patients with early-stage NSCLC treated with stereotactic body radiotherapy. Clin Lung Cancer. 2014;15(4):287–93.
28. Crabtree TD, Denlinger CE, Meyers BF, El Naqa I, Zoole J, Krupnick AS, Kreisel D, Patterson GA, Bradley JD. Stereotactic body radiation therapy versus surgical resection for stage I non-small cell lung cancer. J Thorac Cardiovasc Surg. 2010;140(2):377–86.
29. Parashar B, Patel P, Monni S, Singh P, Sood N, Trichter S, Sabbas A, Wernicke AG, Nori D, Chao KS. Limited resection followed by intraoperative seed implantation is comparable to stereotactic body radiotherapy for solitary lung cancer. Cancer. 2010;116(21):5047–53.
30. Grills IS, Mangona VS, Welsh R, Chmielewski G, McInerney E, Martin S, Wloch J, Ye H, Kestin LL. Outcomes after stereotactic lung radiotherapy or wedge resection for stage I non-small-cell lung cancer. J Clin Oncol. 2010;28(6):928–35.
31. Stanic S, Paulus R, Timmerman RD, Michalski JM, Barriger RB, Bezjak A, Videtic GM, Bradley J. No clinically significant changes in pulmonary function following stereotactic body radiation therapy for early-stage peripheral non-small cell lung cancer: an analysis of RTOG 0236. Int J Radiat Oncol Biol Phys. 2014;88(5):1092–9.
32. Crabtree T, Puri V, Timmerman R, Fernando H, Bradley J, Decker PA, Paulus R, Putnum JB Jr, Dupuy DE, Meyers B. Treatment of stage I lung cancer in high-risk and inoperable patients: comparison of prospective clinical trials using stereotactic body radiotherapy (RTOG 0236), sublobar resection (ACOSOG Z4032), and radiofrequency ablation (ACOSOG Z4033). J Thorac Cardiovasc Surg. 2013;145(3):692–9.

33. Haasbeek CJ, Senan S, Smit EF, Paul MA, Slotman BJ, Lagerwaard FJ. Critical review of nonsurgical treatment options for stage I non-small cell lung cancer. Oncologist. 2008;13(3):309–19.
34. Lagerwaard FJ, Verstegen NE, Haasbeek CJ, Slotman BJ, Paul MA, Smit EF, Senan S. Outcomes of stereotactic ablative radiotherapy in patients with potentially operable stage I non-small cell lung cancer. Int J Radiat Oncol Biol Phys. 2012;83(1):348–53.
35. Onishi H, Araki T. Stereotactic body radiation therapy for stage I non-small-cell lung cancer: a historical overview of clinical studies. Jpn J Clin Oncol. 2013;43(4):345–50.
36. Varlotto J, Fakiris A, Flickinger J, Medford-Davis L, Liss A, Shelkey J, Belani C, DeLuca J, Recht A, Maheshwari N, et al. Matched-pair and propensity score comparisons of outcomes of patients with clinical stage I non-small cell lung cancer treated with resection or stereotactic radiosurgery. Cancer. 2013;119(15):2683–91.
37. Yoshitake T, Nakamura K, Shioyama Y, Sasaki T, Ohga S, Shinoto M, Terashima K, Asai K, Matsumoto K, Matsuo Y, et al. Stereotactic body radiation therapy for primary lung cancers clinically diagnosed without pathological confirmation: a single-institution experience. Int J Clin Oncol. 2015;20(1):53–8.
38. Solda F, Lodge M, Ashley S, Whitington A, Goldstraw P, Brada M. Stereotactic radiotherapy (SABR) for the treatment of primary non-small cell lung cancer; systematic review and comparison with a surgical cohort. Radiother Oncol. 2013;109(1):1–7.
39. Zheng X, Schipper M, Kidwell K, Lin J, Reddy R, Ren Y, Chang A, Lv F, Orringer M, Spring Kong FM. Survival outcome after stereotactic body radiation therapy and surgery for stage I non-small cell lung cancer: a meta-analysis. Int J Radiat Oncol Biol Phys. 2014;90(3):603–11.
40. Chang JY, Senan S, Paul MA, Mehran RJ, Louie AV, Balter P, Groen HJ, McRae SE, Widder J, Feng L, et al. Stereotactic ablative radiotherapy versus lobectomy for operable stage I non-small-cell lung cancer: a pooled analysis of two randomised trials. Lancet Oncol. 2015;16(6):630–7.
41. Yalman D, Selek U. Stereotactic ablative radiotherapy (SABR) in operable early stage non-small cell lung cancer (NSCLC) patients: challenge to claim being undisputed gold standard. Ann Transl Med. 2015;3(11):150.
42. Moghanaki D, Chang JY. Is surgery still the optimal treatment for stage I non-small cell lung cancer? Transl Lung Cancer Res. 2016;5(2):183–9.
43. Yu XJ, Dai WR, Xu Y. Survival outcome after stereotactic body radiation therapy and surgery for early stage non-small cell lung cancer: a meta-analysis. J Invest Surg. 2017:1–8.
44. Li M, Yang X, Chen Y, Yang X, Dai X, Sun F, Zhang L, Zhan C, Feng M, Wang Q. Stereotactic body radiotherapy or stereotactic ablative radiotherapy versus surgery for patients with T1-3N0M0 non-small cell lung cancer: a systematic review and meta-analysis. Onco Targets Ther. 2017;10:2885–92.
45. Rodrigues G, Choy H, Bradley J, Rosenzweig KE, Bogart J, Curran WJ Jr, Gore E, Langer C, Louie AV, Lutz S, et al. Definitive radiation therapy in locally advanced non-small cell lung cancer: executive summary of an American Society for Radiation Oncology (ASTRO) evidence-based clinical practice guideline. Pract Radiat Oncol. 2015;5(3):141–8.
46. Rodrigues G, Choy H, Bradley J, Rosenzweig KE, Bogart J, Curran WJ Jr, Gore E, Langer C, Louie AV, Lutz S, et al. Adjuvant radiation therapy in locally advanced non-small cell lung cancer: executive summary of an American Society for Radiation Oncology (ASTRO) evidence-based clinical practice guideline. Pract Radiat Oncol. 2015;5(3):149–55.
47. Bezjak A, Temin S, Franklin G, Giaccone G, Govindan R, Johnson ML, Rimner A, Schneider BJ, Strawn J, Azzoli CG. Definitive and adjuvant radiotherapy in locally advanced non-small-cell lung cancer: American Society of Clinical Oncology clinical practice guideline endorsement of the American Society for Radiation Oncology evidence-based clinical practice guideline. J Clin Oncol. 2015;33(18):2100–5.
48. Lee PC, Port JL, Korst RJ, Liss Y, Meherally DN, Altorki NK. Risk factors for occult mediastinal metastases in clinical stage I non-small cell lung cancer. Ann Thorac Surg. 2007;84(1):177–81.

49. De Leyn P, Lardinois D, Van Schil P, Rami-Porta R, Passlick B, Zielinski M, Waller D, Lerut T, Weder W. European trends in preoperative and intraoperative nodal staging: ESTS guidelines. J Thorac Oncol. 2007;2(4):357–61.
50. Wang EH, Corso CD, Rutter CE, Park HS, Chen AB, Kim AW, Wilson LD, Decker RH, Yu JB. Postoperative radiation therapy is associated with improved overall survival in incompletely resected stage II and III non-small-cell lung cancer. J Clin Oncol. 2015;33(25):2727–34.
51. Douillard JY, Rosell R, De Lena M, Carpagnano F, Ramlau R, Gonzales-Larriba JL, Grodzki T, Pereira JR, Le Groumellec A, Lorusso V, et al. Adjuvant vinorelbine plus cisplatin versus observation in patients with completely resected stage IB-IIIA non-small-cell lung cancer (Adjuvant Navelbine International Trialist Association [ANITA]): a randomised controlled trial. Lancet Oncol. 2006;7(9):719–27.
52. Douillard JY, Rosell R, De Lena M, Riggi M, Hurteloup P, Mahe MA. Impact of postoperative radiation therapy on survival in patients with complete resection and stage I, II, or IIIA non-small-cell lung cancer treated with adjuvant chemotherapy: the adjuvant Navelbine International Trialist Association (ANITA) randomized trial. Int J Radiat Oncol Biol Phys. 2008;72(3):695–701.
53. Lee JH, Machtay M, Kaiser LR, Friedberg JS, Hahn SM, McKenna MG, McKenna WG. Non-small cell lung cancer: prognostic factors in patients treated with surgery and postoperative radiation therapy. Radiology. 1999;213(3):845–52.
54. Rodrigus P. The impact of surgical adjuvant thoracic radiation for different stages of non-small cell lung cancer: the experience from a single institution. Lung Cancer. 1999;23(1):11–7.
55. Lee SW, Choi EK, Chung WK, Shin KH, Ahn SD, Kim JH, Kim SW, Suh C, Lee JS, Kim WS, et al. Postoperative adjuvant chemotherapy and radiotherapy for stage II and III non-small cell lung cancer (NSCLC). Lung Cancer. 2002;37(1):65–71.
56. El-Sherif A, Fernando HC, Santos R, Pettiford B, Luketich JD, Close JM, Landreneau RJ. Margin and local recurrence after sublobar resection of non-small cell lung cancer. Ann Surg Oncol. 2007;14(8):2400–5.
57. Sawabata N, Maeda H, Matsumura A, Ohta M, Okumura M. Clinical implications of the margin cytology findings and margin/tumor size ratio in patients who underwent pulmonary excision for peripheral non-small cell lung cancer. Surg Today. 2012;42(3):238–44.
58. Tomaszek SC, Kim Y, Cassivi SD, Jensen MR, Shen KH, Nichols FC, Deschamps C, Wigle DA. Bronchial resection margin length and clinical outcome in non-small cell lung cancer. Eur J Cardiothorac Surg. 2011;40(5):1151–6.
59. Gomez DR, Komaki R. Postoperative radiation therapy for non-small cell lung cancer and thymic malignancies. Cancers. 2012;4:307–22.
60. The Lung Cancer Study Group. Effects of postoperative mediastinal radiation on completely resected stage II and stage III epidermoid cancer of the lung. N Engl J Med. 1986;315(22):1377–81.
61. Mayer R, Smolle-Juettner FM, Szolar D, Stuecklschweiger GF, Quehenberger F, Friehs G, Hackl A. Postoperative radiotherapy in radically resected non-small cell lung cancer. Chest. 1997;112(4):954–9.
62. Dautzenberg B, Arriagada R, Chammard AB, Jarema A, Mezzetti M, Mattson K, Lagrange JL, Le Pechoux C, Lebeau B, Chastang C. A controlled study of postoperative radiotherapy for patients with completely resected nonsmall cell lung carcinoma. Groupe d'Etude et de Traitement des Cancers Bronchiques. Cancer. 1999;86(2):265–73.
63. Feng QF, Wang M, Wang LJ, Yang ZY, Zhang YG, Zhang DW, Yin WB. A study of postoperative radiotherapy in patients with non-small-cell lung cancer: a randomized trial. Int J Radiat Oncol Biol Phys. 2000;47(4):925–9.
64. Trodella L, Granone P, Valente S, Valentini V, Balducci M, Mantini G, Turriziani A, Margaritora S, Cesario A, Ramella S, et al. Adjuvant radiotherapy in non-small cell lung cancer with pathological stage I: definitive results of a phase III randomized trial. Radiother Oncol. 2002;62(1):11–9.
65. Le Pechoux C, Dunant A, Pignon JP, De Ruysscher D, Mornex F, Senan S, Casas F, Price A, Milleron B. Need for a new trial to evaluate adjuvant postoperative radiotherapy

in non-small-cell lung cancer patients with N2 mediastinal involvement. J Clin Oncol. 2007;25(7):e10–1.

66. Le Pechoux C. Role of postoperative radiotherapy in resected non-small cell lung cancer: a reassessment based on new data. Oncologist. 2011;16(5):672–81.

67. Spoelstra FO, Senan S, Le Pechoux C, Ishikura S, Casas F, Ball D, Price A, De Ruysscher D, van Sornsen de Koste JR. Variations in target volume definition for postoperative radiotherapy in stage III non-small-cell lung cancer: analysis of an international contouring study. Int J Radiat Oncol Biol Phys. 2010;76(4):1106–13.

68. Lally BE, Zelterman D, Colasanto JM, Haffty BG, Detterbeck FC, Wilson LD. Postoperative radiotherapy for stage II or III non-small-cell lung cancer using the surveillance, epidemiology, and end results database. J Clin Oncol. 2006;24(19):2998–3006.

69. PORT Meta-analysis Trialists Group. Postoperative radiotherapy in non-small-cell lung cancer: systematic review and meta-analysis of individual patient data from nine randomised controlled trials. Lancet. 1998;352(9124):257–63.

70. Burdett S, Stewart L. Postoperative radiotherapy in non-small-cell lung cancer: update of an individual patient data meta-analysis. Lung Cancer. 2005;47(1):81–3.

71. Burdett S, Rydzewska L, Tierney JF, Fisher DJ. A closer look at the effects of postoperative radiotherapy by stage and nodal status: updated results of an individual participant data meta-analysis in non-small-cell lung cancer. Lung Cancer. 2013;80(3):350–2.

72. Billiet C, Decaluwe H, Peeters S, Vansteenkiste J, Dooms C, Haustermans K, De Leyn P, De Ruysscher D. Modern post-operative radiotherapy for stage III non-small cell lung cancer may improve local control and survival: a meta-analysis. Radiother Oncol. 2014;110(1):3–8.

73. Mikell JL, Gillespie TW, Hall WA, Nickleach DC, Liu Y, Lipscomb J, Ramalingam SS, Rajpara RS, Force SD, Fernandez FG, et al. Postoperative radiotherapy is associated with better survival in non-small cell lung cancer with involved N2 lymph nodes: results of an analysis of the National Cancer Data Base. J Thorac Oncol. 2015;10(3):462–71.

74. Robinson CG, Patel AP, Bradley JD, DeWees T, Waqar SN, Morgensztern D, Baggstrom MQ, Govindan R, Bell JM, Guthrie TJ, et al. Postoperative radiotherapy for pathologic N2 non-small-cell lung cancer treated with adjuvant chemotherapy: a review of the National Cancer Data Base. J Clin Oncol. 2015;33(8):870–6.

75. Matsuguma H, Nakahara R, Ishikawa Y, Suzuki H, Inoue K, Katano S, Yokoi K. Postoperative radiotherapy for patients with completely resected pathological stage IIIA-N2 non-small cell lung cancer: focusing on an effect of the number of mediastinal lymph node stations involved. Interact Cardiovasc Thorac Surg. 2008;7(4):573–7.

76. Saji H, Tsuboi M, Yoshida K, Kato Y, Nomura M, Matsubayashi J, Nagao T, Kakihana M, Usuda J, Kajiwara N, et al. Prognostic impact of number of resected and involved lymph nodes at complete resection on survival in non-small cell lung cancer. J Thorac Oncol. 2011;6(11):1865–71.

77. Urban D, Bar J, Solomon B, Ball D. Lymph node ratio may predict the benefit of postoperative radiotherapy in non-small-cell lung cancer. J Thorac Oncol. 2013;8(7):940–6.

78. Lopez Guerra JL, Gomez DR, Lin SH, Levy LB, Zhuang Y, Komaki R, Jaen J, Vaporciyan AA, Swisher SG, Cox JD, et al. Risk factors for local and regional recurrence in patients with resected N0-N1 non-small-cell lung cancer, with implications for patient selection for adjuvant radiation therapy. Ann Oncol. 2013;24(1):67–74.

79. Hui Z, Dai H, Liang J, Lv J, Zhou Z, Feng Q, Xiao Z, Chen D, Zhang H, Yin W, et al. Selection of proper candidates with resected pathological stage IIIA-N2 non-small cell lung cancer for postoperative radiotherapy. Thorac Cancer. 2015;6(3):346–53.

80. Pless M, Stupp R, Ris HB, Stahel RA, Weder W, Thierstein S, Gerard MA, Xyrafas A, Fruh M, Cathomas R, et al. Induction chemoradiation in stage IIIA/N2 non-small-cell lung cancer: a phase 3 randomised trial. Lancet. 2015;386(9998):1049–56.

81. Shah AA, Berry MF, Tzao C, Gandhi M, Worni M, Pietrobon R, D'Amico TA. Induction chemoradiation is not superior to induction chemotherapy alone in stage IIIA lung cancer. Ann Thorac Surg. 2012;93(6):1807–12.

82. Auperin A, Le Pechoux C, Rolland E, Curran WJ, Furuse K, Fournel P, Belderbos J, Clamon G, Ulutin HC, Paulus R, et al. Meta-analysis of concomitant versus sequential radiochemotherapy in locally advanced non-small-cell lung cancer. J Clin Oncol. 2010;28(13):2181–90.
83. Albain KS, Rusch VW, Crowley JJ, Rice TW, Turrisi AT 3rd, Weick JK, Lonchyna VA, Presant CA, McKenna RJ, Gandara DR, et al. Concurrent cisplatin/etoposide plus chest radiotherapy followed by surgery for stages IIIA (N2) and IIIB non-small-cell lung cancer: mature results of Southwest Oncology Group phase II study 8805. J Clin Oncol. 1995;13(8):1880–92.
84. Burkes RL, Shepherd FA, Blackstein ME, Goldberg ME, Waters PF, Patterson GA, Todd T, Pearson FG, Jones D, Farooq S, et al. Induction chemotherapy with mitomycin, vindesine, and cisplatin for stage IIIA (T1-3, N2) unresectable non-small-cell lung cancer: final results of the Toronto phase II trial. Lung Cancer. 2005;47(1):103–9.
85. Weiden PL, Piantadosi S. Preoperative chemotherapy (cisplatin and fluorouracil) and radiation therapy in stage III non-small-cell lung cancer: a phase II study of the Lung Cancer Study Group. J Natl Cancer Inst. 1991;83(4):266–73.
86. Albain KS, Swann RS, Rusch VW, Turrisi AT 3rd, Shepherd FA, Smith C, Chen Y, Livingston RB, Feins RH, Gandara DR, et al. Radiotherapy plus chemotherapy with or without surgical resection for stage III non-small-cell lung cancer: a phase III randomised controlled trial. Lancet. 2009;374(9687):379–86.
87. van Meerbeeck JP, Kramer GW, Van Schil PE, Legrand C, Smit EF, Schramel F, Tjan-Heijnen VC, Biesma B, Debruyne C, van Zandwijk N, et al. Randomized controlled trial of resection versus radiotherapy after induction chemotherapy in stage IIIA-N2 non-small-cell lung cancer. J Natl Cancer Inst. 2007;99(6):442–50.
88. Eberhardt WE, Pottgen C, Gauler TC, Friedel G, Veit S, Heinrich V, Welter S, Budach W, Spengler W, Kimmich M, et al. Phase III study of surgery versus definitive concurrent chemoradiotherapy boost in patients with resectable stage IIIA(N2) and selected IIIB non-small-cell lung cancer after induction chemotherapy and concurrent chemoradiotherapy (ESPATUE). J Clin Oncol. 2015;33(35):4194–201.
89. Curran WJ Jr, Paulus R, Langer CJ, Komaki R, Lee JS, Hauser S, Movsas B, Wasserman T, Rosenthal SA, Gore E, et al. Sequential vs. concurrent chemoradiation for stage III non-small cell lung cancer: randomized phase III trial RTOG 9410. J Natl Cancer Inst. 2011;103(19):1452–60.
90. Topkan E, Parlak C, Topuk S, Guler OC, Selek U. Outcomes of aggressive concurrent radiochemotherapy in highly selected septuagenarians with stage IIIB non-small cell lung carcinoma: retrospective analysis of 89 patients. Lung Cancer. 2013;81(2):226–30.
91. Antonia SJ, Villegas A, Daniel D, Vicente D, Murakami S, Hui R, Yokoi T, Chiappori A, Lee KH, de Wit M, et al. Durvalumab after chemoradiotherapy in stage III non-small-cell lung cancer. N Engl J Med. 2017;377(20):1919–29.
92. Sezen D, Bolukbasi Y, Topkan E, Selek U. Selection criteria for definitive treatment approach in thoracic malignancies: radiation oncology perspective. In: Ozyigit G, Selek U, Topkan E, editors. Principles and practice of radiotherapy techniques in thoracic malignancies. Cham: Springer International; 2016.
93. Seppenwoolde Y, Shirato H, Kitamura K, Shimizu S, van Herk M, Lebesque JV, Miyasaka K. Precise and real-time measurement of 3D tumor motion in lung due to breathing and heartbeat, measured during radiotherapy. Int J Radiat Oncol Biol Phys. 2002;53(4):822–34.
94. Shirato H, Suzuki K, Sharp GC, Fujita K, Onimaru R, Fujino M, Kato N, Osaka Y, Kinoshita R, Taguchi H, et al. Speed and amplitude of lung tumor motion precisely detected in four-dimensional setup and in real-time tumor-tracking radiotherapy. Int J Radiat Oncol Biol Phys. 2006;64(4):1229–36.
95. Liu HH, Balter P, Tutt T, Choi B, Zhang J, Wang C, Chi M, Luo D, Pan T, Hunjan S, et al. Assessing respiration-induced tumor motion and internal target volume using four-dimensional computed tomography for radiotherapy of lung cancer. Int J Radiat Oncol Biol Phys. 2007;68(2):531–40.

96. Keall PJ, Mageras GS, Balter JM, Emery RS, Forster KM, Jiang SB, Kapatoes JM, Low DA, Murphy MJ, Murray BR, et al. The management of respiratory motion in radiation oncology report of AAPM Task Group 76. Med Phys. 2006;33(10):3874–900.

97. Chavaudra J, Bridier A. Definition of volumes in external radiotherapy: ICRU reports 50 and 62. Cancer Radiother. 2001;5(5):472–8.

98. Underberg RW, Lagerwaard FJ, Slotman BJ, Cuijpers JP, Senan S. Use of maximum intensity projections (MIP) for target volume generation in 4DCT scans for lung cancer. Int J Radiat Oncol Biol Phys. 2005;63(1):253–60.

99. Rietzel E, Liu AK, Chen GT, Choi NC. Maximum-intensity volumes for fast contouring of lung tumors including respiratory motion in 4DCT planning. Int J Radiat Oncol Biol Phys. 2008;71(4):1245–52.

100. Ahnesjo A. Collapsed cone convolution of radiant energy for photon dose calculation in heterogeneous media. Med Phys. 1989;16(4):577–92.

101. Aarup LR, Nahum AE, Zacharatou C, Juhler-Nottrup T, Knoos T, Nystrom H, Specht L, Wieslander E, Korreman SS. The effect of different lung densities on the accuracy of various radiotherapy dose calculation methods: implications for tumour coverage. Radiother Oncol. 2009;91(3):405–14.

102. Bragg CM, Conway J. Dosimetric verification of the anisotropic analytical algorithm for radiotherapy treatment planning. Radiother Oncol. 2006;81(3):315–23.

103. Bush K, Gagne IM, Zavgorodni S, Ansbacher W, Beckham W. Dosimetric validation of Acuros XB with Monte Carlo methods for photon dose calculations. Med Phys. 2011;38(4):2208–21.

104. Vanderstraeten B, Reynaert N, Paelinck L, Madani I, De Wagter C, De Gersem W, De Neve W, Thierens H. Accuracy of patient dose calculation for lung IMRT: a comparison of Monte Carlo, convolution/superposition, and pencil beam computations. Med Phys. 2006;33(9):3149–58.

105. Bortfeld T, Jokivarsi K, Goitein M, Kung J, Jiang SB. Effects of intra-fraction motion on IMRT dose delivery: statistical analysis and simulation. Phys Med Biol. 2002;47(13):2203–20.

106. Lynch R, Pitson G, Ball D, Claude L, Sarrut D. Computed tomographic atlas for the new international lymph node map for lung cancer: a radiation oncologist perspective. Pract Radiat Oncol. 2013;3(1):54–66.

107. Giraud P, Antoine M, Larrouy A, Milleron B, Callard P, De Rycke Y, Carette MF, Rosenwald JC, Cosset JM, Housset M, et al. Evaluation of microscopic tumor extension in non-small-cell lung cancer for three-dimensional conformal radiotherapy planning. Int J Radiat Oncol Biol Phys. 2000;48(4):1015–24.

108. Asamura H, Nakayama H, Kondo H, Tsuchiya R, Naruke T. Lobe-specific extent of systematic lymph node dissection for non-small cell lung carcinomas according to a retrospective study of metastasis and prognosis. J Thorac Cardiovasc Surg. 1999;117(6):1102–11.

109. Gomez DR, Chang JY. Adaptive radiation for lung cancer. J Oncol. 2011;2011.

110. Chang JY, Bezjak A, Mornex F. Stereotactic ablative radiotherapy for centrally located early stage non-small-cell lung cancer: what we have learned. J Thorac Oncol. 2015;10(4):577–85.

111. Zhao L, Zhou S, Balter P, Shen C, Gomez DR, Welsh JD, Lin SH, Chang JY. Planning target volume D95 and mean dose should be considered for optimal local control for stereotactic ablative radiation therapy. Int J Radiat Oncol Biol Phys. 2016;95(4):1226–35.

112. Machtay M, Bae K, Movsas B, Paulus R, Gore EM, Komaki R, Albain K, Sause WT, Curran WJ. Higher biologically effective dose of radiotherapy is associated with improved outcomes for locally advanced non-small cell lung carcinoma treated with chemoradiation: an analysis of the Radiation Therapy Oncology Group. Int J Radiat Oncol Biol Phys. 2012;82(1):425–34.

113. Ramella S, Trodella L, Mineo TC, Pompeo E, Stimato G, Gaudino D, Valentini V, Cellini F, Ciresa M, Fiore M, et al. Adding ipsilateral V20 and V30 to conventional dosimetric constraints predicts radiation pneumonitis in stage IIIA-B NSCLC treated with combined-modality therapy. Int J Radiat Oncol Biol Phys. 2010;76(1):110–5.

114. Jin H, Tucker SL, Liu HH, Wei X, Yom SS, Wang S, Komaki R, Chen Y, Martel MK, Mohan R, et al. Dose-volume thresholds and smoking status for the risk of treatment-related

pneumonitis in inoperable non-small cell lung cancer treated with definitive radiotherapy. Radiother Oncol. 2009;91(3):427–32.

115. Kalemkerian GP. Staging and imaging of small cell lung cancer. Cancer Imaging. 2011;11:253–8.

116. Schneider BJ, Saxena A, Downey RJ. Surgery for early-stage small cell lung cancer. J Natl Compr Canc Netw. 2011;9(10):1132–9.

117. NCCN. Clinical practice guidelines in oncology. Small Cell Lung Cancer. https://www.nccn. org/professionals/physician_gls/pdf/sclc.pdf.

118. Yang CF, Chan DY, Speicher PJ, Gulack BC, Wang X, Hartwig MG, Onaitis MW, Tong BC, D'Amico TA, Berry MF, et al. Role of adjuvant therapy in a population-based cohort of patients with early-stage small-cell lung cancer. J Clin Oncol. 2016;34(10):1057–64.

119. Brock MV, Hooker CM, Syphard JE, Westra W, Xu L, Alberg AJ, Mason D, Baylin SB, Herman JG, Yung RC, et al. Surgical resection of limited disease small cell lung cancer in the new era of platinum chemotherapy: its time has come. J Thorac Cardiovasc Surg. 2005;129(1):64–72.

120. Warde P, Payne D. Does thoracic irradiation improve survival and local control in limited-stage small-cell carcinoma of the lung? A meta-analysis. J Clin Oncol. 1992;10(6):890–5.

121. Pignon JP, Arriagada R, Ihde DC, Johnson DH, Perry MC, Souhami RL, Brodin O, Joss RA, Kies MS, Lebeau B, et al. A meta-analysis of thoracic radiotherapy for small-cell lung cancer. N Engl J Med. 1992;327(23):1618–24.

122. Pignon JP, Arriagada R. Role of thoracic radiotherapy in limited-stage small-cell lung cancer: quantitative review based on the literature versus meta-analysis based on individual data. J Clin Oncol. 1992;10(11):1819–20.

123. De Ruysscher D, Pijls-Johannesma M, Bentzen SM, Minken A, Wanders R, Lutgens L, Hochstenbag M, Boersma L, Wouters B, Lammering G, et al. Time between the first day of chemotherapy and the last day of chest radiation is the most important predictor of survival in limited-disease small-cell lung cancer. J Clin Oncol. 2006;24(7):1057–63.

124. De Ruysscher D, Pijls-Johannesma M, Vansteenkiste J, Kester A, Rutten I, Lambin P. Systematic review and meta-analysis of randomised, controlled trials of the timing of chest radiotherapy in patients with limited-stage, small-cell lung cancer. Ann Oncol. 2006;17(4):543–52.

125. Turrisi AT 3rd, Kim K, Blum R, Sause WT, Livingston RB, Komaki R, Wagner H, Aisner S, Johnson DH. Twice-daily compared with once-daily thoracic radiotherapy in limited small-cell lung cancer treated concurrently with cisplatin and etoposide. N Engl J Med. 1999;340(4):265–71.

126. Miller KL, Marks LB, Sibley GS, Clough RW, Garst JL, Crawford J, Shafman TD. Routine use of approximately 60 Gy once-daily thoracic irradiation for patients with limited-stage small-cell lung cancer. Int J Radiat Oncol Biol Phys. 2003;56(2):355–9.

127. Roof KS, Fidias P, Lynch TJ, Ancukiewicz M, Choi NC. Radiation dose escalation in limited-stage small-cell lung cancer. Int J Radiat Oncol Biol Phys. 2003;57(3):701–8.

128. Bogart JA, Herndon JE 2nd, Lyss AP, Watson D, Miller AA, Lee ME, Turrisi AT, Green MR. 70 Gy thoracic radiotherapy is feasible concurrent with chemotherapy for limited-stage small-cell lung cancer: analysis of cancer and Leukemia Group B study 39808. Int J Radiat Oncol Biol Phys. 2004;59(2):460–8.

129. Fried DB, Morris DE, Poole C, Rosenman JG, Halle JS, Detterbeck FC, Hensing TA, Socinski MA. Systematic review evaluating the timing of thoracic radiation therapy in combined modality therapy for limited-stage small-cell lung cancer. J Clin Oncol. 2004;22(23):4837–45.

130. Huncharek M, McGarry R. A meta-analysis of the timing of chest irradiation in the combined modality treatment of limited-stage small cell lung cancer. Oncologist. 2004;9(6):665–72.

131. Komaki R, Paulus R, Ettinger DS, Videtic GM, Bradley JD, Glisson BS, Langer CJ, Sause WT, Curran WJ Jr, Choy H. Phase II study of accelerated high-dose radiotherapy with concurrent chemotherapy for patients with limited small-cell lung cancer: Radiation Therapy Oncology Group protocol 0239. Int J Radiat Oncol Biol Phys. 2012;83(4):e531–6.

132. Faivre-Finn C, Snee M, Ashcroft L, Appel W, Barlesi F, Bhatnagar A, Bezjak A, Cardenal F, Fournel P, Harden S, et al. Concurrent once-daily versus twice-daily chemoradiotherapy in patients with limited-stage small-cell lung cancer (CONVERT): an open-label, phase 3, randomised, superiority trial. Lancet Oncol. 2017;18(8):1116–25.
133. Slotman BJ, van Tinteren H, Praag JO, Knegjens JL, El Sharouni SY, Hatton M, Keijser A, Faivre-Finn C, Senan S. Use of thoracic radiotherapy for extensive stage small-cell lung cancer: a phase 3 randomised controlled trial. Lancet. 2015;385(9962):36–42.
134. Zhu H, Zhou Z, Wang Y, Bi N, Feng Q, Li J, Lv J, Chen D, Shi Y, Wang L. Thoracic radiation therapy improves the overall survival of patients with extensive-stage small cell lung cancer with distant metastasis. Cancer. 2011;117(23):5423–31.
135. Giuliani ME, Atallah S, Sun A, Bezjak A, Le LW, Brade A, Cho J, Leighl NB, Shepherd FA, Hope AJ. Clinical outcomes of extensive stage small cell lung carcinoma patients treated with consolidative thoracic radiotherapy. Clin Lung Cancer. 2011;12(6):375–9.
136. Jeremic B, Shibamoto Y, Nikolic N, Milicic B, Milisavljevic S, Dagovic A, Aleksandrovic J, Radosavljevic-Asic G. Role of radiation therapy in the combined-modality treatment of patients with extensive disease small-cell lung cancer: a randomized study. J Clin Oncol. 1999;17(7):2092–9.
137. Palma DA, Warner A, Louie AV, Senan S, Slotman B, Rodrigues GB. Thoracic radiotherapy for extensive stage small-cell lung cancer: a meta-analysis. Clin Lung Cancer. 2016;17(4):239–44.
138. Gore EM, Hu C, Sun AY, Grimm DF, Ramalingam SS, Dunlap NE, Higgins KA, Werner-Wasik M, Allen AM, Iyengar P, et al. Randomized phase II study comparing prophylactic cranial irradiation alone to prophylactic cranial irradiation and consolidative extracranial irradiation for extensive-disease small cell lung cancer (ED SCLC): NRG Oncology RTOG 0937. J Thorac Oncol. 2017;12(10):1561–70.
139. Auperin A, Arriagada R, Pignon JP, Le Pechoux C, Gregor A, Stephens RJ, Kristjansen PE, Johnson BE, Ueoka H, Wagner H, et al. Prophylactic cranial irradiation for patients with small-cell lung cancer in complete remission. Prophylactic Cranial Irradiation Overview Collaborative Group. N Engl J Med. 1999;341(7):476–84.
140. Le Pechoux C, Dunant A, Senan S, Wolfson A, Quoix E, Faivre-Finn C, Ciuleanu T, Arriagada R, Jones R, Wanders R, et al. Standard-dose versus higher-dose prophylactic cranial irradiation (PCI) in patients with limited-stage small-cell lung cancer in complete remission after chemotherapy and thoracic radiotherapy (PCI 99-01, EORTC 22003-08004, RTOG 0212, and IFCT 99-01): a randomised clinical trial. Lancet Oncol. 2009;10(5):467–74.
141. Gondi V, Pugh SL, Tome WA, Caine C, Corn B, Kanner A, Rowley H, Kundapur V, DeNittis A, Greenspoon JN, et al. Preservation of memory with conformal avoidance of the hippocampal neural stem-cell compartment during whole-brain radiotherapy for brain metastases (RTOG 0933): a phase II multi-institutional trial. J Clin Oncol. 2014;32(34):3810–6.
142. Slotman BJ, Faivre-Finn C, Kramer GW, Rankin E, Snee M, Hatton M, Postmus PE, Collette L, Musat E, Senan S. Prophylactic cranial irradiation in patients with extensive disease caused by small-cell lung cancer responsive to chemotherapy: fewer symptomatic brain metastases and improved survival. Ned Tijdschr Geneeskd. 2008;152(17):1000–4.
143. Takahashi T, Yamanaka T, Seto T, Harada H, Nokihara H, Saka H, Nishio M, Kaneda H, Takayama K, Ishimoto O, et al. Prophylactic cranial irradiation versus observation in patients with extensive-disease small-cell lung cancer: a multicentre, randomised, open-label, phase 3 trial. Lancet Oncol. 2017;18(5):663–71.
144. van Loon J, De Ruysscher D, Wanders R, Boersma L, Simons J, Oellers M, Dingemans AM, Hochstenbag M, Bootsma G, Geraedts W, et al. Selective nodal irradiation on basis of (18) FDG-PET scans in limited-disease small-cell lung cancer: a prospective study. Int J Radiat Oncol Biol Phys. 2010;77(2):329–36.
145. Shirvani SM, Komaki R, Heymach JV, Fossella FV, Chang JY. Positron emission tomography/computed tomography-guided intensity-modulated radiotherapy for limited-stage small-cell lung cancer. Int J Radiat Oncol Biol Phys. 2012;82(1):e91–7.

Breast Cancer

4

Yasemin Bolukbasi, Duygu Sezen, Yucel Saglam,
and Ugur Selek

4.1   Noninvasive Disease (Ductal Carcinoma In Situ)

Overview

Epidemiology

Noninvasive (In situ) breast disease represents more than 20% of all breast malignancies. Ductal carcinoma in situ (DCIS) compromises 85% whereas lobular carcinoma in situ (LCIS) represents about 15% of these noninvasive cancers. LCIS is multicentric in up to 90% of patients and bilateral in up to 60%. Similar to invasive breast cancer; the risk increases with age while family history of breast cancer, nulliparity, older age at first full term birth early menarche, late menopause, obesity, germ-line mutation are the other risk factors.

Pathology

DCIS refers to noninfiltrating lesions composed of malign epithelial cells confined to the ductal lumens of the breast. DCIS is a precursor to invasive disease and one third of cases is expected progress to invasive cancer if it is not treated. Three pathologic grades as low, intermediate and high are defined for DCIS. Approximately %70 of DCIS cases are ER positive, and expression rate is higher in low-grade lesions.

Y. Bolukbasi (✉) · U. Selek
Department of Radiation Oncology, Faculty of Medicine, Koç University, Istanbul, Turkey

Department of Radiation Oncology, The University of Texas MD Anderson Cancer Center, Houston, TX, USA
e-mail: yaseminb@ameriaknhastanesi.org

D. Sezen · Y. Saglam
Department of Radiation Oncology, School of Medicine, Koç University, Istanbul, Turkey
e-mail: yucels@amerikanhastanesi.org

© Springer Nature Switzerland AG 2019
G. Ozyigit, U. Selek (eds.), *Radiation Oncology*,
https://doi.org/10.1007/978-3-319-97145-2_4

LCIS is defined as a noninvasive lobular proliferation in the terminal ductal lobular units that composed of neoplastic cells filling the acini. Estrogen receptor (ER) and/or progesterone receptor (PR) are frequently positive for LCIS. Human epidermal growth factor receptor 2 (HER2) is almost always negative except pleomorphic LCIS. Loss of E-cadherin is characteristic for LCIS and routinely used to distinguish lobular and ductal lesions.

Diagnosis

Mammography remains the most critical component of diagnostic imaging in noninvasive lesions. DCIS is usually recognized with micro calcifications on mammograms. However LCIS is most commonly mammographically occult and diagnosed as incidental finding. Nevertheless pleomorphic LCIS and LCIS with central necrosis may be diagnosed with calcifications. MRI is increasingly being used to detect multicentric disease and consider surgical technique.

Definitive Treatment

Breast conserving surgery with radiotherapy is the mainstay of the treatment for DCIS. Radiotherapy is almost always recommended in order to increase local control. However, for low-risk disease with negative margins with >1 cm or in older patients with small lesions local excision only may be an option. Mastectomy may be chosen for high-risk disease (i.e., diffuse disease with positive margins despite re-excision), multicentric disease or patient decision.

Treatment usually consists of observation for LCIS. The rate of in-breast failure at 12 years is less than 15%. LCIS has a minimal impact on survival rates. Tamoxifen or bilateral mastectomy is the other options for high-risk patients.

Keywords: Ductal carcinoma in situ, Radiotherapy

4.1.1 Case Presentation

A 51 year old woman with no significant past medical history had her scanning mammogram which revealed microcalcifications in the upper outer quadrant of the right breast.

Her breast examination was unremarkable without any palpable lesion or lymphadenomegaly. She was nulliparous and never used oral contraceptives. Age of menarche was 11 and she was still premenopausal. She had a history of social alcohol consumption for nearly 20 years but no cigarette smoking. She was in good physical status with body mass index of 27 kg/m^2 and she had no family history of cancer.

A core needle biopsy revealed a low grade ductal carcinoma in situ (DCIS), ER (+), PR(+), HER 2. A bilateral breast MRI did not reveal any pathological axillary lymph nodes and she was staged as cTisN0M0.

The patient underwent lumpectomy. Operation pathology confirmed the previous diagnoses of low grade DCIS among a site of 22 mm with at least 6 mm surgical margins. Immunohistochemically workup confirmed ER and PR positivity. Her 2 amplification was absent.

Regarding her ductal carcinoma in situ with negative margins, staged as pT1is pN0, and had no evidence of distant metastasis, hypofractionated whole breast tangent were planned as 40 Gy in 15 fractions.

4.1.1.1 Case Evaluation

The main factors to question during the consultation:

- The most important risk factor for DCIS and breast cancer development is age as well as age at menarche, first pregnancy, menopause, family history, obesity, and mammographic breast density [1, 2].
- The use of hormone treatment—especially progesterone and estrogen combination increases the risk
- Prior radiotherapy exposure to chest was also a well-established risk factor [3, 4].
- Family history and age at the diagnosis, would be the most valuable clue for genetic mutations [5]. BRCA germline mutations seem to occur frequently in triple-negative breast carcinomas, whereas an association with ductal carcinoma in situ (DCIS) is rare [6].
- If the patient has genetic mutations, prophylactic mastectomy eradicates approximately the risk of breast cancers, nevertheless has no effect on the risk of ovarian/fallopian tube cancer development. Prophylactic bilateral salpingo-oophorectomy should be offered as the risk of ovarian/fallopian tube cancers decreases by 80% and breast cancers by 50% [7]

4.1.1.2 Physical Examination

- Firstly, perform physical examination especially examine breast in sitting and supine position and perform bilateral node examination. Arm extension and ability of arm movement has to be checked as during the simulation arm has to be at least 90° abducted.
- Skin edema (peau d'orange) or erythema, nipple retraction are very important to define locally advanced stages.

4.1.1.3 Routine Work Up

- Labs: Routine CBC, chemistry with liver and renal functions
- Please make sure that you have seen Mammogram (shows asymmetry, clustered microcalcification, mass, and architectural distortion) and/or ultrasound of breast and lymph node basins

- Tissue diagnosis could be provided by either fine needle aspiration (FNA), Tru-Cut biopsy or vacuum-assisted biopsy—via sonography, MRI, or stereotactic-guided procedure
- Report of the path specimen should include size, grade, margin, estrogen receptor (ER)/progesterone receptor (PR)/Her2neu status
- Breast MRI is optional: Firstly it could be helpful for pre-op staging and surgical planning [8]. American Cancer Society recommends annual MR screening for especially women with a BRCA 1 or 2 mutation, who had a first-degree relative with a BRCA 1 or 2 mutation and had a lifetime risk of breast cancer of 20–25% or more using standard risk assessment models (BRCAPRO, Claus, Tyrer-Cuzick), whom received radiation treatment to the chest between ages 10 and 30, such as for Hodgkin's disease, does carry or have a first-degree relative who carries a genetic mutation in the TP53 or PTEN genes (Li-Fraumeni syn- drome and Cowden and Bannayan-Riley-Ruvalcaba syndromes) [9].
- The use of breast MRI continues to evolve as recent reported high false-positive rates blurred the routine use, but it may have a role in selected cases

4.1.1.4 Pathology

DCIS refers to non infiltrating lesions composed of malign epithelial cells confined to the ductal lumens of the breast. Historically, a classification has been used dividing tumors into cribriform, comedo, solid, papillary, and papillary subtypes [10]. Comedo subtype has the worst prognosis. However; the above-mentioned classification has some disadvantages in practical use. Firstly, because of the heterogeneity of the lesions, more than one subtype may be frequently defined. As well, it is not always convenient with the clinical behavior [11].

Three pathologic grades as low, intermediate and high are defined for DCIS. Approximately %70 of DCIS cases are ER positive, and expression rate is higher in low-grade lesions.

LCIS is defined as a noninvasive lobular proliferation in the terminal ductal lobular units that composed of neoplastic cells filling the acini. Estrogen receptor (ER) and/or progesterone receptor (PR) are frequently positive for LCIS. Human epidermal growth factor receptor 2 (HER2) is almost always negative except pleomorphic LCIS. Loss of E-cadherin is characteristic for LCIS and routinely used to distinguish lobular and ductal lesions.

4.1.1.5 Genetic Evaluation of Recurrence

12-gene Oncotype DX DCIS Score: The Oncotype DX breast cancer assay was performed for patients with DCIS treated with surgery without radiation in the Eastern Cooperative Oncology Group (ECOG) E5194 study. The association of the prospectively defined DCIS Score (calculated from seven cancer-related genes and five reference genes) with the risk of developing an IBE was evaluated in 327 patients with adequate tissue for analysis. For the prespecified DCIS risk groups of low, intermediate, and high, the 10-year risks of developing an ipsilateral breast event (IBE; local recurrence of DCIS or invasive carcinoma) were 10.6%, 26.7%, and 25.9%, respectively, and for an invasive IBE, 3.7%, 12.3%, and 19.2%, respectively (both log rank P ≤ 0.006). In multivariable analyses, factors associated with IBE risk were DCIS Score, tumor size, and menopausal status (all P ≤ 0.02) [12].

MD Anderson Cancer Center DCIS Nomogram: The DCIS nomogram integrates clinicopathologic variables to provide an individualized risk estimate of ipsilateral breast tumor recurrence (IBTR) in a woman with DCIS treated with breast conserving surgery. Therefore for this nomogram, 1868 consecutive patients were evaluated. Ten clinical, pathologic, and treatment variables were built into a nomogram estimating probability of IBTR at 5 and 10 years after breast conserving surgery. Factors with the greatest influence on risk of IBTR in the model were adjuvant RT or endocrine therapy, age, margin status, number of excisions, and treatment time period. This nomogram may be usefull for individual decision making and help avoid over or undertreatment of noninvasive breast cancer [13].

4.1.1.6 Staging

Noninvasive breast lesions are named as Tis (carcinoma in situ) with subgroups Tis (DCIS) and Tis (LCIS) in American Joint Committee on Cancer (AJCC) Cancer Staging System. In the eight edition; Lobular carcinoma in situ (LCIS) is removed as a pathologic tumor in situ (pTis) category for T categorization. LCIS is a benign entity and is removed from TNM staging [14].

4.1.2   Evidence Based Treatment Recommendations

Treatment strategy is constituted on extention of DCIS and excluding any invasive process. Following the confirmation of DCIS, mastectomy is the outstanding treatment option [15]. However in local disease; breast conserving surgery followed by whole breast radiotherapy is the recommended treatment.

4.1.2.1 Mastectomy in DCIS

Mastectomy can be an option in ductal carcinoma in situ treatment with excellent disease control rates [16–19]. While conservative options have come to the fore front for invasive carcinoma, breast conserving surgery has been increasingly used as an option for in situ carcinomas although there is no randomized data comparing two surgical techniques for DCIS [19].

Recently, total mastectomy is administered to patients with diffuse multicentric lesions or who is not eligible for radiation therapy because of medical contraindication. Additionally, it may be an option in case of local recurrence after breast conserving surgery [18].

4.1.2.2 Breast Conserving Surgery With/Without Whole Breast Radiotherapy in DCIS

The addition of radiotherapy after breast conserving surgery was first shown to reduce the risk of ipsilateral recurrence in the treatment of invasive breast cancer.

Breast conserving surgery routinely also used with adjuvant whole breast radiotherapy in DCIS same as invasive carcinoma regarding sufficient retrospective and prospective evidence supporting this treatment concept.

The European Organization for Research and Treatment of Cancer investigated the role of radiotherapy (RT) after local excision (LE) of ductal carcinoma-in-situ (DCIS) of the breast in a randomized trial [20]. One thousand ten women with DCIS who underwent local excision, were randomly assigned to observation versus RT (50 Gy). The risk of DCIS and invasive local recurrence was reduced by 48% (P = 0.0011) and 42% (P = 0.0065) respectively. Both groups had similar low risks of metastases and death. At multivariate analysis, factors significantly associated with an increased local recurrence risk were young age (≤40 year), symptomatic detection, intermediately or poorly differentiated DCIS (as opposed to well-differentiated DCIS, cribriform or solid growth pattern, doubtful margins, and treatment by LE alone. All patient subgroups benefited from RT. With long-term follow-up, RT after LE for DCIS continued to reduce the risk of LR, with a 47% reduction at 10 years.

Additionally, Wapnir et al. evaluated long-term outcomes of invasive ipsilateral breast tumor recurrences (IBTR) after lumpectomy in NSABP B-17 and B-24 randomized clinical trials for DCIS [21]. In the NSABP B-17 trial, patients with localized DCIS were randomly assigned to the lumpectomy group or to the lumpectomy followed by radiotherapy group. In the NSABP B-24 double-blinded, placebo-controlled trial all patients were randomly assigned to LRT+ placebo, or LRT + tamoxifen. Median follow-up was 207 months for the B-17 trial (N = 813 patients) and 163 months for the B-24 trial (N = 1799 patients). Of 490 IBTR events, 53.7% were invasive. Radiation reduced invasive IBTR by 52% in the LRT group compared with lumpectomy only. LRT + tamoxifen reduced invasive IBTR by 32% compared with LRT + placebo. The 15-year cumulative incidence of invasive IBTR was 19.4% for lumpectomy only, 8.9% for LRT (B-17), 10.0% for LRT + placebo (B-24), and 8.5% for LRT + TAM. The 15-year cumulative incidence of all contralateral breast cancers was 10.3% for LO, 10.2% for LRT (B-17), 10.8% for LRT + placebo (B-24), and 7.3% for LRT + tamoxifen. Invasive IBTR was associated with increased mortality risk, whereas recurrence of DCIS was not. Among all patients (with or without invasive IBTR), the 15-year cumulative incidence of breast cancer death was 3.1% for LO, 4.7% for LRT (B-17), 2.7% for LRT + placebo (B-24), and 2.3% for LRT + TAM. Although invasive IBTR increased the risk for breast cancer-related death, radiation therapy and tamoxifen reduced I-IBTR, and long-term prognosis remained excellent after breast-conserving surgery for DCIS.

The United Kingdom Coordinating Committee on Cancer Research (UKCCCR) DCIS Working Group and investigators from Australia and New Zealand have also investigated the role of radiotherapy for DCIS in a randomized trial [22]. Within a 2 × 2 factorial protocol design, four treatment regimens were compared: excision alone, excision plus tamoxifen, excision plus radiotherapy, and excision plus radiotherapy and tamoxifen. Tamoxifen as prescribed as 20 mg/day and radiotherapy was delivered through whole-breast tangential fields to a total dose of 50 Gy without boost. With a median follow-up of 12.7 years, radiotherapy was associated with a reduction in ipsilateral invasive (HR 0.32, p < 0.0001) and noninvasive recurrences (HR 0.38, p < 0.0001). The addition of tamoxifen to radiotherapy offered minimal benefit toward the overall ipsilateral local control rates; however, it did appear to reduce the ipsilateral recurrence rate of DCIS (HR 0.70, p = 0.03) and contralateral events (HR 0.44, p = 0.005).

Twenty years of follow-up data for the SweDCIS trial was also confirmed the efficacy of radiotherapy in DCIS patients who had breast conserving surgery [23]. There were 129 in situ and 129 invasive ipsilateral breast events. RT reduced 20-year recurrence by 12% (10% for in situ and 2% for invasive). There was a no statistically significantly increased number of contralateral events in the RT arm (67 vs. 48 events; hazard ratio, 1.38; 95% CI, 0.95 to 2.00). Breast cancer-specific death and overall survival were not different between groups. Younger women experienced a relatively higher risk of invasive ipsilateral breast event and lower effect of RT.

Randomized controlled trials have shown that RT following breast conserving surgery is effective in reducing local failure for DCIS, but potential long-term complications from addition of RT is also an issue in such patients with long life expectancy. Cochrane met analysis aimed to determine the balance between the benefits and harms [24]. Four randomized controlled trials involving 3925 women were included in this review. Three trials compared the addition of RT to BCS. One trial was a two by two factorial design comparing the use of RT and tamoxifen, each separately or together, in which participants were randomized in at least one arm. Analysis confirmed a statistically significant benefit from the addition of radiotherapy on all ipsilateral breast events (P < 0.00001), ipsilateral invasive recurrence (p = 0.001) and ipsilateral DCIS recurrence (P = 0.03). Radiotherapy was effective in all subgroups. No significant long-term toxicity from radiotherapy was found.

Another issue is the selection of DCIS cases that radiotherapy can be omitted. In this context The Radiation Therapy Oncology Group conducted a prospective randomized trial in identified good-risk (mammographically detected low- or intermediate-grade DCIS, measuring less than 2.5 cm with margins ≥3 mm) patients in order to evaluate the contribution of radiotherapy after breast-conserving surgery compared with observation [25]. Six hundred thirty-six patients were enrolled and tamoxifen use (62%) was optional among patients. During median 7.17 year follow-up time; 2 local failures in the RT arm, and 19 in the observation arm were reported. At 7 years, the LF rate was 0.9% in the RT arm versus 6.7% in the observation arm (P < 0.001). Grade 1 to 2 acute toxicities occurred in 30% and 76% of patients in the observation and RT arms, respectively; grade 3 or 4 toxicities occurred in 4.0% and 4.2% of patients, respectively. Although longer follow-up is planned in this setting, local failure rate was decreased significantly with the addition of RT.

4.1.2.3 Tamoxifen in DCIS

Approximately %70 of DCIS cases are ER positive. Two randomized phase III trials reported that Tamoxifen reduces local recurrence and contralateral events by about % 30 although absolute benefit diminishes with increased follow-up. The NSABP B-24 was conducted as a double-blinded, placebo- controlled trial of DCIS patients with breast conserving surgery [21]. Patients were randomly assigned to radiotherapy + placebo versus radiotherapy + tamoxifen. When compared with radiotherapy only arm, incidence of ipsilateral invasive recurrence was reduced by %32 in radiotherapy with tamoxifen arm. Fifteen year-cumulative incidence of all contralateral breast cancers was %8.5 for radiotherapy and tamoxifen arm, while %10 for radiation only arm. Invasive recurrence was associated with increased mortality risk, whereas recurrence of DCIS was not. On secondary analysis, benefit only seen for ER+ patients while no benefit was seen with tamoxifen in ER negative DCIS [26].

In another phase III trial, 1071 women were randomly assigned to radiotherapy alone, radiotherapy + tamoxifen, tamoxifen alone and no adjuvant treatment after breast conserving surgery [22]. After 12.7 year follow up, 376 (197 DCIS and 163 invasive cancers, 16 of unknown invasiveness) breast cancers were occurred. Tamoxifen reduced ipsilateral DCIS recurrences (HR 0.7) and contralateral tumors (HR 0.44) while no effect on ipsilateral invasive disease. In summary, breast conserving strategy of lumpectomy following radiotherapy was accepted a standard approach for DCIS in the first phase while adjuvant tamoxifen improve the outcomes.

4.1.3 Treatment Planning

4.1.3.1 Radiation Dose and Scheme for DCIS

In randomized DCIS studies, commonly used radiotherapy dose was 50 Gy for whole breast. However, radiation boost to operation bed was mentioned rarely. Although there is some data supporting boost, the effect of boost in patients with DCIS is controversial [27–29]. Boost recommended for age ≤50 years (any grade), high-grade, positive margin, or close (<2 mm) margin. For other DCIS pts, boost decision making should be individualized according to age, grade and surgical margins. Therefore optimal negative margins are still question debate. Society of Surgical Oncology (SSO), the American Society for Radiation Oncology (ASTRO) and the American Society of Clinical Oncology (ASCO) a 2 mm margin is considered adequate in DCIS treated with WBI [30]. Several phase III studies are also ongoing in order the evaluate the benefit of boost in DCIS.

The most recent and important approach for early stage breast cancers was the hypofractionation (dose per fraction >2 Gy, shorter overall RT time) that was proven by four randomized Canadian and United Kingdom trials. Currently, there is no available randomized data on hypofractionated RT in DCIS. However, retrospective data and a meta-analysis reported no significant difference between hypofraction-ated and conventional radiotherapy [27, 31–34].

4.1.3.2 Simulation and Field Design

Patient is positioned supine, ipsilateral arm above head, on an angled breast board or on a Vac-Lok™ cradle, face moved towards the contralateral side. Lumpectomy bed scar and the borders of breast are outlined with wire (Fig. 4.1). CT scans with 3 mm slice thickness, were obtained starting form chin to at least 3 cm lower to the inframammary fold of breast.

Borders are usually located 2 cm above and below palpable breast tissue, medial is at midline and lateral is at mid axillary line. When tangent field is placed encompassing all of breast, posterior of the borders must not exceed >2–3 cm in lung. Usually minimum 2 cm extension was designed to encompass the breathing motion and movement of breast anteriorly. Wedges or field-in-field

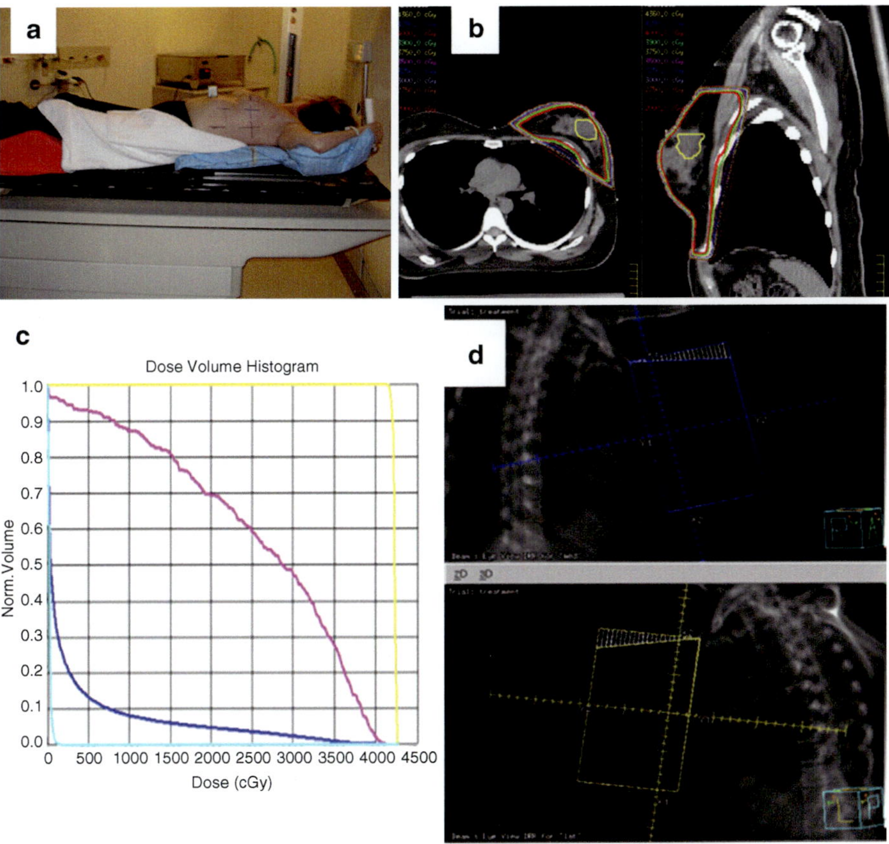

Fig. 4.1 Patient with DCIS. (**a**) Set-up photographs. (**b**) Lateral and sagittal dose distribution (**c**) DVH −40 Gy in 15 fractions were planned for this patients. (**d**) DRR's of tangent fields

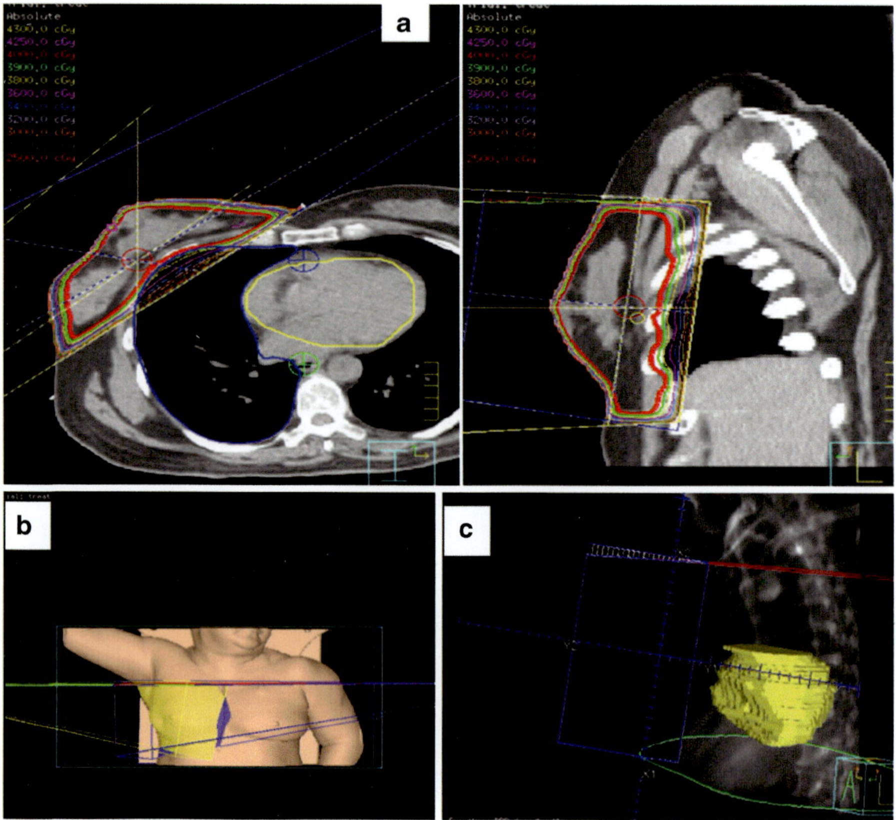

Fig. 4.2 Right breast planning CT images (**a**) shows isodose lines and DVH with hot spots of less than 7%, heart and lung dose is v20 = 5% respectively. (**b**) Skin rendering view of field design (**c**) DRR of lateral field

technique are used to improve dose homogeneity and to keep hot spots <10% (Fig. 4.2).

In case of boost planning, operation bed is outlined in breast tissue for boost with 1–2 cm margin. The boost may be given with electron or photon. For electron boost, energy is elected based on the depth of the tumor bed, with 90% isodose line covering the target.

4.1.3.3 Target Volumes

GTV = None (after lumpectomy)

CTV1 = The palpable whole breast as outlined by the skin wire + 1.5 cm margins superiorly and inferiorly, and modified to exclude 0.5 cm near the skin of the breast and pectoralis muscle and chest wall are excluded + draining LNs

CTV2 = Lumpectomy bed and any surgical clips + 1 to 2 cm margins respecting the CTV1 anteriorly and posteriorly; pectoralis muscle and chest wall are excluded

PTV = CTV + 0.5 cm

4.1.3.4 Radiotherapy Doses

Conventional doses: 1.8–2 Gy × 25 fractions to 45–50 Gy

Hypofractionation doses: 2.67 Gy × 15 fraction to 40 Gy

4.1.3.5 Dose Constraints

- Ipsilateral lung = V20 to <10–20% Contralateral lung = V10 to <5%
- Total lung = V20 to <10%, mean dose <13 Gy
- Heart = V5 to <10%; V25 to <5%, mean less than 4 Gy
- Contralateral breast = max dose <3 Gy, V10 to <5%
- Spinal cord = 45–50 Gy (if treating supraclavicular field)

4.1.4   Follow Up

There is no evidence from randomize trials supporting any particular follow up sequence or protocol [15]. Physical examination is recommended every 6 months for the first 5 years and then annually. Annual bilateral mammogram, or in the case of unilateral mastectomy, annual mammogram of the contralateral breast is warranted. Patients should be educated to do Breast self-exams.

In the absence of clinical signs or positive physical findings, blood work including tumor marker, chest X-rays, bone scans or other special investigations are not recommended.

Side effects of hormonal therapy should be explained. Vitamin D and calcium could be advised as nutritional supplements. A dual energy X-ray absorption scan (DEXA) is recommended to allow early treatment of osteoporosis. Bisphosphonates could be used in patients with iatrogenic premature menopause and in post-menopausal patients treated with AIs to prevent bone mineral loss. Hot flashes should be managed without hormonal therapy. Vaginal dryness and atrophy is usually overcome with non-hormonal lubricants and if needed, low dose vaginal estrogen therapy can be used after discussing the risks with patients.

Patients on Tamoxifen are at higher risk of developing endometrial cancer so pelvic exam and PAP smear every 12 months for patients with intact uterus.

4.2   Early Stage Breast Cancer

Overview
Epidemiology

Breast cancer is the most frequent diagnosed cancer in women. Primarily due to the screening studies, breast cancer incidence is increasing. Established risk factors are: Older age, germ-line mutation, personal history of breast cancer, high radiation exposure to chest, family history, early menarche, late menopause, older age at first full term birth, not having children, using menopause hormone therapy, obesity after menopause.

Pathology

The most common histopathological type is infiltrating ductal (76%) cancer, followed by invasive lobular (8%), mucinous (colloid) (2.4%), tubular (1.5%), medullary (1.2%), and papillary (1%) cancers. Other subtypes, including metaplastic breast cancer and invasive micropapillary breast cancer, all account for less than 5 percent of cases.

Diagnosis

The majority of patients with T1 and T2 breast cancers presents with a painless or slightly tender breast mass or have an abnormal screening mammogram. Mammography remains the most critical component of diagnostic imaging in breast cancer patients. The other routine radiographic studies include breast ultrasound and Magnetic resonance (MRI) The evaluation for distant metastases includes contrast-enhanced computed tomography (CT) of chest, and abdomen, bone scintigraphy.

Definitive Treatment

Approximately 70–80% of patients with stage I or II invasive breast cancers are technically candidates for breast conserving surgery. Careful pathological evaluation is mandatory. It is critical to have estrogen receptor, progesterone receptor, ki 67 percentage, HER2 status, surgical margin with, histological type, intraductal component of lymphovascular invasion, grade in details. The use of "no ink on tumor" as the standard for an adequate margin in invasive cancer in the era of multidisciplinary therapy is related with low rates of IBTR. Positive margins (ink on invasive carcinoma or ductal carcinoma in situ) are associated with a two-fold increase in the risk of IBTR compared with negative margins.

All the patients with breast conserving surgery had an adjuvant whole breast radiotherapy indication with either hypo fractionated or conventional fractionation. To guide the decision of chemotherapy, Genomic testing is suitable for early-stage, estrogen-receptor-positive breast cancers. If ER and/PR positivity is present in pathological evaluation, the patient is a candidate for hormonal treatment.

Keywords: Early stage breast cancer, Radiotherapy

## 4.2.1	Case Presentation

A 53 year old woman had her yearly scanning mammogram which revealed an abnormal density in the upper outer quadrant of the right breast. The size of the density was 16 mm.

Her breast examination revealed palpable 1.8 cm mobile hard mass but no axillary lymph nodes. She had two full-term pregnancies at age 23 and 28, breast fed for about 1 year, and never used oral contraceptives. She was still premenopausal. She denied any previous radiation exposure. She had no history of any other disease.

She had been smoking at least 5 cigarettes per day for the last 30 years and reported occasional alcohol intake for about 3–4 glasses of red wine per week. She had no family history of cancer.

A core needle biopsy revealed a high grade invasive ductal carcinoma (IDC), ER (+), PR(+), HER 2 (2+). Ki-67 was 12%. FISH was negative for HER2 amplification. A PET-CT scan for metastatic work-up reported no sign of dissemination. A breast ultrasound did not reveal any pathological axillary lymph nodes and she was staged as cT1cN0M0.

The patient underwent lumpectomy and sentinel lymh node dissection. Operation pathology confirmed the previous diagnoses of high grade IDC, tumor size 17 mm with at least 6 mm surgical margins. There was no peritumoral lymphovascular invasion or necrosis. None of the two sentinel lymph nodes showed any evidence of metastatic disease. Immunohistochemical workup confirmed ER and PR positivity and Ki-67 score was 17%. Her 2 amplification was absent. She requested to have an Oncotype Dx test and the result revealed a recurrence Score of 20.

Although she had early breast cancer, staged as pT1c pN0, and had no evidence of distant metastasis, she had an Oncotype DX recurrence score at the high-intermediate range and therefore, elected to proceed with chemotherapy. Four cycles of chemotherapy with docetaxel and cyclophosphamide (TC) protocol was administered and she was then referred for adjuvant radiotherapy. Hypofractionated whole breast tangent were planned for 15 fractions and 10 Gy boost to operation cavity. Deep breath hold technique was not found to be beneficial as no elective nodal irradiation was advised.

4.2.1.1 Case Evaluation

The main factors to question during the consultation:

- The most important risk factor for breast cancer development is age as well as age at menarche, first pregnancy, menopause, family history, obesity, and mammographic breast density [1, 2].
- The use of hormone treatment—especially progesterone and estrogen combination increases the risk
- Prior radiotherapy exposure to chest was also a well-established risk factor [3, 4].
- Gene mutation is noted in 5–10% of breast cancers. Family history and age at the diagnosis, would be the most valuable clue for genetic mutations [5]. The literature of germ line testing has been activity increasing. According to guidelines, consider BRCA 1, 2 testing if breast cancer diagnosis was before 40 years of age, presence of bilateral breast cancer, a family history of breast and ovarian cancer, presence of breast cancer in one or more male family members, multiple cases of breast cancer in the family, one or more family members with two primary types of BRCA-related cancer, and being from Ashkenazi Jewish ethnicity [5, 35].
- If the patient has genetic mutations, prophylactic mastectomy eradicates approximately the risk of breast cancers, nevertheless has no effect on the risk of

ovarian/fallopian tube cancer development. Prophylactic bilateral salpingo-oophorectomy should be offered as the risk of ovarian/fallopian tube cancers decreases by 80% and breast cancers by 50% [7]

4.2.1.2 Physical Examination

- Firstly, perform physical examination especially examine breast in sitting and supine position and perform bilateral node examination. Arm extension and ability of arm movement has to be checked as during the simulation arm has to be at least 90° abducted.
- Skin edema (peau d'orange) or erythema, nipple retraction is very important to define locally advanced stages.

4.2.1.3 Routine Work Up

- Labs: Routine CBC, chemistry with liver and renal functions
- Please make sure that you have seen Mammogram (shows asymmetry, clustered microcalcification, mass, and architectural distortion) and/or ultrasound of breast and lymph node basins
- Tissue diagnosis could be provided by either fine needle aspiration (FNA), Tru-Cut biopsy or vacuum-assisted biopsy—via sonography, MRI, or stereotactic-guided procedure
- Report of the path specimen should include size,
- grade, margin, estrogen receptor (ER)/progesterone receptor (PR)/Her2neu status
- Breast MRI is optional: Firstly it could be helpful for pre-op staging and surgical planning [8]. American Cancer Society recommends annual MR screening for especially women with a BRCA 1 or 2 mutation, who had a first-degree relative with a BRCA 1 or 2 mutation and had a lifetime risk of breast cancer of 20–25% or more using standard risk assessment models (BRCAPRO, Claus, Tyrer-Cuzick), whom received radiation treatment to the chest between ages 10 and 30, such as for Hodgkin's disease, does carry or have a first-degree relative who carries a genetic mutation in the TP53 or PTEN genes (Li-Fraumeni syn- drome and Cowden and Bannayan-Riley-Ruvalcaba syndromes) [9].
- The use of breast MRI continues to evolve as recent reported high false-positive rates blurred the routine use, but it may have a role in selected clinical scenarios such as invasive lobular cancers, axillary adenopathy with occult breast primary, evaluating response to neoadjuvant chemotherapy, and also if more information is needed for dense breast [9, 36].
- Metastatic work-up: Chest x-ray, CT of the abdomen and pelvis is still recommended. Bone scan is recommended for locally advanced disease or bony symptoms, or increased alkaline phosphatase, PET scan is widely available but still considered as optional.

4.2.1.4 Pathology

The invasive breast carcinomas comprise several histological subtypes; such as ductal carcinoma, lobular carcinoma, tubular, medullary, and mucinous carcinomas. The estimated percentages from a population-based series of 135,157 women with breast cancer reported to the Surveillance, Epidemiology, and End Results (SEER) database of the National Cancer Institute between 1992 and 2001, are 76% infiltrating ductal and 8% invasive lobular carcinoma. Tubular, medullary, and mucinous carcinomas generally were proven to have better prognosis.

The pathology report should include ER/PR receptor status, ki 67 percentages and HER status.

Molecular subtypes approximated by receptor status include:
Luminal A: ER/PR+ Her2neu−
Luminal B: ER/PR+ Her2neu +
Basal-like: ER/PR− Her2neu− (triple negative)
Her2neu+: ER/PR− Her2neu+

4.2.1.5 Genetic Evaluation of Recurrence

First-generation prognostic signatures: Oncotype DX, MammaPrint, Genomic Grade Index.

Newer tests: Prosigna, EndoPredict, Breast Cancer Index.

Oncotype Dx for early stage ER+, LN- invasive breast cancer is a diagnostic test that analyzes a panel of 21 genes within a breast tumor to determine a recurrence score between 0 and 100 that predicts a recurrence risk within the next 10 years [37]. Score 0–17 is low risk- the benefit of chemotherapy is small, score 18–30 is intermediate risk- unclear whether the benefit of chemo outweighs the side effect, score >30 is high risk- the benefits of chemo is greater than the side effects. A fixed pathology specimen could be used for testing [38].

MammaPrint score: MammaPrint (Agilent, Amsterdam, and the Netherlands) is a microarray-based prognostic score performed by a central laboratory for breast cancer patients younger than 61 years of age with stage I/II, lymph node-negative or one to three lymph node-positive disease. MammaPrint measures the mRNA expression of 70 genes and stratifies patients into low-risk or high-risk prognostic groups. Fresh–frozen tissue (and on-site) is essential for processing [39, 40].

PAM50/risk of recurrence/Prosigna kit: Nanostring technology to quantify mRNA expression of 50 genes was used in the PAM50 molecular classification algorithm. The risk of recurrence score was calculated, different form the other tests, it does not obviously report the subtype of breast cancer and is approved to assess the distant recurrence-free survival for stage I/II (including one to three positive nodes), ER-positive breast cancer in postmenopausal women treated with adjuvant endocrine therapy [37]. A very important fact of this test is that it can be performed by local hospital pathology laboratories with a special device named as the Nanostring nCounter Dx Analysis System (Nanostring Technologies) [41].

4.2.2 Staging: Breast Cancer

At the beginning of 2018, a new breast cancer staging has been released which has included genetic evaluation and tumor subtypes into the grouping different from the previous AJCC staging (Table 4.1) [14].

Table 4.1 Staging of breast cancer (AJCC 8th ed.)

T category	T criteria
Definition of primary tumor (T)—clinical and pathological	
TX	Primary tumor cannot be
T0	No evidence of primary tumor
Tis (DCIS)[a]	Ductal carcinoma in situ
Tis (Paget)	Paget disease of the nipple NOT associated with invasive carcinoma and/or ductal carcinoma in situ (DCIS) in the underlying breast parenchyma. Carcinomas in the breast parenchyma associated with Paget disease are categorized based on the size and characteristics of the parenchymal disease, although the presence of Paget disease should still be noted
T1	Tumor $\leq$20 mm in greatest dimension
T1mi	Tumor $\leq$1 mm in greatest dimension
T1a	Tumor >1 mm but $\leq$5 mm in greatest dimension (round any measurement 1.0–1.9 mm to 2 mm)
T1b	Tumor >5 mm but $\leq$10 mm in greatest dimension
T1c	Tumor >10 mm but $\leq$20 mm in greatest dimension
T2	Tumor >20 mm but $\leq$50 mm in greatest dimension
T3	Tumor >50 mm in greatest dimension
T4	Tumor of any size with direct extension to the chest wall and/or to the skin (ulceration or macroscopic nodules); invasion of the dermis alone does not qualify as T4
T4a	Extension to the chest wall; invasion or adherence to pectoralis muscle in the absence of invasion of chest wall structures does not qualify as T4
T4b	Ulceration and/or ipsilateral macroscopic satellite nodules and/or edema (including peau d'orange) of the skin that does not meet the criteria for inflammatory carcinoma
T4c	Both T4a and T4b are present
T4d	Inflammatory carcinoma (see "rules for classification")

cN category	cN criteria
Definition of regional lymph nodes—clinical (CN)	
cNX[b]	Regional lymph nodes cannot be assessed (e.g., previously removed)
cN0	No regional lymph node metastases (by imaging or clinical examination)
cN1	Metastases to movable ipsilateral levels I and II axillary lymph node(s)
cN1mi[c]	Micrometastases (approximately 200 cells, larger than 0.2 mm, but not larger than 2.0 mm)
cN2	Metastases in ipsilateral levels I and II axillary lymph nodes that are clinically fixed or matted *or* in ipsilateral internal mammary nodes in the absence of axillary lymph node metastases
cN2a	Metastases in ipsilateral levels I and II axillary lymph nodes fixed to one another (matted) or to other structures

Table 4.1 (continued)

cN category	cN criteria
cN2b	Metastases only in ipsilateral internal mammary nodes in the absence of axillary lymph node metastases
cN3	Metastases in ipsilateral infraclavicular (level III axillary) lymph node(s) with or without levels I and II axillary lymph node involvement, in ipsilateral internal mammary lymph node(s) with levels I and II axillary lymph node metastases, or in ipsilateral supraclavicular lymph node(s) with or without axillary or internal mammary lymph node involvement
cN3a	Metastases in ipsilateral infraclavicular lymph node(s)
cN3b	Metastases in ipsilateral internal mammary lymph node(s) and axillary lymph node(s)
cN3c	Metastases in ipsilateral supraclavicular lymph node(s)

pN category	pN criteria
Definition of regional lymph nodes—pathological (PN)	
pNX	Regional lymph nodes cannot be assessed (e.g., not removed for pathological study or previously removed)
pN0	No regional lymph node metastasis identified or ITCs only pN0(i+) ITCs only (malignant cell clusters not larger than 0.2 mm) in regional lymph node(s)
pN0(mol+)	Positive molecular findings by reverse transcriptase polymerase chain reaction (RT-PCR); no ITCs detected
pN1	Micrometastases or metastases in 1–3 axillary lymph nodes and/or clinically negative internal mammary nodes with micrometastases or macrometastases by sentinel lymph node biopsy
pN1mi	Micrometastases (approximately 200 cells, larger than 0.2 mm, but not larger than 2.0 mm)
pN1a	Metastases in 1–3 axillary lymph nodes, at least one metastasis larger than 2.0 mm
pN1b	Metastases in ipsilateral internal mammary sentinel nodes, excluding ITCs
pN1c	pN1a and pN1b combined
pN2	Metastases in 4–9 axillary lymph nodes or positive ipsilateral internal mammary lymph nodes by imaging in the absence of axillary lymph node metastases
pN2a	Metastases in 4–9 axillary lymph nodes (at least one tumor deposit larger than 2.0 mm)
pN2b	Metastases in clinically detected internal mammary lymph nodes with or without microscopic confirmation; with pathologically negative axillary nodes
pN3	Metastases in 10 or more axillary lymph nodes, in infraclavicular (level III axillary) lymph nodes, positive ipsilateral internal mammary lymph nodes by imaging in the presence of one or more positive levels I and II axillary lymph nodes, in more than three axillary lymph nodes and micrometastases or macrometastases by sentinel lymph node biopsy in clinically negative ipsilateral internal mammary lymph nodes, *or* in ipsilateral supraclavicular lymph nodes
pN3a	Metastases in 10 or more axillary lymph nodes (at least one tumor deposit larger than 2.0 mm) *or* metastases to the infraclavicular (level III axillary) lymph nodes
pN3b	pN1a or pN2a in the presence of cN2b (positive internal mammary nodes by imaging) *or* pN2a in the presence of pN1b
pN3c	Metastases in ipsilateral supraclavicular lymph nodes

(continued)

Table 4.1 (continued)

M category	M criteria
Definition of distant metastasis (M)	
M0	No clinical or radiographic evidence of distant metastases[d]
cM0(i+)	No clinical or radiographic evidence of distant metastases in the presence of tumor cells or deposits not larger than 0.2 mm detected microscopically or by molecular techniques in circulating blood, bone marrow, or other nonregional nodal tissues in a patient without symptoms or signs of metastases
M1	Distant metastases detected by clinical and radiographic means (cM) and/or histologically proven metastases larger than 0.2 mm (pM)

When T is…	And N is…	And M is…	Then the stage group is…
AJCC anatomic and prognostic stage groups AJCC anatomic stage groups			
Tis	N0	M0	0
T1	N0	M0	IA
T0	N1mi	M0	IB
T1	N1mi	M0	IB
T0	N1	M0	IIA
T1	N1	M0	IIA
T2	N0	M0	IIA
T2	N1	M0	IIB
T3	N0	M0	IIB
T0	N2	M0	IIIA
T1	N2	M0	IIIA
T2	N2	M0	IIIA
T3	N1	M0	IIIA
T3	N2	M0	IIIA
T4	N0	M0	IIIB
T4	N1	M0	IIIB
T4	N2	M0	IIIB
Any T	N3	M0	IIIC
Any T	Any N	M1	IV

T	N	M	G	HER2 status[e]	ER	PR	Prognostic stage group
Prognostic stage group							
Tis	N0	M0	1–3	Any	Any	Any	0
T1	N0	M0	1	Positive	Any	Any	IA
T1	N0	M0	1–2	Negative	Positive	Positive	IA
T1	N0	M0	2	Positive	Positive	Positive	IA
T1	N0	M0	3	Positive	Positive	Any	IA
T0–1	N1mi	M0	1	Positive	Any	Any	IA
T0–1	N1mi	M0	1–2	Negative	Positive	Positive	IA
T0–1	N1mi	M0	2	Positive	Positive	Positive	IA
T0–1	N1mi	M0	3	Positive	Positive	Any	IA

Table 4.1 (continued)

T	N	M	G	HER2 status[e]	ER	PR	Prognostic stage group
Multigene panel[f]—oncotype DX® recurrence score less than 11							
T1–2	N0	M0	1–3	Negative	Positive	Any	IA
T1	N0	M0	1	Negative	Positive	Negative	IB
T1	N0	M0	1	Negative	Negative	Positive	IB
T1	N0	M0	2	Positive	Positive	Negative	IB
T1	N0	M0	2	Positive	Negative	Any	IB
T1	N0	M0	2	Negative	Negative	Positive	IB
T1	N0	M0	3	Positive	Negative	Any	IB
T1	N0	M0	3	Negative	Positive	Positive	IB
T0–1	N1mi	M0	1	Negative	Positive	Negative	IB
T0–1	N1mi	M0	1	Negative	Negative	Positive	IB
T0–1	N1mi	M0	2	Positive	Positive	Negative	IB
T0–1	N1mi	M0	2	Positive	Negative	Any	IB
T0–1	N1mi	M0	2	Negative	Negative	Positive	IB
T0–1	N1mi	M0	3	Positive	Negative	Any	IB
T0–1	N1mi	M0	3	Negative	Positive	Positive	IB
T2	N0	M0	1–3	Positive	Positive	Positive	IB
T2	N0	M0	1,2	Negative	Positive	Positive	IB
T1	N1	M0	1–3	Positive	Positive	Positive	IB
T1	N1	M0	1–2	Negative	Positive	Positive	IB
T2	N1	M0	1	Negative	Positive	Positive	IB[g]
T2	N1	M0	2	Positive	Positive	Positive	IB[g]
T0–2	N2	M0	1–2	Positive	Positive	Positive	IB[g]
T0–2	N2	M0	1	Negative	Positive	Negative	IIIA
T0–2	N2	M0	1	Negative	Negative	Positive	IIIA
T0–2	N2	M0	2	Positive	Positive	Negative	IIIA
T0–2	N2	M0	2	Positive	Negative	Any	IIIA
T3	N1–2	M0	1	Positive	Positive	Negative	IIIA
T3	N1–2	M0	1	Positive	Negative	Any	IIIA
T3	N1–2	M0	1	Negative	Positive	Negative	IIIA
T3	N1–2	M0	1	Negative	Negative	Positive	IIIA
T3	N1–2	M0	2	Positive	Positive	Negative	IIIA
T3	N1–2	M0	2	Positive	Negative	Any	IIIA
T4	N0–2	M0	1	Negative	Positive	Positive	IIIA
Any	N3	M0	1	Negative	Positive	Positive	IIIA[g]
T2	N1	M0	1–2	Negative	Negative	Negative	IIIB[g]
T2	N1	M0	3	Negative	Positive	Negative	IIIB[g]
T3	N0	M0	1–2	Negative	Negative	Negative	IIIB
T3	N0	M0	3	Negative	Positive	Negative	IIIB
T0–2	N2	M0	2	Negative	Positive	Negative	IIIB
T0–2	N2	M0	2	Negative	Negative	Positive	IIIB
T0–2	N2	M0	3	Positive	Positive	Negative	IIIB
T0–2	N2	M0	3	Positive	Negative	Any	IIIB
T0–2	N2	M0	3	Negative	Positive	Positive	IIIB

(continued)

Table 4.1 (continued)

T	N	M	G	HER2 status[e]	ER	PR	Prognostic stage group
T3	N1–2	M0	2	Negative	Positive	Negative	IIIB
T3	N1–2	M0	2	Negative	Negative	Positive	IIIB
T3	N1–2	M0	3	Positive	Positive	Negative	IIIB
T3	N1–2	M0	3	Positive	Negative	Any	IIIB
T3	N1–2	M0	3	Negative	Positive	Positive	IIIB
T4	N0–2	M0	1	Positive	Any	Any	IIIB
T4	N0–2	M0	2	Positive	Positive	Positive	IIIB
T4	N0–2	M0	2	Negative	Positive	Positive	IIIB
T4	N0–2	M0	3	Positive	Positive	Positive	IIIB
Any	N3	M0	1	Positive	Any	Any	IIIB
Any	N3	M0	2	Positive	Positive	Positive	IIIB
Any	N3	M0	2	Negative	Positive	Positive	IIIB
Any	N3	M0	3	Positive	Positive	Positive	IIIB
T2	N1	M0	3	Negative	Negative	Any	IIIC[g]
T3	N0	M0	3	Negative	Negative	Any	IIIC
T0–2	N2	M0	2	Negative	Negative	Negative	IIIC[g]
T0–2	N2	M0	3	Negative	Positive	Negative	IIIC[g]
T0–2	N2	M0	3	Negative	Negative	Any	IIIC[g]
T3	N1–2	M0	2	Negative	Negative	Negative	IIIC[g]
T3	N1–2	M0	3	Negative	Positive	Negative	IIIC[g]
T3	N1–2	M0	3	Negative	Negative	Any	IIIC[g]
T4	N0–2	M0	1	Negative	Positive	Negative	IIIC
T4	N0–2	M0	1	Negative	Negative	Any	IIIC
T4	N0–2	M0	2	Positive	Positive	Negative	IIIC
T4	N0–2	M0	2	Positive	Negative	Any	IIIC
T4	N0–2	M0	2	Negative	Positive	Negative	IIIC
T4	N0–2	M0	2	Negative	Negative	Any	IIIC
T4	N0–2	M0	3	Positive	Positive	Negative	IIIC
T4	N0–2	M0	3	Positive	Negative	Any	IIIC
T4	N0–2	M0	3	Negative	Any	Any	IIIC
Any	N3	M0	1	Negative	Positive	Negative	IIIC
Any	N3	M0	1	Negative	Negative	Any	IIIC
Any	N3	M0	2	Positive	Positive	Negative	IIIC
Any	N3	M0	2	Positive	Negative	Any	IIIC
Any	N3	M0	2	Negative	Positive	Negative	IIIC
Any	N3	M0	2	Negative	Negative	Any	IIIC
Any	N3	M0	3	Positive	Positive	Negative	IIIC
Any	N3	M0	3	Positive	Negative	Any	IIIC
Any	N3	M0	3	Negative	Any	Any	IIIC
AnyT	AnyN	M1	1–3	Any	Any	Any	IV

(sn) and (f) suffixes should be added to the N category to denote confirmation of metastasis by sentinel node biopsy and fine-needle aspiration/core needle biopsy, respectively

(sn) and (f) suffixes should be added to the N category to denote confirmation of metastasis by sentinel node biopsy or FNA/core needle biopsy, respectively, with N0 further resection of nodes

Table 4.1 (continued)

The prognostic value of these prognostic stage groups is based on the populations of persons with breast cancer that have been offered and mostly treated with appropriate endocrine and/or systemic chemotherapy

Used with permission of the American Joint Committee on Cancer (AJCC), Chicago, Illinois. The original and primary source for this information is the AJCC Cancer Staging Manual, Eighth Edition (2017) published by Springer International Publishing

[a]Lobular carcinoma in situ (LCIS) is a benign entity and is removed from TNM staging in the AJCC Cancer Staging Manual, Eighth Edition

[b]The cNX category is used sparingly in cases where regional lymph nodes have previously been surgically removed or where there is no documentation of physical examination of the axilla

[c]cN1mi is rarely used but may be appropriate in cases where sentinel node biopsy is Performed before tumor resection, most likely to occur in cases treated with neoadjuvant therapy

[d]Note that imaging studies are not required to assign the cM0 category

[e]For cases where HER2 is determined to be "equivocal" by ISH (FISH or CISH) testing under the 2013 ASCO/CAP HER2 testing guidelines, HER2 "negative" category should be used for staging in the prognostic stage group table

[f]If Oncotype DX® is not performed or not available or if the Oncotype DX® score is 11 or greater for patients with T1–2 N0 M0 HER2-negative ER-positive cancer, then the prognostic stage group is assigned based on the anatomic and biomarker categories shown above. Oncotype DX® is the only multigene panel included to classify prognostic stage because prospective level I data supports this use for patients with a score <11. Future updates may include results from other multigene panels to assign cohorts of patients to prognostic stage groups when there are high level data to support these assignments

[g]Denotes a stage group for which the use of grade and prognostic factors changed the group, more than one stage group from the anatomic stage group (e.g., from anatomic stage group IIB to prognostic stage group IB)

Main differences could be listed as:

- There are two stage group tables presented in this chapter. First one is the anatomic stage group table that is based solely on anatomic extent of cancer as defined by the T, N, and M categories. Secondly, the prognostic stage group table is based on populations of persons with breast cancer that have been offered—and mostly treated with—appropriate endocrine and/or systemic chemotherapy, which includes anatomic T, N, and M plus tumor grade and the status of the biomarkers human epidermal growth factor receptor 2 (HER2), estrogen receptor (ER), and progesterone receptor (PR) [42].
- Lobular carcinoma in situ (LCIS) is removed as a pathologic tumor in situ (pTis) category for T categorization. LCIS is a benign entity and is removed from TNM staging. Also it is confirmed that the maximum invasive tumor size (T) is a reasonable estimate of tumor volume. Small, microscopic satellite foci of tumor

around the primary tumor do not appreciably alter tumor volume and are not added to the maximum tumor size.

- The T categorization of multiple synchronous tumors is simplified. These are identified clinically and/or by macroscopic pathologic examination, and their presence documented using the (m) modifier for the T category. This new edition specifically continues using only the maximum dimension of the largest tumor for clinical (cT) and pathological (pT) T classification; the size of multiple tumors is not added [42].

4.2.3 Evidence Based Treatment Recommendations

4.2.3.1 Lumpectomy vs. Mastectomy

Breast conserving strategy of lumpectomy and surgical axillary staging following radiotherapy was accepted a standard approach for early stage breast cancer (stage I-II) in the first phase. Even for node negative patients, the absolute risk reduction was 15.4% (95% CI 13.2–17.6) for any breast recurrences as well as the improvement of 15 year breast cancer related mortality from 17.2% to 20.5% [43]. Also total mastectomy with surgical axillary staging ± RT as indicated could serve as a second choice [44]. Mastectomy reserved for patients ineligible for breast conserving surgery + radiotherapy due to medical or surgical contraindications, or patient preference. Contraindications to breast conserving surgery include multicentricity, ratio of tumor size to breast, diffuse microcalcifications, persistent close/positive margins after multiple number of re-excisions, previous breast RT, pregnancy, and scleroderma (lupus is a relative contraindication). Axillary lymph node involvement is not a contraindication to breast conserving surgery + radiotherapy.

4.2.3.2 Axillary Dissection vs. Radiotherapy

Surgical evaluation/treatment of axilla could be either axillary LN dissection (ALND) or Sentinel lymph node biopsy (SLNbx). The first study to evaluated the value of radiotherapy in axillary local control was NSABP B-04 which evaluated the role of radiotherapy instead of axillary radiotherapy for clinically negative breast cancer patients. Even systemic therapy was administrated to the patients, among cN0 patients, axillary failure was <4% if addressed surgically or with RT vs. 19% in TM alone arm [45]. In 2004, Louis-Sylvestre published a study, randomized to ALND or axillary RT for 658 cN0 patients with <3 cm primary and twenty-one percent of the patients in the axillary dissection group were pN+ [46]. Even a decrement in isolated axillary recurrences in ALND group at 15 years (1 vs. 3%; p = 0.04) were reported, identical OS and breast, supraclavicular, and distant recurrence at 15 years (73.8 vs. 75.5%) were recorded, [46]. This results were confirmed by NSABP B-32 randomized trial with similar outcome in 8-year OS, DFS, or sites of first treatment failure for upfront ALND vs.

SLNBx [46]. The following ACOSOG Z-11 trial randomized 856 patients with positive SLN randomized to lumpectomy + SLND with or without completion ALND. Of the patients, 89% received whole breast RT. The results revealed no significant difference in LR (2.8% SLND vs. 4.1% completion ALND) [47]. Radiotherapy filed details were analyzed in another publication where most patients were treated with tangents alone (n = 540), 15% received radiation directed at the SCV, which were more likely to be patients with higher numbers of involved LN [48].

AMAROS trial also randomized 1425 patients with + SLN to receive either ALND or axillary RT and reported that 5-year rate of axillary recurrence was not significantly different (0.43% for ALND vs. 1.19% for axillary RT) [49]. Importantly, patients with ALND had higher rates of clinical lymphedema and increase in arm circumference >10% [49].

In the eight year update of OTOASOR (Optimal Treatment Of the Axilla—Surgery Or Radiotherapy) trial, that compared completion of axillary lymph node dissection to regional nodal irradiation (RNI) in patients with sentinel lymph node metastasis (pN1sn) in stage I-II breast cancer, axillary recurrence was 2.0% in ALND arm vs. 1.7% in RNI arm (p = 1.00). Overall survival at 8 years was 77.9% vs. 84.8% (p = 0.060), and DFS was 72.1% in ALND arm and 77.4% after RNI (p = 0.51). The results also proved that radiotherapy for axillary management is statistically not inferior to surgical approach [50, 51].

4.2.3.3 Hypofractionation

The most recent and important approach for early stage breast cancers was the hypofractionation (>2 Gy per fraction) that was proven by four randomized Canadian and United Kingdom trials. All of them reported encouraging long-term data on local control, toxicity profile and cosmetic outcomes (Table 4.2) [52–54]. Whelan et al. evaluated whether a hypofractionated 3-week schedule of whole-breast irradiation was as effective as a 5-week schedule and stated no difference between the two fractionation schedules with regard to adverse effects, cosmetic outcome, local recurrence, or overall survival [53]. No boost was delivered and Large-breasted patients over >25 cm separation were not allowed. Of the patients, 11% received chemotherapy in each arm and 25% was <50 years old [53]. The UK Standardization of Breast Radiotherapy (START) Trialists' Group also randomized women with early-stage breast cancer treated with primary surgery to either traditional WBRT or one of two hypofractionated schedules (41.6 Gy in 13 fractions or 39.0 Gy in 13 fractions). At 5-year follow-up, they established similar outcomes in terms of local recurrence [52]. The START Trialists' Group also performed START B, randomizing early stage breast cancer patients to conventional (50 Gy in 25 fractions) versus hypofractionated WBRT (40 Gy in 15 fractions) after lumpectomy. At 6-year follow-up, similar to recent studies, they stated no difference in local recurrence with reduced late adverse effects, fewer distant metastases, greater disease-free survival, and greater overall survival in hypofractionated arm

Table 4.2 Randomized trials of hypofactionation schemas

Trial	Schema	Number of patients	stage	Median follow up	Local recurrence	Overall survival	Adverse cosmesis (%)
RHM/GOC	50Gy/25/2Gy	470	T1–3	9.7 y	12%	NR	40
1986–1998	42.9Gy/13/3.3 Gy	466	N0–1		10%		46
	39Gy/13/3 Gy	474			15%		30
Canadian	50Gy/25/2Gy	612	Pt1–2	12 y	8%	84%	29
1993–1996	42.5Gy/16/2.6 Gy	622	PN0		7%	85%	30
START A	50Gy/25/2 Gy	749	PT1–3a	9.3 y	7%	80%	42
1998–2002	41.6Gy/13/3.2 Gy	750	Pn0–1		6%	82%	42
START B	50Gy/25/2 Gy	1105	pT1–3a	9.9 y	6%	81%	40
1999–2002	40Gy/15/2.67 Gy	1110	pN0–1		4%	84%	30

[52]. Moreover, the benefits of the hypofractionated schedules in the START A and B trials were maintained at 10-year follow-up [52]. Photographic and patient-assessed late adverse effects were lower with 39 vs. 50 Gy and with 40 vs. 50 Gy. Estimated α/β was 4.6 Gy for tumor control and 3.4 Gy for late breast appearance change. In the Canadian trial by Owen et al. 1410 T1–3 N01 patients randomized to 50 Gy in 25, 39 Gy in 13, or 42.9 Gy in 13 fractions over 5 weeks. Thirty percent of patients were <50 year old and boost was delivered 75% of the patients. Ten-year ipsilateral breast recurrence rates of 12.1%, 14.8%, and 9.6% (6.7–12.6) in each arm, respectively.

Depending on these trials, the preferred worldwide dose-fractionation scheme of hypofractionated WBI were 4000 cGy in 15 fractions or 4250 cGy in 16 fractions for early stage invasive breast cancer receiving WBI with or without inclusion of the low axilla [55]. On the other hand, the American Society for Radiation Oncology (ASTRO) evidence-based guideline supports the use of hypofractionated WBRT for patients aged $\geq$50 years, stage pT1-T2 pN0M0, as long as the hypofractionated radiation plan can achieve radiation dose heterogeneity of $\leq$7%. Overall, the hypofractionated schedules seemed safe and would decrease the number of days required and at the same time drawing resource utilization.

4.2.3.4 Boost Dose to Surgical Bed

Using boost to surgical bed has been an important discussion topic. The EORTC "boost vs no boost trial" (22,881/10882) had exposed that 16 Gy in 8 fraction boost dose had dropped the incidence of local recurrences from 10.2% to 6.2% compared to no additional dose with an increment of severe fibrosis form 1.6% to 4.4% in 10 years [56]. All age groups benefited from boost, although benefit was small if >60 years old. In another trial from Lyon, also confirmed that the local recurrences were decreased by adding additional boost dose to cavity with a cost of higher grade 1 telangiectasia (12.4% vs. 5.9%) [57]. Ongoing RTOG 1005 trial has been matching standard conventionally fractionated (50 Gy/25 fr) or hypo-fractionated (42.7/16 fraction) WBI, followed by a sequential boost of 12–14 Gy/6–7 fr versus hypofractionated accelerated WBI delivering 40 Gy/15 fr with a concomitant boost of 3.2 Gy to the tumor bed (up to 48 Gy/15 fr). This trial has been closed to accrual and results were awaited [58]. The IMPORT HIGH trial also randomized the standard arm—40.5 Gy/15 fr and a sequential tumor bed boost of 16 Gy/8 fraction for adjunctive 1.6 weeks (23 fractions for a total of 4.6 weeks) to two different experimental arm: in addition to 2.4 Gy × 15 fractions to the whole breast and 2.67 Gy × 15 fractions to the index quadrant, the first arm receives 3.2 Gy × 15 fractions (up to 48 Gy), while the second arm gets 3.53 Gy × 15 fractions (up to 53 Gy) to the tumor bed [59]. As a summary of additional boost was mainly recommended for selected patients, such as younger than 50 years old, age 51–70 with pathological features like close surgical margin, hormone negativity and extensive intraductal component to balance the gain and the rate of side effects.

4.2.3.5 Accelerated Partial Breast Irradiation (APBI)

APBI decreases the size of radiotherapy fields with an anatomy based target volume contouring, which usually defined as lumpectomy cavity plus 1–2 cm margin. Also this method had been using hypo fractionated schemes in range from 30.3 Gy to 40 Gy/15 fractions which lessened the number of days that patients spends in hospital [60–62]. The main two randomized trials from Hungary and GEC-ESRTO has established similar and low local recurrence rates (Hungarian NIO trial: 10 years follow up-5.1% vs 5.9%, GEC-ESTRO 5 years follow-up- 0.9% vs 1.4%) with acceptable adverse cosmetic rates [61, 62]. The basics of APBI technique has been established with interstitial applications, which requires experience, more specific equipment and physics support. As administration of APBI is easier and more accessible with external radiotherapy devices, a recent published Phase 3 IMPORT low trial has assessed the role of partial breast radiotherapy compared to whole breast radiotherapy and primarily proven that this external APBI technique was easily adapted in daily practice as 30 radiotherapy centers in the UK have participated in this trail. Women aged 50 years or older who had undergone breast-conserving surgery for unifocal invasive ductal adenocarcinoma of grade 1–3, with a tumour size of 3 cm or less (pT1–2), none to three positive axillary nodes (pN0–1), and minimum microscopic margins of non-cancerous tissue of 2 mm or more, were recruited and were randomly assigned to receive 40 Gy whole-breast radiotherapy (control), 36 Gy whole-breast radiotherapy and 40 Gy to the partial breast (reduced-dose group), or 40 Gy to the partial breast only (partial-breast group) in 15 daily treatment fractions. The results has not been inferior with a 5 year absolute difference in local relapse of −0.38% and announced hypofractionated external APBI as new standard clinical approach [60]. Moreover, the improvement in RT techniques has been resulted in lesser side effects in the published series. The results of phase 3 trial using various APBI techniques- NSABP-B39/RTPG 0413 has been awaiting [63]. Similarly, the intraoperative radiotherapy approach has been tested in ELIOT and TARGIT-A trials [64, 65]. In the ELIOT trial, IORT was prescribed by 6–9 MeV electron beams to 90% isodose line at the tumor bed and after 5.8 median follow-up, the 5 years ipsilateral breast tumor recurrence rate were 4.4% for IORT and 0.4% for WBRT [64]. In the TARGIT trial, APBI was delivered by low-energy X-rays (50 Kv maximum) at the tip of a 3.2 mm diameter tube placed at the center of a spherical tumor bed applicator. A dose of 20 Gy was delivered at the surface of tumor bed, lowering to 5–7 Gy approximately at 1 cm depth [65]. The 5 years local recurrence rate was 3.3% for TARGIT and 1.3% for WBRT [65]. Even there are many ongoing many debates about APBI, longer term follow-up results have been waiting about the results of toxicity [65]. APBI could be offered to very highly selected patients outside trials.

4.2.3.6 Radiotherapy for Elderly Patients

In a selected group of patient categorized as "low risk" (elderly (≥65–70 years), small tumors (<2 cm), node negative axilla, estrogen positive receptors), radiation therapy (RT) after local excision and adjuvant endocrine treatment has been demonstrated to have a limited absolute benefit in terms of local control and no benefit in overall survival [66–68]. In the Cancer and Leukemia Group B (CALGB) 9343 study, women aged ≥70 years with estrogen receptor-positive (ER+) early-stage breast cancer were randomized to lumpectomy plus tamoxifen with or without WBRT [66]. A small improvement in local recurrence (10% vs 2%) and no difference in breast preservation, distant metastasis, and overall survival had been reported at the 10-year follow-up [66]. The BASO II study was a randomized patients aged ≤ 70 with node-negative low-grade breast cancer sized ≤20 mm and no evidence of lympho-vascular invasion to a 2 × 2 factorial design, evaluating the effect of the addition of WBI or tamoxifen or both after wide local excision on free margins and axillary sampling or clearance. The four available treatment arms included surgery only, surgery + WBI, surgery + tamoxifen or surgery + WBI + tamoxifen. At a median observation time of 121 months, the cumulative incidence of ipsilateral breast tumor recurrence was 10.2% for patients not receiving radiation, 3.9% for those receiving radiotherapy, 11.7% for those not receiving tamoxifen and 4.2% for patients receiving tamoxifen. Even the risk of local recurrence was reduced by the addition of WBI or tamoxifen, this is not linked with a significant improvement in OS [69].

Adjuvant hormonal therapy was suggested for all ER-positive tumors. This recommendation was independent from patient's age, menopausal status, node status, or chemotherapy administration [68, 70].

Tamoxifen could be used for all ages and all patients. Aromatase inhibitors consisting anastrozole, letrozole, exemestane are indicated for specifically postmenopausal patients [70]. Side effects include hot flashes, night sweats, vaginal dryness, musculoskeletal symptoms/arthralgia, and osteoporosis [68].

4.2.3.7 Radiotherapy Timing

Radiotherapy usually started within 2–6 weeks of surgery, if the patients receives chemotherapy, RT begins 3–4 weeks after the last chemotherapy session. Timing of chemotherapy and radiotherapy was evaluated in 244 post lumpectomy patients with stage I/II breast cancer [71]. All the patients were randomized either to adjuvant doxorubicin-based chemo followed by RT or adjuvant RT followed by four cycles of same chemo. After 11-year follow-up, overall survival, distant metastases, time to any event, or site of first failure were similar. The only major difference was for patients with close margins (<1 mm) where LR was 32% with chemo first vs. 4% with RT first; for + margins [71].

4.2.4 Treatment Planning

4.2.4.1 Simulation and Field Design

Patient is positioned supine, ipsilateral arm above head, on an angled breast board or on a Vac-Lok™ cradle, face moved towards the contralateral side. Lumpectomy bed scar and the borders of breast are outlined with wire. CT scans with 3 mm slice thickness, were obtained starting form chin to at least 3 cm lower to the inframammary fold of breast.

Target Volumes (Fig. 4.3)
GTV = None (after lumpectomy)
   CTV1 = The palpable whole breast as outlined by the skin wire +1.5 cm margins superiorly and inferiorly, and modified to exclude 0.5 cm near the skin of the breast and pectoralis muscle and chest wall are excluded + draining LNs
   CTV2 = Lumpectomy bed and any surgical clips +1 to 2 cm margins respecting the CTV1 anteriorly and posteriorly; pectoralis muscle and chest wall are excluded.
   PTV = CTV + 0.5 cm

Borders are usually located 2 cm above and below palpable breast tissue, medial is at midline and lateral is at mid axillary line (Fig. 4.4). When tangent field is placed encompassing all of breast, posterior of the borders must not exceed >2–3 cm in lung (Fig. 4.5). Usually minimum 2 cm extension was designed to encompass the breathing motion and movement of breast anteriorly. Wedges or field-in-field technique are used to improve dose homogeneity and to keep hot spots <10%.

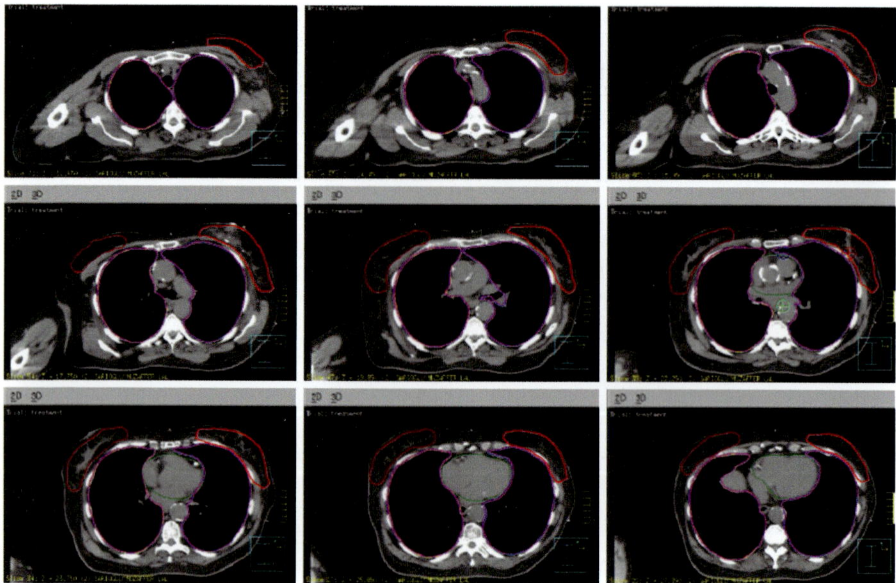

Fig. 4.3 Delineation of treatment volumes for cT1bN0M0 breast cancer patient. Red; CCTV breast, maroon; contralateral breast, green: heart PTV

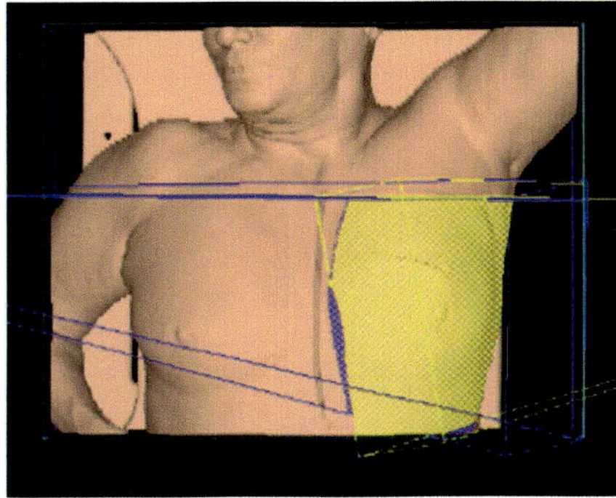 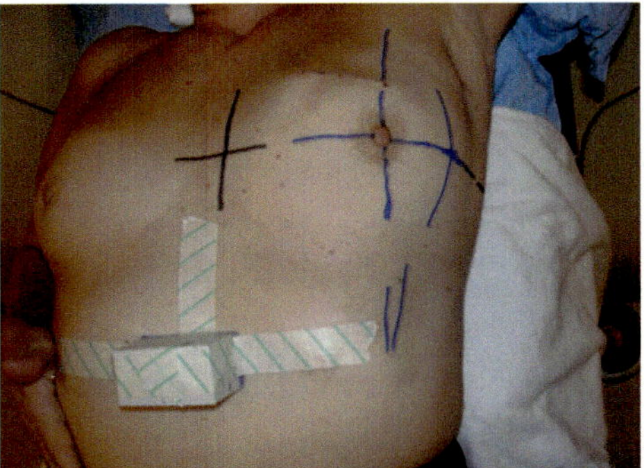

Fig. 4.4 Set-up for left breast cancer with RPM device. The place of the box has to be marked at the time of simulation

Fig. 4.5 If Caudal edge of the field extended within the 2 cm of humeral head, "high" tangent fields covers the level I and a portion of level II lymph nodes

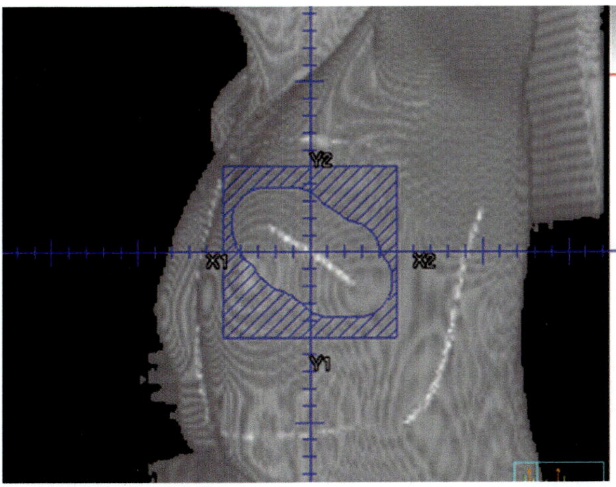

Tumor bed is outlined in breast tissue for boost with 1–2 cm margin (Fig. 4.6). The boost may be given with electron or photon. For electron boost, energy is elected based on the depth of the tumor bed, with 90% isodose line covering the target (Fig. 4.7).

Recommended Doses
Breast
Conventional doses: 1.8–2 Gy × 25 fractions to 45–50 Gy
Hypofractionation doses: 2.67 Gy × 15 fraction to 40 Gy
Boost dose: 10 Gy in 4–5 fractions
Positive margin/young age/close margin: 14–16 Gy in 7–8 fractions or 12.5 Gy in 5 fractions may be used.

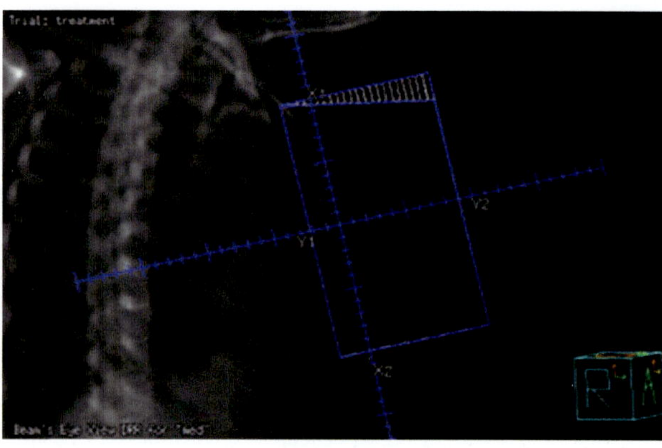

Fig. 4.6 Boost volume covers operation cavity and incision with 2 cm margin. Usually electrons were used for treatment delivery

4.2.4.2 Dose Constraints

- Ipsilateral lung = V20 to <10–20% Contralateral lung = V10 to <5%
- Total lung = V20 to <10%, mean dose <13 Gy
- Heart = V5 to <10%; V25 to <5%, mean less than 4 Gy
- Contralateral breast = max dose <3 Gy, V10 to <5%
- Spinal cord = 45–50 Gy (if treating supraclavicular field)

4.2.5 Treatment Algorithm

Treatment algorithm of early stage breast cancer is summarized in Fig. 4.8.

4.2.6 Follow Up

There is no evidence from randomize trials supporting any particular follow up sequence or protocol [15].

Physical examination is recommended every 6 months for the first 5 years and then annually. Long term follow up was recommended for especially hormone positive patients as median time to breast cancer recurrence is 5–7 years for patients receiving hormonal treatment.

Annual bilateral mammogram, or in the case of unilateral mastectomy, annual mammogram of the contralateral breast is warranted.

4.2.6.1 Patients were Educated to do Breast Self-Exams

In the absence of clinical signs or positive physical findings, blood work including tumor marker, chest X-rays, bone scans or other special investigations are not recommended.

Although chemotherapy can stop menstrual periods, this doesn't necessarily mean a woman can't become pregnant during treatment. It's important to use

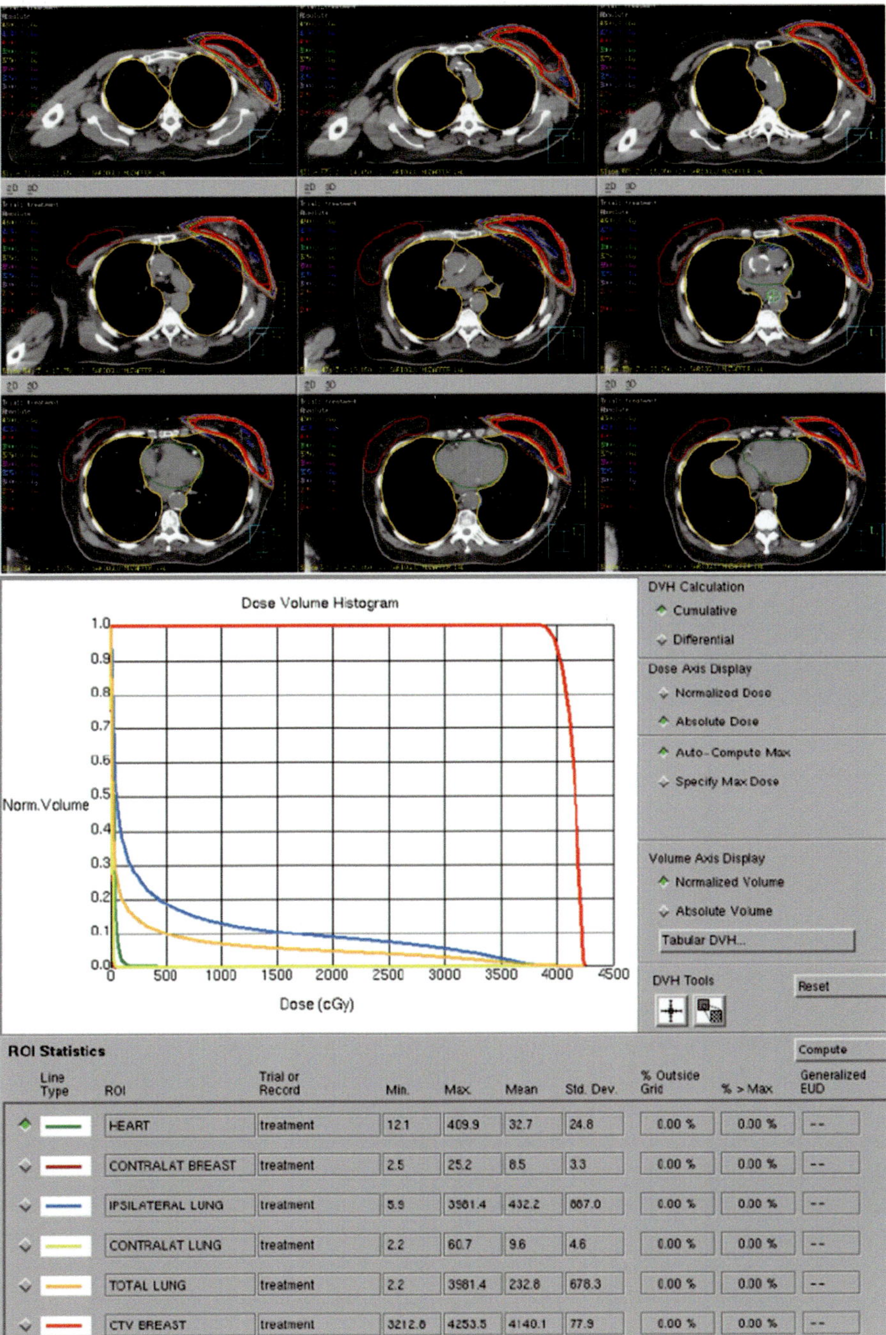

Fig. 4.7 Tangential whole breast radiotherapy. Axial dose distributions were presented. Total dose of 40 Gy in 2.67 Gy/fraction was delivered. 95% isodose coverage (red) and dose-volume histogram are shown. Heart: green, Contralateral breast: Maroon, Ipsilateral lung: light blue, Contralateral lung: yellow, Total lung: orange, CTV breast: red

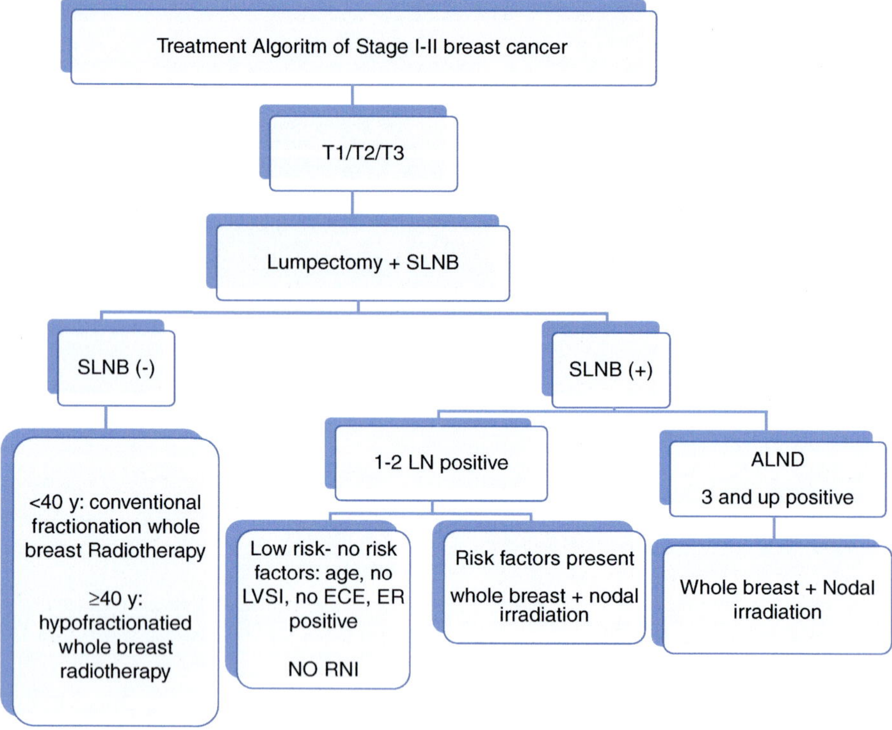

Fig. 4.8 Treatment algorithm of early stage breast cancer

contraception during and after breast cancer treatment. Non-hormonal forms of contraception, such as condoms, diaphragms, intrauterine contraceptive devices (IUDs) or male or female sterilization are usually preferred.

Side effects of hormonal therapy has to be explained. Vitamin D and calcium could be advised as nutritional supplements. A dual energy X-ray absorption scan (DEXA) is recommended to allow early treatment of osteoporosis. Bisphosphonates could be used in patients with iatrogenic premature menopause and in post-menopausal patients treated with AIs to prevent bone mineral loss. Hot flashes should be managed without hormonal therapy. Vaginal dryness and atrophy is usually overcame with non-hormonal lubricants and if needed, low dose vaginal estrogen therapy can be used after discussing the risks with patients.

Patients on Tamoxifen are at higher risk of developing endometrial cancer so pelvic exam and pap smear every 12 months for patients with intact uterus.

4.3   Locally Advanced Stage Breast Cancer

Overview
Epidemiology
The incidence of breast cancer is increased by approximately 4% every year by the use of more widely screening mammography. Almost 7% of the new breast cancer have primary tumors larger more than 5 cm and 30% of them have positive lymph node metastases.

Pathology
Usually invasive ductal and lobular carcinoma were the most commonly seen histopathologies. It is unusual to present as locally advanced cancer for histologically "favorable "tumors such as tubular, medullary carcinomas.

Diagnosis
Patients usually admit to medical centers with palpable breast mass. As the disease grows within breast, tumor could infiltrate the dermis or pectoral muscle. Skin retraction could be seen due to the attachment of Cooper's ligament. Also the infiltration of dermal lymphatics, edema can occur and this clinical sign is called "peau d'orange". The evaluation for distant metastases includes contrast-enhanced computed tomography (CT) of chest, and abdomen, bone scintigraphy or whole-body integrated fluorodeoxyglucose positron emission tomography.

Definitive Treatment
Locally advanced breast cancer consists of a wide range of breast cancer patients, both operable and inoperable. The current standard of treatment usually depends on the biological factors of the primary tumor. The multidisciplinary evaluation of the patients is crucial. As a primary choice, the multimodal therapy could start with neoadjuvant chemotherapy for patients with high grade tumor, triple negative biology, HER2 positive and high lymph node tumor load. Approximately %80–90 of the patients demonstrated partial or complete response to chemotherapy. Administrating surgery first could be a suitable option for stage IIIA patients. Patients having Estrogen and/or progesterone receptor positivity in pathology examination, they are candidates for hormonal treatment.

Keywords: Locally advanced stage breast cancer, Radiotherapy

4.3.1   Case Presentation

A 36 year old woman presented with a self-palpated left breast mass. Her detailed physical breast examination revealed a 7 cm palpable mobile hard mass located under areolar region and several large axillary lymph nodes with limited mobility. Her mammogram revealed multiple areas of heterogeneity, disseminated microcalcifications and ultrasound revealed several enlarged left axillary lymph nodes, the largest measuring 29 mm by 22 mm with a thickened cortices, and replaced hilar fat. She had no history of pregnancy and used hormonal contraception for the last 5 years. She denied previous radiation exposure. She was premenopausal. She had no additional history of any other disease. She did not smoke or consume alcohol. She had no family history of cancer.

A Core needle biopsy confirmed a high grade invasive ductal carcinoma (IDC), which was ER (+), PR(+), HER 2 (3+) and Ki 67 25%. A PET-CT scan revealed almost 8 cm an FDG avid mass (SUV max: 9.3) that measured almost 8 cm located at the lower part of breast and multiple axillary FGD positive lymph nodes. She had no evidence of distant metastatic disease and was staged as cT3N2M0.

Neoadjuvant chemotherapy with dose-dense AC protocol followed by paclitaxel and trastuzumab with pertuzumab was administrated. She had excellent clinical response and the primary mass and the axillary lymph nodes were completely undetectable by physical examination at the end of the treatment although the breast ultrasound still showed heterogeneous areas of increased echogenicity. Afterwards, she underwent left mastectomy and expander placement and axillary lymph node dissection after the sentinel node revealed a 1.7 mm micrometastasis. Postoperative pathology revealed no cancer cells but a fibrous area with a denser stroma which measured 80 mm by 24 mm. Apart from the single metastatic lymph node detected by the sentinel lymph node biopsy, there were no other lymph nodes with breast cancer metastasis. However, there was evidence of prior involvement with metastatic disease as evidenced by hyalinized stromal scars in 3 other lymph nodes (1mic/10). She was staged as ypT0ypN0mic.

Conventional fractionated whole chest wall tangent, MI, Supraclavicular field were planned for 25 fractions. Deep breath hold technique was used to spare heart. She will continue Herceptin and start Tamoxifen.

4.3.1.1 Patient Evaluation

Patients with locally advanced breast cancer, frequently admits to hospital after detecting a breast mass on self-examination. Mostly, regional lymphadenopathy is present at the time of diagnosis of T3 or T4 primary breast cancers. Pain, limited range of motion, edema, and weakness or numbness of the arm could be a part of presentation of disease due to an advanced axillary or supraclavicular adenopathy. The history of presenting signs and symptoms is the critical to classify a breast cancer as inflammatory. All patients has to be evaluated with a comprehensive initial history and physical examination to distinguish inflammatory breast cancer from other T4 tumors. The breast examination should include breast asymmetry, mass size, skin erythema or edema, and skin or nipple retraction. Mobility of the primary mass should be experienced. Skin edema is best evaluated with the patient in the supine position. Edema of the skin causes thickening, which makes the hair follicles more prominent, resulting in the classic "peau d'orange" appearance. The axilla and infraclavicular and supraclavicular fossae should be examined with the patient upright, and regional adenopathy should be described to include the size, consistency, and mobility of axillary, infraclavicular, and supraclavicular lymph nodes.

In addition to breast symptoms, the history should include questions related to the changes in general health and to symptoms possibly due to metastases such as persistent bone pain, or neurological changes. Incontrast to the general approach of early-stage disease, the patients with T3 or T4 tumors are usually treated with neoadjuvant chemotherapy, so careful pretreatment evaluation of disease is important to lead locoregional therapies.

4.3.2 Evidence Based Treatment Recommendations

Locally advanced stage III-IV breast cancer patients are usually treated with a combined-modality approach where SEER data have revealed that patients with advanced-stage disease, treated with a combination treatment approach have 5-year survival rates of approximately 70% [72]. Multidisciplinary evaluation of the patients is crucial [73]. Even mastectomy followed by adjuvant chemotherapy and radiation therapy is standard therapeutic approach, the neoadjuvant use of chemotherapy before surgery is rising in especially cases, reduction in the size of the primary tumor and nodal metastases is essential [74]. The advantage of neoadjuvant chemotherapy is the evaluation of the tumor's response to chemotherapy and providing complete response which individual prognosis change. The two largest trials that compared neoadjuvant and adjuvant chemotherapy found that delivering chemotherapy before surgery provided no overall survival advantage compared to delivering chemotherapy after surgery [75, 76]. The National Surgical Adjuvant Breast and Bowel Project (NSABP) B-18 randomized 1523 patients with early-stage, operable breast cancer to receive four cycles of doxorubicin/cyclophosphamide (AC) either before or after surgical treatment [75]. The overall survival and disease-free survival rates were nearly identical between the two groups [77]. The increasing use of neoadjuvant chemotherapy has raised many questions concerning the surgical and radiotherapeutic management of patients with locally advanced breast cancer. Especially the use of sentinel lymph node and use of postmastectomy radiotherapy are the main clinical questions that have been debated.

4.3.2.1 Recommended Treatment Options

Stage IIB (T3N0) and IIIA patients, could be either neoadjuvant chemo followed by surgery (mastectomy or breast conserving surgery) and RT as indicated, or surgery with following adjuvant chemo, HT, and/or trastuzumab RT as indicated.

Stage IIIB–IIIC patients, usually treatment starts with neoadjuvant chemo followed by surgery (mastectomy or breast conserving surgery and radiotherapy.

4.3.2.2 Post Mastectomy Radiotherapy

A modified radical mastectomy (resection of the breast, pectoralis fascia, and levels I and II axillary lymph nodes) remains the most common surgical treatment for patients with locally advanced breast cancer. Postmastectomy radiation therapy (PMRT) aids this cohort of patients by decreasing locoregional recurrence and improving overall survival. Historically, it was looked into whether the benefits of postmastectomy radiation were blurred by its long term cardiac toxicity. First meta-analysis in 1987 came from Cusik et al., reporting a poorer survival with PMRT [78]. Later, the Early Breast Cancer Trialists' Collaborative Group (EBCTCG) has performed a more broad meta-analyses of trials investigating postmastectomy radiation therapy [79]. This analysis included 9933 patients treated on clinical trials with mastectomy, axillary clearance with or without PMRT. The results clearly established that PMRT reduced isolated locoregional recurrence rate for patients with lymph node-positive disease treated with mastectomy (15-year isolated locoregional recurrence rate 29% vs 8%). Improvement of locoregional control also reduced the 15-year breast cancer mortality rate from 60% to 55% with radiation [79]. Many of the trials included in meta-analyses included patients at low risk for locoregional recurrence, used unconventional radiation doses, fractionation patterns, and radiation field designs, and enrolled patients of earlier era where systemic therapies were either less effective or entirely omitted. Van de Steene et al. steered a similar meta-analysis excluding trials that began before 1970, trials with small number of patients, and trials that used unconventional fractionation schedules. The analysis revealed that overall survival improved reducing odds of death by 12.4% by PMRT [80]. In addition, Whelan et al performed a meta-analysis of the published PMRT trials that included systemic therapy in both treatment arms, showed that the use of radiation after mastectomy was also shown to reduce the risk of any recurrence and mortality [81].

Practice changing studies have come from The Danish Breast Cancer Cooperative Group. In (DBCCG) 82b and 82c studies, patients randomized to receive radiation therapy in these studies had a lower 18-year rate of locoregional recurrence and a higher 18-year overall survival rate (Table 4.3) [82, 83]. Also Vancouver, British Columbia trial randomized 318 women who are premenopausal with lymph node-positive disease to receive mastectomy and CMF chemotherapy with or without PMRT and confirmed the promising results of PMRT use [84]. Randomized PMRT trials are summarized in Table 4.3.

The guidelines recommend radiation after mastectomy for patients with 1–3 positive lymph nodes who have had axillary node surgery. Still, some of these women have such a low risk of recurrence that the side effects of radiation overshadow its benefits. For this group of patients, factors that could decrease the risk of

Table 4.3 Randomized trials evaluating post mastectomy radiotherapy after mastectomy

Trial	No of patients	Locoregional recurrences(%)	Distant metastases rates	Overall survival(%)
Danish 82b	1708	9		54
Radiation no radiation		32		45
Danish 82c	1375	8		45
Radiation no radiation		35		36
Danish 82b /82 c	3083	14		37
Radiation no radiation		49		27
Vancouver	318	10		47
		26		37

Consensus indications for PMRT [85]
T3/4 (T3N0 controversial)
≥4+ nodes
Close/positive margins.
1–3 positive lymph nodes (controversial)

recurrence or increase the risk of radiation side effects such as being older than 45, other medical conditions that could limit a woman's life expectancy, other medical conditions that could increase the risk of side effects, having only 1 positive lymph node, luminal A subtype, the presence of extracapsular extension greater than 2 mm, tumor size larger than 4 cm, positive or close (<2 mm) surgical margins, lymphovascular space invasion, invasion of the skin, nipple, or pectoralis muscle could impact the choice of treatment [85]. The going SUPREMO trial randomized about 1600 pts with high-risk node-negative or 1–3 positive nodes to PMRT or not [86]. Results would help clarify the clinical approach to this topic.

4.3.2.3 Postmastectomy Radiation Therapy after Neoadjuvant Chemotherapy

Neoadjuvant chemotherapy changes the extent of pathological disease in 80% to 90% of cases. 3088 patients treated on NSABP B-18 and B-27 treated with neoadjuvant chemotherapy and radiation therapy was not allowed [75]. The findings revealed that the response to neoadjuvant chemotherapy correlated with risk of loco regional recurrence, meaning that chemotherapy response may also predict which patients require radiation therapy. In detail, patients who had pathologic complete response in both the primary tumor and the axillary nodes had the lowest risk of locoregional recurrence, whereas patients with residual invasive disease in the breast who were pathologically node-negative had an intermediate risk of locoregional recurrence and patients with residual positive lymph nodes had the highest risk of locoregional recurrence [75]. M. D. Anderson compared the outcomes of 579 patients who received neoadjuvant chemotherapy, mastectomy, and radiation therapy with those of 136 patients who were treated with neoadjuvant chemotherapy and mastectomy alone on prospective clinical trials. Despite the imbalances in both T and N clinical stage, the locoregional recurrence rate was significantly lower in the patients treated with PMRT than in those treated with neoadjuvant chemotherapy and mastectomy alone (10-year locoregional recurrence rates were 8% and 22%, respectively, p = 0.001) [87]. In multivariate analysis, PMRT was showed to be associated with improved cause-specific survival, (HR = 0.49; 95% CI, 0.34 to 0.71; p < 0.001) and locoregional recurrence-free survival (HR = 0.21; 95% CI, 0.12 to 0.37; p < 0.001). Patients with clinical stage III breast cancer who achieve a pathologic complete response to neoadjuvant chemotherapy still had high locoregional recurrence rate (3%—PMRT vs 33% no PMRT (p = 0.006)).

On the basis of MD Anderson data, PMRT is usually recommend for all patients with clinical T3 or T4 tumors or clinical stage III disease regardless of their response to neoadjuvant chemotherapy [88]. In clinical stage I or II breast cancer scenario, PMRT should be advised for patients with four or more positive lymph nodes after chemotherapy and for the unusual patient in whom the disease progresses and the primary tumor exceeds 5 cm in diameter [89].

4.3.2.4 Regional Lymphatic Irradiation

Two large radiation oncology studies (the National Cancer Institute of Canada (NCIC) MA.20 trial and the European Organization for Research and Treatment of Cancer (EORTC) 22,922 trial) evaluated whether more extensive lymphatic treatment benefited patients with higher-risk lymph node-negative, or lower risk lymph node-positive disease [90]. The NCIC MA.20 trial enrolled women diagnosed with early-stage, node-positive (pN1–3) or high-risk, node-negative breast cancer treated with BCS and adjuvant chemotherapy [90, 91]. High-risk features are listed as pT3N0 or pT2N0 with fewer than 10 axillary lymph nodes removed and a least one of the following: grade 3 histology, estrogen-receptor negativity, or lymphovascular invasion. Patients were randomized to either whole breast irradiation ± RNI. Approximately 85% of the patients had 1–3 positive lymph nodes. At 10-years, RNI was linked with a statistically significant improvement in DFS from 77% to 82% (P: 0.01) [90]. The EORTC 22922, consists more than 4000 breast cancer patients with a central/medially located tumor or a peripherally located tumor with axillary involvement, randomized patients to ± RNI (defined as radiotherapy to the IMC and medial SCV) after BCS or mastectomy. A significant decrease in breast cancer mortality with RNI (12.5% vs. 14.4%, P: 0.02) was demonstrated in addition to improved DFS (72.1% vs. 69.1%, P: 0.04) and distant- DFS (78% vs 75.5%; P: 0.02) [91]. None of the trials proved a long-term OS benefit after RNI [92].

A meta-analysis of these two studies proposed that the addition of regional nodal irradiation (RNI) to the level III axillary, supraclavicular and upper internal mammary lymph nodes provide an improvement in disease free survival and distant metastasis free survival as well as a 1–2% overall survival advantage [93]. Despite all these findings, patients with 1–3 positive lymph nodes or high-risk, node negative stage II breast cancer require customized field design based on clinical and pathological findings when considering RNI. These factors could be listed as favorable histology, luminal A/B subtypes, low Oncotype DX score, and none or micrometastatic nodal involvement after a SLN dissection only [92].

4.3.2.5 RNI Field Design Recommendation

- Low risk stage II: Inclusion of the level I/II axilla within the tangent fields were recommended.
- High risk stage II disease: consider RT to all ipsilateral
- Lymphatic stations, which are the level I-III axilla, supraclavicular
- Fossa, and the internal mammary nodes. If an ALND (defined as 10 or more lymph nodes resected) was performed, the level I/II axilla can be excluded from the fields.
- Neoadjuvant chemotherapy: Comprehensive radiotherapy to all regional lymphatics

4.3.2.6 Postmastectomy and Reconstruction

The role of adjuvant radiotherapy and reconstruction in the treatment of breast cancer are evolving. The most common used options are either two stages of the reconstruction procedure or permanent implant. There were no prospective randomized controlled trials, and all were retrospective cohorts or controlled groups studies. Up to date, there are eight studies evaluating the two stages of reconstruction methods either with expander or permanent implants. A metaanalysis of all studies, representing 899 cases, reported that the risks for reconstruction failure and major complication requiring reoperation tended to be higher in the group with tissue expanders compared to implants but the differences were not significant. Importantly, the group of tissue expanders had a significantly lower risk of severe capsular contracture (relative risk, 0.44; P < 0.001).

Another metaanalysis comprising 5314 patients, reported the complications and satisfaction of patients who received PMRT or not after mastectomy and an immediate prosthetic breast reconstruction (1069 PMRT vs 4245 non-PMRT). Primary outcomes revealed a statistically significant increase in overall complications [odds ratio (OR) 3.45; 95% confidence interval (95% CI) 2.62–4.54; P < 0.00001], reconstruction failure (OR: 2.59; 95% CI 1.46–4.62; P = 0.001), and capsular contracture (OR: 5.26, 95% CI: 2.73–10.13, P < 0.00001) after receiving PMRT. Even PMRT for patients who underwent immediate implant-based breast reconstruction led to higher risks of reconstruction failure, to preserve body health, breast both immediate or delayed reconstruction are commonly preferred surgical methods. Due to the low level of evidence and insufficient sample sizes, further studies are needed to support evidence-based decision making, especially to distinguish the patients characteristics and treatment factors that effects failure and contracture rates.

4.3.2.7 Breath Hold-Cardiac Sparing Methods

Breast cancer radiotherapy reduces the risk of cancer recurrence and death demonstrated by randomized trials, but as meta-analyses also have found an increase in cardiac deaths following breast cancer radiotherapy associated with the volume of the heart receiving 5 Gy or more [79]. Darby et al. directed a population-based case-control study reporting major coronary events, that includes 2168 women treated with radiotherapy for breast cancer between 1958 and 2001 in Sweden and Denmark. The overall average of the mean doses to the whole heart was 4.9 Gy (range, 0.03–27.72) and the rates of major coronary events were linked with a 7% increase in risk of ischemic events per gray increase in mean heart dose with no apparent threshold [94]. This effect of radiation on heart was growing within the first 5 years after therapy and cardiac risk factors before radiotherapy was not significantly associated with those changes.

In clinical practice, there are two commercially available devices: active breathing coordinator™ (ABC_DIBH) (Elekta, Crawley, UK) and Varian RPM system guiding patients to hold their breath while radiotherapy is delivered, which pushes the heart down and away from the radiotherapy field. This technique requires additional cost, education of staff and time consuming procedure depending on patient's capacity and therapist's experience. In a dosimetric analysis, free and breath hold technique were planned with both forward and inverse IMRT presenting a significant decrease of radiation exposure to the contralateral breast, left and right ventricles, as well as proximal and especially distal LAD by breath hold with forward IMRT, as inverse IMRT provided no additional advantage [95]. Another positive study reported that deep inspiration breath hold plans proven large reductions of dose to the heart compared with left-sided FB plans; V20Gy of the heart is reduced from 7.8% to 2.3%, V40Gy from 3.4% to 0.3% and mean dose from 5.2 to 2.7 Gy (−48%, p < 0.0001) [96].

Besides the routine use of deep breath old techniques for left breast cancer patients, Essers et al. showed that the gain of this technique for right breast treatment without IMN, the average mean lung dose reduced from 6.5 to 5.4 Gy for the total lung and from 11.2 to 9.7 Gy for the ipsilateral lung while if internal mammaria lymph node irradiation is added, significant gain will continue for lung doses [97]. A multicenter study conducted at the Royal Marsden Hospital (Sutton, UK) to evaluate the feasibility and heart-sparing ability of the voluntary breath-hold (VBH) technique. Mean cardiac doses (Gy) for free-breathing and VBH techniques, respectively, were: heart 1.8 and 1.1, LAD 12.1 and 5.4, maximum LAD 35.4 and 24.1 (all

P < 0.001). Median CT and treatment session times were reported as 21 and 22 min, respectively. The UK HeartSpare Study, has confirmed that interfraction reproducibility with the voluntary breath hold technique is analogous to the performed with the spirometry-based device [98].

As a conclusion, to date, there is only retrospective or dosimetric studies were presented and no data studying the clinical benefits and oncological outcomes for patients treated with this technique. Especially the cardiac data will be presented in 15–20 years.

Treatment recommendations for locally advanced breast cancer according to NCCN guidelines are summarized in Table 4.4 [99].

Table 4.4 NCCN guidelines for locally advanced breast cancer

Large primary ± regional adenopathy			
Preoperative systemic treatment	Response	Mastectomy and surgical staging+ reconstruction or lumpectomy with axillary staging	• Complete planned chemotherapy if not completed before surgery • Consider adjuvant capecitabine in patients with triple negative breast cancer and residual invasive cancer following standard neoadjuvant treatment with taxane and anthracycline based chemotherapy • Adjuvant radiation therapy to the breast/chest wall, infraclavicular area, internal mammary nodes and any part of the axillary bed at risk • Adjuvant endocrine therapy if RE positive and /or PR positive • If HER-2 positive, complete up to 1 year of HER-2 targeted therapy with trastuzumab ± pertuzumab. İt could be given concurrently with radiation therapy and with endocrine therapy if indicated.
	No response	Consider additional systemic chemotherapy and / or preoperative radiation	• If there is response—see above • No response- individualized treatment
Early- locally advanced tumor or Resectable	Mastectomy Lumpectomy SLNB±ALND	Adjuvant chemotherapy	• Adjuvant radiation therapy to the breast/chest wall, infraclavicular area, internal mammary nodes and any part of the axillary bed at risk • Adjuvant endocrine therapy if RE positive and /or PR positive • If HER-2 positive, complete up to 1 year of HER-2 targeted therapy with trastuzumab ± pertuzumab. İt could be given concurrently with radiation therapy and with endocrine therapy if indicated

4.3.2.8 Postmastectomy Radiation Technique

Radiation treatment plays a critical role in the management of locally advanced breast cancer. Generally the initial target volume should include the breast and chest wall and draining lymphatics such as the undissected axillary apex and the supraclavicular fossa lymph nodes.

4.3.2.9 Steps of Simulation

1. Patients should be immobilized with their ipsilateral arm abducted (90° to 120°) and externally rotated. Please check the soft tissues of the arm cranial to the junction of the tangent and supraclavicular fossa field to avoid unnecessary irradiation of the proximal arm. Also skin folds within the supraclavicular fossa should be flattened as much as possible (Fig. 4.9).

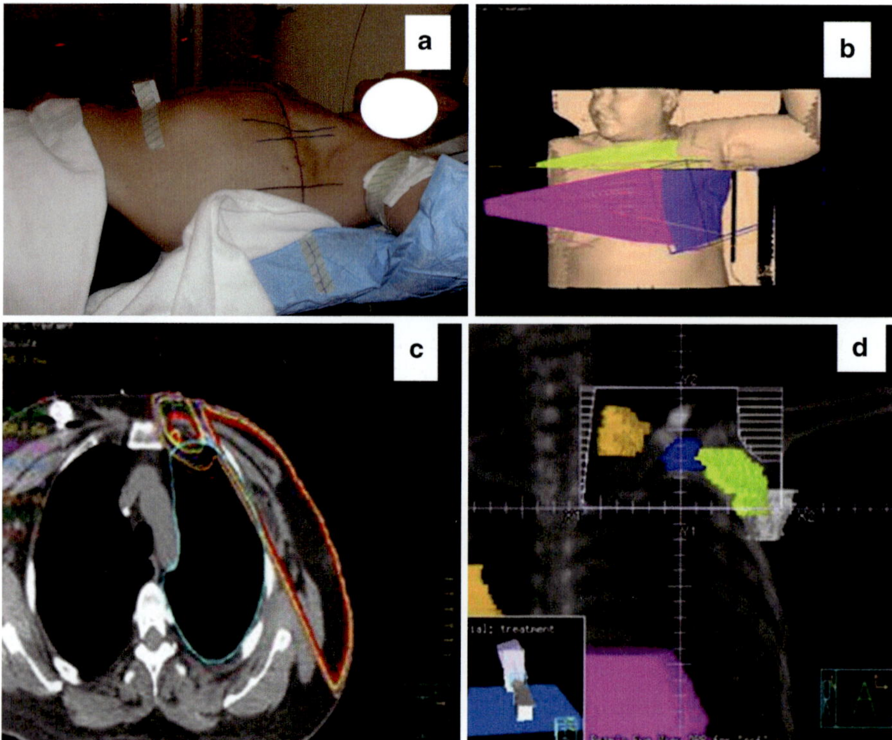

Fig. 4.9 (**a**) Set-up position of the patients (breast elevated board- blue med-tec). Head was turned to the contralateral side. In order to keep upper part of the supraclavicular field flat, arm is abducted almost with 90°. If soft tissue of the arm hangs down, we usually tape the arm to make sure that it is not effected from the tangent field as shown in (**b**) Field arrangement on skin rendering view (**c**) Axial view of dose distribution (**d**) Levels of axillary region are presented. Orange: supraclavicular, blue: level 3, green: level 2, white: level 1

2. Patients are placed on a 5° to 15° angle board to flatten the slope of the chest wall in the region of the sternum.

3. Radiopaque wires are placed on the surgical scar(s), drain sites, and clinical treatment borders. The border between the chest wall/breast field and the supraclavicular field is typically placed at the bottom of the clavicular head.

4. Please check anterior view of the supraclavicular field to estimate the lung volume. IF the volume seems larger, the angle of the board could be lowered or the border between supraclavicular and tangents could be raised.

5. 3 mm CT images are obtained and isocenters are marked.

6. On CT images, tumor bed (for cases of breast conservation), the internal mammary artery and vein in the upper three interspaces (i.e., from the caudal edge of the first rib to the cranial edge of the fourth rib), and the dissected level III axillary apex lymph nodes are delineated. Tangent fields are created with matched, nondivergent deep and cranial borders by using a kick of the couch. The nondivergent deep border is typically achieved by the gantry rotation or the use of a half-beam block. The collimators are rotated to match the chest wall slope, and any volume that extends cranially above the match line into the supraclavicular field is blocked. (Fig. 4.10)

7. Internal mammary could be covered by tangents or separate AP fields.

8. A supraclavicular field is rotated 10° to −20° to be off the spinal cord and esophagus.

9. For patients with advanced disease, we typically place the fields to encompass axillary nodal groups at least with a dose of 45 Gy

10. The medial chest wall and internal mammary lymph nodes are treated with a medial electron field that includes the contoured internal mammary vessels and is angled 15 to 30 or more degrees. The angle is selected to minimize the cold triangle at the junction between the electron and tangent fields, with coverage ≥35 Gy at the cold triangle considered acceptable (Fig. 4.11).

11. Accept coverage of contoured nodal targets with the 90% isodose line.

12. Field-in-field technique using static forward-planned IMRT often used to optimize dose distribution.(Fig. 4.3)

13. Ipsilateral lung V20 is limited to ≤10% with two- field tangents and ≤20% with three-field (SCV) technique.

14. Left ventricle and combined bilateral ventricle limits: V5 ≤10% and V25 ≤5%. Also record and attempt to minimize whole heart dose (less than 4 Gy). Deep inspiration breath hold respiratory gating, prone positioning, and/or MLC blocking may be used to minimize dose to lung and heart. (Fig. 4.12)

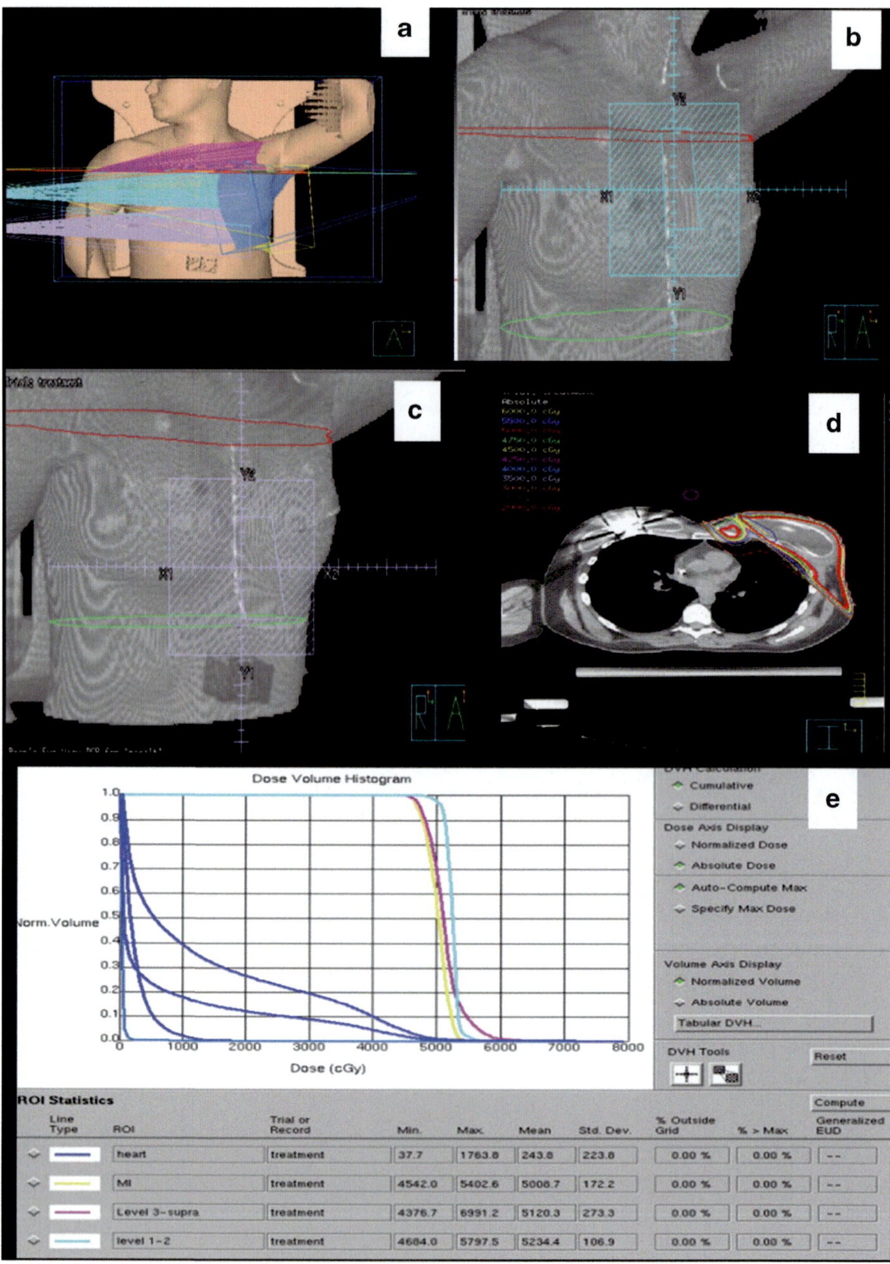

Fig. 4.10 (**a**) Set-up of fields on patient body (**b**) and (**c**). Blocks of upper and lower MI electron fields. The energy of upper electron field is higher than the lower field. The aim with this is to cover IMC nodes with at least 45 Gy while minimizing the dose to heart and coronary arteries. (**d**) Axial view of dose distribution. We maintain at least 39 Gy isodose line as continuous. (**e**) DVH evaluation

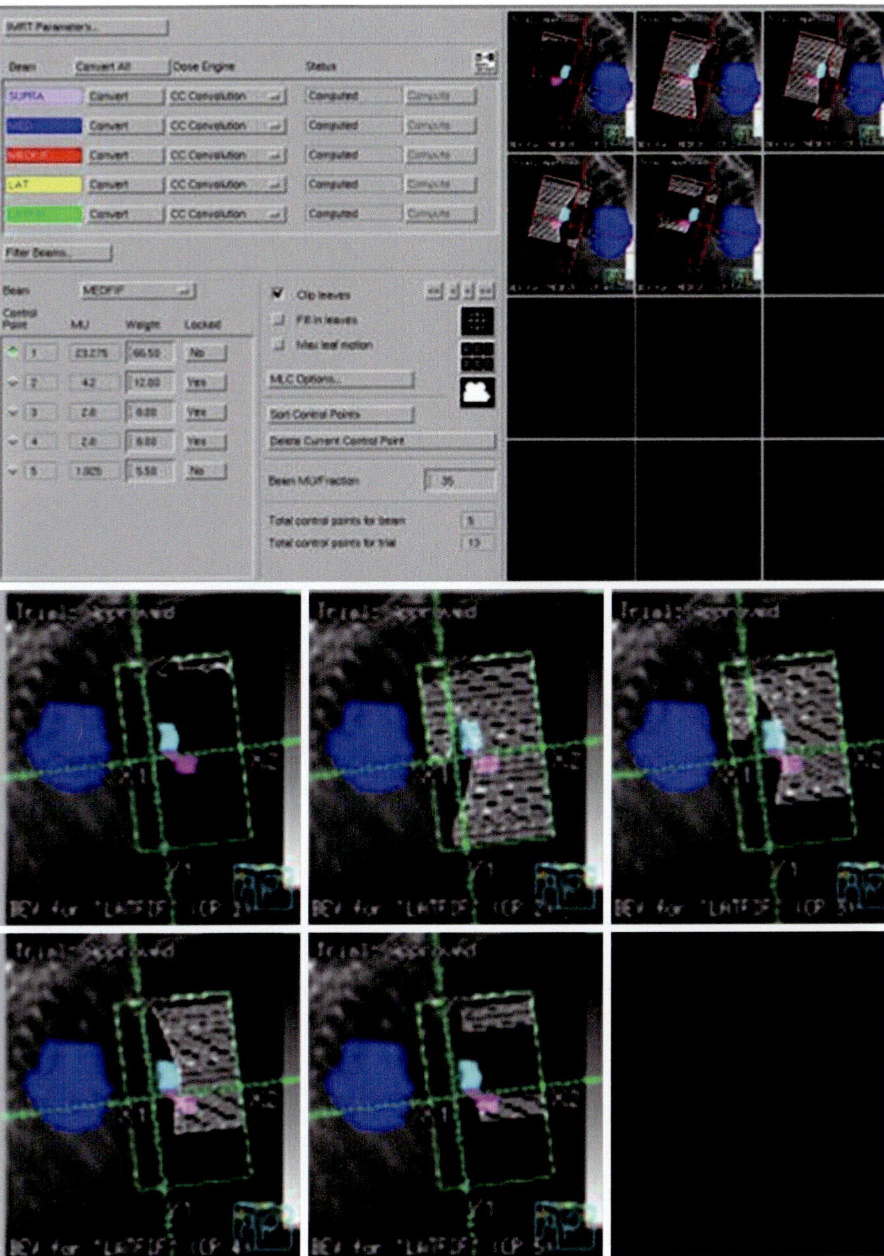

Fig. 4.11 Field and field—Forward IMRT technique for locally advanced breast planning. Tumor bed: light blue, incision: pink, heart: blue

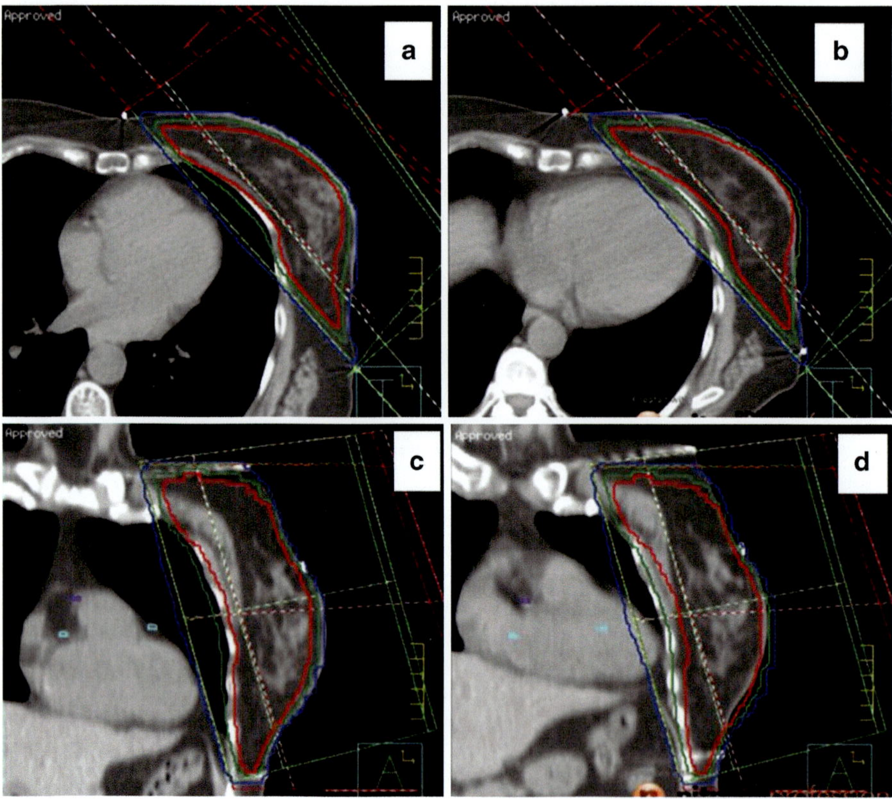

Fig. 4.12 Field arrangements for (**a**) Forward IMRT with Breath hold, (**b**) Forward IMRT with free breathing, (Red line—50 Gy, Green line—47.5 G, Blue line—25 Gy.). (**c**) Forward IMRT with Breath hold, (**d**) Forward IMRT with free breathing, Coronal view of isodose distribution; Red line—50 Gy, Green line—47.5 G, Blue line—25 Gy

Breast borders: superior Clinical reference + 2nd rib insertion; inferior Clinical reference + loss of CT apparent breast; anterior skin; posterior Excludes pectoralis m., chest wall, ribs; medial Sternal-rib junction; lateral Clinical reference + mid axillary line typically excluded latissimus dorsi m.

Chest wall borders: superior Caudal border of the clavicular head; inferior Clinical reference + loss of CT apparent contralateral breast; anterior skin; posterior Rib-pleural interface; included pectoralis m., chest wall, ribs; medial Sternal-rib junction; lateral Clinical reference + mid axillary line typically excluded latissimus dorsi m.

Axilla level I borders: superior Axillary vessels cross lateral edge of pec minor m.; inferior Pec major m. insert into ribs; anterior Plane defined by: anterior surface of pec major m and latissimus dorsi m.; posterior Ant surface of subscapularis m.; medial Lat border of pec minor m.; lateral Med border of latissimus dorsi m.

Axilla level II borders: superior Axillary vessels cross medial edge of pec minor m.; inferior Axillary vessels cross lateral edge of pec minor m.; anterior Ant surface of pec minor m.; posterior Ribs and intercostal m.; medial Med border of pec minor m.; lateral Lat border of pec minor m

Axilla level III borders: superior Pec minor m. insert on coracoid; inferior Axillary vessels cross medial edge of pec minor m.; anterior Post surface of pec major m.; posterior Ribs and intercostal m.; medial Thoracic inlet; lateral Med border of pec minor m.

Supraclavicular borders: superior Caudal to coracoid cartilage; inferior Junction of brachioceph-axillary vn./caudal edge clavicular head; anterior Sternocleidomastoid m.; posterior Ant aspect of the scalene m.; medial Excludes thyroid and trachea; lateral Cranial: lat edge of SCM m. caudal: junction first rib and clavicle.

Internal mammary borders: superior Sup aspect of the medial first rib; inferior Cranial aspect of the fourth rib.

References

1. Kamińska M, et al. Breast cancer risk factors. Prz Menopauzalny. 2015;14(3):196–202.
2. Nelson HD, et al. Risk factors for breast Cancer for women age 40 to 49: a systematic review and meta-analysis. Ann Intern Med. 2012;156(9):635–48.
3. Land CE. Radiation and breast cancer risk. Prog Clin Biol Res. 1997;396:115–24.
4. Lahham A, ALMasri H, Kameel S. Estimation of female radiation doses and breast Cancer risk from chest Ct examinations. Radiat Prot Dosimetry. 2017;179:303–9.
5. U.S. Preventive Services Task Force. Risk assessment, genetic counseling, and genetic testing for brca-related cancer in women: recommendation statement. Am Fam Physician. 2015;91(2):118A–E.
6. Lax SF. Hereditary breast and ovarian cancer. Pathologe. 2017;38(3):149–55.
7. Rebbeck TR, Kauff ND, Domchek SM. Meta-analysis of risk reduction estimates associated with risk-reducing salpingo-oophorectomy in BRCA1 or BRCA2 mutation carriers. J Natl Cancer Inst. 2009;101(2):80–7.
8. Schenberg T, et al. MRI screening for breast cancer in women at high risk; is the Australian breast MRI screening access program addressing the needs of women at high risk of breast cancer? J Med Radiat Sci. 2015;62(3):212–25.
9. Saslow D, et al. American Cancer Society guidelines for breast screening with MRI as an adjunct to mammography. CA Cancer J Clin. 2007;57(2):75–89.
10. Page DL, Rogers LW. Combined histologic and cytologic criteria for the diagnosis of mammary atypical ductal hyperplasia. Hum Pathol. 1992;23(10):1095–7.
11. Silverstein MJ, et al. Prognostic classification of breast ductal carcinoma-in-situ. Lancet. 1995;345(8958):1154–7.
12. Solin LJ, et al. A multigene expression assay to predict local recurrence risk for ductal carcinoma in situ of the breast. J Natl Cancer Inst. 2013;105(10):701–10.
13. Rudloff U, et al. Nomogram for predicting the risk of local recurrence after breast-conserving surgery for ductal carcinoma in situ. J Clin Oncol. 2010;28(23):3762–9.
14. Giuliano AE, Edge SB, Hortobagyi GN. Eighth edition of the AJCC Cancer staging manual: breast cancer. Ann Surg Oncol. 2018;25(7):1783–5.
15. Gradishar WJ, et al. Breast cancer, version 4.2017, NCCN clinical practice guidelines in oncology. J Natl Compr Cancer Netw. 2018;16(3):310–20.

16. Tunon-De-Lara C, et al. Analysis of 676 cases of ductal carcinoma in situ of the breast from 1971 to 1995: diagnosis and treatment—the experience of one institute. Am J Clin Oncol. 2001;24(6):531–6.
17. Vargas C, et al. Factors associated with local recurrence and cause-specific survival in patients with ductal carcinoma in situ of the breast treated with breast-conserving therapy or mastectomy. Int J Radiat Oncol Biol Phys. 2005;63(5):1514–21.
18. Hassett MJ, et al. Treating second breast events after breast-conserving surgery for ductal carcinoma in situ. J Natl Compr Cancer Netw. 2018;16(4):387–94.
19. Frank S, et al. Ductal carcinoma in situ (DCIS) treated by mastectomy, or local excision with or without radiotherapy: a monocentric, retrospective study of 608 women. Breast. 2016;25:51–6.
20. EORTC Breast Cancer Cooperative Group, et al. Breast-conserving treatment with or without radiotherapy in ductal carcinoma-in-situ: ten-year results of European Organisation for Research and Treatment of Cancer randomized phase III trial 10853—a study by the EORTC Breast Cancer Cooperative Group and EORTC Radiotherapy Group. J Clin Oncol. 2006;24(21):3381–7.
21. Wapnir IL, et al. Long-term outcomes of invasive ipsilateral breast tumor recurrences after lumpectomy in NSABP B-17 and B-24 randomized clinical trials for DCIS. J Natl Cancer Inst. 2011;103(6):478–88.
22. Cuzick J, et al. Effect of tamoxifen and radiotherapy in women with locally excised ductal carcinoma in situ: long-term results from the UK/ANZ DCIS trial. Lancet Oncol. 2011;12(1):21–9.
23. Warnberg F, et al. Effect of radiotherapy after breast-conserving surgery for ductal carcinoma in situ: 20 years follow-up in the randomized SweDCIS trial. J Clin Oncol. 2014;32(32):3613–8.
24. Goodwin A, et al. Post-operative radiotherapy for ductal carcinoma in situ of the breast. Cochrane Database Syst Rev. 2013;11:CD000563.
25. McCormick B, et al. RTOG 9804: a prospective randomized trial for good-risk ductal carcinoma in situ comparing radiotherapy with observation. J Clin Oncol. 2015;33(7):709–15.
26. Allred DC, et al. Adjuvant tamoxifen reduces subsequent breast cancer in women with estrogen receptor-positive ductal carcinoma in situ: a study based on NSABP protocol B-24. J Clin Oncol. 2012;30(12):1268–73.
27. Lazzeroni M, et al. Adjuvant therapy in patients with ductal carcinoma in situ of the breast: the Pandora's box. Cancer Treat Rev. 2017;55:1–9.
28. Omlin A, et al. Boost radiotherapy in young women with ductal carcinoma in situ: a multicentre, retrospective study of the rare cancer network. Lancet Oncol. 2006;7(8):652–6.
29. Wong P, et al. Ductal carcinoma in situ—the influence of the radiotherapy boost on local control. Int J Radiat Oncol Biol Phys. 2012;82(2):e153–8.
30. Morrow M, et al. Society of Surgical Oncology-American Society for Radiation Oncology-American Society of Clinical Oncology consensus guideline on margins for breast-conserving surgery with whole-breast irradiation in ductal carcinoma in situ. Pract Radiat Oncol. 2016;6(5):287–95.
31. Oar AJ, et al. Hypofractionated versus conventionally fractionated radiotherapy for ductal carcinoma in situ (DCIS) of the breast. J Med Imaging Radiat Oncol. 2016;60(3):407–13.
32. Williamson D, et al. Local control with conventional and hypofractionated adjuvant radiotherapy after breast-conserving surgery for ductal carcinoma in-situ. Radiother Oncol. 2010;95(3):317–20.
33. Hathout L, et al. Hypofractionated radiation therapy for breast ductal carcinoma in situ. Int J Radiat Oncol Biol Phys. 2013;87(5):1058–63.
34. Nilsson C, Valachis A. The role of boost and hypofractionation as adjuvant radiotherapy in patients with DCIS: a meta-analysis of observational studies. Radiother Oncol. 2015;114(1):50–5.
35. Berliner JL, et al. NSGC practice guideline: risk assessment and genetic counseling for hereditary breast and ovarian Cancer. J Genet Couns. 2013;22(2):155–63.
36. Wellings E. Breast cancer screening for high-risk patients of different ages and risk—which modality is most effective? Cureus. 2016;8(12):e945.

37. Dowsett M, et al. Comparison of PAM50 risk of recurrence score with oncotype DX and IHC4 for predicting risk of distant recurrence after endocrine therapy. J Clin Oncol. 2013;31(22):2783–90.
38. Penault-Llorca F, et al. The 21-gene recurrence score(R) assay predicts distant recurrence in lymph node-positive, hormone receptor-positive, breast cancer patients treated with adjuvant sequential epirubicin- and docetaxel-based or epirubicin-based chemotherapy (PACS-01 trial). BMC Cancer. 2018;18(1):526.
39. Beumer IJ, et al. Prognostic value of MammaPrint(®) in invasive lobular breast Cancer. Biomark Insights. 2016;11:139–46.
40. Cuadros M, Llanos A. Validation and clinical application of MammaPrint(R) in patients with breast cancer. Med Clin (Barc). 2011;136(14):627–32.
41. Aggarwal S, et al. Practical consensus recommendations on management of HR + ve early breast cancer with specific reference to genomic profiling. South Asian J Cancer. 2018;7(2):96–101.
42. Cserni G, et al. The new TNM-based staging of breast cancer. Virchows Arch. 2018;472(5):697–703.
43. Early Breast Cancer Trialists' Collaborative Group, et al. Effect of radiotherapy after breast-conserving surgery on 10-year recurrence and 15-year breast cancer death: meta-analysis of individual patient data for 10,801 women in 17 randomised trials. Lancet. 2011;378(9804):1707–16.
44. Veronesi U, et al. Twenty-year follow-up of a randomized study comparing breast-conserving surgery with radical mastectomy for early breast cancer. N Engl J Med. 2002;347(16):1227–32.
45. Fisher B, et al. Twenty-year follow-up of a randomized trial comparing total mastectomy, lumpectomy, and lumpectomy plus irradiation for the treatment of invasive breast cancer. N Engl J Med. 2002;347(16):1233–41.
46. Louis-Sylvestre C, et al. Axillary treatment in conservative management of operable breast cancer: dissection or radiotherapy? Results of a randomized study with 15 years of follow-up. J Clin Oncol. 2004;22(1):97–101.
47. Krag DN, et al. Sentinel-lymph-node resection compared with conventional axillary-lymph-node dissection in clinically node-negative patients with breast cancer: overall survival findings from the NSABP B-32 randomised phase 3 trial. Lancet Oncol. 2010;11(10):927–33.
48. Jagsi R, et al. Radiation field design in the ACOSOG Z0011 (alliance) trial. J Clin Oncol. 2014;32(32):3600–6.
49. Donker M, et al. Radiotherapy or surgery of the axilla after a positive sentinel node in breast cancer (EORTC 10981-22023 AMAROS): a randomised, multicentre, open-label, phase 3 non-inferiority trial. Lancet Oncol. 2014;15(12):1303–10.
50. Savolt A, et al. Eight-year follow up result of the OTOASOR trial: the optimal treatment of the axilla - surgery or radiotherapy after positive sentinel lymph node biopsy in early-stage breast cancer: a randomized, single Centre, phase III, non-inferiority trial. Eur J Surg Oncol. 2017;43(4):672–9.
51. Savolt A, et al. Does the result of completion axillary lymph node dissection influence the recommendation for adjuvant treatment in sentinel lymph node-positive patients? Clin Breast Cancer. 2013;13(5):364–70.
52. Haviland JS, et al. The UK standardisation of breast radiotherapy (START) trials of radiotherapy hypofractionation for treatment of early breast cancer: 10-year follow-up results of two randomised controlled trials. Lancet Oncol. 2013;14(11):1086–94.
53. Whelan TJ, et al. Long-term results of hypofractionated radiation therapy for breast cancer. N Engl J Med. 2010;362(6):513–20.
54. Owen JR, et al. Effect of radiotherapy fraction size on tumour control in patients with early-stage breast cancer after local tumour excision: long-term results of a randomised trial. Lancet Oncol. 2006;7(6):467–71.
55. Smith BD, et al. Radiation therapy for the whole breast: executive summary of an American Society for Radiation Oncology (ASTRO) evidence-based guideline. Pract Radiat Oncol. 2018;8(3):145–52.

56. Bartelink H, et al. Impact of a higher radiation dose on local control and survival in breast-conserving therapy of early breast cancer: 10-year results of the randomized boost versus no boost EORTC 22881-10882 trial. J Clin Oncol. 2007;25(22):3259–65.
57. Romestaing P, et al. Role of a 10-Gy boost in the conservative treatment of early breast cancer: results of a randomized clinical trial in Lyon, France. J Clin Oncol. 1997;15(3):963–8.
58. Chen GP, et al. A planning comparison of 7 irradiation options allowed in RTOG 1005 for early-stage breast cancer. Med Dosim. 2015;40(1):21–5.
59. Tsang Y, et al. Clinical impact of IMPORT HIGH trial (CRUK/06/003) on breast radiotherapy practices in the United Kingdom. Br J Radiol. 2015;88(1056):20150453.
60. Coles CE, et al. Partial-breast radiotherapy after breast conservation surgery for patients with early breast cancer (UK IMPORT LOW trial): 5-year results from a multicentre, randomised, controlled, phase 3, non-inferiority trial. Lancet. 2017;390(10099):1048–60.
61. Strnad V, et al. 5-year results of accelerated partial breast irradiation using sole interstitial multicatheter brachytherapy versus whole-breast irradiation with boost after breast-conserving surgery for low-risk invasive and in-situ carcinoma of the female breast: a randomised, phase 3, non-inferiority trial. Lancet. 2016;387(10015):229–38.
62. Polgar C, et al. Breast-conserving therapy with partial or whole breast irradiation: ten-year results of the Budapest randomized trial. Radiother Oncol. 2013;108(2):197–202.
63. NSABP B-39, RTOG 0413: a randomized phase III study of conventional whole breast irradiation versus partial breast irradiation for women with stage 0, I, or II breast cancer. Clin Adv Hematol Oncol. 2006;4(10):719–21.
64. Veronesi U, et al. Intraoperative radiotherapy versus external radiotherapy for early breast cancer (ELIOT): a randomised controlled equivalence trial. Lancet Oncol. 2013;14(13):1269–77.
65. Vaidya JS, et al. Risk-adapted targeted intraoperative radiotherapy versus whole-breast radiotherapy for breast cancer: 5-year results for local control and overall survival from the TARGIT-A randomised trial. Lancet. 2014;383(9917):603–13.
66. Hughes KS, et al. Lumpectomy plus tamoxifen with or without irradiation in women age 70 years or older with early breast cancer: long-term follow-up of CALGB 9343. J Clin Oncol. 2013;31(19):2382–7.
67. Kunkler IH, et al. Breast-conserving surgery with or without irradiation in women aged 65 years or older with early breast cancer (PRIME II): a randomised controlled trial. Lancet Oncol. 2015;16(3):266–73.
68. Potter R, et al. Lumpectomy plus tamoxifen or anastrozole with or without whole breast irradiation in women with favorable early breast cancer. Int J Radiat Oncol Biol Phys. 2007;68(2):334–40.
69. Blamey RW, et al. Radiotherapy or tamoxifen after conserving surgery for breast cancers of excellent prognosis: British Association of Surgical Oncology (BASO) II trial. Eur J Cancer. 2013;49(10):2294–302.
70. Buzdar AU. 'Arimidex' (anastrozole) versus tamoxifen as adjuvant therapy in postmenopausal women with early breast cancer—efficacy overview. J Steroid Biochem Mol Biol. 2003;86(3–5):399–403.
71. Bellon JR, et al. Sequencing of chemotherapy and radiation therapy in early-stage breast cancer: updated results of a prospective randomized trial. J Clin Oncol. 2005;23(9):1934–40.
72. Narod SA, Iqbal J, Miller AB. Why have breast cancer mortality rates declined? J Cancer Policy. 2015;5:8–17.
73. Rajan S, et al. Multidisciplinary decisions in breast cancer: does the patient receive what the team has recommended? Br J Cancer. 2013;108(12):2442–7.
74. Chapman CH, Jagsi R. Postmastectomy radiotherapy after Neoadjuvant chemotherapy: a review of the evidence. Oncology (Williston Park). 2015;29(9):657–66.
75. Rastogi P, et al. Preoperative chemotherapy: updates of National Surgical Adjuvant Breast and bowel project protocols B-18 and B-27. J Clin Oncol. 2008;26(5):778–85.
76. Haddad TC, Goetz MP. Landscape of neoadjuvant therapy for breast cancer. Ann Surg Oncol. 2015;22(5):1408–15.
77. Teshome M, Hunt KK. Neoadjuvant therapy in the treatment of breast cancer. Surg Oncol Clin N Am. 2014;23(3):505–23.

78. Cuzick J, et al. Overview of randomized trials of postoperative adjuvant radiotherapy in breast cancer. Cancer Treat Rep. 1987;71(1):15–29.
79. Clarke M, et al. Effects of radiotherapy and of differences in the extent of surgery for early breast cancer on local recurrence and 15-year survival: an overview of the randomised trials. Lancet. 2005;366(9503):2087–106.
80. Van de Steene J, Soete G, Storme G. Adjuvant radiotherapy for breast cancer significantly improves overall survival: the missing link. Radiother Oncol. 2000;55(3):263–72.
81. Whelan TJ, et al. Does locoregional radiation therapy improve survival in breast cancer? A meta-analysis. J Clin Oncol. 2000;18(6):1220–9.
82. Overgaard M, et al. Evaluation of radiotherapy in high-risk breast cancer patients: report from the Danish breast Cancer cooperative group (DBCG 82) trial. Int J Radiat Oncol Biol Phys. 1990;19(i):1121–4.
83. Overgaard M, Nielsen HM, Overgaard J. Is the benefit of postmastectomy irradiation limited to patients with four or more positive nodes, as recommended in international consensus reports? A subgroup analysis of the DBCG 82 b&c randomized trials. Radiother Oncol. 2007;82(3):247–53.
84. Ragaz J, et al. Locoregional radiation therapy in patients with high-risk breast cancer receiving adjuvant chemotherapy: 20-year results of the British Columbia randomized trial. J Natl Cancer Inst. 2005;97(2):116–26.
85. Recht A, et al. Postmastectomy radiotherapy: an American Society of Clinical Oncology, American Society for Radiation Oncology, and Society of Surgical Oncology focused guideline update. Ann Surg Oncol. 2017;24(1):38–51.
86. Thomas JS, et al. The BIG 2.04 MRC/EORTC SUPREMO trial: pathology quality assurance of a large phase 3 randomised international clinical trial of postmastectomy radiotherapy in intermediate-risk breast cancer. Breast Cancer Res Treat. 2017;163(1):63–9.
87. Huang EH, et al. Postmastectomy radiation improves local-regional control and survival for selected patients with locally advanced breast cancer treated with neoadjuvant chemotherapy and mastectomy. J Clin Oncol. 2004;22(23):4691–9.
88. McGuire SE, et al. Postmastectomy radiation improves the outcome of patients with locally advanced breast cancer who achieve a pathologic complete response to neoadjuvant chemotherapy. Int J Radiat Oncol Biol Phys. 2007;68(4):1004–9.
89. Buchholz TA, et al. Predictors of local-regional recurrence after Neoadjuvant chemotherapy and mastectomy without radiation. J Clin Oncol. 2002;20(1):17–23.
90. Whelan TJ, et al. Regional nodal irradiation in early-stage breast cancer. N Engl J Med. 2015;373(4):307–16.
91. Poortmans PM, et al. Internal mammary and medial supraclavicular irradiation in breast cancer. N Engl J Med. 2015;373(4):317–27.
92. Moreno AC, Shaitelman SF, Buchholz TA. A clinical perspective on regional nodal irradiation for breast cancer. Breast. 2017;34(Suppl 1):S85–s90.
93. Budach W, et al. Adjuvant radiotherapy of regional lymph nodes in breast cancer—a meta-analysis of randomized trials. Radiat Oncol. 2013;8:267.
94. Darby SC, et al. Risk of ischemic heart disease in women after radiotherapy for breast cancer. N Engl J Med. 2013;368(11):987–98.
95. Bolukbasi Y, et al. Reproducible deep-inspiration breath-hold irradiation with forward intensity-modulated radiotherapy for left-sided breast cancer significantly reduces cardiac radiation exposure compared to inverse intensity-modulated radiotherapy. Tumori. 2014;100(2):169–78.
96. Nissen HD, Appelt AL. Improved heart, lung and target dose with deep inspiration breath hold in a large clinical series of breast cancer patients. Radiother Oncol. 2013;106(1):28–32.
97. Essers M, et al. Should breathing adapted radiotherapy also be applied for right-sided breast irradiation? Acta Oncol. 2016;55(4):460–5.
98. Bartlett FR, et al. The UK HeartSpare study (stage II): multicentre evaluation of a voluntary breath-hold technique in patients receiving breast radiotherapy. Clin Oncol (R Coll Radiol). 2017;29(3):e51–6.
99. NCCN guideline/breast cancer. 2018. Last accessed May 2018.

Gastrointestinal System Cancers

5

Pervin Hurmuz, Gozde Yazici, Melis Gultekin,
Sezin Yuce Sari, Mustafa Cengiz, and Gokhan Ozyigit

5.1 Esophagus Cancer

Overview

Epidemiology: Mainly seen in Northern Iran, central Asia and China. Major risk factors are poor nutritional status, low intake of fruits and vegetables, and drinking beverages at high temperatures. In Western countries, obesity, smoking and excessive alcohol consumption account for most cases.

Pathology: Squamous cell carcinoma (SCC) and adenocarcinoma constitute more than 95% of esophageal malignant tumors. Although the incidence of SCC is decreasing in the United States, the incidence of adenocarcinoma arising out of Barrett's esophagus is rising dramatically in the recent decades.

Diagnosis: Patients usually present with progressive dysphagia and weight loss. The diagnosis requires a histologic examination by upper gastrointestinal endoscopy. Endoscopic ultrasound is preferred for locoregional staging. The evaluation for distant metastases includes contrast-enhanced computed tomography (CT) of the neck, chest, and abdomen or whole-body integrated fluorodeoxyglucose positron emission tomography.

Definitive Treatment: Surgery is the mainstay of treatment however combined modality therapy is recommended rather than surgery alone, for patients with locally advanced disease. Trimodality scheme is the treatment of choice for patients with operable stage II or above esophageal cancer. For patients

P. Hurmuz (✉) · G. Yazici · M. Gultekin · S. Y. Sari · M. Cengiz · G. Ozyigit
Department of Radiation Oncology, Faculty of Medicine, Hacettepe University,
Ankara, Turkey

© Springer Nature Switzerland AG 2019
G. Ozyigit, U. Selek (eds.), *Radiation Oncology*,
https://doi.org/10.1007/978-3-319-97145-2_5

with cervical esophageal cancer, inoperable disease or not fit for surgery definitive chemo radiation is an effective treatment option. The delineation of the treatment volumes and the radiation doses depends on the location of the tumor.

Keywords: Esophagus cancer; Radiotherapy

5.1.1 Case Presentation

Our patient was a 57 year-old gentleman with KPS of 100. He applied to the clinics with gradually increasing swallowing difficulty and painful swallowing in last 3 months. Physical examination revealed normal vital signs and systemic physical examination. He had medical history of type 2 DM which is under control for 5 years with oral anti-diabetics. He had a previous history of smoking 30 packs/year, but quitted 2 years ago. He declared drinking alcohol occasionally. His whole blood count, and kidney and liver function tests were normal. Esophago-gastro-duedonoscopy (EGD) revealed ulserovegetative mass located within the 25–35th cm of esophagus covering 1/2 of the lumen. Contrast-enhanced thorax and abdominal computed tomography (CT) showed 85 mm esophageal lesion starting from the level of carina and extending inferiorly. There was suspicion of bronchial invasion by the esophageal mass. However, bronchoscopy showed no evidence of invasion of bronchus. Whole body fluorodeoxyglucose (FDG) positron emission tomography (PET)/CT demonstrated accumulation of FDG in esophagus between the levels of thoracic fifth and eighth vertebras with SUVmax of 13.3 (Fig. 5.1). Biopsy from the esophageal lesion revealed squamous cell carcinoma (SCC). According to 8th edition AJCC/UICC staging system, patient has stage II (cT2N0M0) esophageal SCC located at the mid thoracic level (Tables 5.1 and 5.2) [1].

5.1.2 Evidence Based Treatment Recommendations

Pretreatment staging for esophageal cancer includes an evaluation for locoregional disease extent and an evaluation for distant metastases. Patients should have contrast-enhanced CT of the neck, chest, and abdomen, EGD, endoscopic ultrasound (EUS), FDG-PET/CT, and bronchoscopy for upperand middle-third lesions. The tumor, node, metastasis (TNM) staging system of the combined American Joint Committee on Cancer (AJCC)/Union for International Cancer Control (UICC) for esophageal cancer is used for staging [1].

Surgery has been the standard of care for early-stage esophageal cancer. However multimodal treatment approaches are preferred for locally advanced disease. Neoadjuvant chemoradiation is the preferred treatment option for non-metastatic locally advanced disease, if the patient is medically fit for surgery. If the patient is

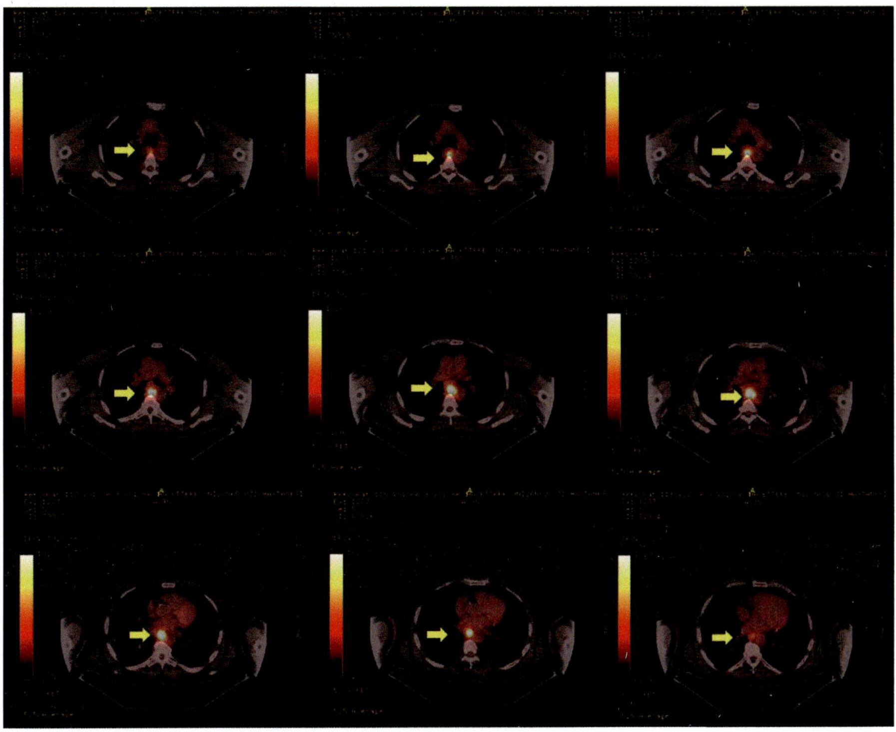

Fig. 5.1 Whole body fluorodeoxyglucose (FDG) positron emission tomography (PET)/CT demonstrated accumulation of FDG in esophagus between the levels of thoracic fifth and eighth vertebras with SUVmax of 13.3

Table 5.1 Esophagus and esophagogastric junction cancers—TNM staging AJCC UICC, 2017

Primary tumor (T), squamous cell carcinoma and adenocarcinoma	
T category	*T criteria*
TX	Tumor cannot be assessed
T0	No evidence of primary tumor
Tis	High-grade dysplasia, defined as malignant cells confined to the epithelium by the basement membrane
T1	Tumor invades the lamina propria, muscularis mucosae, or submucosa
T1a	Tumor invades the lamina propria or muscularis mucosae
T1b	Tumor invades the submucosa
T2	Tumor invades the muscularis propria
T3	Tumor invades adventitia
T4	Tumor invades adjacent structures
T4a	Tumor invades the pleura, pericardium, azygos ven, diaphragm, or peritoneum
T4b	Tumor invades other adjacent structures, such as the aorta, vertebral body, or airway

(continued)

Table 5.1 (continued)

Regional lymph nodes (N), squamous cell carcinoma and adenocarcinoma	
N *category*	N *criteria*
NX	Regional lymph nodes cannot be assessed
N0	No regional lymph node metastasis
N1	Metastasis in one or two regional lymph nodes
N2	Metastasis in three to six regional lymph nodes
N3	Metastasis in seven or more regional lymph nodes
Distant metastasis (M), squamous cell carcinoma and adenocarcinoma	
M *category*	M *criteria*
M0	No distant metastasis
M1	Distant metastasis
Histologic grade (G), squamous cell carcinoma and adenocarcinoma	
G	G *definition*
GX	Grade cannot be assessed
G1	Well differentiated
G2	Moderately differentiated
G3	Poorly differentiated, undifferentiated
Location (L), squamous cell carcinoma[a]	
Location in the stage grouping of esophageal squamous cancers	
Location category	*Location criteria*
X	Location unknown
Upper	Cervical esophagus to lower border of azygos vein
Middle	Lower border of azygos vein to lower border of inferior pulmonary vein
Lower	Lower border of inferior pulmonary vein to stomach, including gastroesophageal junction

[a]Location is defined by the position of the epicenter of the tumor in the esophagus
Used with permission of the American College of Surgeons, Chicago, Illinois. The original and primary source for this information is the AJCC Cancer Staging Manual, Eighth Edition (2017) published by Springer International Publishing

Table 5.2 Clinical stage groups for squamous cell carcinoma—TNM staging AJCC UICC, 2017

Clinical (cTNM)			
cT	cN	M	Stage
Tis	N0	M0	0
T1	N0–1	M0	I
T2	N0–1	M0	II
T3	N0	M0	II
T3	N1	M0	III
T1–3	N2	M0	III
T4	N0–2	M0	IVA
Any T	N3	M0	IVA
Any T	Any N	M1	IVB

Used with permission of the American College of Surgeons, Chicago, Illinois. The original and primary source for this information is the AJCC Cancer Staging Manual, Eighth Edition (2017) published by Springer International Publishing

not fit for surgery, have a lesion located in the cervival esophagus or decline surgery, definitive chemoradiation is used for treatment (https://www.nccn.org/professionals/physician_gls/pdf/esophageal.pdf3. Accessed May 2018).

5.1.2.1 Literature Review

Surgery has been the standard of care for localized esophageal cancer. However several randomized studies showed the benefit of adding neoadjuvant chemoradiation to improve treatment results (Table 5.3) [2–8].

The Trans-Tasman Radiation Oncology Group (TROG) randomized 256 patients but failed to find a progression-free survival or OS improvement with neoadjuvant therapy [5]. CALGB 9781 is one of the recent studies that randomized patients to either esophagectomy with node dissection alone or cisplatin 100 mg/m^2 and fluorouracil 1000 mg/m^2/day for 4 days on weeks 1 and 5 concurrent with radiation therapy (50.4 Gy total: 1.8 Gy/fraction over 5.6 weeks) followed by esophagectomy with node dissection. The trial was closed due to poor accrual however, with a median follow-up was 6 years, 5-year survival was 39% (95% CI, 21–57%) versus 16% (95% CI, 5–33%) in favor of trimodality therapy [6].

Long term results of the 'ChemoRadiotherapy for Oesophageal cancer followed by Surgery Study' (CROSS) comparing neoadjuvant chemoradiotherapy plus

Table 5.3 Phase III studies of preoperative chemoradiotherapy plus surgery versus surgery alone for esophageal cancer

Study	Pathology	No	Arms	Median F/U (year)	pCR %	3 years OS %	p (OS)
Urba et al. [2]	SCC+adeno	50	FVC/45 Gy/Sx	8.2	28	30	0.15
		50	Sx		–	16	
EORTC [3]	SCC	143	Cisp/37 Gy/Sx	4.6	20	33	NS
		138	Sx		–	36	
Walsh et al. [4]	Adeno	58	CF/40 Gy/Sx	1.5	22	32	0.01
		55	Sx		–	6	
TROG [5]	SCC+adeno	128	CF/35 Gy/Sx	5.4	16	35	NS
		128	Sx		–	31	
CALGB 9871 [6]	SCC+adeno	30	CF/50 Gy/Sx	6	40	39 (5 years)	0.008
		26	Sx		–	16 (5 years)	
CROSS [7]	SCC+adeno	180	Pac-Carbo/41.4 Gy/	7	29	49 months	0.001
		188	Sx		–	24 months	
			Sx				
FFCD [8]	SCC+adeno	97	CF/45 Gy/Sx	7.8	33	47.5	NS
		98	Sx		–	53	

SCC squamous cell carcinoma, *Adeno* adenocarcinoma, *Sx* surgery, *FVC* 5-flourouracil, vinblastine, cisplatin, *Pac* paclitaxel, *Carbo* carboplatin, *F/U* follow up, *pCR* pathological complete response, *OS* overall survival, *NS* not significant

surgery versus surgery alone in patients with SCC and adenocarcinoma of the esophagus or esophagogastric junction showed overall survival benefits for neoadjuvant chemoradiotherapy [7]. In this study patients were randomized to receive either weekly administration of five cycles of neoadjuvant chemoradiotherapy (intravenous carboplatin [AUC 2 mg/mL/min] and intravenous paclitaxel [50 mg/m^2 of body-surface area] for 23 days) with concurrent radiotherapy (41.4 Gy, given in 23 fractions of 1.8 Gy on 5 days/week) followed by surgery, or surgery alone. With a median follow-up time of 84.1 months median overall survival was 48.6 months (95% CI 32.1–65.1) in the neoadjuvant chemoradiotherapy plus surgery group and 24.0 months (14.2–33.7) in the surgery alone group (HR 0.68 [95% CI 0.53–0.88]; log-rank p = 0.003). There was no difference between SCC and adenocarcinoma histopathology. After these modern studies neoadjuvant chemoradiotherapy has become the standard of care for patients with operable esophageal cancer.

Neoadjuvant chemoradiotherapy plus surgery (trimodality treatment) is associated with improved survival compared to surgery alone in operable patients regardless of the primary histopathologic subtype [2, 4, 6, 7]. A meta-analysis showed a strong evidence for a survival benefit of neoadjuvant chemoradiotherapy or chemotherapy over surgery alone in patients with oesophageal carcinoma, however a clear advantage of neoadjuvant chemoradiotherapy over neoadjuvant chemotherapy has not been established yet [9]. Patients who are not fit for surgery or who declines surgery definitive chemoradiation (bimodality treatment) is an effective strategy. Compared to definitive chemoradiation, trimodality treatment has better local/regional control rates with increased toxicity rates. In case of trimodality treatment patient is re-assessed within 5–8 weeks after chemoradiation preferably by PET-CT or chest/abdomen/pelvic contrast enhanced CT and upper GI endoscopy for surgery. All patients should be evaluated for nutritional status before the commence of treatment, and enteric feeding tube or PEG tube should be considered in necessary cases.

Postoperative therapy has the advantage of knowing the exact pathological stage and extend of the disease. However studies of adjuvant therapy have not demonstrated a clear survival benefit. Adjuvant radiotherapy has been shown to improve local control in the setting of T3–T4 disease, nodal positivity or R1/R2 resection [10]. In the United States, a standard of care is postoperative chemoradiation for resected GE junction adenocarcinomas, based on the results of the Intergroup 116 trial [11]. This trial randomized 556 patients with gastric adenocarcinomas (20% of whom had tumors that involved the GE junction) to adjuvant chemotherapy and chemoradiation with bolus 5-fluorouracil (5-FU)/leucovorin versus observation alone following surgery. Patients who received adjuvant chemoradiation had an improvement in relapse-free survival (RFS) (3-year RFS 48% vs 31%, p < 0.001) and OS (3-year OS 51% vs 40%, p < 0.005).

Perioperative chemotherapy is the predominant approach in Europe and also in the United States, based primarily on the phase III MAGIC (Medical Research Council Adjuvant Gastric Infusional Chemotherapy) trial [12]. This trial randomized 503 patients with gastric adenocarcinomas (26% of tumors located in the lower esophagus/GE junction) to 3 cycles each of preoperative and postoperative ECF and surgery, or surgery alone. The resected tumors were significantly smaller and less advanced in the perioperative-chemotherapy group. Compared with the surgery group, the perioperative-chemotherapy group had a higher likelihood of overall survival (p = 0.009; 5-year survival rate, 36% vs. 23%) and of progression-free survival (p < 0.001). However, evidence of benefit for preoperative chemotherapy in SCC histology is very limited. The metaanalysis by Sjoquist et al. did not show a clear improvement in survival for preoperative chemotherapy in patients with SCC (HR 0.92, 95% CI 0.81–1.04; p = 0.18) [9].

RTOG 85-01 is a phase III study that compared RT alone (64 Gy in 32 fractions over 6.5 weeks) versus concurrent chemoradiotherapy (two cycles of infusional FU [1000 mg/m^2/day, days 1–4, weeks 1 and 5] plus cisplatin [75 mg/m^2 day 1 of weeks 1 and 5] and RT [50 Gy in 25 fractions over 5 weeks]) in patients with locoregional thoracic esophageal cancer. 90% patients had SCC. The chemoradiotherapy group received two additional chemotherapy courses, after RT [13]. The median survival was 8.9 months in the radiotherapy arm, as compared with 12.5 months in the patients treated with chemo radiation. In the long term results of the same study, persistence of disease was the most common mode of treatment failure; however, it was less common in the groups receiving chemoradiotherapy than in the group treated with RT only (26% vs. 37%). Severe acute toxic effects also were greater in the combined therapy groups. There were no significant differences in severe late toxic effects between the groups [14]. As a result of this trial, definitive chemoradiotherapy became the standard of care for patients with inoperable disease. In the US Intergroup Study 0123 (INT 0123), 236 patients with nonmetastatic esophageal SCC or adenocarcinoma received concurrent cisplatin and FU (as in RTOG 85-01), but they were randomly assigned to one of two different radiotherapy doses: 50.4 Gy or 64.8 Gy [15]. Higher radiotherapy doses were not associated with better survival or locoregional control rates but was significantly more toxic. However, this study was conducted before the era of 3D-CRT. At present, 50 Gy of RT plus concurrent cisplatin and FU remains a standard treatment regime for definitive chemoradiotherapy.

5.1.3 Treatment Recommendations

Treatment recommendations for non-metastatic esophageal cancer according to NCCN guidelines are summarized in Table 5.4.

Table 5.4 NCCN guidelines version 1.2018 (https://www.nccn.org/professionals/physician_gls/pdf/esophageal.pdf3. Accessed May 2018)

Stage	Recommended treatment
pTis, pT1a	Endoscopic therapies or esophagectomy
pT1bN0	Esophagectomy
cT1b-T4a, N0-N+	Preoperative chemoradiation (non-cervical esophagus) (RT, 41.4–50.4 Gy + concurrent chemotherapy) or Definitive chemoradiation (only for patients who decline surgery) (recommended for cervical esophagus) (RT, 50–50.4 Gy + concurrent chemotherapy) or Esophagectomy (non-cervical esophagus) (T1b/T2, N0 low risk lesions: <2 cm, well differentiated)
cT4b	Definitive chemoradiation (only for patients who decline surgery) (recommended for cervical esophagus) (RT, 50–50.4 Gy + concurrent chemotherapy) Consider chemotherapy alone in the setting of invasion of trachea, great vessels, or heart
R0 resection—SCC (p AnyT, Any N)	Surveillance
R0 resection—adenocarcinoma	**N0**: pTis-pT1-pT2 → Surveillance pT3, pT4a → Surveillance or Adjuvant chemoradiation **N+**: Adjuvant chemoradiation (flouropyrimidine based) or chemotherapy
R1 resection	Adjuvant chemoradiation (flouropyrimidine based)
R2 resection	Adjuvant chemoradiation (flouropyrimidine based) Or Palliative treatment

R0 no residual disease, *R1* microscopic residual disease, *R2* macroscopic residual disease, *SCC* squamous cell carcinoma

5.1.4 Treatment Planning

5.1.4.1 Simulation

Patients should be immobilized according to the location of esophageal cancer. For tumors located at the cervical or upper-third of thoracic esophagus, patients should ideally be immobilized with head–neck–shoulder thermoplastic masks. For tumors located at the thoracic esophagus or esophagogastric junction, patients should ideally be immobilized with their arms above their head in a vacuum bag. For tumors located at the lower part of esophagus patients should be advised to avoid having meal 2–4 h before simulation and each treatment to limit differences in gastric filling. Intravenous contrast can be considered during simulation to visualize vascular structures and delineate lymph nodes better. A CT slice thickness of 3 mm is recommended. Planning CT should encompass the entire thoracic cavity starting from thoracic inlet to a point below the bottom of both kidneys (especially for distal esophageal tumors). Consideration of 4 dimensional CT is recommended.

5.1.4.2 Contouring

The gross tumor volume (GTV) consists of primary esophageal tumor (EGD, CT, EUS, or FDG-PET) and involved lymph nodes. Lymph nodes with biopsy, increased FDG uptake, or enlarged short- axis diameter are delineated as GTV. There is no consensus about elective nodal coverage for esophageal cancer. The principles of contouring are summarized in Table 5.5. Entire esophagus from cricoid cartilage to EGJ, spinal cord and bilateral lungs should be contoured. In upper esophageal tumors, the brachial plexus and larynx, in lower esophagus tumors, the heart, liver, stomach, duodenum and bilateral kidneys should be delineated.

Case Contouring Delineation of target volumes for the case is shown in Fig. 5.2.

Case Plan The patient presented here has stage II (cT2N0M0) esophageal SCC located at the mid thoracic level. The case was discussed in the multidisciplinary meeting and neoadjuvant chemoradiation was planned. Patient received neoadjuvant radiotherapy (total 50.4 Gy in 1.8 Gy/fraction) with concurrent chemotherapy (weekly Paclitaxel (50 mg/m^2)-Carboplatin (AUC 2) utilizing IMRT technique. Treatment planning details are seen in Figs. 5.3 and 5.4.

5.1.4.3 Dose Recommendations

Neoadjuvant: 40–50.4 Gy in 1.8–2 Gy/fraction

Definitive: 50.4 Gy (up to 66 Gy for tumor at cervical esophagus) in 1.8–2 Gy/fraction

Postoperative: 45–50.4 Gy in 1.8–2 Gy/fraction

Higher doses may be appropriate in cases where the tumor is located in the cervical region and surgery is not planned.

Concomitant Chemotherapy Weekly Paclitaxel (50 mg/m^2)-Carboplatin (AUC 2) or 2 cycles of infusional fluorouracil (1000 mg/m^2/day, 4 days)-Cisplatin (100 mg/m^2, day 1)

Table 5.5 Definition of target volumes for radiotherapy for esophageal cancer [16–18]

Definition	GTV-CTV margin	CTV-PTV margin	Elective nodal coverage
Cervical esophagus	Primary: 3–5 cm longitudinally; 0.5–1 cm circumferentially	No IGRT: 0.5–1 cm	Supraclavicular, higher echelon
Proximal esophagus		IGRT: 0.5 cm	Supraclavicular, periesophageal
Middle esophagus	Involved lymph node: 0.5–1 cm in all directions		Periesophageal, mediastinal
Lower esophagus			Periesophageal, perigastric, celiac

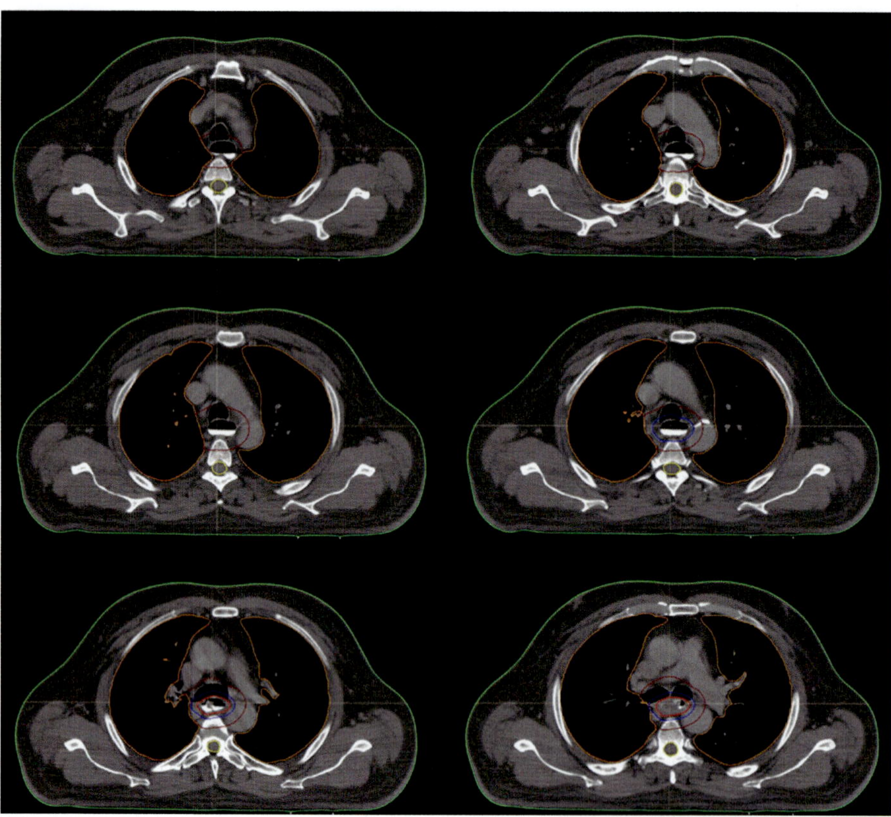

Fig. 5.2 Delineation of treatment volumes for cT2N0M0 mid-thoracic esophageal SCC patient. Periesophageal and adjacent mediastinal lymph nodes are included electively in the target. **Red; GTV, blue; CTV, brown: PTV**

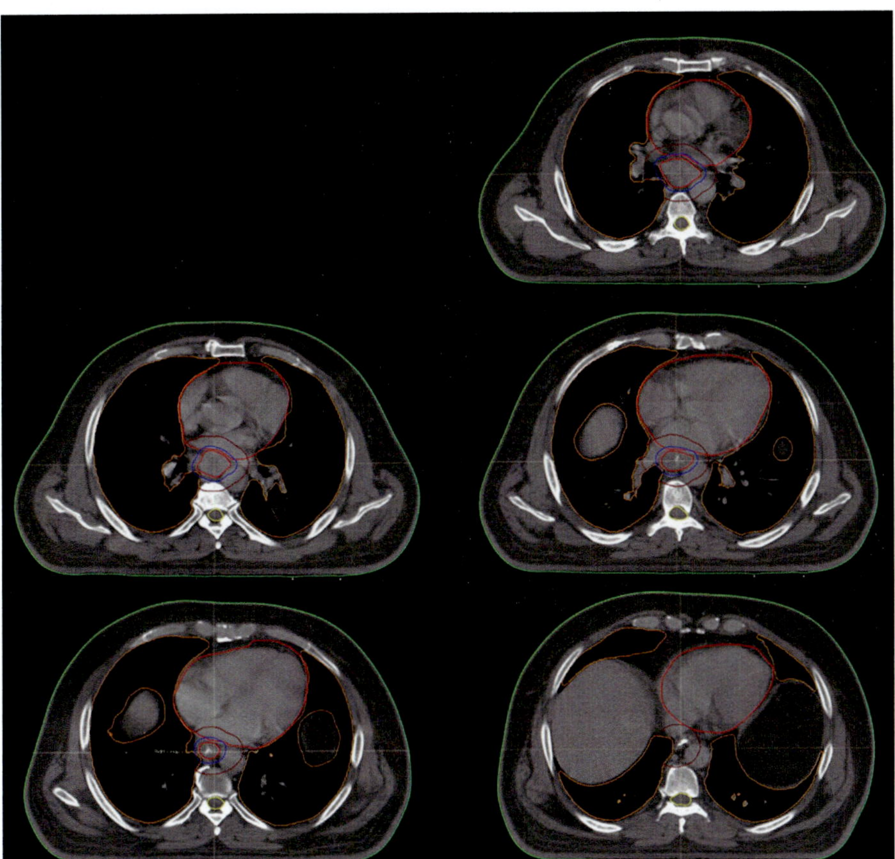

Fig. 5.2 (continued)

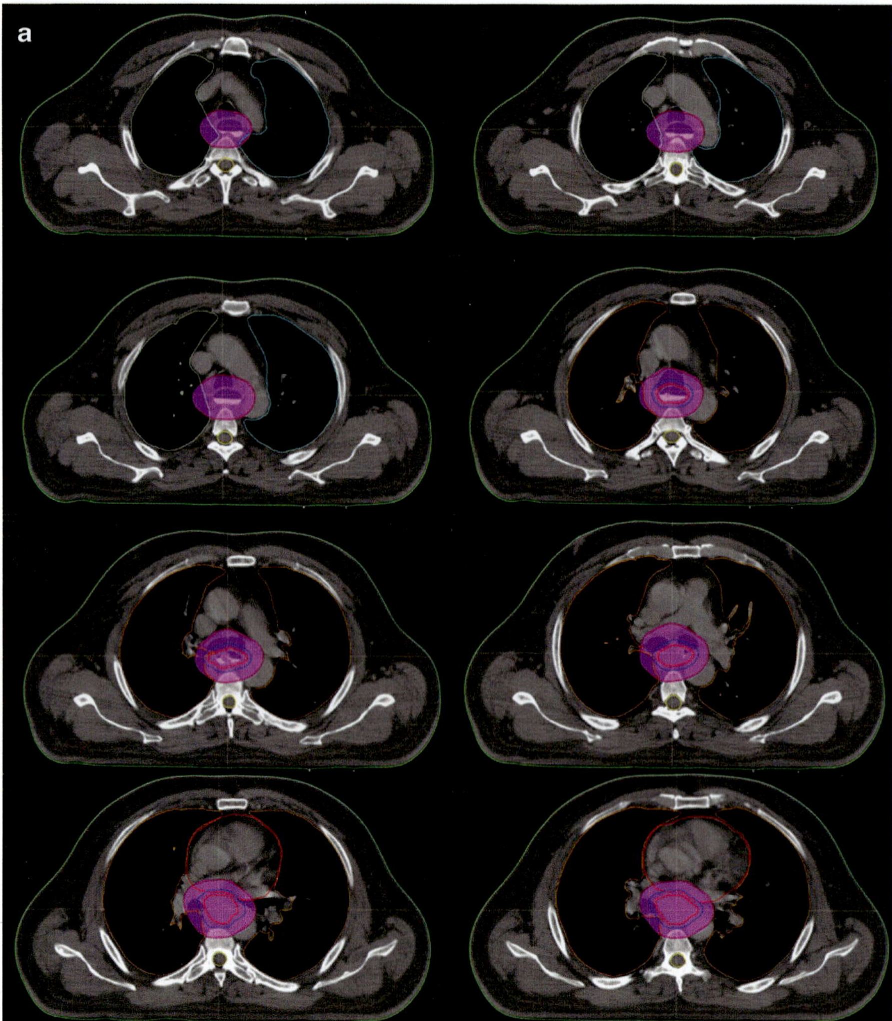

Fig. 5.3 Three dimensional conformal radiotherapy planning in the neoadjuvant setting of cT2N0M0 disease. Total dose of 45 Gy in 1.8 Gy/fraction was delivered. (**a, b**) 95% isodose coverage (pink) and (**c**) dose-volume histogram are shown. Left Lung: cyan, Heart: red, Body: green, Right Lung: light green, Spinal Cord: yellow, Total Lung: orange, GTV: red, CTV: blue, PTV: claret red

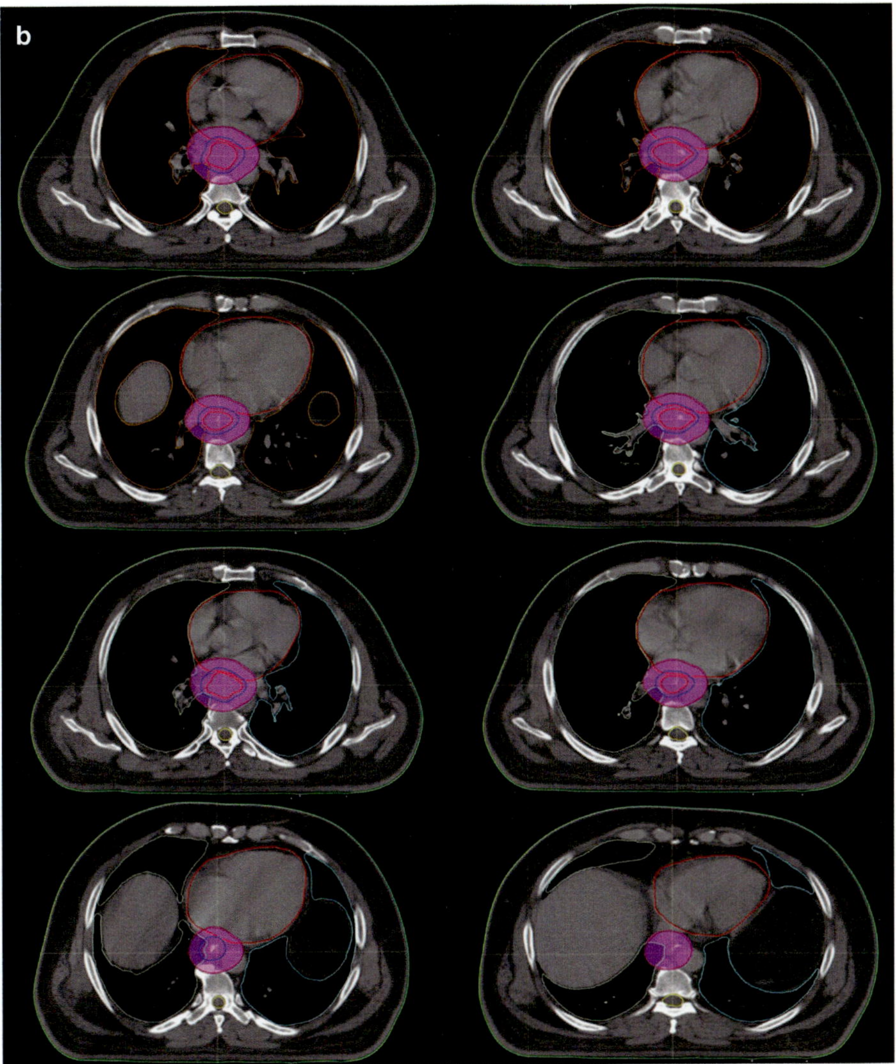

Fig. 5.3 (continued)

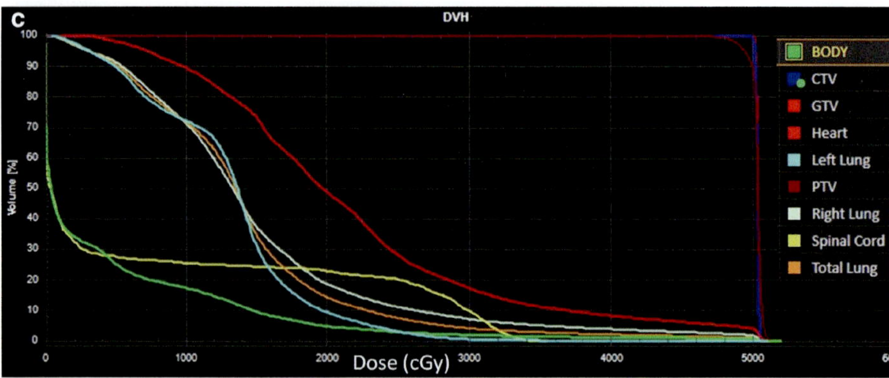

Fig. 5.3 (continued)

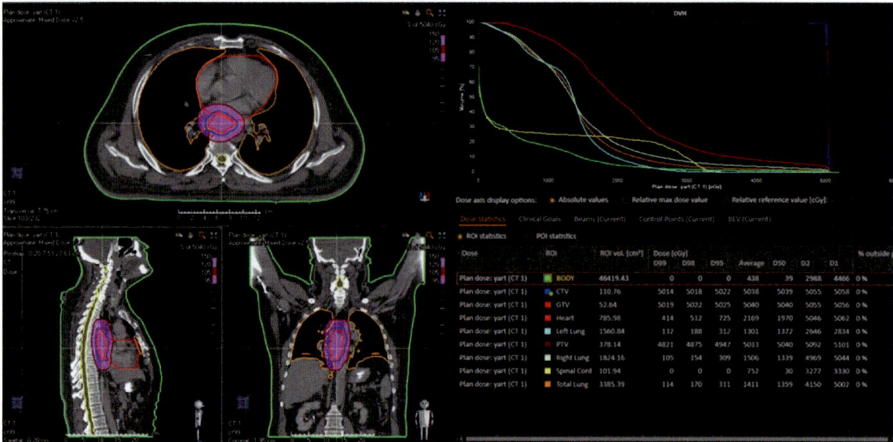

Fig. 5.4 IMRT plan of the patient

Treatment Delivery Techniques 3D-CRT is recommended over 2D-RT for better coverage of the target volume while protecting the surrounding normal organs. IMRT provides a better RT plan than 3D-CRT. However, no trial has compared IMRT plus concurrent chemotherapy with the same chemotherapy regimen plus standard fractionation 3D-CRT, and thus, the safety and efficacy of IMRT compared with standard 3D-CRT remains undefined.

5.1.4.4 Dose Constraints for Critical Structures

Table 5.6 shows dose-volume constraints for treatment planning.

5.1.5　Follow-Up (F/U) Recommendations

Bimodality therapy (definitive chemoradiation): Literature suggests that local/regional relapses are common after bimodality therapy. Most of the relapses (95%) occur within 24 months, thus surveillance for at least 24 months is recommended.

Table 5.6 Dose-volume considerations for treatment planning [19]

Organ	Constraints
Lung	V20 $\leq$ 30% V10 < 40% Mean < 20 Gy
Spinal cord	Dmax (0.03 cc) $\leq$ 50 Gy
Heart	Max dose (0.03 cc) $\leq$ 52 Gy V40 < 50% Mean < 26 Gy
Liver	Mean dose $\leq$ 28 Gy
Kidneys (bilateral combined kidneys)	Mean < 15–18 Gy Max dose (0.03 cc) $\leq$ 45 Gy V20 $\leq$ 32% V23 < 30% V28 < 20%

Imaging (CT chest/abdomen with contrast) should be considered every 6–9 months at least for the first 2 years. EGD every 3–6 months for first 2 years, and then every 6 months for the third year is recommended (https://www.nccn.org/professionals/physician_gls/pdf/esophageal.pdf3. Accessed May 2018).

Trimodality therapy (neoadjuvant chemoradiation plus surgery): Local/regional relapses are uncommon, therefore EGD surveillance is not recommended. However, 90% of the relapses occur within 36 months after surgery thus 36 months of surveillance is preferred (https://www.nccn.org/professionals/physician_gls/pdf/esophageal.pdf3. Accessed May 2018).

5.2 Gastric Cancer

Overview

Epidemiology: Gastric cancers most commonly are seen in Eastern Asia, Eastern Europe and South America, with lower rates in North America and Western Europe.

Pathology: There are two distinct types of gastric adenocarcinoma; intestinal and diffuse types. Diffuse type cancers are highly metastatic and characterized by poor prognosis.

Diagnosis: Weight loss and epigastric pain are the most common presenting symptoms of gastric cancer. Upper endoscopy with biopsy is the main diagnostic study. Contrast-enhanced computed tomography (CT) of the thorax-abdomen-pelvic region is recommended to see the local and distant extend of the disease. Endoscopic ultrasonography (EUS) is a reliable nonsurgical method available for evaluating the depth of invasion.

Definitive Treatment: Endoscopic resection is appropriate for selected very early tumors. For stage IB–III gastric cancer, radical gastrectomy is indicated and perioperative therapy is recommended.

Keywords: Gastric cancer; Radiotherapy

5.2.1   Case Presentation

He was a 57 year-old gentleman with a KPS of 100 applied to hospital with gradually increasing dyspepsia and weight loss over the last 6 months. His physical examination revealed normal vital signs and systemic findings. He had medical history of left nephrectomy due to trauma 27 years ago. He had no smoking or alcohol history. His whole blood count, and kidney and liver function tests were normal. Esophago-gastro-duedonoscopy (EGD) revealed malignant tumoral mass starting from antrum and extending to the pylorus. Contrast-enhanced thorax- abdomen computed tomography (CT) showed tumoral mass located at the antrum (Fig. 5.5). Biopsy from the tumoral mass was consistent with adenocarcinoma. Patient had total gastrectomy and D2 lymph node dissection with pathology of; adenocarcinoma, grade III, intestinal type. Tumor was 7.5 × 7 cm, located at the lesser curvature and invading the whole layers of stomach including serosa. Lymphovascular and perineural invasion was positive. Surgical margins are clear. Among 21 of 35 lymph node dissected were metastatic (15 in lesser curvature, 6 in greater curvature).

Patient applied to our clinics after 4 cycles of Docetaxel- Oxaliplatin-5FU chemotherapy. According to the 8th edition AJCC/UICC staging system, patient has pT4aN3b (Stage IIIC) disease (Tables 5.7 and 5.8) [20].

5.2.2   Evidence Based Treatment Recommendations

Weight loss and epigastric pain are the most common presenting symptoms of gastric cancer. Upper endoscopy with biopsy is the main diagnostic study. Contrast-enhanced computed tomography (CT) of the thorax-abdomen-pelvic region is recommended to see the local and distant extend of the disease. Endoscopic ultrasonography (EUS) is a reliable nonsurgical method available for evaluating the depth of invasion.

Endoscopic resection is appropriate for selected very early tumors. For stage IB–III gastric cancer, radical gastrectomy is indicated and perioperative therapy is recommended for these patients. Medically fit patients should undergo D2 resections in high-volume surgical centers [21].

5.2.2.1 Literature Review

Surgery is the primary treatment of localized gastric cancer. Adjuvant chemoradiation remains a rational standard therapy for curatively resected gastric cancer with primaries T3 or greater and/or positive LNs. In this group of patients, chemoradiation is associated with improved relapse free survival and

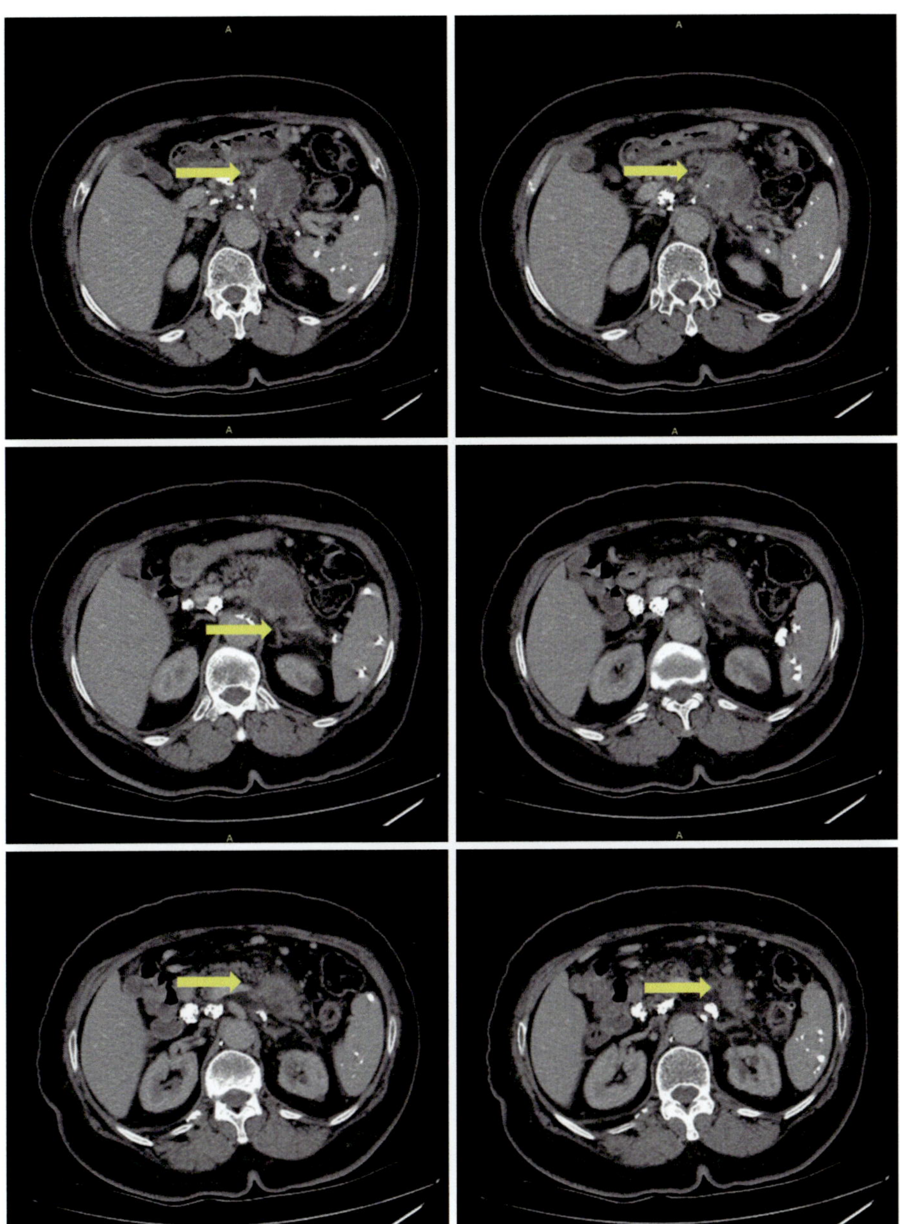

Fig. 5.5 Tumoral mass located at the antral region of the stomach and extending into pylorus

Table 5.7 Gastric cancer pathological TNM staging, AJCC UICC, 2017

Primary tumor (T)	
T category	T criteria
TX	Primary tumor cannot be assessed
T0	No evidence of primary tumor
Tis	Carcinoma in situ: Intraepithelial tumor without invasion of the lamina propria, high-grade dysplasia
T1	Tumor invades the lamina propria, muscularis mucosae, or submucosa
T1a	Tumor invades the lamina propria or muscularis mucosae
T1b	Tumor invades the submucosa
T2	Tumor invades the muscularis propria[a]
T3	Tumor penetrates the subserosal connective tissue without invasion of the visceral peritoneum or adjacent structures[b,c]
T4	Tumor invades the serosa (visceral peritoneum) or adjacent structures[b,c]
T4a	Tumor invades the serosa (visceral peritoneum)
T4b	Tumor invades adjacent structures/organs
Regional lymph nodes (N)	
N category	N criteria
NX	Regional lymph node(s) cannot be assessed
N0	No regional lymph node metastasis
N1	Metastasis in one or two regional lymph nodes
N2	Metastasis in three to six regional lymph nodes
N3	Metastasis in seven or more regional lymph nodes
N3a	Metastasis in 7–15 regional lymph nodes
N3b	Metastasis in 16 or more regional lymph nodes
Distant metastasis (M)	
M category	M criteria
M0	No distant metastasis
M1	Distant metastasis

Used with permission of the American College of Surgeons, Chicago, Illinois. The original and primary source for this information is the AJCC Cancer Staging Manual, Eighth Edition (2017) published by Springer International Publishing

[a]A tumor may penetrate the muscularis propria with extension into the gastrocolic or gastrohepatic ligaments, or into the greater or lesser omentum, without perforation of the visceral peritoneum covering these structures. In this case, the tumor is classified as T3. If there is perforation of the visceral peritoneum covering the gastric ligaments or the omentum, the tumor should be classified as T4

[b]The adjacent structures of the stomach include the spleen, transverse colon, liver, diaphragm, pancreas, abdominal wall, adrenal gland, kidney, small intestine, and retroperitoneum

[c]Intramural extension to the duodenum or esophagus is not considered invasion of an adjacent structure, but is classified using the depth of the greatest invasion in any of these sites

Table 5.8 Pathological TNM Stage groups, AJCC UICC, 2017

T	N	M	Stage
Tis	N0	M0	0
T1	N0	M0	IA
T1	N1	M0	IB
T2	N0	M0	IB
T1	N2	M0	IIA
T2	N1	M0	IIA
T3	N0	M0	IIA
T1	N3a	M0	IIB
T2	N2	M0	IIB
T3	N1	M0	IIB
T4a	N0	M0	IIB
T2	N3a	M0	IIIA
T3	N2	M0	IIIA
T4a	N1	M0	IIIA
T4a	N2	M0	IIIA
T4b	N0	M0	IIIA
T1	N3b	M0	IIIB
T2	N3b	M0	IIIB
T3	N3a	M0	IIIB
T4a	N3a	M0	IIIB
T4b	N1	M0	IIIB
T4b	N2	M0	IIIB
T3	N3b	M0	IIIC
T4a	N3b	M0	IIIC
T4b	N3a	M0	IIIC
T4b	N3b	M0	IIIC
Any T	Any N	M1	IV

Used with permission of the American College of Surgeons, Chicago, Illinois. The original and primary source for this information is the AJCC Cancer Staging Manual, Eighth Edition (2017) published by Springer International Publishing

overall survival, regardless of the extend of lymph node dissection. Table 5.9 summarizes the important adjuvant chemoradiation studies for resected gastric cancer.

Intergroup 0116 trial randomized 556 patients to observation alone or adjuvant chemoradiotherapy (one cycle of FU/LV bolus chemotherapy followed by chemoradiotherapy and then two more cycles of chemotherapy) [11]. The median overall survival in the surgery-only group was 27 months, as compared with 36 months in the chemoradiotherapy group (p < 0.005). The median duration of relapse-free survival was 30 months in the chemoradiotherapy group and 19 months in the

Table 5.9 Randomized adjuvant chemoradiation studies

Study	Patients	Surgery	Adjuvant treatment	Overall survival	Local control	Relapse free survival
SWOG9008/ INT-0116 [11, 22]	Resected Stage IB–IV (M0) 556	D0 = 54% D1 = 36% D2 = 10%	Observation vs 5FU/ LV → chemoRT (45 Gy w 2 × 5FU/ LV) → 2 × 5FU/LV	41% vs 50% (3 years) Median 27 months vs 35 months (p = 0.0046) (10 years)	64% vs 76% (3 years)	Median 19 months vs 27 months (p < 0.001) (10 years)
Kim et al. [23]	Resected Stage III–IV (M0) ChemoRT: 544 Surgery alone: 446	R0, D2	Observation vs 5FU/ LV → chemoRT (45 Gy w 2 × 5FU/ LV) → 2 × 5FU/LV	51.1% vs 57% (p = 0.019) (5 years)		47.9% vs 54.5% (p = 0.016) (5 years)
ARTIST trial [24]	Resected Stage IB–IV (M0) 458	R0, D2	Postoperative • 6 chemo (capecitabine/ cisplatin) • 2 chemo → ChemoRT (45 Gy+capecitabine) → 2 chemo	All patients 74% vs 78% (NS) DFS: LN (+) → 72% vs 77% (p = 0.03)		

ChemoRT chemoradiotherapy, *chemo* chemotherapy, *5FU* 5 flouro-uracil, *LV* leucovorine, *ECF* epirubicin, cisplatin, and fluorouracil, *LN* lymph node, *DFS* disease free survival

surgery-only group (p < 0.001). Long term follow-up demonstrates strong persistent significant benefit from adjuvant chemoradiotherapy [22]. Main criticism about this trial was the limited extent of the surgical procedure in most cases. Although D2 lymph node resection was recommended, 54% of patients had less than D1 resection. This leads to questioning the role of adjuvant chemoradiotherapy in case of D2 resection.

Kim et al. investigated the effect of postoperative chemoradiotherapy on the relapse rate and survival rate of 544 patients with D2 resected gastric cancer [23]. The results were compared with 446 patients received surgery without further adjuvant treatment. Chemoradiotherapy and adjuvant chemotherapy regime was the same as the Intergroup 0116 trial. The median duration of overall survival was significantly longer in the chemoradiotherapy group than in the comparison group (95.3 months vs. 62.6 months; p = 0.0200). The 5-year survival rates were consistently longer in the chemoradiotherapy group than those in the comparison group. Chemoradiotherapy was associated with increases in the median duration of relapse-free survival (75.6 months vs. 52.7 months; p = 0.0160).

CALGB 80101 trial (Alliance; Phase III Intergroup Trial of Adjuvant Chemoradiation After Resection of Gastric or Gastroesophageal Adenocarcinoma) assessed whether a postoperative chemoradiotherapy regimen that replaced FU/LV (as in Intergroup 0116 trial) with a potentially more active systemic therapy could further improve overall survival [25]. In this study 546 patients who had undergone a curative resection of stage IB–IV (M0) gastric or gastroesophageal junction adenocarcinoma were randomly assigned to receive either postoperative FU plus LV before and after combined FU and radiotherapy (FU plus LV arm) or postoperative epirubicin, cisplatin, and infusional FU (ECF) before and after combined FU and radiotherapy (ECF arm). With a median follow-up duration of 6.5 years, 5-year overall survival rates were 44% in the FU plus LV arm and 44% in the ECF arm and 5-year disease-free survival rates were 39% in the FU plus LV arm and 37% in the ECF arm. The effect of treatment seemed to be similar across all examined patient subgroups.

There is also question of omitting radiotherapy and continue with adjuvant chemotherapy. ARTIST trial randomized 458 patients with completely resected gastric cancer and a D2 lymph node dissection to either six courses of postoperative capecitabine/cisplatin or to two courses of postoperative capecitabine/cisplatin followed by chemoradiotherapy (45 Gy RT with concurrent daily capecitabine [825 mg/m^2 twice daily]) and two additional courses of capecitabine/cisplatin [24]. With 7 years of follow-up, disease free survival and overall survival remained similar between treatment The significant effect of the addition of radiotherapy on outcomes differed by Lauren classification and lymph node. Subgroup analyses also showed that chemoradiotherapy significantly improved disease free survival in patients with lymph node positive disease and with intestinal-type.

Preoperative combined chemotherapy and radiation therapy is more commonly used for esophageal, EGJ, and gastric cardia cancers but there are no randomized trials investigating the role of preoperative chemoradiotherapy for noncardia gastric cancers. German POET trial comparing neoadjuvant chemoradiotherapy with induction chemotherapy alone was limited to patients with EGJ adenocarcinoma. The results revealed that patients in the preoperative chemoradiotherapy arm had a significant higher probability of showing pathologic complete response (15.6% vs 2.0%) or tumor-free lymph nodes (64.4% vs 37.7%) at resection. Preoperative radiation therapy improved 3-year survival rate from 27.7% to 47.4% (p = 0.07) with no difference in postoperative mortality rates [26].

CRITICS trial compared perioperative chemotherapy with preoperative chemotherapy and postoperative chemoradiotherapy in patients with resectable gastric adenocarcinoma [27]. Seven-hundred-eighty-eight patients were enrolled to the study. Surgery consisted of a radical resection of the primary tumour and at least a D1+ lymph node dissection. Postoperative treatment started within 4–12 weeks after surgery. Chemotherapy consisted of three preoperative 21-day cycles and three postoperative cycles of intravenous epirubicin (50 mg/m^2 on day 1), cisplatin (60 mg/m^2 on day 1) or oxaliplatin (130 mg/m^2 on day 1), and capecitabine

(1000 mg/m^2 orally as tablets twice daily for 14 days in combination with epirubicin and cisplatin, or 625 mg/m^2 orally as tablets twice daily for 21 days in combination with epirubicin and oxaliplatin), received once every 3 weeks. Chemoradiotherapy consisted of 45 Gy in 25 fractions of 1.8 Gy, for 5 weeks, five daily fractions per week, combined with capecitabine (575 mg/m^2 orally twice daily on radiotherapy days) and cisplatin (20 mg/m^2 intravenously on day 1 of each 5 weeks of radiation treatment). At a median follow-up of 61.4 months, median overall survival was 43 months in the chemotherapy group and 37 months in the chemoradiotherapy group (p = 0.90). Postoperative toxicity was similar in the chemotherapy and chemoradiotherapy groups but neutropenia (including grade 3–4 neutropenia) was more frequent in the chemotherapy group.

5.2.2.2 Treatment Recommendations

Treatment recommendations according to ESMO guidelines are summarized in Table 5.10 [21].

For patients with potentially resectable noncardia gastric cancer, randomized trials and meta-analyses provide support for the use of adjuvant chemoradiotherapy, adjuvant chemotherapy or perioperative chemotherapy. For most patients with potentially resectable gastric cancer beyond the submucosa and high likelihood of developing distant metastasis, neoadjuvant therapy over initial surgery is preferred.

Table 5.10 Treatment recommendations according to ESMO guidelines [21]

Stage	Treatment recommendations
Operable T1N0	Consider endoscopic/limited resection
Operable >T1N0	• Preoperative chemotherapy → Surgery → Postoperative chemotherapy • Surgery → Adjuvant chemoradiation → Adjuvant chemotherapy
Inoperable or metastatic	Palliative chemotherapy • Her2 negative • Platinum+ fluoropyrimidine-based doublet or triplet regimen • HER2-positive: Trastuzumab + CF/CX • Clinical trials Best supportive care if unfit for treatment

5.2.3   Treatment Planning

5.2.3.1 Simulation

Patients should ideally be immobilized with their arms above their head in a vacuum bag and should avoid having meal 2–4 h before simulation and each treatment to limit differences in gastric filling. CT simulation using ≤3 mm thickness is recommended. Intravenous contrast can be considered during simulation to visualize vascular structures and delineate lymph nodes better.

5.2.3.2 Contouring

Preoperative CT scans should be used for identification of preoperative tumour volume. CTV for postoperative radiation therapy for gastric cancer depends on the location of the primary disease and the status of lymph node metastasis [28]. Three areas must be identified as CTV for adjuvant radiotherapy: the gastric tumour bed, the anastomosis or stumps and the regional lymphatics. Duedenal stump should preferably be covered in patients who have had a partial gastrectomy for distal/antral tumours. However, it should not be covered in patients with proximal/cardia tumours who have had a total gastrectomy. Para-aortic nodes should be included for the entire length of the CTV. A 4 cm margin of the oesophagus should be included in the CTV for tumours of the gastrooesophageal junction Hepatogastric ligament should preferably be treated in all cases as it is at high risk of recurrence. Table 5.11 shows the description of the target volumes.

Case Contouring   Target volume delineation of current case is seen in Fig. 5.6.

Table 5.11   Target volume definitions

Target volume	Description
GTV	Gross residual disease after surgery
PTVresidual	GTV + 1.5 cm
CTV45	Coverage of nodal groups according to subsite. Also includes remnant stomach, Anastomosis (gastrojejunal, oesophagojejunal), and duodenal stump
PTV45	CTV 45 + 1 cm margin

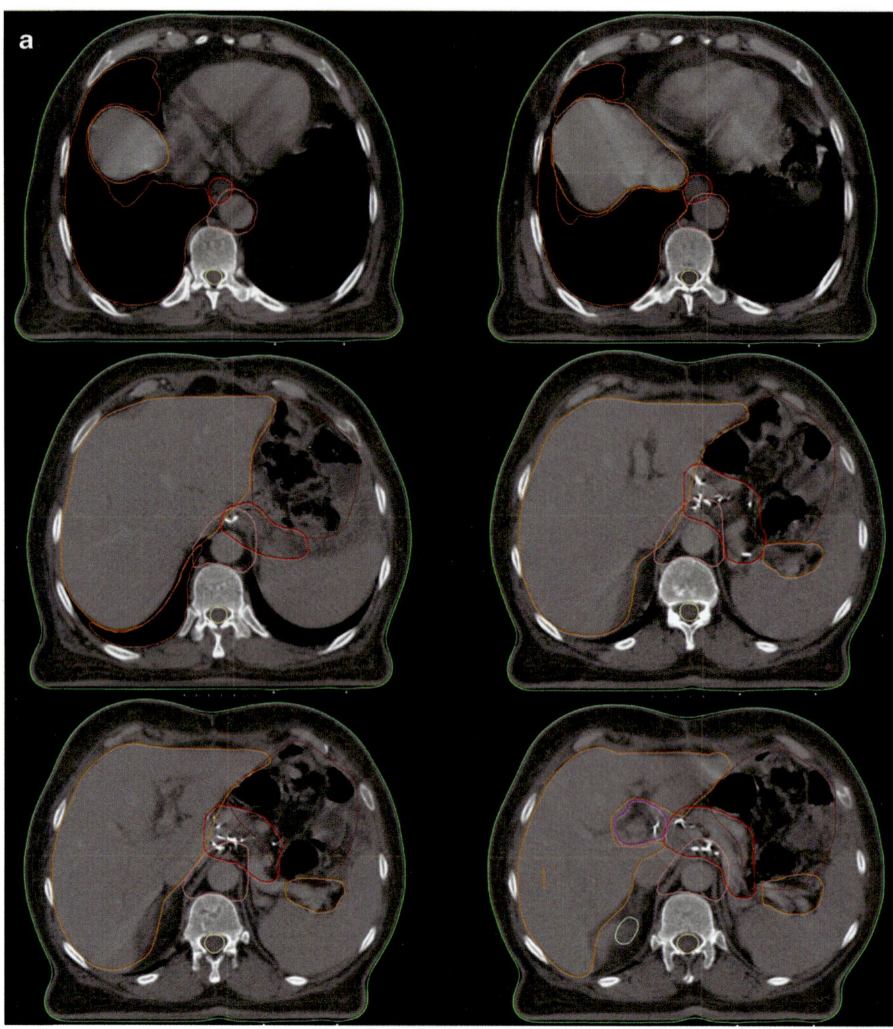

Fig. 5.6 (**a**, **b**) Patient has pT4N3b disease located at the antral region. Green = CTVtotal; Orange = CTVsplenic hilus; Pink = CTVpara-aortic; Red = CTVprimer; Blue = CTVceliac; Lila = CTVportalHilus

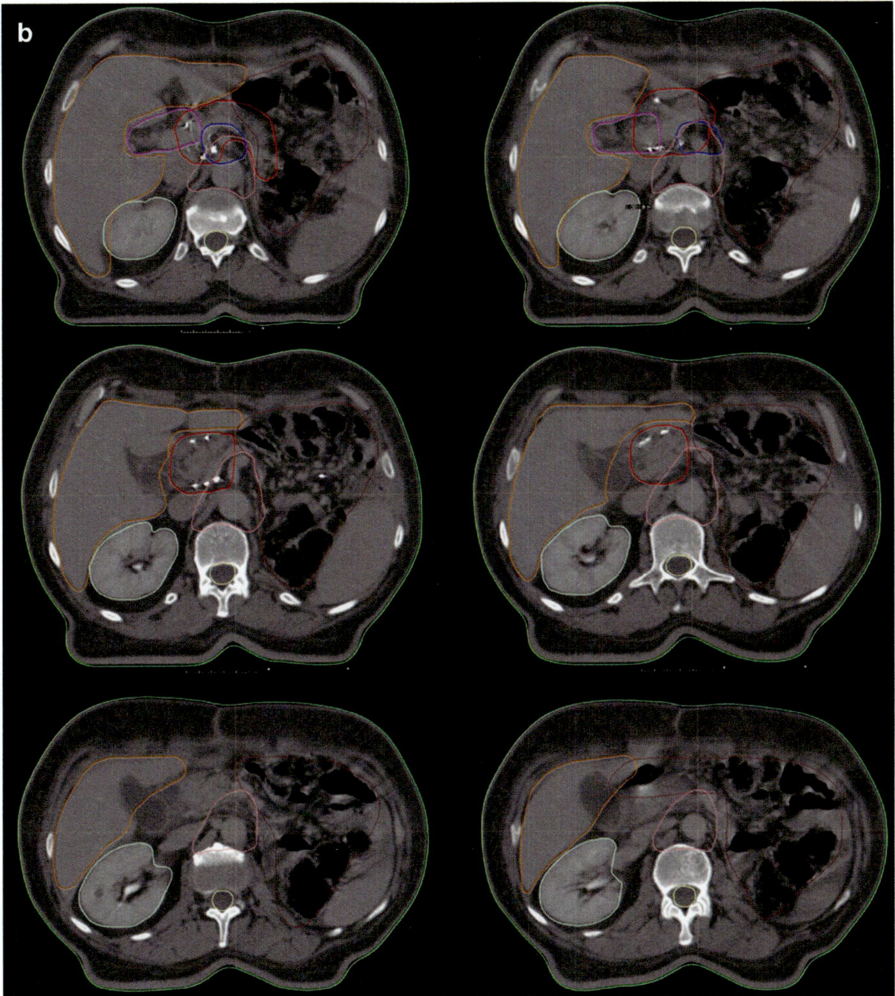

Fig. 5.6 (continued)

Case Plan Patient had pT4aN3b (Stage IIIC) disease, thus he received 45 Gy in 1.8 Gy/fraction with concomitant capecitabine. 3DCRT planning of the case is shown in Figs. 5.7 and 5.8.

Dose Recommendations Postoperative: 45 Gy in 1.8 Gy/fraction

Concomitant   Chemotherapy Flouropyrimidine (Infusional   fluorouracil   or Capecitabine)

5.2.3.3 Dose Constraints for Critical Structures
Table 5.12 shows the recommended dose constraints for organs at risk.

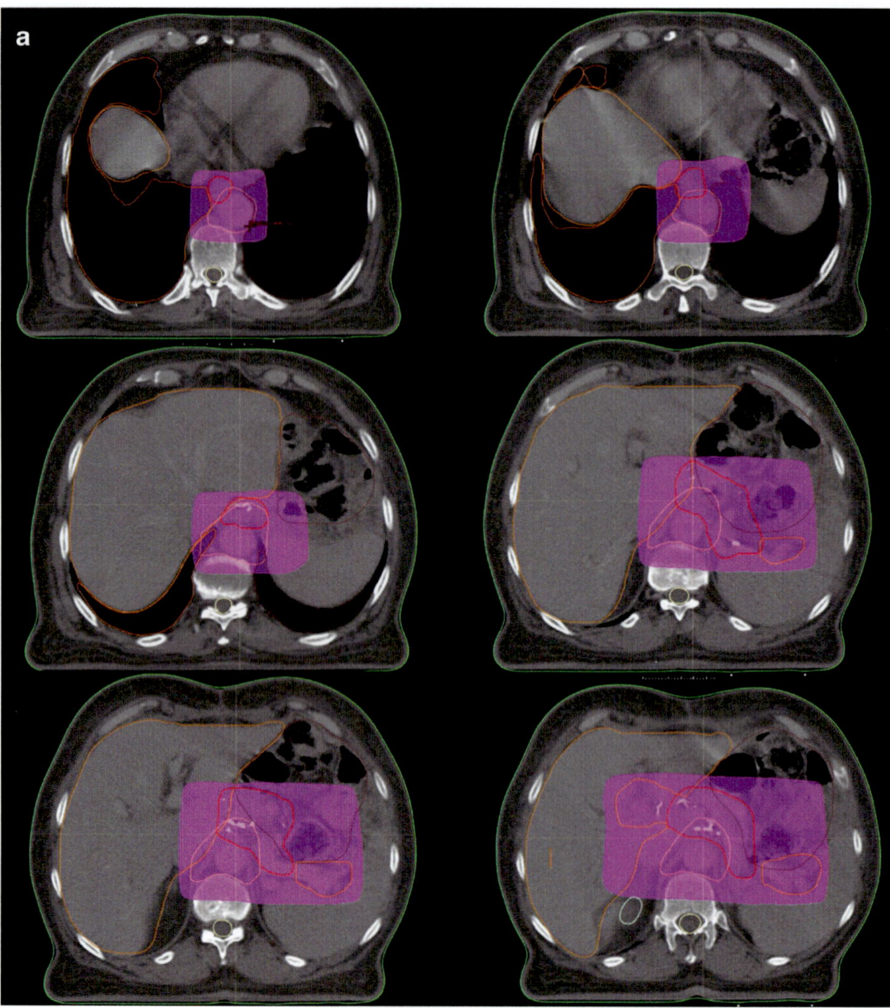

Fig. 5.7 Patient received 45 Gy in 1.8 Gy/fraction with three dimensional conformal radiotherapy technique. (**a**, **b**) 95% isodose coverage (pink) and (**c**) dose-volume histogram are shown

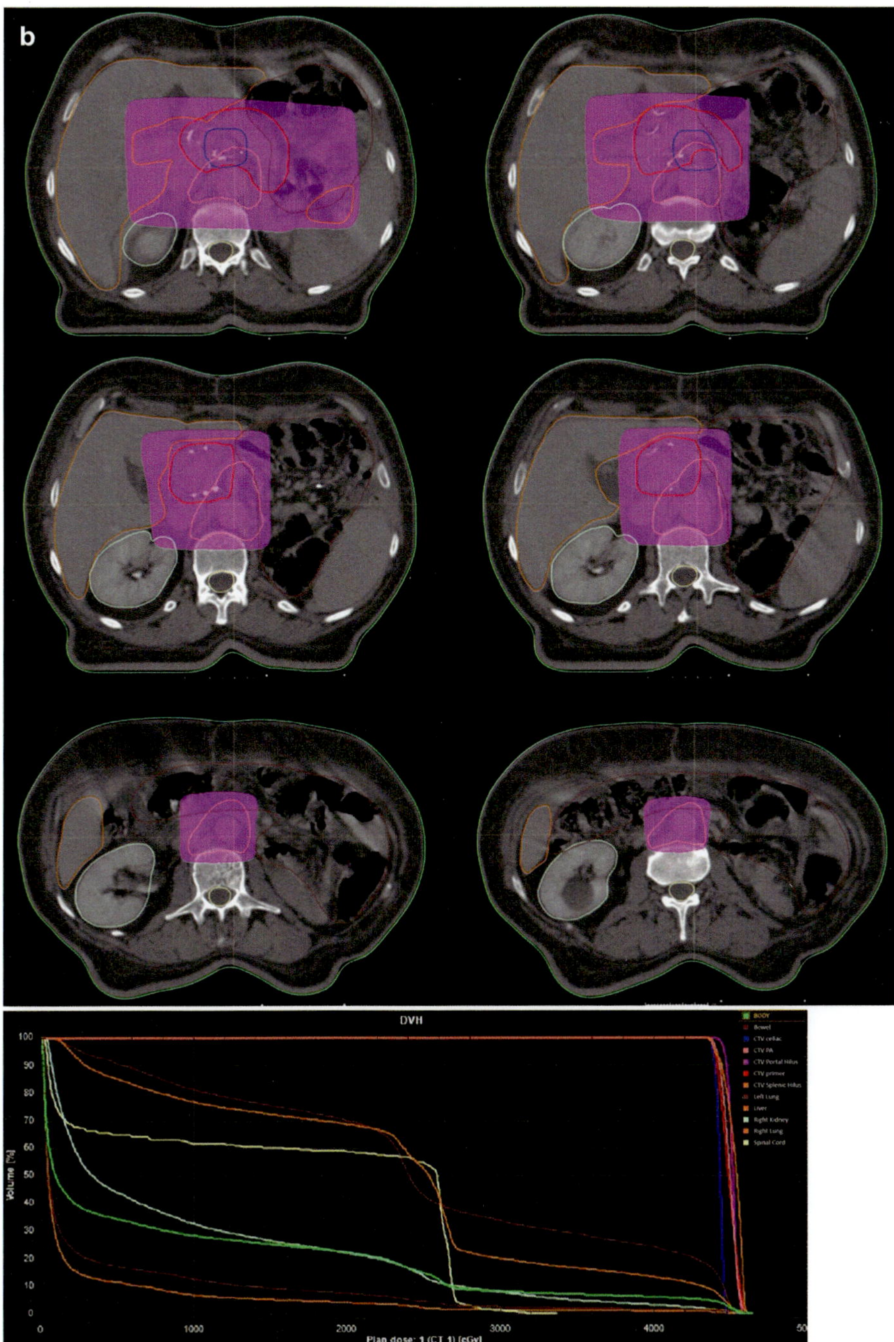

Fig. 5.7 (continued)

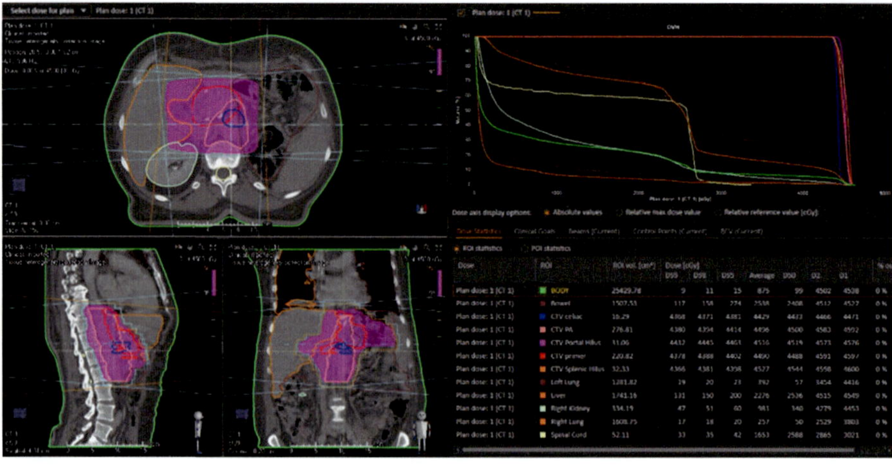

Fig. 5.8 Treatment plan of the patient

Table 5.12 Recommended dose constraints for organs at risk [19]

Organ	Constraints
Liver	Mean dose 30–32 Gy
Kidney	V18 < 33% V15 < 30% (each kidney evaluated separately)
Spinal cord	D max < 50 Gy
Small intestine	V45 < 195 cc (entire potential space within the peritoneal cavity)
Bowel	Mean < 18 Gy
Heart	V30 < 46% (pericardium) V25 < 10% (whole heart) Mean dose <26 (pericardium)

5.2.4 Follow-Up (F/U) Recommendations

According to ESMO Guidelines [21]: A regular follow-up may allow investigation and treatment of symptoms, psychological support and early detection of recurrence, though there is no evidence that it improves survival outcomes Follow-up should be tailored to the individual patient and the stage of the disease. Dietary support is recommended for patients on either a radical or a palliative pathway, with reference to vitamin and mineral deficiencies

In the advanced disease setting, identification of patients for second-line chemotherapy and clinical trials requires regular follow-up to detect symptoms of disease progression before significant clinical deterioration. If relapse/disease progression is suspected, then a clinical history, physical examination and directed blood tests should be carried out. Radiological investigations should be carried out in patients who are candidates for further chemotherapy or RT.

5.3   Pancreas Cancer

Overview

Epidemiology: Pancreatic cancer is the fourth leading cause of cancer mortality in the United States with the overall 5-year survival of only 5%. The major risk factors are high body mass and lack of physical activity, nonhereditary chronic pancreatitis and hereditary risk factors, such as hereditary pancreatitis.

Pathology: More than 95% of malignant neoplasms of the pancreas are adenocarcinoma arising from the exocrine elements of the pancreas.

Diagnosis: The most common presenting symptoms are pain, jaundice, and weight loss. Endoscopic ultrasonography (EUS) with biopsy should be considered to obtain diagnosis. Pancreatic protocol computed tomography (CT) provides an assessment of local and regional extent of the disease and gives information about the resectability of the disease. Chest and pelvic CT are used to demonstrate distant metastasis. Serum CA 19-9 might be used in the follow up if elevated at the time of diagnosis.

Definitive Treatment: Surgery is the mainstay of treatment however most of the patients are unresectable at the time of diagnosis due to presence of distant metastasis or vascular invasion. Treatment decision is made according to the resectability of the tumor. Chemotherapy is typically used in all stages of the disease; however the role of adjuvant chemoradiotherapy is controversial and is usually considered for patients with margin positive or lymph node positive disease.

Keywords: Pancreas cancer; Radiotherapy

5.3.1   Case Presentation

K.O. is a 74 year-old female with KPS of 90. She applied to the clinics with gradually increasing abdominal pain in last 6 months. Physical examination was normal. She had medical history of type 2 DM which is under control for 10 years with oral anti-diabetics. He had neither smoking nor alcohol history. His whole blood count, kidney and liver function tests were normal. Contrast-enhanced thorax and abdominal computed tomography (CT) revealed 54 × 50 mm mass located in the tail of pancreas and invading splenic artery. Periportal, periceliac and gastrohepatic calcific lymph nodes consistent with sequel of granulomatous disease (Fig. 5.9). Endoscopic biopsy revealed adenocarcinoma. Patient had distal subtotal pancreate ctomy+splenectomy+celiac   lymph   nodedissection.   Pathology   was: Adenocarcinoma, tumor 5.2 × 4 × 4 cm. in diameter. Eight metastatic lymph nodes and 5 reactive lymph nodes. Congestive spleen. Chronic cholecystitis. Clear surgical margins.

According to 8th edition AJCC/UICC staging system, patient has stage III (pT3N2M0) adenocarcinoma of the pancreas (Table 5.13) [29].

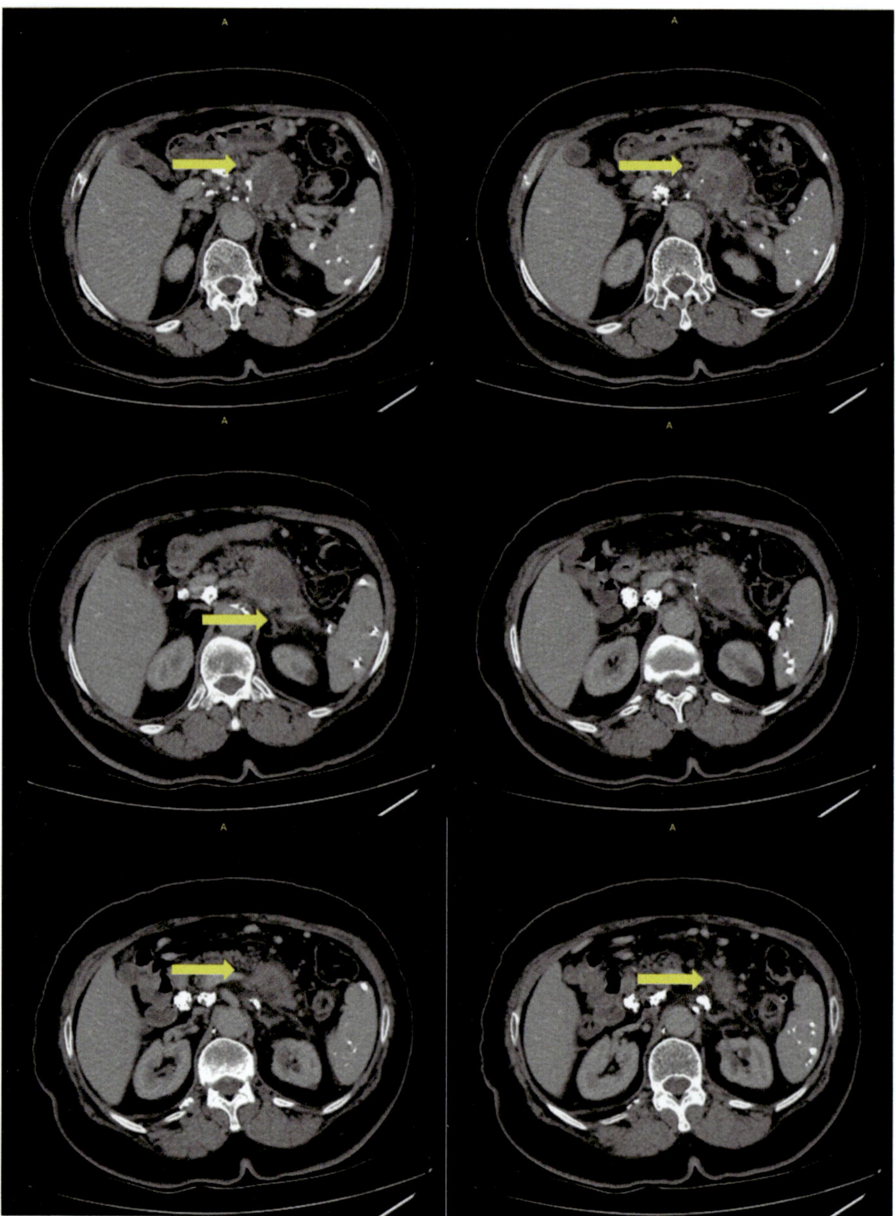

Fig. 5.9 Contrast-enhanced thorax and abdominal computed tomography (CT) revealed 54 × 50 mm mass located in the tail of pancreas and invading splenic artery. Periportal, periceliac and gastrohepatic calcific lymph nodes consistent with sequel of granulomatous disease

Table 5.13 Pancreatic cancers—TNM staging AJCC UICC, 2017 [29]

Primary tumor (T)	
T category	*T criteria*
TX	Primary tumor cannot be assessed
T0	No evidence of primary tumor
Tis	Carcinoma in situ This includes high-grade pancreatic intraepithelial neoplasia (PanIn-3), intraductal papillary mucinous neoplasm with high-grade dysplasia, intraductal tubulopapillary neoplasm with high-grade dysplasia, and mucinous cystic neoplasm with high-grade dysplasia
T1	Tumor $\leq$2 cm in greatest dimension
T1a	Tumor $\leq$0.5 cm in greatest dimension
T1b	Tumor >0.5 cm and <1 cm in greatest dimension
T1c	Tumor 1–2 cm in greatest dimension
T2	Tumor >2 cm and $\leq$4 cm in greatest dimension
T3	Tumor >4 cm in greatest dimension
T4	Tumor involves celiac axis, superior mesenteric artery, and/or common hepatic artery, regardless of size

Regional lymph nodes (N)	
N category	*N criteria*
NX	Regional lymph nodes cannot be assessed
N0	No regional lymph node metastases
N1	Metastasis in one to three regional lymph nodes
N2	Metastasis in four or more regional lymph nodes

Distant metastasis (M)	
M category	*M criteria*
M0	No distant metastasis
M1	Distant metastasis

Stage groups			
T	*N*	*M*	*Stage*
Tis	N0	M0	0
T1	N0	M0	IA
T1	N1	M0	IIB
T1	N2	M0	III
T2	N0	M0	IB
T2	N1	M0	IIB
T2	N2	M0	III
T3	N0	M0	IIA
T3	N1	M0	IIB
T3	N2	M0	III
T4	Any N	M0	III
Any T	Any N	M1	IV

Used with permission of the American College of Surgeons, Chicago, Illinois. The original and primary source for this information is the AJCC Cancer Staging Manual, Eighth Edition (2017) published by Springer International Publishing

5.3.2 Evidence Based Treatment Recommendations

The most common presenting symptoms are pain, jaundice, and weight loss. Endoscopic ultrasonography (EUS) with biopsy should be considered to obtain diagnosis. Pancreatic protocol computed tomography (CT) provides an assessment of local and regional extent of the disease and gives information about the resectability of the disease. MRI may be used if patient has iodinated contrast allergy. Chest and pelvic CT are used to demonstrate distant metastasis. Laboratory workup should include complete blood count, CEA, CA 19-9, glucose, amylase, lipase, bilirubin, ALP, LDH, ALT, and AST. Serum CA 19-9 might be used in the follow up if elevated at the time of diagnosis. Endoscopic retrograde cholangiopancreatography (ERCP) is indicated if there is suspicion in the diagnosis or in case of need for biliary decompression. The tumor, node, metastasis (TNM) staging system of the combined American Joint Committee on Cancer (AJCC)/Union for International Cancer Control (UICC) for pancreatic cancer is used for staging [29].

Complete surgical resection is considered as the potentially curative treatment. However, only 15–20% of patients have potentially resectable disease at diagnosis [30]. A pancreatic cancer is unresectable if there is distant metastases or vascular invasion. Local unresectability is usually due to vascular invasion, particularly of the superior mesenteric artery (SMA). The NCCN consensus report guidelines define a staging system based on tumor extent and offer treatment recommendations accordingly (Table 5.14) (https://www.nccn.org/professionals/physician_gls/pdf/pancreatic.pdf. Accessed May 2018). However, even after complete (R0) resection both systemic and local recurrence rates are high; thus systemic chemotherapy, radiotherapy, and chemoradiotherapy have been used in addition to surgery to improve treatment results. For patients with unresectable disease, initial chemotherapy followed by local treatment (surgery or chemoradiation/SBRT) is preferred (https://www.nccn.org/professionals/physician_gls/pdf/pancreatic.pdf. Accessed May 2018).

5.3.2.1 Literature Review

Treatment decisions should ideally be made in multidisiplinary setting.

Resectable Disease Upfront surgery is typically recommended. Major patterns of failure after surgical resection are locoregional or distant relapses. Patients with lymph node positive disease and margin positive disease have high risk of locoregional relapse. Adjuvant chemotherapy and chemoradiotherapy (5FU or gemcitabine based) have improved survival over surgery alone. Chemotherapy is typically used in all stages of the disease; however the role of adjuvant chemoradiotherapy is controversial and is usually considered for patients with margin positive or lymph node positive disease. Neoadjuvant therapy may be considered in patients with high risk features (very high CA 19-9, large primary tumors, large regional lymph nodes, excessive weight loss and extreme pain) (https://www.nccn.org/professionals/physician_gls/pdf/pancreatic.pdf. Accessed May 2018) [31].

Table 5.14 NCCN definitions for resectability (https://www.nccn.org/professionals/physician_gls/pdf/pancreatic.pdf. Accessed May 2018)

	Arterial	Venous
Resectable	No arterial tumor contact around CA, SMA, and CHA	No tumor contast with SMV or PV or ≤180° contact without vein contour irregularity
Borderline resectable	**Pancreatic head/uncinate process:** • Solid tumor contact with CHA without extension to CA or hepatic artery (HA) bifurcation allowing for safe and complete resection and reconstruction • Solid tumor contact with the SMA of ≤180° • Solid tumor contact with variant arterial anatomy and the presence and degree of tumor contact should be noted if present, as it may affect surgical planning **Pancreatic body/tail:** • Solid tumor contact with the CA of ≤180° • Solid tumor contact with the CA of >180° without involvement of the aorta and with intact and uninvolved gastroduedonal artery	• Solid tumor contact with the SMV or PV >180°, contact of ≤180° with contour irregularity of the vein but with suitable vessel proximal and distal to the site of involvement allowing for safe and complete resection and vein reconstruction • Solid tumor contact with IVC
Unresectable	• Distant metastasis (including non-regional LN metastasis) **Pancreatic head/uncinate process:** • Solid tumor contact with SMA >180° • Solid tumor contact with CA >180° **Pancreatic body/tail:** • Solid tumor contact of >180° with the SMA or CA • Solid tumor contact with the CA and aortic involvement	**Pancreatic head/uncinate process:** • Unreconstructable SMV/PV due to tumor involvement or occlusion (can be due to tumor or bland thrombus) • Contact with most proximal draining jejunal branch into SMV **Body and tail:** • Unreconstructable SMV/PV due to tumor involvement or occlusion (can be due to tumor or bland thrombus)

CA celiac artery, *SMA* superior mesenteric artery, *CHA* common hepatic artery, PV portav vein, *SMV* superior mesenteric vein, *IVC* inferior vena cava

Table 5.15 Adjuvant chemoradiation or chemotherapy randomized studies in pancreatic cancer

Study	No	Treatment	Median survival (months)
GITSG [32]	22	Observation	11
	21	40.0 Gy RT + bolus 5-FU	20
EORTC 40891 [33]	54	Observation	12.6
	60	40.0 Gy RT + CI 5-FU	17.1
ESPAC-1 [34]	69	Observation	16.9
	73	40.0 Gy split-course RT + bolus 5-FU/LV	13.9
	72	40.0 Gy split-course RT + bolus	19.9
	75	5-FU → 5-FU/LV	21.6
		Bolus 5-FU/LV	
EORTC 40013/FFCD	45	Gemcitabine	24.4
9203/GERCOR [35]	45	Gemcitabine → Gemcitabine + RT (50.4 Gy)	24.3

RT radiotherapy, *No* number

The role of adjuvant chemoradiotherapy is controversial in pancreatic cancer and its use differs among Europe and United States. However; it should be kept in mind that there is lack of standardization in the treatment protocols in the studies published before (Table 5.15).

GITSG study randomized patients with resected pancreatic cancer to either observation or radiotherapy (40 Gy) plus concurrent bolus fluorouracil (FU; 500 mg/m^2/day on the first 3 and last 3 days of radiotherapy), followed by maintenance chemotherapy (FU 500 mg/m^2/day for three days monthly) for 2 years or until disease progression [32]. Patients receiving postoperative chemoradiotherapy had significantly longer median overall survival (20 vs 11 months) and higher 2 year survival rate (20% vs 10%). Following closure of the study, an additional 30 patients were registered on the combined modality arm, and the latest report including confirmed the initial survival benefit [36].

Following this study, EORTC conducted a study that randomized 114 patients with resected pancreatic cancer to postoperative concurrent FU (25 mg/kg/day by continuous infusion) plus radiotherapy (40 Gy in split courses) or observation [33]. The median duration of survival was 19.0 months for the observation group and 24.5 months in the treatment group (p = 0.208). The 2-year survival estimates were 41% and 51%, respectively. There was no reduction in locoregional recurrence with combined modality therapy. The major criticisms of the two studies are the status of surgical margins, suboptimal radiotherapy dose and the method of split-course of delivery. Furthermore, in the EORTC study, 20% of patients randomized to treatment never received it because of postoperative complications or patient refusal.

European Study for Pancreatic Cancer (ESPAC)-1 trial initially set out to randomize patients to a 2 × 2 factorial design in which the relative benefits of adjuvant chemotherapy, chemoradiotherapy, or chemoradiotherapy followed by chemotherapy would be compared with observation alone. After resection, 541 patients were randomized to adjuvant chemoradiotherapy (20 Gy/10 fraction over 2 weeks with 500 mg/m^2 fluorouracil intravenously on days 1–3, repeated after 2 weeks) or chemotherapy (intravenous fluorouracil 425 mg/m^2 and folinic acid 20 mg/m^2 daily for 5 days, monthly for 6 months). Initial results of the study showed no benefit for adjuvant chemoradiotherapy (median survival = 15.5 months vs 16.1 months, p = 0.24). There was evidence of a survival benefit for adjuvant chemotherapy (median survival = 19.7 months with chemotherapy vs 14.0 months without chemotherapy, p = 0.0005) [37]. Long term results of ESPAC, with a median follow-up of 47 months, demonstrated that 5 year survival rate was 10% among patients assigned to receive chemoradiotherapy and 20% among patients who did not receive chemoradiotherapy (p = 0.05). The five-year survival rate was 21% among patients who received chemotherapy and 8% among patients who did not receive chemotherapy (p = 0.009). The benefit of chemotherapy persisted after adjustment for major prognostic factors [34]. However there are several criticisms about this trial; radiotherapy dose in this trial is suboptimal, split-course radiotherapy might lead to tumor repopulation, no adjuvant chemotherapy in the chemoradiation group, and the analyses in the chemotherapy group were not "intent-to-treat" analysis. However after this trial many European centers prefer to use chemotherapy rather than chemoradiotherapy in the adjuvant setting.

ESPAC-3 trial randomized 985 patients with resected pancreatic cancer to 6 months of postoperative adjuvant treatment with either gemcitabine (1000 mg/m^2 weekly for three of every 4 weeks) or leucovorin-modulated fluorouracil (leucovorin 20 mg/m^2 followed by fluorouracil 425 mg/m^2 IV bolus days 1–5 every 28 days) [38]. With a median follow-up of 34 months, median survival was similar (23.6 vs 23 months). However, the patients assigned to FU/leucovorin had more grade 3 to 4 treatment-related toxicity, and more treatment-related hospitalizations.

EORTC-40013-22012/FFCD-9203/GERCOR is a phase II study of postoperative gemcitabine versus gemcitabine-based chemoradiotherapy. In this study patients were randomized to receive either four cycles of gemcitabine or gemcitabine for two cycles followed by weekly gemcitabine with concurrent radiation (50.4 Gy). The results showed that local recurrence alone at first progression in the chemoradiotherapy group was notably lower (11% vs 24%), as was the rate of local and distant progression (13% vs 20%). Two-year overall survival rates were similar (50.2% vs. 50.6%) [35].

Adjuvant Chemoradiation or Chemotherapy randomized studies in Pancreatic Cancer are summarized in Table 5.15.

Unresectable Disease There is no consensus as to the best approach for patients with locally advanced, unresectable pancreatic cancer. Neoadjuvant chemotherapy of FOLFIRINOX is the widely used treatment option for these patients followed by re-evaluation for surgery. If the patient is not proper for surgery chemoradiation/SBRT are considered for treatment in patients with good performance status. For patients who are not considered candidates for surgery or radiotherapy, continued chemotherapy is a rational approach.

Borderline Resectable Disease A meta-analysis of phase II trials showed that neoadjuvant treatment have some activity in patients with borderline/unresectable pancreatic adenocarcinoma. One third of tumors were able to be ultimately resected after treatment [39]. Median survival in this patients was 22.3 months. FOLFIRINOX and gemcitabine combinations are the widely used neoadjuvant treatment regimes.

5.3.2.2 Treatment Recommendations

Treatment recommendations for non-metastatic pancreatic cancer according to NCCN guidelines are summarized in Table 5.16.

5.3.3 Treatment Planning

5.3.3.1 Simulation

Patients should be immobilized with their arms above their head in a vacuum bag. For tumors located at the lower part of esophagus patients should be advised to

Table 5.16 NCCN guidelines version 1.2018 (https://www.nccn.org/professionals/physician_gls/pdf/pancreatic.pdf. Accessed May 2018) and ASCO guidelines [40, 41]

Stage	Recommended treatment
Resectable	Surgery → Adjuvant treatment • All patients with resected pancreatic cancer who did not receive preoperative therapy should be offered 6 months of adjuvant chemotherapy with either gemcitabine or fluorouracil plus folinic acid in the absence of medical or surgical contraindications • Adjuvant treatment should be initiated within 8 weeks of surgical resection, assuming complete recovery. There are currently no data to support combination chemotherapy regimens in the adjuvant setting, and the panel recommends against such use unless used as part of a clinical trial • Adjuvant chemoradiation may be offered to patients who did not receive preoperative therapy and present after resection with microscopically positive margins (R1) and/or node-positive disease after completion of 4–6 months of systemic adjuvant chemotherapy • For patients with pancreatic cancer who received preoperative therapy, there are no RCT data to guide the administration of postoperative therapy. A total of 6 months of adjuvant therapy (including preoperative regimen) is offered based on extrapolation from adjuvant therapy trials
Borderline resectable	Neoadjuvant treatment → Surgery • If there is local disease progression after induction chemotherapy, but without evidence of systemic spread, then CRT or SBRT may be offered • If there is systemic spread systemic treatments should be considered
Unresectable	Neoadjuvant treatment (chemotherapy, Chemoradiotherapy, induction chemotherapy → chemoradiotherapy or SBRT) → Surgery • If there is local disease progression after induction chemotherapy, but without evidence of systemic spread, then CRT or SBRT may be offered • If there is systemic spread systemic treatments should be considered

avoid having meal 2–4 h before simulation and each treatment to limit differences in gastric filling. Intravenous-oral contrast can be considered during simulation to visualize vascular structures and delineate lymph nodes better. A CT slice thickness of 3 mm is recommended. Planning CT should encompass the entire abdomen. Considerations of four dimensional CT or active-breathing control techniques are recommended due to the significant tumor and normal tissue motion with respiration.

5.3.3.2 Contouring

Definitive Chemoradiotherapy

According to RTOG 1102 (https://www.rtog.org/clinicaltrials/protocoltable/studydetails.aspx?study=1102. Accessed May 2018) protocol:

The gross tumor volume (GTV): Primary tumor and the lymph node >10 mm (after reviewing the diagnostic CT, pancreas protocol CT, PET-CT, and/or MR abdomen if applicable). The CTV includes a 1 cm expansion off the GTV and should encompass all relevant nodal regions

The clinical target volume (CTV): GTV plus a 10 mm expansion for microscopic extension in regions at risk (e.g., vertebral body to be excluded). Uninvolved regional nodes will NOT be included in the CTV.

The planning target volume (PTV): CTV plus a 20 mm expansion in the cranial and caudal directions and a 10 mm expansion in the radial (lateral, anterior and posterior and oblique dimensions).

Elective nodal irradiation is controversial for locally advanced, unresectable and borderline resectable pancreatic cancer.

Postoperative Chemoradiotherapy

According to RTOG 0848 (https://www.rtog.org/LinkClick.aspx?fileticket=CLd1-1PWZek%3d&tabid=237. Accessed May 2018) protocol:

CTV includes

Post-operative bed: Based on location of initial tumor from pre-operative imaging and pathology reports pathology reports

Anastomoses: Pancreaticojejunostomy (PJ), Choledochal or hepaticojunostomy

Lymph node coverage: Peripancreatic, celiac, superior mesenteric, porta hepatis, para-aortic lymph nodes

Para-aortic nodes extends from the top of the uppermost CTV slice to the bottom of L2 or L3 if there is a low-lying tumor. It is recommended to expand 2.5 cm to the right, 1 cm to the left, 0.2 cm posteriorly, and 2 cm anteriorly from aorta. Superior mesenteric lymph node is the proximal 2.5–3.0 cm of the vessel. Celiac axis is the most proximal 1.0–1.5 cm of the vessel. Postoperative bed is expanded by 1 cm to form CTV. Porta hepatis can be omitted in case of body or tail lesions.

PTV includes CTV + 0.5 cm.

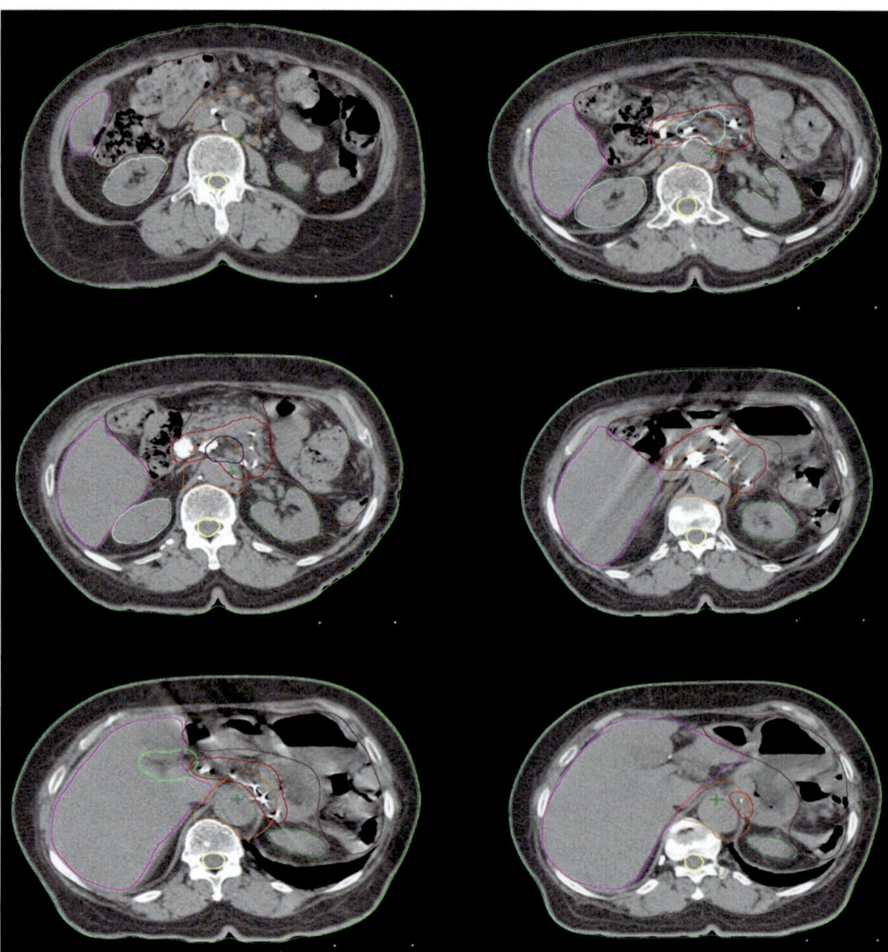

Fig. 5.10 Delineation of treatment volumes Red = CTVprimary, blue = CTVceliac, orange = CTVparaaortic, navy = CTVsuperior mesenteric, green = CTVportal

Case Contouring Delineation of target volumes for the case in the adjuvant setting is shown in Fig. 5.10.

Case Plan The case presented here has stage III pancreatic adenocarcinoma located at the tail. The patient received adjuvant chemoradiation following 6 cycles of adjuvant chemotherapy (capecitabine-gemcitabine). Patient received adjuvant radiotherapy (total 50.4 Gy in 1.8 Gy/fraction) with concurrent chemotherapy (weekly gemcitabine) utilizing 3DCRT technique. Treatment planning details are seen in Figs. 5.11 and 5.12.

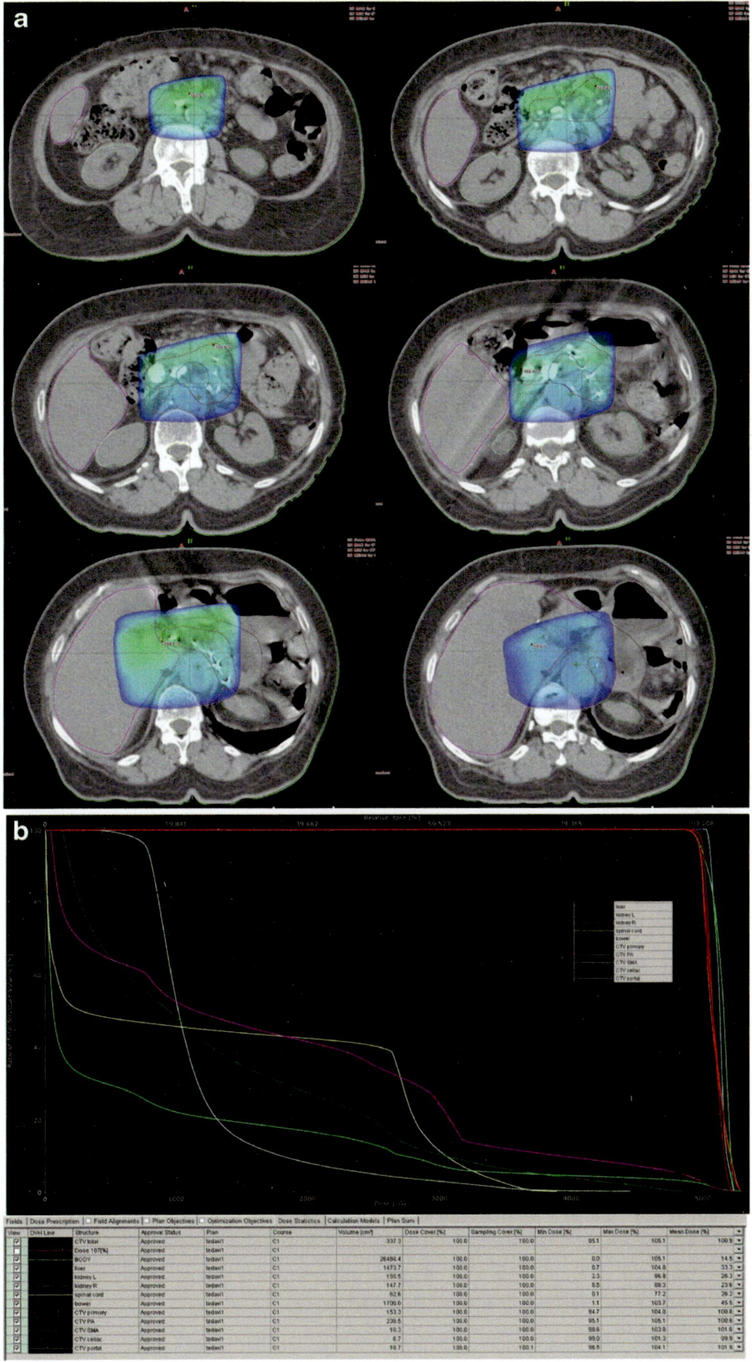

Fig. 5.11 Three dimensional conformal radiotherapy planning of the patient with pancreatic cancer after surgery. Total dose of 50.4 Gy in 1.8 Gy/fraction was delivered by 3DCRT technique (**a**) 95% isodose coverage (blue) and (**b**) dose-volume histogram are shown. Red = CTVprimary, light blue = CTVceliac, orange = CTVparaaortic, navy = CTVsuperior mesenteric, green = CTVportal

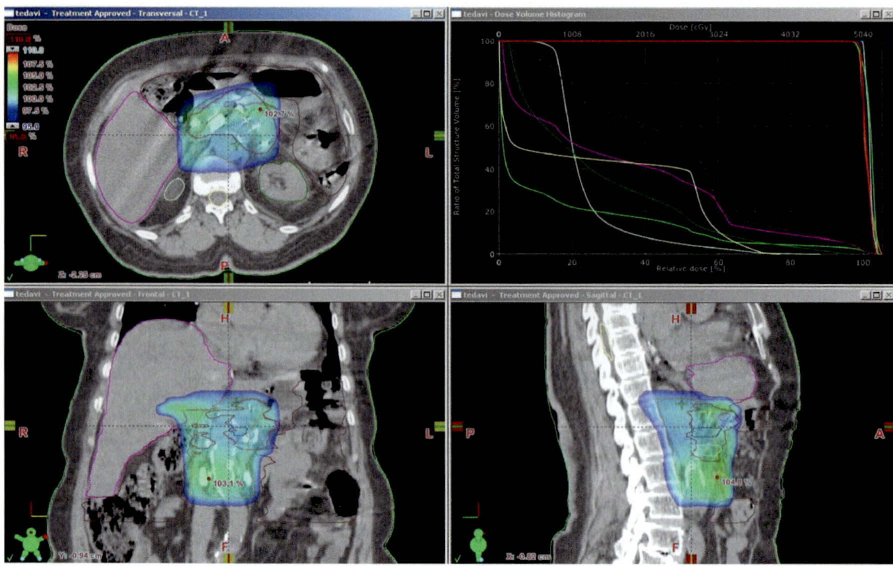

Fig. 5.12 Treatment plan of the patient showing the 95% isodose line blue in color

5.3.3.3 Dose Recommendations

Definitive: 45–54 Gy in 1.8–2 Gy/fraction, stereotactic body RT (SBRT) may be used as a part of a clinical trial 30–35 Gy/3 fractions or 25–45 Gy in 5 fractions)

Postoperative: 45–50.4 Gy in 1.8–2 Gy/fraction ±5–9 Gy boost to tumor bed and anastomosis, if clinically appropriate.

Concomitant Chemotherapy Flouropyrimidine (CI-5FU or capecitabine) or Gemcitabine

Treatment Delivery Techniques 3D-CRT and IMRT should be used. Where available, SBRT is an alternative to chemoradiotherapy, although there are no trials establishing the comparable efficacy of SBRT and standard fractionation radiotherapy in this setting.

5.3.3.4 Dose Constraints for Critical Structures

Table 5.17 shows dose-volume constraints for treatment planning.

5.3.3.5 Follow-Up (F/U) Recommendations

A follow-up visit every 3–4 months that includes a physical examination, and liver and renal function tests for 2 years, after which time intervals can be increased to every 6 months.

Table 5.17 Dose constraints for chemoradiatiotherapy (file:///C:/Users/USER/Downloads/1102.pdf. Accessed May 2018; https://www.rtog.org/LinkClick.aspx?fileticket=CLd1-1PWZek%3d&tabid=237. Accessed May 2018)

Organ	Unresectable disease	Adjuvant treatment
Kidneys (left and right)	Not more than 30% of the total volume can receive ≥18 Gy. If only one kidney is functional, not more than 10% of the volume can receive ≥18 Gy	For 3D conformal plans in patients with two normally functioning kidneys, at least 50% of the right kidney and at least 65% of the left kidney must receive <18 Gy. For IMRT planning, mean dose to bilateral kidneys must be <18 Gy. If only one kidney is present, not more than 15% of the volume of that kidney can receive ≥18 Gy and no more than 30% can get ≥14 Gy
Stomach, duodenum, jejunum	Max dose 55 Gy	Max dose <54 Gy; <10% of each organ volume can receive between 50 and 53.99 Gy, <15% of the volume of each organ can receive between 45 and 49.99 Gy
Liver	Mean dose cannot exceed 30 Gy	Mean liver dose must be ≤25 Gy
Spinal cord	Max dose to a volume of at least 0.03 cc must be ≤45 Gy	Max dose ≤45 Gy

Testing for serum CA 19-9 (if initially elevated) and CT scanning) at least every three to four months during the first 2 years, and then every 6 months once disease stability is comfortably established.

Routine use of positron emission tomography (PET) imaging is not recommended [42].

5.4   Rectum Cancer

Overview

Epidemiology: Rectal cancer is a common disease influenced by both environmental and genetic factors.

Pathology: Adenocarcinoma is the most common histopathology.

Diagnosis: Rectal bleeding is the most common symptom. In addition to digital clinical examination and rigid proctoscopy, patients should undergo preoperative either rectal MRI or transrectal ultrasound, chest-abdomen-pelvic CT.

Definitive Treatment: Surgery remains the main treatment in patients with rectal cancer. However radiotherapy also remains a standard component of management of locally advanced rectal cancer. Preoperative chemoradiation is associated with improved local control, sphincter preservation and lower treatment related toxicity rates compared to postoperative radiotherapy.

Keywords: Rectum cancer; Radiotherapy

5.4.1 Case Presentation

She is a 65 year-old female with a KPS of 100 applied to the clinics with rectal bleeding. Physical examination was normal. She does not have a smoking or alcohol utilization history. Her whole blood count, and kidney and liver function tests were normal. Rectosigmoidoscopy revealed ulsero-vegetan mass located within the 5–12th cm of rectum. Contrast-enhanced thorax-abdomen computed tomography (CT) showed asymmetrical thickening of the rectal wall starting 4 cm proximal to anal canal and extending 7 cm proximally. Peri-rectal lymph nodes and specular extensions into para-rectal fatty tissue (Fig. 5.13). Pelvic magnetic resonance imaging (MRI) with contrast-diffusion MRI revealed rectal mass circumferentially covering the lumen, starting from the proximal anorectal ring and extending 7 cm proximally (Fig. 5.14). Tumor has specular extensions into mesorectum. There are several pathological lymph nodes in the para-rectal area. Biopsy of the mass was adenocarcinoma. According to AJCC Cancer Staging System, the patient has cT3N1c (Stage IIIB) mid-rectum cancer (Table 5.18) (https://www.nccn.org/professionals/physician_gls/pdf/rectal.pdf. Accessed 10 May 2018). Neoadjuvant chemoradiation is planned with concomitant daily capecitabine. Surgery was planned 6 weeks after chemoradiation.

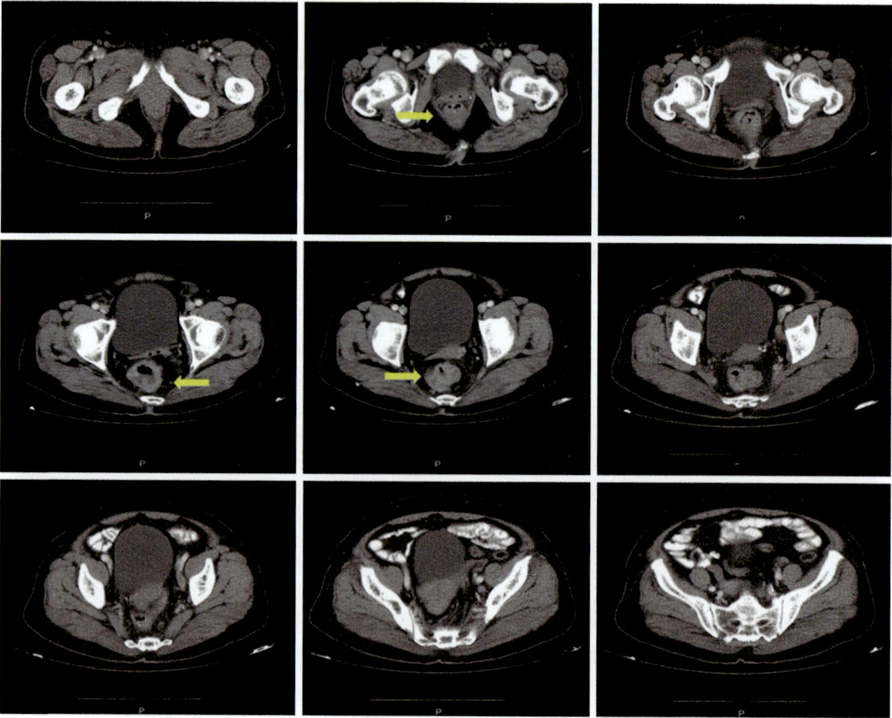

Fig. 5.13 CT images showing asymmetrical thickening of the rectal wall starting 4 cm proximal to anal canal and extending 7 cm proximally. Peri-rectal lymph nodes and spicular extensions into para-rectal fatty tissue

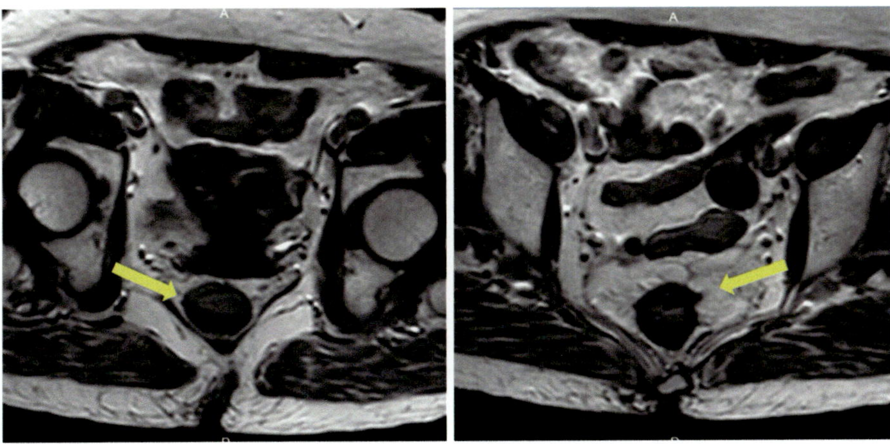

Fig. 5.14 TRA-T1W_TSE-axial images of rectal tumor with spicular extensions to mesorectum

Table 5.18 Rectum cancer TNM staging AJCC UICC, 2017

Primary tumor (T)	
T category	*T criteria*
TX	Primary tumor cannot be assessed
T0	No evidence of primary tumor
Tis	Carcinoma in situ, intramucosal carcinoma (involvement of lamina propria with no extension through muscularis mucosae)
T1	Tumor invades the submucosa (through the muscularis mucosa but not into the muscularis propria)
T2	Tumor invades the muscularis propria
T3	Tumor invades through the muscularis propria into pericolorectal tissues
T4	Tumor invades the visceral peritoneum, or invades or adheres to adjacent organs or structures
T4a	Tumor invades through the visceral peritoneum (including gross perforation of the bowel through tumor and continuous invasion of tumor through areas of inflammation to the surface of the visceral peritoneum)
T4b	Tumor directly invades or adheres to adjacent organs or structures
Regional lymph nodes (N)	
N category	*N criteria*
NX	Regional lymph nodes cannot be assessed
N0	No regional lymph node metastasis
N1	One to three regional lymph nodes are positive (tumor in lymph nodes measuring ≥ 0.2 mm), or any number of tumor deposits are present and all identifiable lymph nodes are negative
N1a	One regional lymph node is positive
N1b	Two or three regional lymph nodes are positive
N1c	No regional lymph nodes are positive, but there are tumor deposits in the: • Subserosa • Mesentery • Nonperitonealized pericolic, or perirectal/mesorectal tissues

(continued)

Table 5.18 (continued)

N2	Four or more regional nodes are positive
N2a	Four to six regional lymph nodes are positive
N2b	Seven or more regional lymph nodes are positive

Distant metastasis (M)

M category	M criteria
M0	No distant metastasis by imaging, etc., no evidence of tumor in distant sites or organs. (This category is not assigned by pathologists)
M1	Metastasis to one or more distant sites or organs, or peritoneal metastasis is identified
M1a	Metastasis to one site or organ is identified without peritoneal metastasis
M1b	Metastasis to two or more sites or organs is identified without peritoneal metastasis
M1c	Metastasis to the peritoneal surface is identified alone or with other site or organ metastases

Stage groups

T	N	M	Stage
Tis	N0	M0	0
T1, T2	N0	M0	I
T3	N0	M0	IIA
T4a	N0	M0	IIB
T4b	N0	M0	IIC
T1–T2	N1/N1c	M0	IIIA
T1	N2a	M0	IIIA
T3–T4a	N1/N1c	M0	IIIB
T2–T3	N2a	M0	IIIB
T1–T2	N2b	M0	IIIB
T4a	N2a	M0	IIIC
T3–T4a	N2b	M0	IIIC
T4b	N1–N2	M0	IIIC
Any T	Any N	M1a	IVA
Any T	Any N	M1b	IVB
Any T	Any N	M1c	IVC

Used with permission of the American College of Surgeons, Chicago, Illinois. The original and primary source for this information is the AJCC Cancer Staging Manual, Eighth Edition (2017) published by Springer International Publishing

5.4.2 Evidence Based Treatment Recommendations

5.4.2.1 Literature Review

Rectal bleeding is the most common symptom. In addition to digital clinical examination and rigid proctoscopy, patients should undergo preoperative either rectal MRI or transrectal ultrasound, chest-abdomen-pelvic CT.

Surgery: Surgery is the curative treatment for rectal cancer. Superficially invasive (T1), small rectal adenocarcinomas may be treated with local excision, however most of the tumors are deeply invasive tumors. Surgical procedure is the total mesorectal excision (TME) that includes resection of local lymph nodes with transabdominal procedures. Tumors located in the upper and middle rectum can be managed with a sphincter-sparing low anterior resection; however tumors in the lower rectum may require an abdominoperineal resection. Preoperative chemoradiotherapy may be used to to spare the sphincters in this group of patients.

Preoperative Chemoradiotherapy: The current standard of care within United States for patients with T3/T4 tumors or lymph node positive disease is neoadjuvant standard fractionated chemoradiation followed by total mesorectal excision (TME) and adjuvant 5-flourouracyl based chemotherapy (https://www.nccn.org/professionals/physician_gls/pdf/rectal.pdf. Accessed 10 May 2018). In the post-TME era Dutch rectal trial which included 1805 patients compared 5 × 5 Gy radiotherapy followed by TME to TME alone. It was shown that 10 year local-regional relapse rate improved with radiotherapy (5% vs. 11%, p < 0.001) with similar overall survival rates [43].

German rectal trial randomized 823 patients with T3/T4N0M0 or lymph node + disease to either surgery followed by chemoradiation (5FU and radiotherapy to 55.8 Gy) and adjuvant 4 cycles of 5FU chemotherapy or chemoradiation (5FU and radiotherapy to 50.4 Gy) followed by surgery and adjuvant 4 cycles of 5FU chemotherapy. Surgery was performed 6 weeks after the completion of chemoradiotherapy [44]. The 10-year cumulative incidence of local relapse was 7.1% and 10.1% in the pre- and postoperative arms, respectively (p = 0.048) At the time of surgery 9% of the patients achieved complete pathological response (pCR). The overall five-year survival rates were 76% and 74%, respectively (p = 0.80). The five-year cumulative incidence of local relapse was 6% for patients assigned to preoperative chemoradiotherapy and 13% in the postoperative-treatment group (p = 0.006). Grade 3 or 4 acute toxic effects occurred in 27% of the patients in the preoperative-treatment group, as compared with 40% of the patients in the post-operative-treatment group (p = 0.001); the corresponding rates of long-term toxic effects were 14% and 24%, respectively (p = 0.01). Preoperative chemoradiation improved sphincter preservation rates [45]. After the results of this trial; preoperative therapy has become the standard of care for T3/T4 or lymph node + rectal cancer cases.

5.4.2.2 Short Course vs. Long Course Preoperative Radiotherapy?

Polish trial randomized 312 patients with T3/T4 resectable rectal cancers to receive either preoperative irradiation (25 Gy in five fractions) and surgery within 7 days or chemoradiation (50.4 Gy in 28 fractions, bolus 5FU and leucovorin) and surgery 4–6 weeks later [46] With a median follow up time of 4 years, this study showed that neoadjuvant chemoradiation did not increase survival, local control or late toxicity compared with short-course radiotherapy alone. Early radiation toxicity was higher in the chemoradiation group (18.2 vs. 3.2%; p < 0.001).

TROG 0104 trial randomized 326 patients with T3N0-2M0 rectal adenocarcinoma within 12 cm from anal verge to either pelvic radiotherapy 5 × 5 Gy in 1 week followed by early surgery, and six courses of adjuvant chemotherapy or long course of chemoradiation (50.4 Gy, 1.8 Gy/fraction, in 5.5 weeks, with continuous infusional fluorouracil 225 mg/m^2/day) followed by surgery in 4–6 weeks, and four courses of chemotherapy [47]. There was no difference in treatment outcomes (overall survival, local relapse and pCR) and toxicities. However recently published Stockholm III trial in terim results showed that short term radiotherapy induces improved downstaging if surgery is delayed 4–8 weeks [48]. But long term follow up is necessary for short term treatment to take place of long term chemoradiation.

5.4.2.3 Postoperative Chemoradiotherapy

For resected stage II or III rectal cancer, data from two randomized GITSG and NCCTG trials demonstrated a significant local control and survival benefit for postoperative combined modality therapy over surgery or postoperative RT alone [49, 50]. Thus in 1990 US (NIH) Consensus Conference recommended postoperative chemotherapy plus pelvic radiotherapy (45–55 Gy) as a standard treatment after resection of a stage II or III rectal cancer [51]. Concomitant use of a fluoropyrimidine as a radiation sensitizer during postoperative RT is preferred over using RT alone.

Treatment Recommendations: Current treatment recommendations for rectal cancer according to NCCN guidelines is shown in Table 5.19 (https://www.nccn. org/professionals/physician_gls/pdf/rectal.pdf. Accessed 10 May 2018).

Table 5.19 Treatment recommendations according to NCCN guidelines version 1.2018 (https://www.nccn.org/professionals/physician_gls/pdf/rectal.pdf. Accessed 10 May 2018)

Clinical stage	Treatment recommendation
T1, N0	Transanal local excision, if appropriate
T1–2, N0	Transabdominal resection
T3, N_{any} with clear circumferential margin (CRM) (by MRI) T1–T2 N1–2	Chemoradiation • Capecitabine/long course radiotherapy or infusional 5FU/long course radiotherapy (category 1) • Bolus 5FU/leucovorine/long course radiotherapy Or Short course radiotherapy Or Chemotherapy • FOLFOX or CAPEOX • 5FU/leucovorin or capecitabine Followed by surgery ± adjuvant systemic treatment
T3, N_{any} with involved CRM (by MRI) T4, N_{any} Locally unresectable or medically inoperable	Chemoradiation • Capecitabine/long course radiotherapy or infusional 5FU/long course radiotherapy (category 1) • Bolus 5FU/leucovorine/long course radiotherapy Followed by restaging at 6 weeks post radiotherapy If clear CRM → Surgery ± systemic therapy If CRM + → Chemotherapy (12–16 weeks) → restaging → surgery±systemic therapy Or Chemotherapy (12–16 weeks) • FOLFOX (preferred) or CAPEOX (preferred) or 5FU/leucovorin or capecitabine → capecitabine/RT (preferred) or infusional 5FU/RT (preferred) or bolus 5FU/leucovorin/ RT → restaging → surgery ± systemic therapy

5.4.3 Treatment Planning

Simulation: Patients may be simulated either in the prone position with the use of a belly board for anterior displacement of the bowel or supine position. If IMRT is planned, then it is recommended that the patient be simulated in the supine position in a body mold or other immobilization device for accurate setup reproducibility. A radiopaque marker should be placed on the anus. Bladder filling/emptying may be considered, especially if IMRT is used. A full bladder may keep bowel from migrating into the pelvis. CT simulation with ≤3 mm thickness with IV contrast should be performed to delineate the pelvic blood vessels and gross tumor volume. The use of oral contrast may be helpful to identify the small bowel, which is an important organ at risk.

Contouring: The primary gross tumor volume (GTV-P) is defined as all gross disease on physical examination and imaging studies (PET-CT, MRI). The nodal GTV (GTV-N) includes all visible perirectal, mesorectal, and involved iliac lymph nodes. The principles of contouring in the preoperative setting are summarized in Table 5.20.

Table 5.20 Description of treatment volumes [52]

Target volume	Description
GTV	GTV-P = all gross disease on physical examination and imaging studies GTV-N = all visible perirectal and uninvolved iliac nodes, any lymph node in doubt as GTV in the absence of biopsy
CTV-high risk (CTV-HR)	CTV-HR = GTV-P and GTV-N + 1.5–2-cm margin expansion superiorly and inferiorly (excluding the uninvolved bone, muscle). This volume should include the entire rectum, mesorectum, and presacral space axially at these levels. A 1–2-cm margin around gross tumor invasion into adjacent organs should be added. Coverage of the entire presacral space and mesorectum should be strongly considered. Any visible mesorectal nodes on CT and PET should also be included To cover the iliac lymphatics, a 0.7-cm margin around the iliac vessels should be drawn (excluding the muscle and bone) To cover the external iliac nodes, an additional 1-cm margin anterolaterally around the vessels is needed Anteriorly, a margin of 1–1.5 cm should be added into bladder to account for changes in bladder and rectal filling
CTV-standard risk (CTV-SR)	Should cover the entire mesorectum and right bilateral internal iliac lymph nodes for T3 tumors. Bilateral external iliac lymph nodes for T4 tumors with anterior organ involvement should also be included A 1–2-cm margin in adjacent organs with gross tumor invasion should be added for T4 lesions Superiorly, the entire rectum and mesorectum should be included (usually up to L5/S1) and at least 2-cm margin superior to gross disease, whichever is most cephalad. Inferiorly, the CTV should extend to the pelvic floor or at least 2 cm below the gross disease, whichever is most caudal To cover the iliac lymphatics, a 0.7-cm margin around the iliac vessels should be drawn (excluding the muscle and bone) To cover the external iliac nodes, an additional 1-cm margin anterolaterally around the vessels is needed Anteriorly, a margin of 1–1.5 cm should be added into bladder to account for changes in bladder and rectal filling
PTV	Each CTV should be expanded by 0.5–1 cm, depending on choice, IGRT

RTOG anorectal contouring atlas shows descriptions of three elective CTVs in patients with rectal and anal cancers [53]. CTV-A includes the perirectal, presacral, and internal iliac regions and should be covered in all patients with rectal cancer. CTV-B includes the external iliac nodes (covered only in rectal cancer cases with T4 disease or for primary rectal tumors that extend inferiorly into the distal anal canal). CTV-C includes the inguinal region (should be considered in rectal cancer cases that extend into the distal anal canal).

Case Contouring Treatment volumes in our case were shown in Fig. 5.15.

Case Plan Total dose of 45 Gy in 1.8 Gy/fraction to the lymphatic CTV and 50.4 Gy in 1.8 Gy/fraction to the primary CTV were delivered by 3DCRT (Figs. 5.16 and 5.17). Patient received concomitant capecitabine. Patient was planned to go to surgery after chemoradiotherapy.

Concomittant Chemotherapy Continous infusional fluorouracil, Capecitabine, or 5-fluorouracil/leucovorin

Dose Recommendations Treatment dose recommendations for rectum cancer are summarized in Table 5.21.

Treatment Delivery Techniques Conventional technique uses opposing PA and lateral fields, however 3D conformal radiotherapy (3DCRT) provides a better target coverage with preservation of normal tissues. Today 3DCRT is the standard of care for radiotherapy. However it is known that with IMRT, there is the chance to decrease treatment related toxicity and deliver simultaneous integrated boosts but the data for the treatment outcomes remains to be elucidated. RTOG 0822 phase II trial showed that the use of IMRT in neoadjuvant chemoradiation for rectal cancer did not reduce the rate of GI toxicity [54]. Thirty-five patients (51.5%) experienced grade ≥2 GI toxicity, 12 patients (17.6%) experienced grade 3 or 4 diarrhea, and pCR was achieved in 10 patients (14.7%). With a median follow-up time of 3.98 years, the 4-year rate of locoregional failure was 7.4% (95% confidence interval [CI]: 1.0–13.7%). The 4-year rates of OS and DFS were 82.9% (95% CI: 70.1–90.6%) and 60.6% (95% CI: 47.5–71.4%), respectively.

Surgery is typically planned 6–8 weeks after chemoradiation.

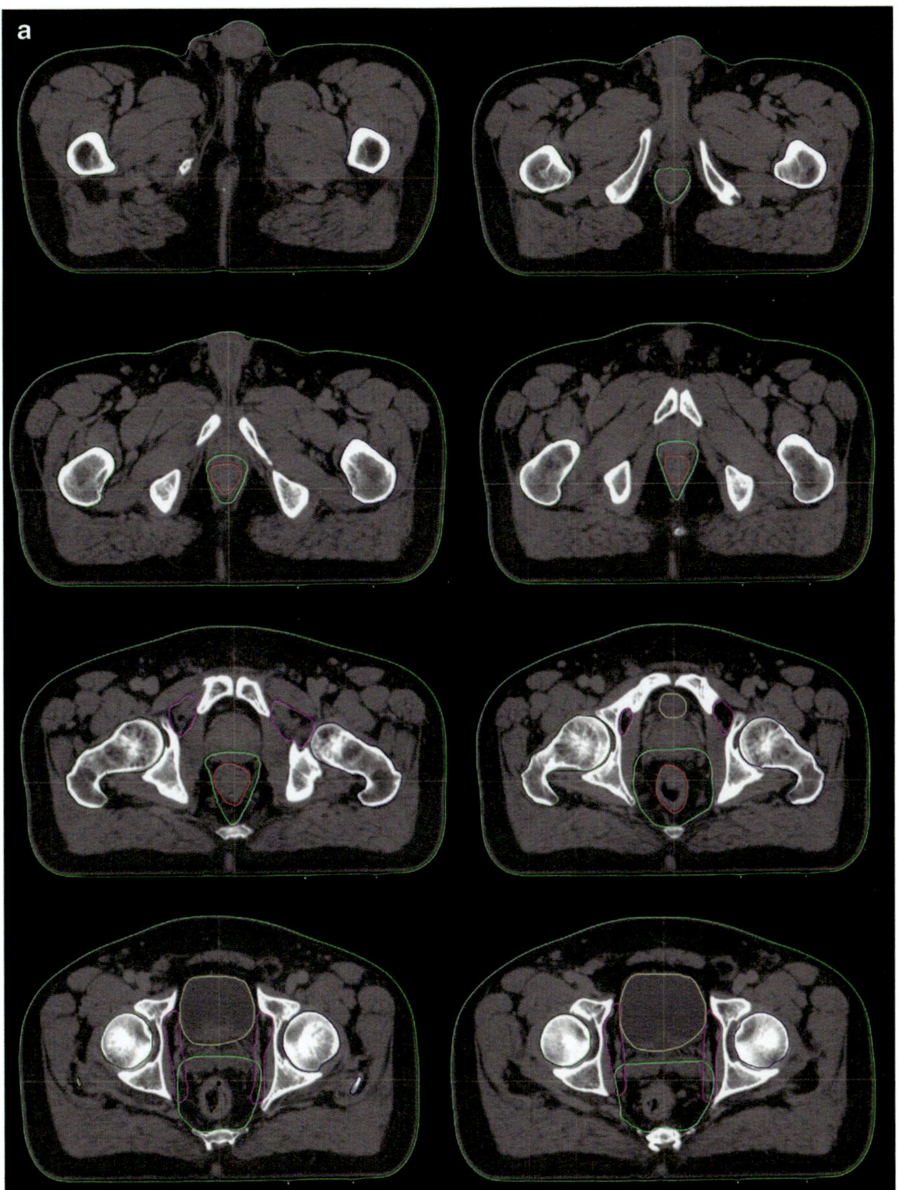

Fig. 5.15 (a, b) Delineation of the target volumes for cT3N1c mid-rectum cancer. Red = GTVrectum, Green = CTVrectum, Magenta = CTVlymphatic

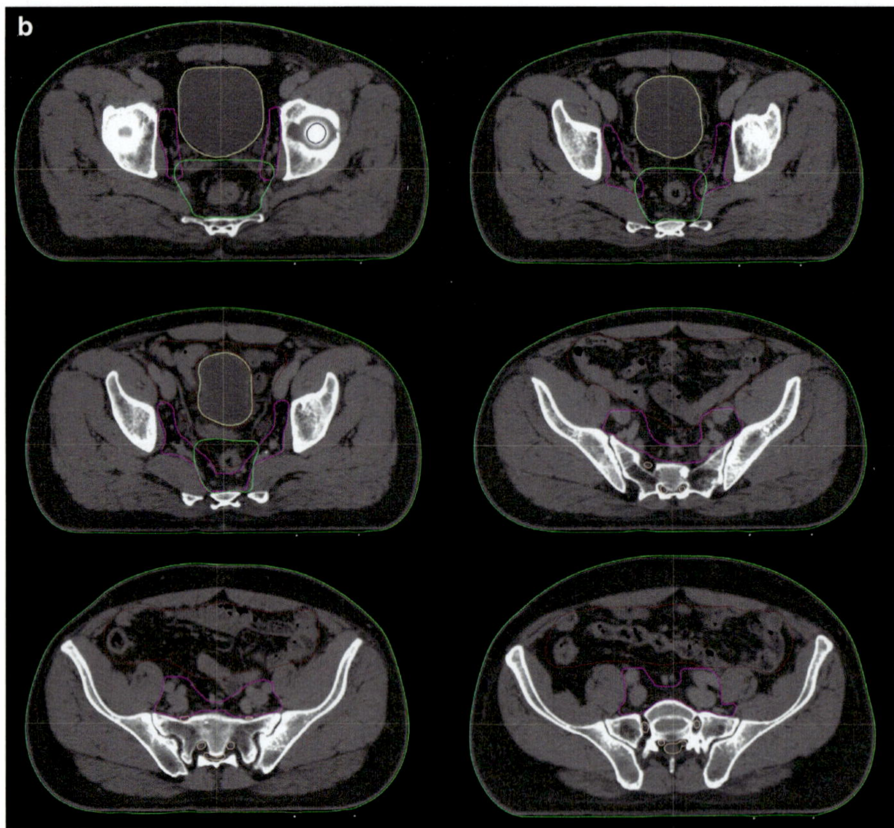

Fig. 5.15 (continued)

5.4.3.1 Dose Constraints for Critical Structures
Recommended dose constraints for critical structures for either 3DCRT or IMRT are summarized in Table 5.22.

5.4.4 Follow-Up (F/U) Recommendations

Clinical assessment: every 6 months for 2 years. History and colonoscopy with resection of colonic polyps every 5 years up to the age of 75 years. A minimum of two CTs of the chest, abdomen and pelvis in the first 3 years and regular serum CEA tests (at least every 6 months in the first 3 years).

High-risk patients (CRM+) may merit more proactive surveillance for local recurrence [57].

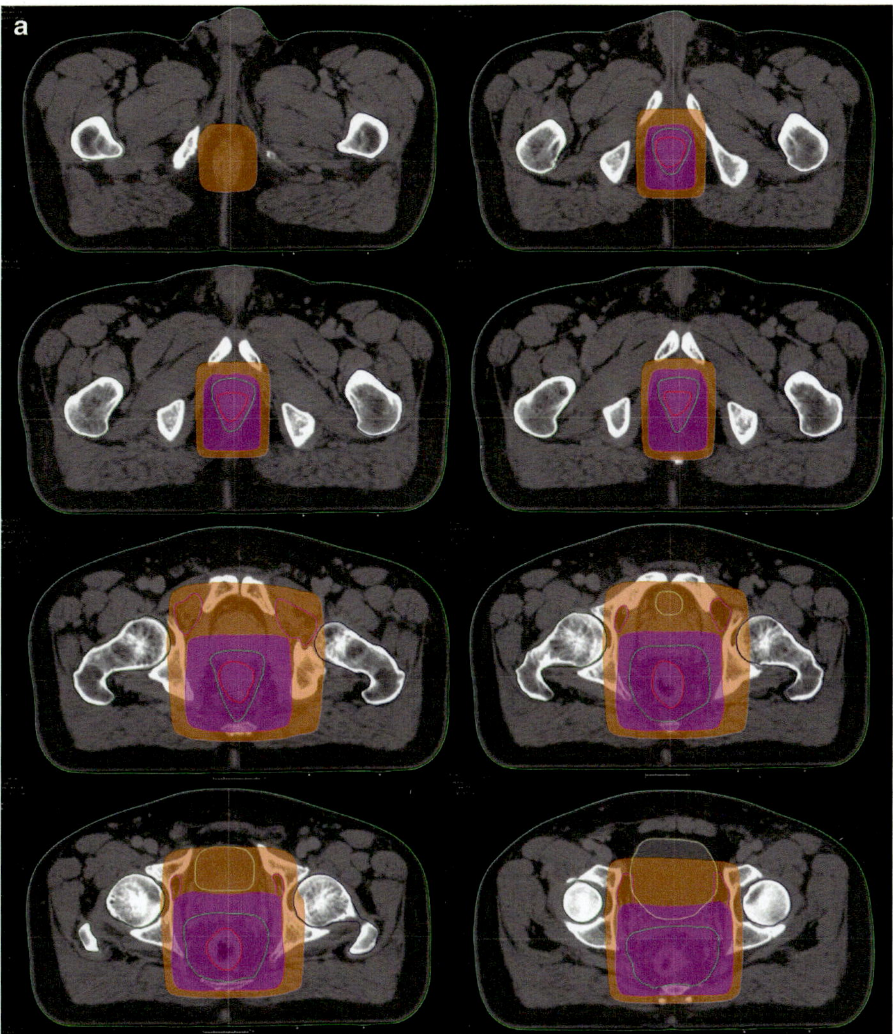

Fig. 5.16 (**a**, **b**) 3DCRT plan of the case orange for 95% isodose for CTV 50.4 Gy and lila for 95% isodose for CTV 45 Gy, (**c**) treatment plan and DVH of the treatment

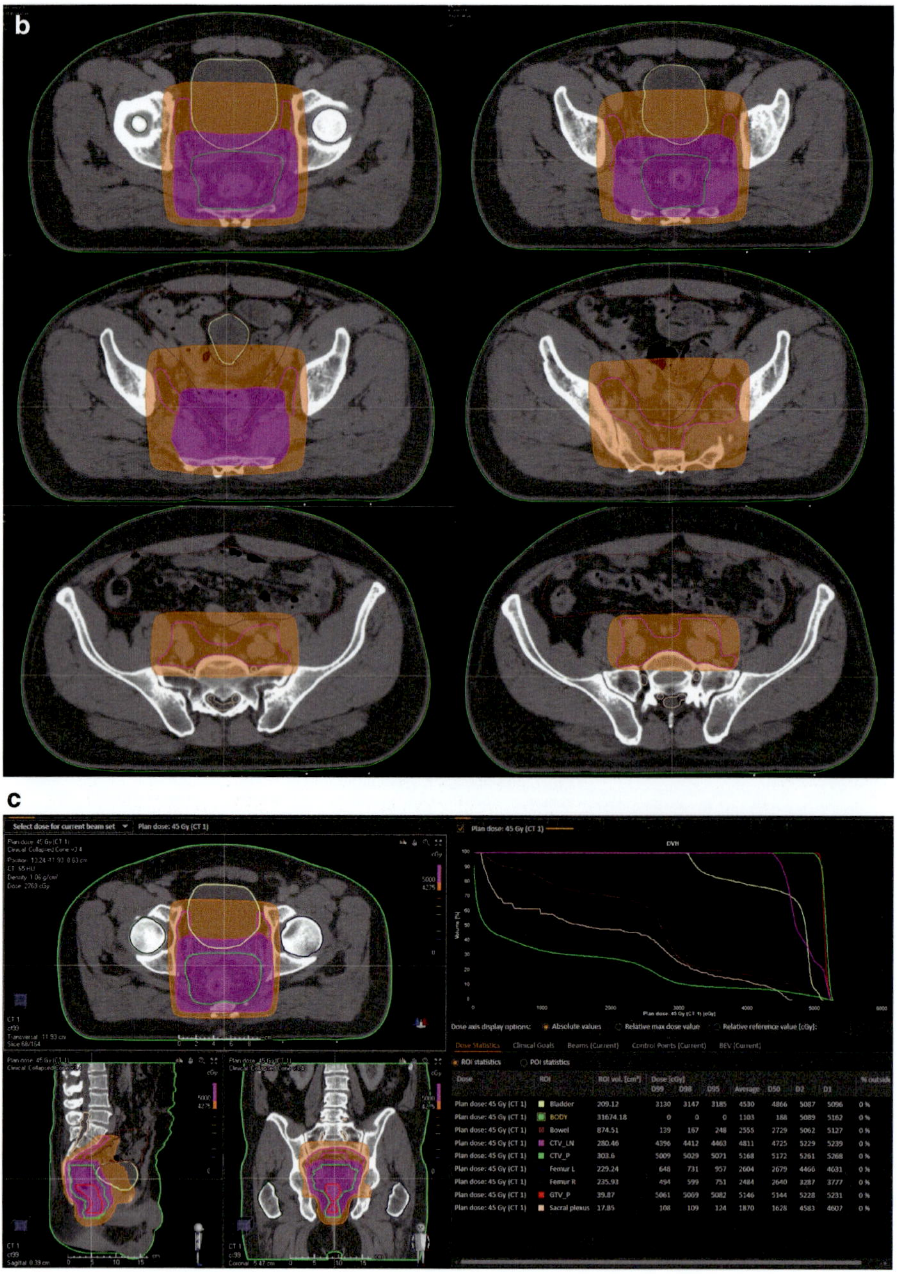

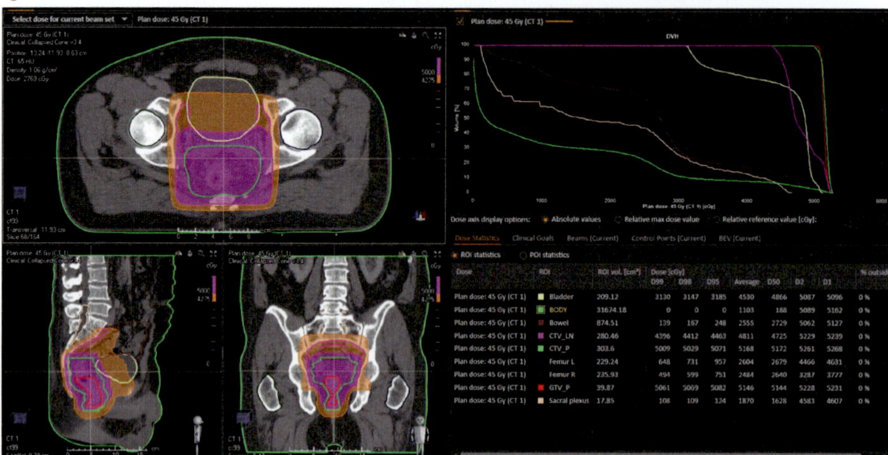

Fig. 5.16 (continued)

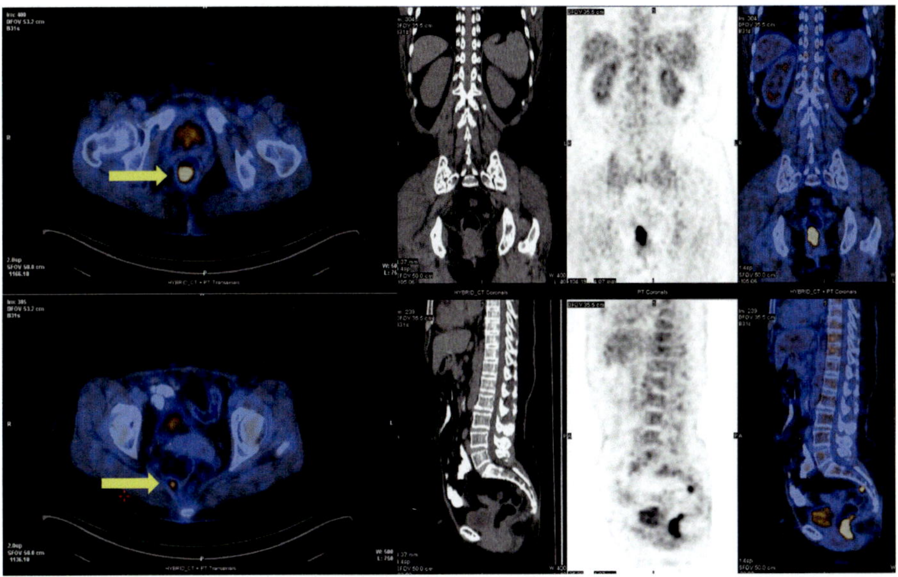

Fig. 5.17 Arrows show accumulation of FDG in anal canal (SUVmax = 13.3) and a metastatic lymph node in the right pararectal region (SUVmax = 6.4)

Table 5.21 Treatment dose recommendations [52]

	PTV-HR	PTV-SR
Preoperative T3 or T1–2 N+	50.4 Gy at 1.8 Gy/fx, or 50 Gy at 2 Gy/fx (SIB)	45 Gy at 1.8 Gy/fx, or 45 Gy at 1.8 Gy/fx (SIB)
Preoperative T4 any N	54–55.8 Gy at 1.8 Gy/fx, or 54 Gy at 2 Gy/fx (SIB)	45 Gy at 1.8 Gy/fx, or 45.9 Gy at 1.7 Gy/fx (SIB)
Preoperative (short course) T3–4 or N+		25 Gy at 5 Gy/fx
Postoperative (negative margins)	54–55.8 Gy at 1.8 Gy/fx, or 54 Gy at 2 Gy/fx (SIB)	45 Gy at 1.8 Gy/fx, or 45.9 Gy at 1.7 Gy/fx (SIB)
Postoperative (gross disease or positive margin)	54–59.4 Gy at 1.8 Gy/fx, or 54–60 Gy at 2 Gy/fx (SIB)	45 Gy at 1.8 Gy/fx, or 45.9 Gy at 1.7 Gy/fx (SIB)

Fx fraction, *SIB* simultaneous integrated boost

Table 5.22 Recommended dose constraints for critical structures for either 3DCRT or IMRT

Organ	Constraints (QUANTEC) [55]	Constraints (RT0G 0822-IMRT) [56]
Small bowel	V15 Gy < 120 cc (individual loops) V45 Gy < 195 cc (entire potential space within peritoneal cavity)	V35 Gy < 180 cc V40 Gy < 100 cc V45 Gy < 65 cc Dmax < 50 Gy
Bladder	Dmax < 65 Gy V65 Gy < 50%	V40 Gy < 40% V45 Gy < 15% Dmax < 50 Gy
Femoral heads		V40 Gy < 40% V45 Gy < 25% Dmax < 50 Gy

5.5 Anal Cancer

> **Overview**
>
> ***Epidemiology***: It has been associated with female gender, infection with human papillomavirus (HPV), lifetime number of sexual partners, genital warts, cigarette smoking, receptive anal intercourse, and infection with HIV.
>
> ***Pathology:*** Squamous cell carcinoma is the most common histopathology (85%) followed by adenocarcinoma (10%). Adenocarcinoma carries poorer prognosis and is treated as rectal adenocarcinoma.
>
> ***Diagnosis:*** Pretreatment clinical staging consists of physical examination and biopsy of the primary tumor, palpation of the groin, computed tomography (CT) of the chest, CT or magnetic resonance imaging of the abdomen and pelvis, and whole body positron emission tomography CT scan.
>
> ***Definitive Treatment:*** Historically the treatment has been surgery with abdominoperineal resection. However, use of concurrent radiotherapy with infusional 5-FU and MMC became the standard of care for patients with SCC with high overall survival, colostomy-free survival and nodal relapse risk reduction rates. There are several radiotherapy techniques for treatment and IMRT shows significant reduction in treatment related toxicities with similar treatment outcomes.
>
> **Keywords**: Anal cancer; Radiotherapy

5.5.1 Case Presentation

She is a 63 year-old female applied to the clinics with rectal bleeding which started 2 months ago. She is a housewife and is married with five children. Patient has a KPS of 90 with normal systemic physical examination findings. Digital rectal examination revealed a crater like irregularity at the level of anal grim. Her gynecological examination was normal. She had no smoking or alcohol consumption but had a past medical history of cholecystectomy (27 years ago) and normal labor of 5 children. She had one brother died of lung cancer. Her whole blood count, and kidney and liver function tests were normal. Rectoscopy showed 2 cm ulcerative lesion with necrotic foci covering the lumen in the anal canal. Whole body fluorodeoxyglucose (FDG) positron emission tomography (PET)/CT demonstrated accumulation of FDG in anal canal (SUVmax = 13.3) consistent with anal cancer and a metastatic lymph node in the right pararectal region less than 11 mm in largest diameter (SUVmax = 6.4) (Fig. 5.17). Biopsy from the anal lesion revealed squamous cell carcinoma (SCC). According to 8th edition AJCC/UICC staging system, patient has stage IIIa (cT1N1aM0) anal SCC (Table 5.23) [58].

Table 5.23 Anal cancer TNM staging AJCC UICC 2017

Primary tumor (T)

T category	T criteria
TX	Primary tumor not assessed
T0	No evidence of primary tumor
Tis	High-grade squamous intraepithelial lesion (previously termed carcinoma in situ, Bowen disease, anal intraepithelial neoplasia II–III, high-grade anal intraepithelial neoplasia)
T1	Tumor $\leq$2 cm
T2	Tumor >2 cm but $\leq$5 cm
T3	Tumor >5 cm
T4	Tumor of any size invading adjacent organ(s), such as the vagina, urethra, or bladder

Regional lymph nodes (N)

N category	N criteria
NX	Regional lymph nodes cannot be assessed
N0	No regional lymph node metastasis
N1	Metastasis in inguinal, mesorectal, internal iliac, or external iliac nodes
N1a	Metastasis in inguinal, mesorectal, or internal iliac lymph nodes
N1b	Metastasis in external iliac lymph nodes
N1c	Metastasis in external iliac with any N1a nodes

Distant metastasis (M)

M category	M criteria
M0	No distant metastasis
M1	Distant metastasis

Stage Groups

T	N	M	Stage
Tis	N0	M0	0
T1	N0	M0	I
T1	N1	M0	IIIA
T2	N0	M0	IIA
T2	N1	M0	IIIA
T3	N0	M0	IIB
T3	N1	M0	IIIC
T4	N0	M0	IIIB
T4	N1	M0	IIIC
Any T	Any N	M1	IV

Used with permission of the American College of Surgeons, Chicago, Illinois. The original and primary source for this information is the AJCC Cancer Staging Manual, Eighth Edition (2017) published by Springer International Publishing

5.5.2 Evidence Based Treatment Recommendations

5.5.2.1 Literature Review

Pretreatment clinical staging consists of physical examination and biopsy of the primary tumor, palpation of the inguinal lymph nodes, computed tomography (CT) of the chest, CT or magnetic resonance imaging (MRI) of the abdomen and pelvis, and whole body positron emission tomography (PET)/CT scan.

Historically the treatment has been surgery with abdominoperineal resection (APR). This resulted in overall survival rates of approximately 50% with permanent colostomy and high loco-regional recurrences [59]. However, in the beginning of eighties, Nigro et al. reported preoperative radiation therapy and chemotherapy results in patients with anal cancer [60]. They delivered 30 Gy, 2 Gy/fraction to the primary tumor with margin and to the pelvic and inguinal lymph nodes. Chemotherapy was given in the form of 5-fluorouracil infusion 1000 mg/m^2 on 1–4 and 29–32 days of the radiation therapy. Mitomycin C was given in the form of intravenous bolus for 15 mg/m^2 on day 1. Surgery was done 4–6 weeks following the last day of radiation treatment. Eighty percent of the patients were found to have pathological complete response. Following these promising results randomized clinical trials support the use of sphincter preserving chemoradiation in this group of patients (Table 5.24).

The Anal Cancer Trial (ACT) Working Party of the United Kingdom Coordination Committee on Cancer Research (UKCCCR) randomly assigned 577 patients with T1–T4 SCC of the anal canal or margin to receive either radiotherapy alone (45 Gy external beam in 20 or 25 fractions over 4–5 weeks plus a 15 Gy external beam or 25 Gy brachytherapy boost), or radiotherapy plus concurrent infusional FU (1000 mg/m^2 for 4 days or 750 mg/m^2 for 5 days during the first and the final weeks of RT) and mitomycin (12 mg/m^2 on day 1 only). After a median follow-up of 42 months 59% radiotherapy patients had a local failure compared with 36% chemoradiotherapy patients (p < 0.0001). The risk of death from anal cancer was also reduced in the chemoradiotherapy arm (p = 0.02). There was no overall survival advantage (p = 0.25). Early morbidity was significantly more frequent in the chemo-radiotherapy arm (p = 0.03), but late morbidity occurred at similar rates [61]. Thirteen year follow up results of the same study showed a 9.1% increase in non-anal cancer deaths in the first 5 years of chemoradiation which disappeared by 10 years. Only 11 patients suffered a locoregional relapse as a first event after 5 years [62].

EORTC 22861 randomly assigned 110 patients with T3–4 or N1–3 anal cancer to receive RT (45 Gy with a 15 or 30 Gy boost) with or without concurrent infusional FU (750 mg/m^2/day on days 1–5 and 29–33) plus mitomycin (15 mg/m^2 day 1 only) [63]. Chemoradiotherapy was associated with a significantly higher pathologic complete remission rate (80% vs 54%), an 18% higher five-year locoregional control rate, a 32% higher colostomy-free rate, and higher event-free and progression-free survival. Overall survival was not significantly different, and the incidence of acute and late side effects and treatment-related mortality did not differ between the groups.

Table 5.24 Important randomized controlled trials in anal cancer

Trial	Patients	No	Median F/U (year)	Arms	LC %	CFS %	DFS %	OS %
ACT-I [61, 62]	T2–T4M0	577	13.1	RT vs chemoRT (5FU-MMC)	41% vs 66%	**20% vs 30%**	**18% vs 30%**	28% vs 33%
EORTC 22861 [63]	T3–T4 or N1–N3M0	103	3.5	RT vs chemoRT (5FU-MMC)	50% vs 68%	40% vs 72%	42% vs 58%	54% vs 58%
RTOG 8704 [64]	Any stage, M0	291	3	ChemoRT (5FU-MMC) vs chemoRT (5FU only)	Negative 6 week biopsy 92% vs 86%	71% vs 59%	73% vs 51%	75% vs 70%
RTOG 9811 [65, 66]	T2–T4M0	649	–	ChemoRT (5FU-MMC) vs 2 cycles 5-FU+CDDP → chemoRT (5FU-CDDP)	80% vs 74%	72% vs 65%	**68% vs 58%**	**78% vs 71%**
ACT-II [67]	Any stage, M0	940	5.1	ChemoRT (5FU-MMC) vs chemoRT (5FU-CDDP) vs chemoRT (5FU-MMC) → maintenance 5FU-MMC vs chemoRT (5FU-CDDP) → maintenance 5FU-CDDP	CR at 26 weeks MMC: 91% vs CDDP: 90%	75% vs 72% vs 73% vs 75%	73% vs 72% vs 73% vs 74%	86% vs 84% vs 82% vs 83%
ACCORD 03 [68]	Primary <4 cm or N1–N3, M0	307	5	ChemoRT (5FU-CDDP) + standard boost vs chemoRT (5FU-CDDP) + high dose boost vs 5FU-CDDP → chemoRT (5FU-CDDP) + standard boost vs 5FU-CDDP → chemoRT (5FU-CDDP) + high dose boost	84% vs 78% vs 72% vs 88%	77% vs 73% vs 70% vs 82%	67% vs 62% vs 64% vs 78%	No NACT: 71% vs NACT: 75%

No number, *5-FU* 5-flourouracyl, *MMC* mitomycin-c, *CDDP* cisplatin, *chemoRT* chemoradiation, *NACT* neo-adjuvant chemotherapy, *F/U* follow-up, *LC* local control, *CFS* colostomy free survival, *OS* overall survival

The role of mitomycin in curative treatment of anal cancer was addressed in a joint trial from the Radiation Therapy Oncology Group (RTOG) and the Eastern Cooperative Oncology Group (ECOG) [64]. In this trial 310 patients with anal cancer of any tumor or nodal stage were randomly assigned to combined modality therapy with or without mitomycin-C. At 4 years, colostomy rates were lower (9% vs 22%; p = 0.002), colostomy-free survival higher (71% vs 59%; p = 0.014), and disease-free survival higher (73% vs 51%; p = 0.0003) in the mitomycin-C arm. A significant difference in overall survival has not been observed and toxicity was greater in the mitomycin-C arm (23% vs 7% grade 4 and 5 toxicity; p < 0.001).

The substitution of cisplatin for mitomycin in the treatment of anal canal cancer was evaluated in 2 randomized trials RTOG 98-11 enrolled 682 non-HIV-infected patients with SCC of the anal canal [65]. It compared induction chemotherapy plus concurrent chemoradiotherapy using cisplatin and FU with the standard regimen of mitomycin, FU, and radiotherapy. In the latest update, there were significant differences favoring FU plus mitomycin in five-year disease-free survival (68% vs 58%, p = 0.006), overall survival (78% vs 71%, p = 0.026) and colostomy-free survival (72% vs 65%, p = 0.05) [66]. Hematologic toxicity was worse in the mitomycin group, but nonhematologic toxicity and late radiotherapy related toxicity were similar in the two groups.

ACT II Trial investigated whether replacing mitomycin with cisplatin in chemoradiation improves response, and whether maintenance chemotherapy after chemoradiation improves survival [67]. Median follow-up was 5.1 years with 940 non-HIV-infected patients with anal SCC. Treatment consisted of radiotherapy in both arms (50.4 Gy in 28 fractions) with concurrent infusion FU (1000 mg/m^2/day on days 1–4 and 29–32) and either cisplatin (60 mg/m^2 on days 1 and 29) or mitomycin (12 mg/m^2 day 1 only). There was a second randomization to receive or not receive maintenance chemotherapy starting 4 weeks after chemoradiotherapy. The complete response rate at 6 months was 90.5% vs 89.6% with mitomycin and cisplatin, respectively, and the 3-year colostomy-free survival rate was similar in patients treated with mitomycin or cisplatin and those treated with and without maintenance treatment. Overall, toxic effects were similar in each group.

UNICANCER ACCORD 03 trial was designed to determine whether dose escalation of the radiation boost or two cycles of induction chemotherapy before concomitant chemoradiotherapy lead to an improvement in colostomy-free survival [67]. Patients with tumors ≥40 mm, or <40 mm and N1-3M0 were randomly assigned to one of four treatment arms: (A) two induction chemotherapy cycles (fluorouracil 800 mg/m^2/day intravenous [IV] infusion, days 1–4 and 29–32; and cisplatin 80 mg/m^2 IV, on days 1 and 29), chemoradiotherapy (45 Gy in 25 fractions over 5 weeks, fluorouracil and cisplatin during weeks 1 and 5), and standard-dose boost (SD; 15 Gy); (B) two induction chemotherapy cycles, chemoradiotherapy, and high-dose boost (HD; 20–25 Gy); (C): RCT and SD boost (reference arm); and (D) chemoradiotherapy and HD boost. With a median follow-up of 50 months, the

5-year colostomy free survival rates were 69.6%, 82.4%, 77.1%, and 72.7% in arms A, B, C, and D, respectively. As a result of these studies it appears that there is no benefit for induction chemotherapy or a continuation of chemotherapy beyond concurrent chemoradiotherapy in anal cancer.

5.5.2.2 Treatment Recommendations

The current recommendation for initial treatment of SCC of the anal canal is definitive chemoradiation using mitomycin-C and 5-fluorouracil-based regimens. Local excision is an option for patients with T1 tumors less than 1 cm in size, although it has never been compared with radiotherapy or chemoradiation and patients should be on close follow up.

Anal cancer radiotherapy is one of the most difficult treatments for patients due to acute side effects effecting skin, bone marrow, gastro intestinal (GI) system, genito urinary (GU) system and sexual organs. Clinical experience using intensity modulated radiotherapy (IMRT) showed relatively low doses to normal structures compared to traditional 2D or 3D techniques. RTOG 0529 is the only prospective phase II trial for the use of IMRT in patients with anal cancer. Compared to the historical control arm of RTOG 9811 trial, patients treated with IMRT had a significant reduction in $\geq$ grad 3 GI and dermatologic toxicity, and $\geq$ grad 2 hematologic toxicity [69]. Call et al. reported that IMRT yielded local control, regional control, distant control, and overall survival rates of 87%, 97%, 91%, and 87%, respectively, at 3 years which is similar to outcomes of 5FU-MMC arm of RTOG 9811 [70]. Thus IMRT based chemo-radiation has become the standard treatment approach with similar treatment outcomes and low toxicity rates.

Treatment response should be initially assessed clinically 8–12 weeks after completion of chemoradiotherapy. For patients with a clinical complete response, re-examination every three to 6 months is recommended. If there is suspicion of persisting disease, a re-evaluation biopsy should be obtained every 4 weeks. Based upon the results from the ACT-II trial, patients with persistent disease can be watched for up to 6 months following completion of chemoradiotherapy as long as there is no progressive disease during this period of follow-up. For patients with evidence of progressive disease at any point, or persisting disease at 26 weeks after completion of combined modality therapy and no evidence of metastatic disease, surgical treatment is recommended. Primary adenocarcinoma of the anal canal is rare, and surgery is recommended rather than initial chemoradiotherapy.

5.5.3 Treatment Planning

5.5.3.1 Simulation

Patient can be simulated in the supine position in a body mold or other immobilization device. Patients may be simulated in frog leg position. Prone position with the use of a belly board can also be used for anterior displacement of the bowel;

however setup reproducibility is more variable. A radiopaque marker should be placed on the anus. A full bladder is recommended as it protects bowel from radiation. CT simulation using ≤3 mm thickness with IV contrast should be performed to delineate the pelvic blood vessels and gross tumor volume (GTV). Other diagnostic imaging studies (PET/CT or MRI) should be used in target volume delineation.

5.5.3.2 Contouring

The primary gross tumor volume (GTV-P) is defined as all gross disease on physical examination and imaging. The nodal GTV (GTV-N) includes all nodes that are ≥1.5 cm, PET positive, or biopsy proven. Detailed contouring atlases available include the RTOG anorectal contouring atlas and the Australasian GI Trials Group Atlas [53, 71]. Table 5.25 shows brief definition of target volumes.

Case Contouring Delineation of target volumes for the case is shown in Fig. 5.18.

Case Plan According to 8th edition AJCC/UICC staging system, patient has stage IIIa (cT1N1aM0) anal SCC and the current standard treatment is definitive chemoradiation. We delivered 40 Gy at 1.6 Gy/fraction to CTV-LR, 45 Gy at 1.8 Gy/fraction to CTV-HR, and a boost dose to total 59.4 Gy to CTV-P and CTV-N, using IMRT. Figures 5.19 and 5.20 shows the treatment planning details for the case. Patient received concomitant chemotherapy.

Table 5.25 Description of target volumes for anal cancer [52, 53, 71–73]

Target volume	Description
GTV	GTV-P: All gross disease on physical examination and imaging GTV-N: All nodes ≥15 mm, PET-positive, or biopsy proven
CTV	CTV-P = GTV-P + 1.5–2.5 cm (excluding uninvolved bone, muscle) CTV-N = CTV-P + 1.0–1.5 cm (excluding uninvolved bone, muscle)
CTV-HR	Entire mesorectum, right and left internal iliac lymph nodes inferior to the inferior most level of sacroiliac joint, inguinal and external iliac lymph nodes Iliac lymph nodes = iliac vessels + 0.7 cm Additional 1.0 cm margin anterolaterally around vessel for external iliac lymph nodes Anteriorly a margin of 1–1.5 cm should be added into the bladder for changes in bladder and rectal filling
CTV-LR	Uninvolved inguinal, external iliac and internal iliac lymph nodes superior to the inferior-most level of the sacroiliac joint Iliac lymph nodes = iliac vessels + 0.7 cm Additional 1.0 cm margin anterolaterally around vessel for external iliac lymph nodes (excluding uninvolved bone, muscle)
PTV	CTV + 0.5–1.0 cm (depending on choice-IGRT)

P primary, *N* node, *IGRT* image guided radiotherapy, *CTV-HR* CTV-high risk, *CTV-LR* CTV-low risk

Concomitant Chemotherapy Two cycles of 5-fluorouracil (1000 mg/m²/day as a 96 h infusion, days 1–5 and 29–33 of radiotherapy) and mitomycin-C (10 mg/m² bolus, days 1 and 29)

Treatment Delivery Techniques There are several techniques and methods of dose prescription for anal cancer, and the exact dose and fractionation will vary based on which technique is used (Table 5.26). However, IMRT yielded significant sparing of acute grade 2+ hematologic and grade 3+ dermatologic and gastrointestinal toxicity compared to conventional radiotherapy.

5.5.3.3 Dose Constraints for Critical Structures

Table 5.27 summarizes the dose constraints for organs at risk for 3DCRT and IMRT.

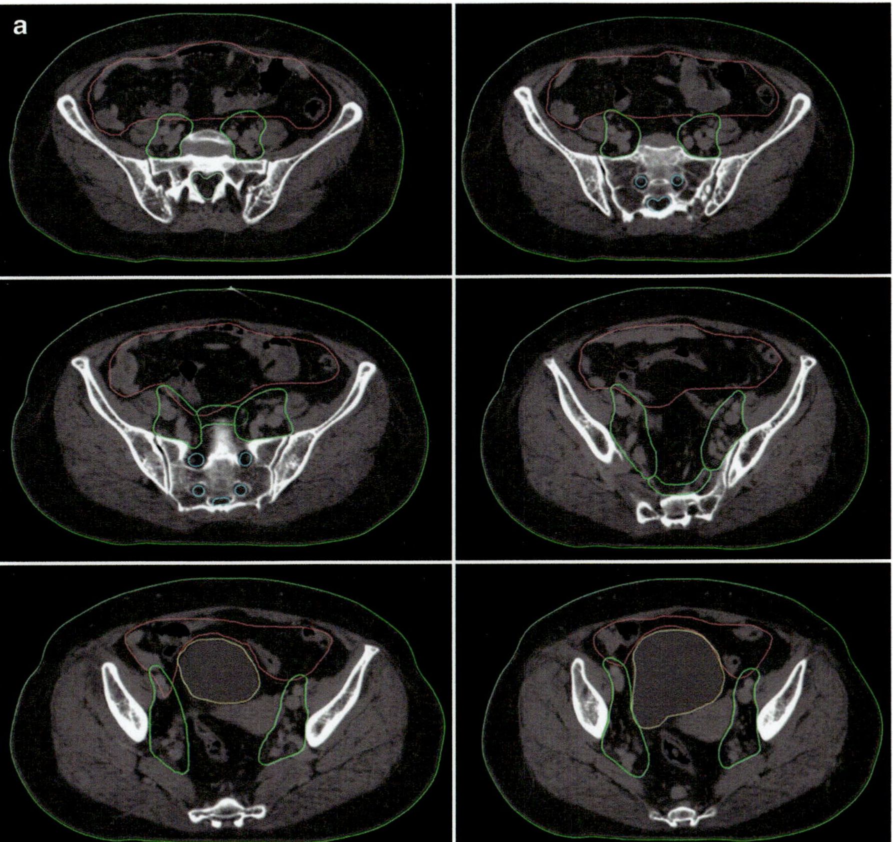

Fig. 5.18 (**a–c**) Delineation of target volumes for T1N1aM0 anal cancer case. Pink = CTV-HR, Purple = CTV-HR (nodal) Orange = CTV-P, Red = CTV-N, Blue = CTV-LR

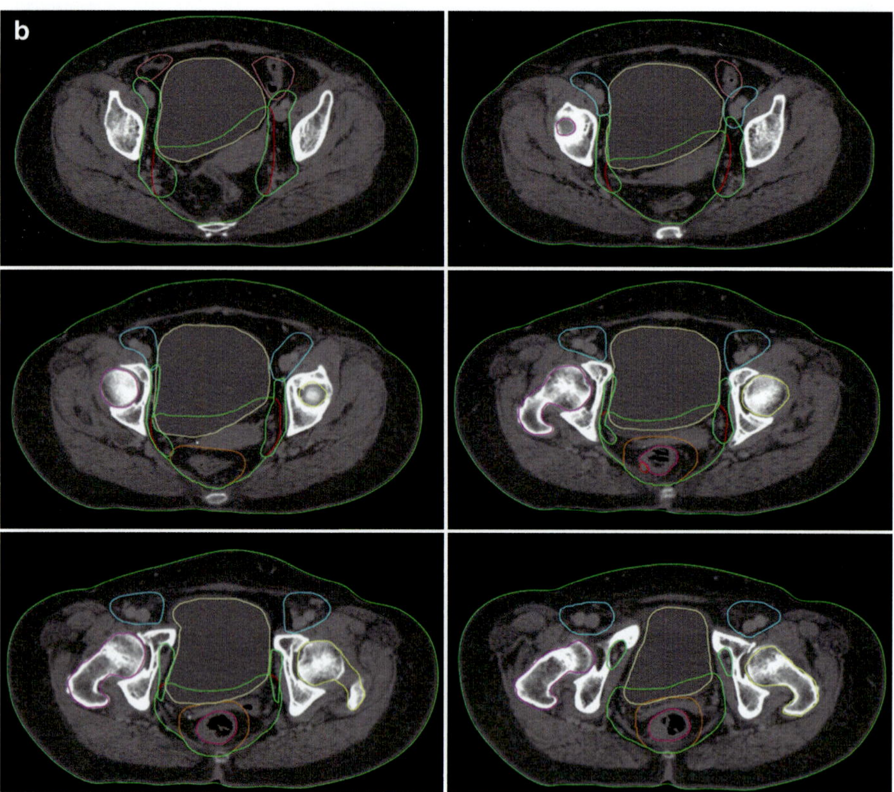

Fig. 5.18 (continued)

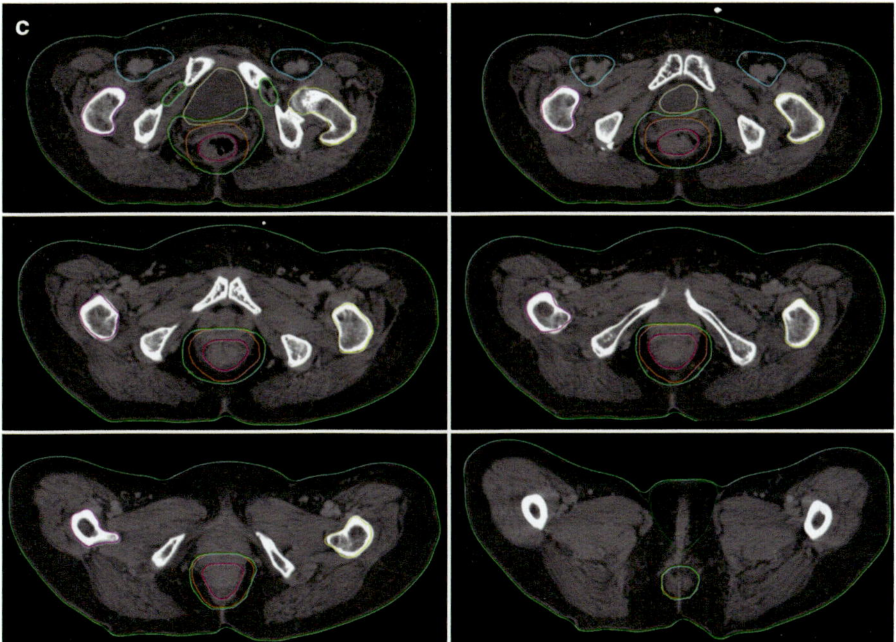

Fig. 5.18 (continued)

5.5.4 Follow-Up (F/U) Recommendations

Patient should be evaluated in eighth to twelfth week with exam and digital rectal examination (DRE). If there is complete remission, DRE every 3–6 months for 5 years, inguinal node palpation every 3–6 months for 5 years, anoscopy every 6–12 months for 3 years, chest/abdomen/pelvic CT with contrast annually for 3 years (if T3–T4 or inguinal lymph nodes positive) is recommended. If there is persistent disease re-evaluation in 4 weeks is recommended. Based on the results of ACT-II study, it may be appropriate to follow patients who have not achieved a complete clinical response with persistent anal cancer up to 6 months following chemoradiation as long as there is no evidence of progressive disease during follow-up period. Persistent disease may continue to regress even at 26th weeks from the start of treatment [67]. However if there is biopsy proven progressive disease restaging and salvage surgery is recommended.

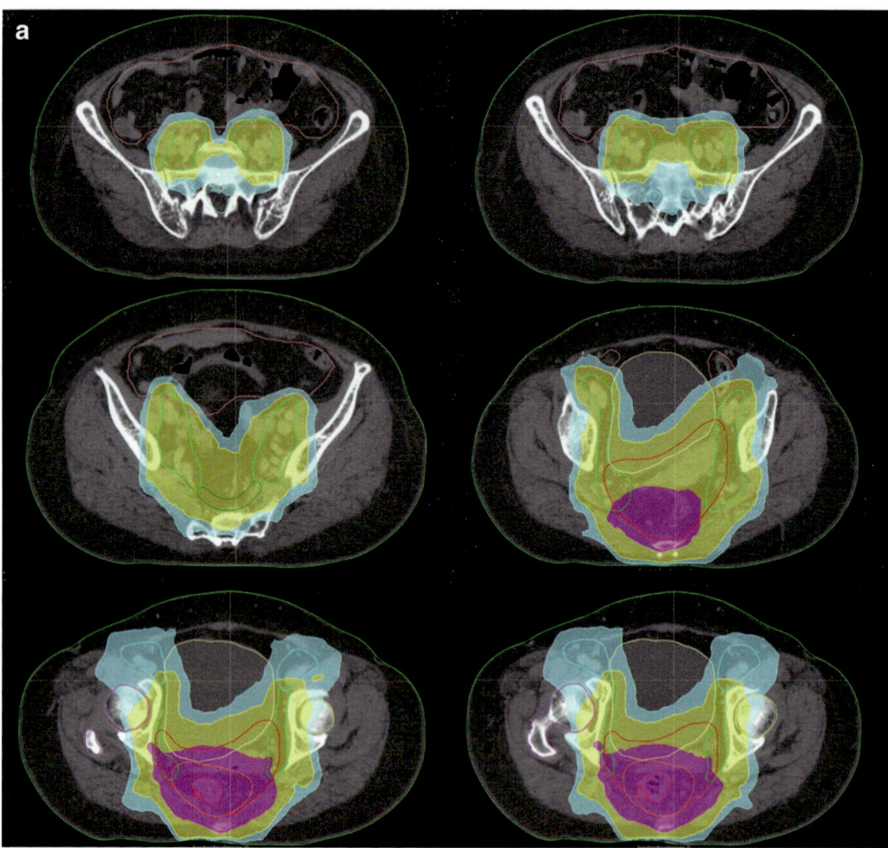

Fig. 5.19 (**a, b**) We delivered 40 Gy at 1.6 Gy/fraction to CTV-LR, 45 Gy at 1.8 Gy/fraction to CTV-HR, and a boost dose to total 59.4 Gy to CTV-P and CTV-N, using IMRT. (**a, b**) 95% isodose for CTV-LR = blue, CTV-HR = yellow and CTV-P + CTV-N = pink in color and dose (**c**) dose-volume histogram for the whole treatment are shown

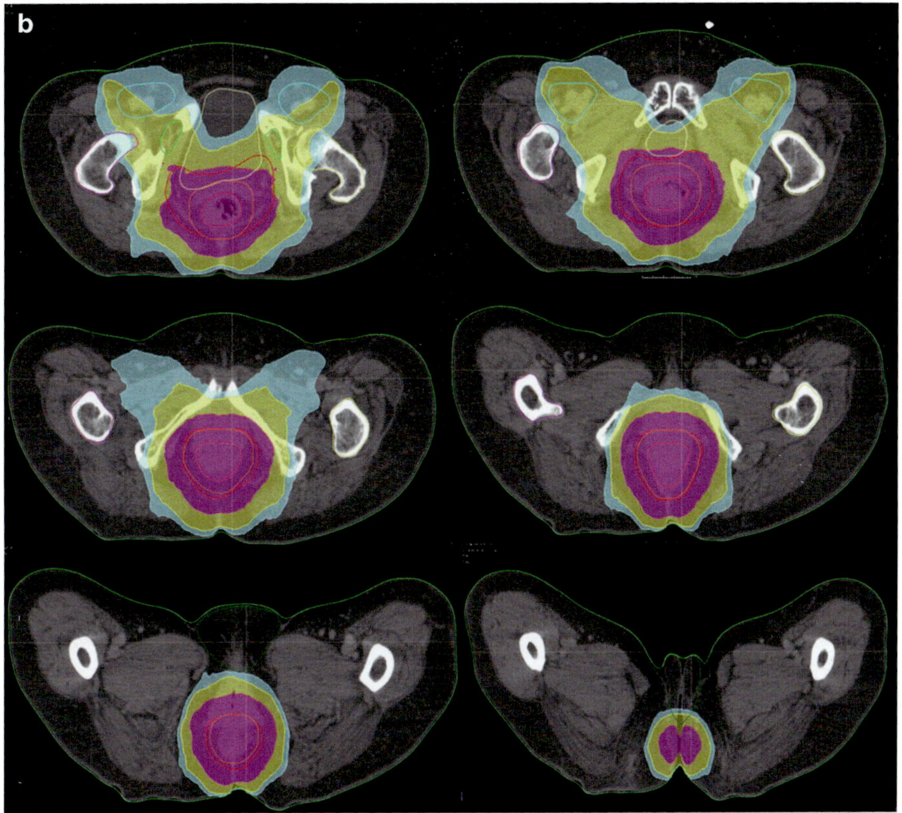

Fig. 5.19 (continued)

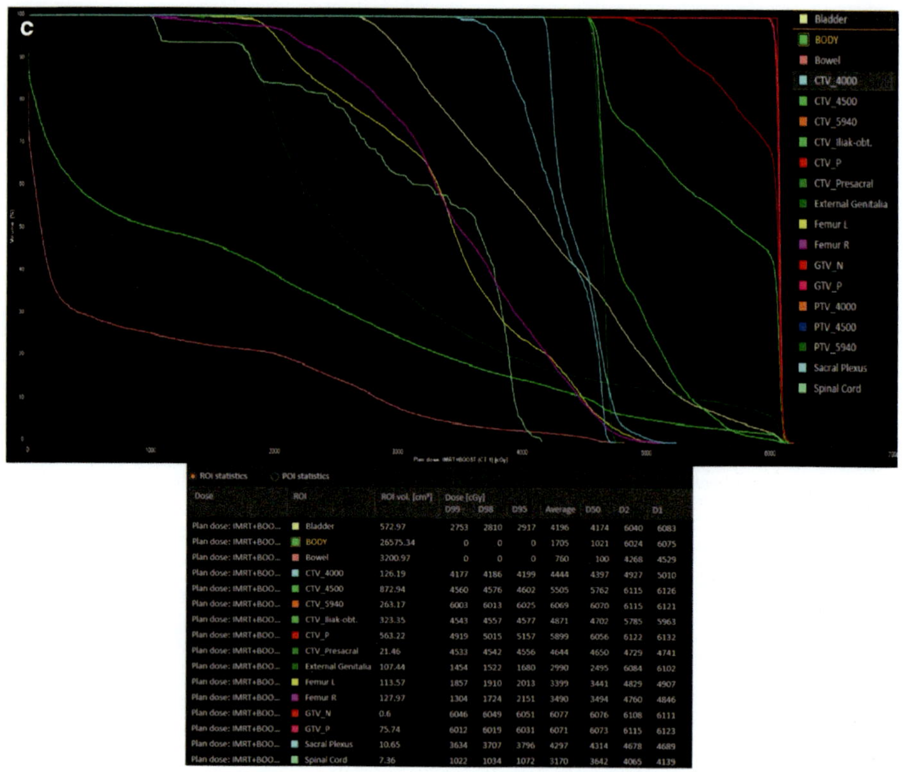

Dose	ROI	ROI vol. [cm³]	Dose [cGy]						
			D99	D98	D95	Average	D50	D2	D1
Plan dose: IMRT+BOO…	Bladder	572.97	2753	2810	2917	4196	4174	6040	6083
Plan dose: IMRT+BOO…	BODY	26575.34	0	0	0	1705	1021	6024	6075
Plan dose: IMRT+BOO…	Bowel	3200.97	0	0	0	760	100	4268	4529
Plan dose: IMRT+BOO…	CTV_4000	126.19	4177	4186	4199	4444	4397	4927	5010
Plan dose: IMRT+BOO…	CTV_4500	872.94	4560	4576	4602	5505	5762	6115	6126
Plan dose: IMRT+BOO…	CTV_5940	263.17	6003	6013	6025	6069	6070	6115	6121
Plan dose: IMRT+BOO…	CTV_Iliak-obt.	323.35	4543	4557	4577	4871	4702	5785	5963
Plan dose: IMRT+BOO…	CTV_P	563.22	4919	5015	5157	5899	6056	6122	6132
Plan dose: IMRT+BOO…	CTV_Presacral	21.46	4533	4542	4556	4644	4650	4729	4741
Plan dose: IMRT+BOO…	External Genitalia	107.44	1454	1522	1680	2990	2495	6084	6102
Plan dose: IMRT+BOO…	Femur L	113.57	1857	1910	2013	3399	3441	4829	4907
Plan dose: IMRT+BOO…	Femur R	127.97	1304	1724	2151	3490	3494	4760	4846
Plan dose: IMRT+BOO…	GTV_N	0.6	6046	6049	6051	6077	6076	6108	6111
Plan dose: IMRT+BOO…	GTV_P	75.74	6012	6019	6031	6071	6073	6115	6123
Plan dose: IMRT+BOO…	Sacral Plexus	10.65	3634	3707	3796	4297	4314	4678	4689
Plan dose: IMRT+BOO…	Spinal Cord	7.36	1022	1034	1072	3170	3642	4065	4139

Fig. 5.19 (continued)

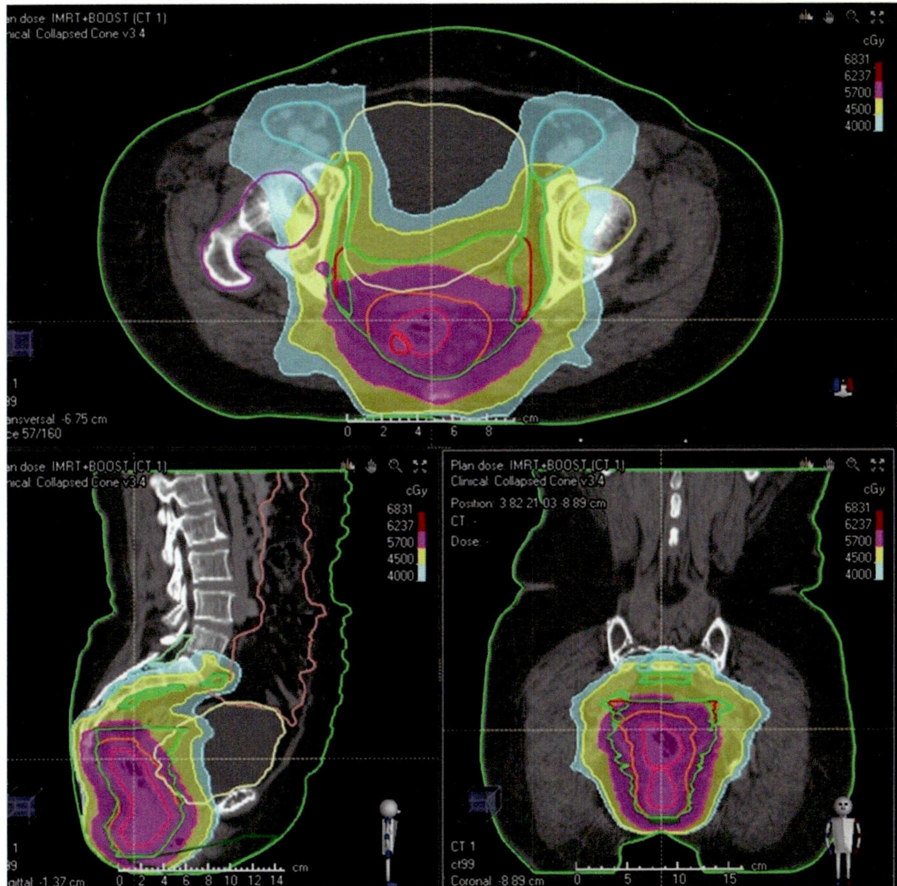

Fig. 5.20 IMRT treatment plan of the patient showing 95% isodose lines; blue = CTV40 Gy, yellow = CTV45 Gy, pink = CTV59.4 Gy

Table 5.26 Recommended treatment dose and fractionation schemes according to two studies

Target volume	RTOG 9811 [74]	RTOG 0529 [69]
CTV-P	T1N0: 45–50.4 Gy at 1.8 Gy/fraction T2N0: 50.4 Gy at 1.8 Gy/fraction N+ or T3–T4: 54–59.4 Gy at 1.8 Gy/fraction	T1N0: not included T2N0: 50.4 Gy at 1.8 Gy/fraction N+ or T3–T4: 54 Gy at 1.8 Gy/fraction
CTV-N	54–59.4 Gy at 1.8 Gy/fraction	If lymph node ≤3 cm: 50.4 Gy at 1.68 Gy/fraction If lymph node ≤3 cm: 54 Gy at 1.8 Gy/fraction
CTV-HR	45 Gy/1.8 Gy/fraction	T2N0: 42 Gy at 1.5 Gy/fraction T2N+ or T3–T4: 45 Gy at 1.5 Gy/fraction
CTV-LR	30.6–36 Gy at 1.8 Gy/fraction (If using IMRT: 40 Gy at 1.6 Gy/fraction)	Not defined, same dose as CTV-HR

P primary, *N* node, *IGRT* image guided radiotherapy, *CTV-HR* CTV-high risk, *CTV-LR* CTV-low risk

Table 5.27 Dose constraints for critical structures based on QUANTEC [55] and RTOG 0529 [69]

Organ	Constraints (QUANTEC) [55]	Constraints [69] (IMRT)
Small bowel	V15 Gy < 120 cc (individual loops) V45 Gy < 195 cc (entire potential space within peritoneal cavity)	V30 Gy < 200 cc V35 Gy < 150 cc V45 Gy < 20 cc Dmax < 50 Gy
Large bowel		V30 Gy < 200 cc V35 Gy < 150 cc V45 Gy < 20 cc
Bladder	Dmax < 65 Gy V65 Gy < 50%	V35 Gy < 50% V40 Gy < 35% V50 Gy < 5%
Femoral heads		V30 Gy < 50% V40 Gy < 35% V44 Gy < 5%
Iliac crest		V30 Gy < 50% V40 Gy < 35% V50 Gy < 5%
External genitalia		V20 Gy < 50% V30 Gy < 35% V40 Gy < 5%

References

1. Rice TW, Patil DT, Blackstone EH. 8th edition AJCC/UICC staging of cancers of the esophagus and esophagogastric junction: application to clinical practice. Ann Cardiothorac Surg. 2017;6(2):119–30. https://doi.org/10.21037/acs.2017.03.14.
2. Urba SG, Orringer MB, Turrisi A, et al. Randomized trial of preoperative chemoradiation versus surgery alone in patients with locoregional esophageal carcinoma. J Clin Oncol. 2001;19(2):305–13.
3. Bosset JF, Gignoux M, Triboulet JP, et al. Chemoradiotherapy followed by surgery compared with surgery alone in squamous-cell cancer of the esophagus. N Engl J Med. 1997;337(3):161–7.
4. Walsh TN, Noonan N, Hollywood D, et al. A comparison of multimodal therapy and surgery for esophageal adenocarcinoma. N Engl J Med. 1996;335(7):462–7.
5. Burmeister BH, Smithers BM, Gebski V, et al. Surgery alone versus chemoradiotherapy followed by surgery for resectable cancer of the oesophagus: a randomised controlled phase III trial. Lancet Oncol. 2005;6(9):659–68.
6. Tepper J, Krasna MJ, Niedzwiecki D, et al. Phase III trial of trimodality therapy with cisplatin, fluorouracil, radiotherapy, and surgery compared with surgery alone for esophageal cancer: CALGB 9781. J Clin Oncol. 2008;26(7):1086–92.
7. Shapiro J, van Lanschot JJB, Hulshof MCCM, et al. Neoadjuvant chemoradiotherapy plus surgery versus surgery alone for oesophageal or junctional cancer (CROSS): long-term results of a randomised controlled trial. Lancet Oncol. 2015;16(9):1090–8.
8. Mariette C, Dahan L, Mornex F, et al. Surgery alone versus chemoradiotherapy followed by surgery for stage I and II esophageal cancer: final analysis of randomized controlled phase III trial FFCD 9901. J Clin Oncol. 2014;32(23):2416–22.
9. Sjoquist KM, Burmeister BH, Smithers BM, et al. Survival after neoadjuvant chemotherapy or chemoradiotherapy for resectable oesophageal carcinoma: an updated meta-analysis. Lancet Oncol. 2011;12(7):681–92.
10. Jabbour SK, Thomas CR. Radiation therapy in the postoperative management of esophageal cancer. J Gastrointest Oncol. 2010;1(2):102–11. https://doi.org/10.3978/j.issn.2078-6891.2010.013.
11. Macdonald JS, Smalley SR, Benedetti J, et al. Chemoradiotherapy after surgery compared with surgery alone for adenocarcinoma of the stomach or gastroesophageal junction. N Engl J Med. 2001;345:725–30.
12. Cunningham D, Allum WH, Stenning SP, et al. Perioperative chemotherapy versus surgery alone for resectable gastroesophageal cancer. N Engl J Med. 2006;355:11–20.
13. Herskovic A, Martz K, al-Sarraf M, et al. Combined chemotherapy and radiotherapy compared with radiotherapy alone in patients with cancer of the esophagus. N Engl J Med. 1992;326(24):1593–8.
14. Cooper JS, Guo MD, Herskovic A, et al. Chemoradiotherapy of locally advanced esophageal cancer: long-term follow-up of a prospective randomized trial (RTOG 85-01). JAMA. 1999;281(17):1623–7.
15. Minsky BD, Pajak TF, Ginsberg RJ, et al. INT 0123 (Radiation Therapy Oncology Group 94-05) phase III trial of combined-modality therapy for esophageal cancer: high-dose versus standard-dose radiation therapy. J Clin Oncol. 2002;20(5):1167–74.
16. Gao XS, Qiao X, Wu F, et al. Pathological analysis of clinical target volume margin for radiotherapy in patients with esophageal and gastroesophageal junction carcinoma. Int J Radiat Oncol Biol Phys. 2007;67(2):389–96.
17. Qiao XY, Wang W, Zhou ZG, et al. Comparison of efficacy of regional and extensive clinical target volumes in postoperative radiotherapy for esophageal squamous cell carcinoma. Int J Radiat Oncol Biol Phys. 2008;70(2):396–402.
18. Hsu FM, Lee JM, Huang PM, et al. Retrospective analysis of outcome differences in preoperative concurrent chemoradiation with or without elective nodal irradiation for esophageal squamous cell carcinoma. Int J Radiat Oncol Biol Phys. 2011;81(4):e593–9.

19. Marks LB, et al. Use of normal tissue complication probability models in the clinic. Int J Radiat Oncol Biol Phys. 2010;76(3 Suppl):S10–9.
20. Sano T, Coit DG, Kim HH, et al. Proposal of a new stage grouping of gastric cancer for TNM classification: International Gastric Cancer Association Staging Project. Gastric Cancer. 2017;20(2):217–25.
21. Smyth EC, Verheij M, Allum W, Cunningham D, Cervantes A, Arnold D, ESMO Guidelines Committee. Gastric cancer: ESMO Clinical Practice Guidelines for diagnosis, treatment and follow-up. Ann Oncol. 2016;27(suppl 5):v38–49.
22. Smalley SR, Benedetti JK, Haller DG, et al. Updated analysis of SWOG-directed intergroup study 0116: a phase III trial of adjuvant radiochemotherapy versus observation after curative gastric cancer resection. J Clin Oncol. 2012;30(19):2327–33.
23. Kim S, Lim d H, Lee J, et al. An observational study suggesting clinical benefit for adjuvant postoperative chemoradiation in a population of over 500 cases after gastric resection with D2 nodal dissection for adenocarcinoma of the stomach. Int J Radiat Oncol Biol Phys. 2005;63:1279–85.
24. Lee J, Lim d H, Kim S, et al. Phase III trial comparing capecitabine plus cisplatin versus capecitabine plus cisplatin with concurrent capecitabine radiotherapy in completely resected gastric cancer with D2 lymph node dissection: the ARTIST trial. J Clin Oncol. 2012;30:268–73.
25. Fuchs CS, Niedzwiecki D, Mamon HJ, et al. Adjuvant chemoradiotherapy with epirubicin, cisplatin, and fluorouracil compared with adjuvant chemoradiotherapy with fluorouracil and leucovorin after curative resection of gastric cancer: results from CALGB 80101 (Alliance). J Clin Oncol. 2017;35(32):3671.
26. Stahl M, Walz MK, Stuschke M, et al. Phase III comparison of preoperative chemotherapy compared with chemoradiotherapy in patients with locally advanced adenocarcinoma of the esophagogastric junction. J Clin Oncol. 2009;27(6):851.
27. Cats A, Jansen EPM, van Grieken NCT, et al. Chemotherapy versus chemoradiotherapy after surgery and preoperative chemotherapy for resectable gastric cancer (CRITICS): an international, open-label, randomised phase 3 trial. Lancet Oncol. 2018;19(5):616–28.
28. Gunderson LL, Tepper JE, editors. Clinical radiation oncology. 2nd ed. Philadelphia: Churchill Livingstone/Elsevier; 2007.
29. Amin MB, Edge S, Greene F, Byrd DR, Brookland RK, Washington MK, Gershenwald JE, Compton CC, Hess KR, Sullivan DC, Jessup JM, Brierley JD, Gaspar LE, Schilsky RL, Balch CM, Winchester DP, Asare EA, Madera M, Gress DM, Meyer LR, editors. AJCC cancer staging manual. 8th ed. New York: Springer; 2017. American Joint Commission on Cancer [cited 2016 Dec 28]. Available from: http://www.springer.com/us/book/9783319406176#aboutBook.
30. Jemal A, Siegel R, Xu J, Ward E. Cancer statistics, 2010. CA Cancer J Clin. 2010;60:277–300.
31. Tzeng CW, Tran Cao HS, Lee JE, et al. Treatment sequencing for resectable pancreatic cancer: influence of early metastases and surgical complications on multimodality therapy completion and survival. J Gastrointest Surg. 2014;18(1):16–24.
32. Kalser MH, Ellenberg SS. Pancreatic cancer. Adjuvant combined radiation and chemotherapy following curative resection. Arch Surg. 1985;120(8):899.
33. Klinkenbijl JH, Jeekel J, Sahmoud T, et al. Adjuvant radiotherapy and 5-fluorouracil after curative resection of cancer of the pancreas and periampullary region: phase III trial of the EORTC gastrointestinal tract cancer cooperative group. Ann Surg. 1999;230(6):776.
34. Neoptolemos JP, Stocken DD, Friess H, et al. A randomized trial of chemoradiotherapy and chemotherapy after resection of pancreatic cancer. N Engl J Med. 2004;350(12):1200.
35. Van Laethem JL, Hammel P, Mornex F, et al. Adjuvant gemcitabine alone versus gemcitabine-based chemoradiotherapy after curative resection for pancreatic cancer: a randomized EORTC-40013-22012/FFCD-9203/GERCOR phase II study. J Clin Oncol. 2010;28(29):4450.
36. Moghanaki D. Further evidence of effective adjuvant combined radiation and chemotherapy following curative resection of pancreatic cancer. Gastrointestinal Tumor Study Group. Cancer. 1987;59(12):2006.
37. Neoptolemos JP, Dunn JA, Stocken DD, et al. Adjuvant chemoradiotherapy and chemotherapy in resectable pancreatic cancer: a randomised controlled trial. Lancet. 2001;358(9293):1576.

38. Valle JW, Palmer D, Jackson R, et al. Optimal duration and timing of adjuvant chemotherapy after definitive surgery for ductal adenocarcinoma of the pancreas: ongoing lessons from the ESPAC-3 study. J Clin Oncol. 2014;32(6):504.

39. Assifi MM, Lu X, Eibl G, Reber HA, et al. Neoadjuvant therapy in pancreatic adenocarcinoma: a meta-analysis of phase II trials. Surgery. 2011;150(3):466–73.

40. Khorana AA, Mangu PB, Berlin J, et al. Potentially curable pancreatic cancer: American Society of Clinical Oncology clinical practice guideline. J Clin Oncol. 2016;34(21):2541–56.

41. Balaban EP, Mangu PB, Yee NS. Locally advanced unresectable pancreatic cancer: American Society of Clinical Oncology clinical practice guideline summary. J Oncol Pract. 2017;13(4):265–9.

42. Khorana MM, Eads JR, Allen P, et al. Locally advanced, unresectable pancreatic cancer: American Society of Clinical Oncology clinical practice guideline. J Clin Oncol. 2016;34(22):2654.

43. van Gijn W, Marijnen CA, Nagtegaal ID, et al. Preoperative radiotherapy combined with total mesorectal excision for resectable rectal cancer: 12-year follow-up of the multicentre, randomised controlled TME trial. Lancet Oncol. 2011;12(6):575–82.

44. Sauer R, Becker H, Hohenberger W, et al. Preoperative versus postoperative chemoradiotherapy for rectal cancer. N Engl J Med. 2004;351(17):1731–40.

45. Sauer R, Liersch T, Merkel S, et al. Preoperative versus postoperative chemoradiotherapy for locally advanced rectal cancer: results of the German CAO/ARO/AIO-94 randomized phase III trial after a median follow-up of 11 years. J Clin Oncol. 2012;30(16):1926–33.

46. Bujko K, Nowacki MP, Nasierowska-Guttmejer A, et al. Long-term results of a randomized trial comparing preoperative short-course radiotherapy with preoperative conventionally fractionated chemoradiation for rectal cancer. Br J Surg. 2006;93(10):1215–23.

47. Ngan SY, Burmeister B, Fisher RJ, et al. Randomized trial of short-course radiotherapy versus long-course chemoradiation comparing rates of local recurrence in patients with T3 rectal cancer: Trans-Tasman Radiation Oncology Group trial 01.04. J Clin Oncol. 2012;30(31):3827–33.

48. Pettersson D, Lörinc E, Holm T, et al. Tumour regression in the randomized Stockholm III Trial of radiotherapy regimens for rectal cancer. Br J Surg. 2015;102(8):972–8.

49. Douglass HO Jr, Moertel CG, Mayer RJ, et al. Survival after postoperative combination treatment of rectal cancer. N Engl J Med. 1986;315(20):1294.

50. Krook JE, Moertel CG, Gunderson LL, et al. Effective surgical adjuvant therapy for high-risk rectal carcinoma. N Engl J Med. 1991;324(11):709.

51. Hall WH. Adjuvant therapy for patients with colon and rectal cancer. JAMA. 1990;264(11):1444–50.

52.   Lee N, Riaz N, Lu J. In: Brady L, Combs S, Lu J, editors. Target volume delineation for conformal and intensity-modulated radiation therapy, Medical radiology: radiation oncology. New York: Springer; 2015.

53. Myerson RJ, Garofalo MC, Naqa IE, et al. Elective clinical target volumes for conformal therapy in anorectal cancer: an RTOG consensus panel contouring atlas. Int J Radiat Oncol Biol Phys. 2009;74(3):824–30.

54. Hong TS, Moughan J, Garofalo MC, et al. NRG Oncology Radiation Therapy Oncology Group 0822: a phase II study of preoperative chemoradiotherapy utilizing intensity modulated radiation therapy (IMRT) in combination with capecitabine and oxaliplatin for patients with locally advanced rectal cancer. Int J Radiat Oncol Biol Phys. 2015;93(1):29–36.

55. Marks LB, Yorke ED, Jackson A, et al. The use of normal tissue complication probability (NTCP) models in the clinic. Int J Radiat Oncol Biol Phys. 2010;76(3):S10–9.

56. Garofalo MC, Hong T, Bendell J, et al. RTOG 0822: a phase II evaluation of preoperative chemoradiotherapy utilizing intensity modulated radiation therapy (IMRT) in combination with capecitabine and oxaliplatin for patients with locally advanced rectal cancer. 2014. http://www.rtog.org/ClinicalTrials/ProtocolTable. Accessed 10 May 2018.

57. Glynne-Jones R, Wyrwicz L, Tiret E, Brown G, Rödel C, Cervantes A, Arnold D, ESMO Guidelines Committee. Rectal cancer: ESMO Clinical Practice Guidelines for diagnosis, treatment and follow-up. Ann Oncol. 2017;28(suppl_4):iv22–40.

58. Welton ML, Steele SR, Goodman KA, et al. Anus. In: Amin MB, editor. AJCC cancer staging manual. 8th ed. Chicago: AJCC; 2017. p. 275.

59. Pintor MP, Northover JM, Nicholls RJ. Squamous cell carcinoma of the anus at one hospital from 1948 to 1984. Br J Surg. 1989;76(8):806–10.

60. Nigro ND, Seydel HG, Considine B, et al. Combined preoperative radiation and chemotherapy for squamous cell carcinoma of the anal canal. Cancer. 1983;51(10):1826–9.

61. Epidermoid anal cancer: results from the UKCCCR randomised trial of radiotherapy alone versus radiotherapy, 5-fluorouracil, and mitomycin. UKCCCR Anal Cancer Trial Working Party. UK Co-ordinating Committee on Cancer Research. Lancet. 1996;348(9034):1049–54.

62. Northover J, Glynne-Jones R, Sebag-Montefiore D, et al. Chemoradiation for the treatment of epidermoid anal cancer: 13-year follow-up of the first randomised UKCCCR Anal Cancer Trial (ACT I). Br J Cancer. 2010;102(7):1123–8.

63. Bartelink H, Roelofsen F, Eschwege F, et al. Concomitant radiotherapy and chemotherapy is superior to radiotherapy alone in the treatment of locally advanced anal cancer: results of a phase III randomized trial of the European Organization for Research and Treatment of Cancer Radiotherapy and Gastrointestinal Cooperative Groups. J Clin Oncol. 1997;15(5):2040–9.

64. Flam M, John M, Pajak TF, et al. Role of mitomycin in combination with fluorouracil and radiotherapy, and of salvage chemoradiation in the definitive nonsurgical treatment of epidermoid carcinoma of the anal canal: results of a phase III randomized intergroup study. J Clin Oncol. 1996;14(9):2527–39.

65. Ajani JA, Winter KA, Gunderson LL, et al. Prognostic factors derived from a prospective database dictate clinical biology of anal cancer: the intergroup trial (RTOG 98-11). Cancer. 2010;116(17):4007. https://doi.org/10.1002/cncr.25188.

66. Gunderson LL, Winter KA, Ajani JA, et al. Long-term update of US GI intergroup RTOG 98-11 phase III trial for anal carcinoma: survival, relapse, and colostomy failure with concurrent chemoradiation involving fluorouracil/mitomycin versus fluorouracil/cisplatin. J Clin Oncol. 2012;30(35):4344–51.

67. James RD, Glynne-Jones R, Meadows HM, et al. Mitomycin or cisplatin chemoradiation with or without maintenance chemotherapy for treatment of squamous-cell carcinoma of the anus (ACT II): a randomised, phase 3, open-label, 2×2 factorial trial. Lancet Oncol. 2013;14(6):516–24.

68. Peiffert D, Tournier-Rangeard L, Gérard JP, et al. Induction chemotherapy and dose intensification of the radiation boost in locally advanced anal canal carcinoma: final analysis of the randomized UNICANCER ACCORD 03 trial. J Clin Oncol. 2012;30(16):1941–8.

69. Kachnic LA, Winter K, Myerson RJ, et al. RTOG 0529: a phase 2 evaluation of dose-painted intensity modulated radiation therapy in combination with 5-fluorouracil and mitomycin-C for the reduction of acute morbidity in carcinoma of the anal canal. Int J Radiat Oncol Biol Phys. 2013;86(1):27–33.

70. Call JA, Prendergast BM, Jensen LG, et al. Intensity-modulated radiation therapy for anal cancer: results from a multi-institutional retrospective cohort study. Am J Clin Oncol. 2016;39(1):8–12.

71. Ng M, Leong T, Chander S, et al. Australasian Gastrointestinal Trials Group (AGITG) contouring atlas and planning guidelines for intensity-modulated radiotherapy in anal cancer. Int J Radiat Oncol Biol Phys. 2012;83(5):1455–62.

72. Taylor A, Rockall AG, Reznek RH, Powell ME. Mapping pelvic lymph nodes: guidelines for delineation in intensity-modulated radiotherapy. Int J Radiat Oncol Biol Phys. 2005;63(5):1604–12.

73. Daly ME, Murphy JD, Mok E, et al. Rectal and bladder deformation and displacement during preoperative radiotherapy for rectal cancer: are current margin guidelines adequate for conformal therapy? Pract Radiat Oncol. 2011;1(2):85–94.

74. Ajani JA, Winter KA, Gunderson LL, et al. Fluorouracil, mitomycin,and radiotherapy vs fl uorouracil, cisplatin, and radiotherapy for carcinoma of the anal canal: a randomized controlled trial. JAMA. 2008;299(16):1914–21.

Genitourinary System Cancers

6

Gokhan Ozyigit, Pervin Hurmuz, Sezin Yuce Sari,
Cem Onal, Fatih Biltekin, Melis Gultekin, Gozde Yazici,
Ozan Cem Guler, and Fadil Akyol

6.1 Bladder Cancer

Overview

Bladder cancer is the fifth most common cancer in males, and the ninth most common cancer in men and women combined. Even though histological types may vary from countries, majority of the patients had urothelial (transitional cell) carcinoma. On the other hand squamous cell carcinoma increases with schistosoma infection. Mostly, bladder cancer has three stages: superficial, muscle-invasive and metastatic disease. Localized bladder cancer is divided into non-muscle invasive and muscle invasive disease. Intravesical therapies are adequate for superficial disease. Treatment strategies basically divided into two group; surgery vs trimodality treatment (TMT) that involves trans-urethral resection (TUR) of tumor tissues and concurrent radiochemotherapy (RCT) for muscle invasive disease. Current 'European Association of Urology' guidelines suggest radical cystectomy as the standard treatment for localized muscle invasive bladder cancer, as radiotherapy (RT) monotherapy

G. Ozyigit (✉) · P. Hurmuz · S. Y. Sari · F. Biltekin · M. Gultekin · G. Yazici · F. Akyol
Department of Radiation Oncology, Faculty of Medicine, Hacettepe University,
Ankara, Turkey
e-mail: gozyigit@hacettepe.edu.tr

C. Onal
Faculty of Medicine, Department of Radiation Oncology, Başkent University, Adana, Turkey

O. C. Guler
Department of Radiation Oncology, Faculty of Medicine, Karadeniz Technical University,
Trabzon, Turkey

© Springer Nature Switzerland AG 2019
G. Ozyigit, U. Selek (eds.), *Radiation Oncology*,
https://doi.org/10.1007/978-3-319-97145-2_6

is not recommended as definitive curative option and multimodality treatment is currently regarded as an alternative in selected, well informed, and compliant patients in whom cystectomy is not considered for clinical reasons.

Key Words: Bladder cancer; Radiotherapy

6.1.1 Case Presentation

He was a 68 years old male patient applied to clinics with gradually increasing hematuria in the last 3 months. He has mild anemia (Hb = 11), but kidney and liver function tests were normal. His physical examination was normal. He has previous history of two transurethral resections (TUR) which revealed non-invasive low grade tumor of the bladder, 2 and 3 years ago. However last cystoscopy done a month ago revealed tumor mass located at the bladder wall, pathology of high grade transitional cell carcinoma (TCC) with muscular invasion. Contrast-enhanced thorax-abdomen-pelvic computed tomography (CT) revealed a tumor mass located at the bladder wall with no pathological pelvic lymph nodes (Fig. 6.1). Gadolinium-enhanced magnetic resonance imaging showed deep muscular invasion of the bladder muscular wall without extra-vesical extensions. Radionuclide bone scan was normal. Patient has T2bN0M0 disease according to AJCC 2017 staging system (Table 6.1).

6.1.2 Evidence Based Treatment Recommendations

Radical cystectomy is still accepted as the gold standard treatment for MIBC [1]. This surgical procedure includes removal of whole bladder and dissection of regional lymph nodes. Additionally, prostate and seminal vesicles are removed in men, and uterus, cervix, ovaries and anterior vagina are removed in women. Despite

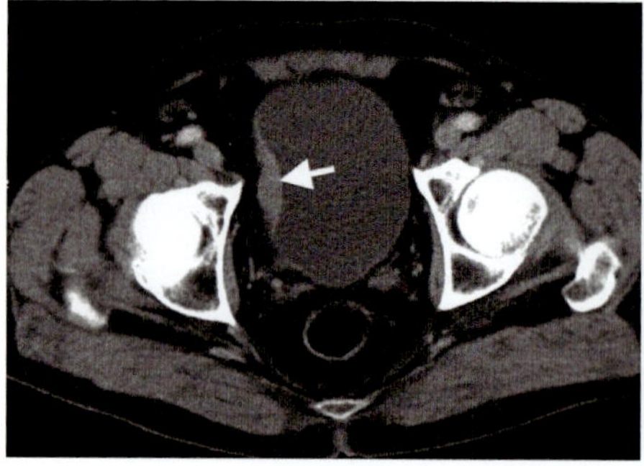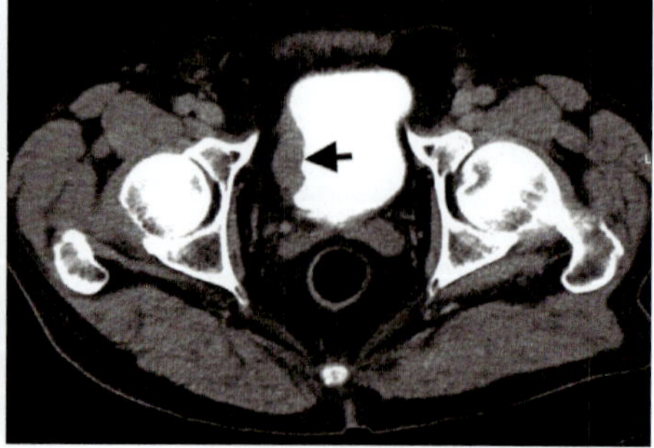

Fig. 6.1 Abdomen-pelvic computed tomography (CT) revealed a tumor mass located at the bladder wall with no pathological pelvic lymph nodes

Table 6.1 Bladder cancer staging

Primary tumor (T)	
T category	T criteria
TX	Primary tumor cannot be assessed
T0	No evidence of primary tumor
Ta	Noninvasive papillary carcinoma
Tis	Urothelial carcinoma in situ: "Flat tumor"
T1	Tumor invades lamina propria (subepithelial connective tissue)
T2	Tumor invades muscularis propria
pT2a	Tumor invades superficial muscularis propria (inner half)
pT2b	Tumor invades deep muscularis propria (outer half)
T3	Tumor invades perivesical soft tissue
pT3a	Microscopically
pT3b	Macroscopically (extravesical mass)
T4	Extravesical tumor directly invades any of the following: Prostatic stroma, seminal vesicles, uterus, vagina, pelvic wall, abdominal wall
T4a	Extravesical tumor invades directly into prostatic stroma, uterus, vagina
T4b	Extravesical tumor invades pelvic wall, abdominal wall
Regional lymph nodes (N)	
N category	N criteria
NX	Lymph nodes cannot be assessed
N0	No lymph node metastasis
N1	Single regional lymph node metastasis in the true pelvis (perivesical, obturator, internal and external iliac, or sacral lymph node)
N2	Multiple regional lymph node metastasis in the true pelvis (perivesical, obturator, internal and external iliac, or sacral lymph node metastasis)
N3	Lymph node metastasis to the common iliac lymph nodes
Distant metastasis (M)	
M category	M criteria
M0	No distant metastasis
M1	Distant metastasis
M1a	Distant metastasis limited to lymph nodes beyond the common iliacs
M1b	Non-lymph-node distant metastases

Used with permission of the American College of Surgeons, Chicago, Illinois. The original and primary source for this information is the AJCC Cancer Staging Manual, Eighth Edition (2017) published by Springer International Publishing

all these techniques, it is not possible to avoid potential morbidity or mortality of RC. Also bladder preservation therapies have a remarkable quality of life (QOL) advantage with similar oncologic outcomes.

Bladder cancer is sensitive to cisplatin-based chemotherapeutics, with survival benefit demonstrated in patients with MIBC. Neoadjuvant chemotherapy only regimen is widely used in perioperative settings in locally advanced patients [2]. However, the benefit of adjuvant RT is still controversial. Although cisplatin based chemotherapy regimens are widely used in patients with MIBC with high risk features after RC, there are no randomized clinical data that has been shown to date.

Bladder preservation therapies basically divided into two groups; single modality and TMT. Single modality treatment consists of TUR alone, partial cystectomy, RT or chemotherapy alone. The results of such treatments have inferior outcomes compared to RC or TMT. Two recently published results of comparative studies have reported similar 5- and 10-year survival rates between radical cystectomy and RT alone [3–5]. In a 10-year retrospective study with 458 patients undergoing RT or cystectomy, no significant difference in 10-year overall survival was observed between RT and radical cystectomy (22% vs. 24%) [6]. In a systematic review, the reported 5-year local control rate ranged between 35 and 45% with a 5-year OS of 25–40% with RT monotherapy [7]. Consequently, RT monotherapy is often reserved for patients deemed unsuitable for cystectomy because of advanced age or comorbidity. There are few studies demonstrating the effectiveness of RT as a treatment option in terms of local control and survival in elderly patients with locally advanced bladder cancer not suitable for cystectomy [8]. Langsenlehner et al. [8] reported complete response rates of 65% and local control rate of 53% after 3 years in 75 bladder cancer patients treated with 50–50.4 Gy course of conformal RT. However, 35% of patients died from bladder cancer.

Optimal bladder preservation therapy is TMT and comprises TUR-BT followed by concurrent RCT. Preliminary studies demonstrated complete response rate to endoscopic resection followed by chemotherapy was nearly twice that achieved by chemotherapy alone and addition of RT further improved disease-free survival with intact bladder [9–11]. The use of bladder-preserving strategies, combining RT and chemotherapy after maximal TUR is alternative to radical cystectomy [12–15]. The extension of TUR-BT is very important in this treatment and it should be as complete as possible in maximal safe procedure.

Since the late 1980s several centers have investigated the bladder preservation strategy as an alternative to radical cystectomy. This strategy is multidisciplinary, entailing maximal TUR-BT, followed by combined RCT [6, 13, 16–24] (Table 6.2). Three centers (University of Erlangen, Germany; Massachusetts General Hospital [MGH], MA, USA; and the University of Paris V, France) together with the Radiation Therapy Oncology Group (RTOG) in a multi-institutional setting have the largest experience. All reached the conclusion that patients who completely respond to TMT (61–87% in different series) are those who shall reap the benefits of long-term survival, while for those who cannot attain CR, cystectomy is the appropriate option. Cystoscopy is performed after a few weeks of RCT to assess the treatment response. If any residual disease (macro- or microscopic) remains, bladder preservation is aborted by cystectomy. On the other hand, if CR is achieved, a consolidation phase of RCT is carried out. Massachusetts General Hospital reported the results of 348 patients with MIBC who were treated with combined RCT [26]. The authors reported complete response (CR) rate of 72%; with 5- and 10-year OS rates of 52% and 35%, respectively. The 5- and 10-year DSS rates were 64% and 59%, respectively. Patients were excluded if they had pathologically proven positive nodes or hydronephrosis. All MGH protocols had in common the use of TUR-BT,

Table 6.2 Bladder preservation trials

Study	N	Fractionation	RT dose (Gy)	OS	Salvage RC (%)
Housset et al. [17][a]	54	Split-course	44 (bid)	3 year, 59%	–
Shipley et al. [14][a]	62	Split-course	64.8	5 year, 49%	25.8
James et al. [18][a]	182	Continuous	55–64	5 year, 48%	11.4
Tunio et al. [19][a]	200	Continuous	65	5 year, 52%	–
Kaufman et al. [25]	34	Split-course	44 (bid)	–	29.4
Hussain et al. [6]	41	Continuous	55 Gy in 20	2 year, 50%	19.5
Peyromaure et al. [20]	43	Split-course	24 Gy in 8 (bid)	–	25.6
Kragelj et al. [21]	84	Continuous	64	9 year, 25%	8.3
Aboziada et al. [22]	50	Split-course	66	1.5 year, 100%	28
Choudhury and Cowan [23]	50	Continuous	52.5 Gy in 20	5 year, 65%	14

RT radiotherapy, *OS* overall survival, *CSS* cause-specific survival, *CR* complete response, *RC* radical cystectomy
[a]Prospective studies

concomitant cisplatin-based RT and cystectomy if complete response was not achieved.

At the University of Erlangen, the authors retrospectively analyzed 415 patients with MIBC. The treatment included TUR-BT followed 4 weeks later by RCT upto a dose of 45–54 Gy to the bladder and pelvic nodes, and then whole bladder dose is boosted to 55.8–59.4 Gy total dose, depending upon the completeness of TUR-BT. Six to 8 weeks after completion of therapy, response is assessed by cystoscopy. If the response is incomplete, cystectomy is indicated. The complete response rates for all patients and radiotherapy alone were 72% and 61%, respectively. The 5- and 10-year OS rates were 51% and 31%, while salvage cystectomy rates were 20% [27].

The Bladder Cancer 2001 (BC2001) study was the first randomized study investigating the role of chemotherapy to TURBT followed by radiotherapy in MIBC [18]. The chemotherapy regimen consisted of 5-FU and MMC. The 2-year DFS was significantly improved in the combined treatment arm compared to RT alone (67% vs. 54%, $p = 0.03$). Also there was a trend favoring RCT arm in 5-year OS rates (48% vs. 35%; $p = 0.16$). National Cancer Institute of Canada (NCIC) investigated the addition of cisplatin chemotherapy to RT for organ sparing treatment modality [12]. There was a statistically significant reduction in pelvic recurrences in patients treated with concurrent RCT compared to RT alone (29% vs. 52%), however no statistically significant difference in OS was observed.

Several investigative protocols were carried out by the 'Radiation Therapy Oncology Group' (RTOG). The first one, RTOG 85-12, consisted of induction RT with cisplatin, thereafter patients with complete response received additional RT and third dose of cisplatin [28]. In RTOG 88-02 study, the toxicity of adding neoadjuvant, cisplatin, methotrexate and vinblastine (CMV) to the combined treatment was evaluated [27]. The good tolerability of the regimen in this study led to RTOG 89-03, a randomized Phase III trial assessing the efficacy of neoadjuvant CMV [28]. However, this study was stopped early due to unacceptably high toxicity rates in the CMV arm. Moreover, the addition of neoadjuvant CMV did not show any benefit in terms of complete response rates, overall survival or bladder-preservation rates. RTOG 95-06 evaluated the accelerated hypofractionated scheme [17]. Although overall survival and bladder-preservation rates were encouraging, grade 3 or more genitourinary toxicity rates were a concern. RTOG 97-06 also evaluated the efficacy of hypofractionated RT scheme [25]. In RTOG 99-06, paclitaxel was added to the concomitant cisplatin and gemcitabine in the adjuvant setting leading to an excellent complete rate of 87% [29].

Radiation dose and schedule varies from countries but the most acceptable fractionation is 40–46 Gy to pelvic lymph nodes and bladder with a boost to tumor a total dose of 60–66 Gy. Cisplatin is the most common concurrent chemotherapy agent. The main goal of this chemotherapy is being a radio sensitizer. After performing TUR-BT, the bladder-preservation protocols usually belong to one of three categories. In the first scheme RT is delivered to patients who attain pathological complete remission after a full dose of chemotherapy. The second scheme includes induction chemotherapy with two to three cycles of CMV, then RCT for the responders. The third scheme entails concomitant RCT either with moderate dose followed by cystoscopy and consolidation RCT, or to give high-dose RCT and to perform cystoscopy after completion of the dose. For all schemes, cystectomy is indicated for those who attained non-complete response. A cystoscopy with re-biopsy should be performed for assessment of therapy response. This evaluation could be done at the end of TMT (continuous course) or before planning to the boost volumes after 40–46 Gy (split course). In the latter, patients responding to the treatment were treated for boost to tumor while non-responders were offered for salvage RC. 5 year overall survival (OS) and cancer specific survival rates range from 36% to 74% and 50% to 82% respectively. Salvage cystectomy rates were 25–30% [30].

Advanced age is not a contraindication for TMT. As older patients are more likely to have significant comorbidities, treatment should be interpreted with carefully. Especially kidney function test (BUN and creatinine), electrolytes and fluid intake should be taken into consideration with attention. RTOG pooled analysis of patients aged 75 or more shoved no significant differences in CR or DSS.

6.1.3 Radiotherapy Techniques

Historically, most of the published data about bladder cancer RT is about two-dimensional conventional RT [31]. Nowadays, 3D-conformal RT is the current standard in most of the clinical trials. IMRT has emerged as an option for image guidance. Advances in RT planning, verification, positioning and delivery provide a means to optimize RT for bladder cancer and overcome difficulties, which have previously limited the success of this treatment. Also, offers the opportunity to reduce the irradiated normal tissue volumes while delivering more intensive and increased RT dose.

Intensity modulated radiotherapy (IMRT), is a new technique which allows more accurate delivery of required doses or beyond to the tumor while protecting adjacent organs or structures [31]. This technique is widely used in radiotherapy and replaced the three dimensional radiotherapy (3D-RT) in the treatment of MIBC. Fractionation schedules and treatment fields varies from centers. There is no randomized trial comparing the conventional fractionation and BID. The most accepted approach is 40–45 Gy to the entire bladder, prostatic/proximal urethra and the lymph nodes in pelvis following by boost 20 Gy to the tumor a total dose of 65–66 Gy. Treating only bladder is for a total dose of 64 Gy in 2 Gy fractions is performed by some groups [31].

6.1.3.1 Clinical Target Volume

CTV1 is the whole bladder, tumor bed (after TUR), proximal urethra, bladder neck and/or prostatic urethra (in case of prostatic fossa involvement), and if existent, extravesical extension with a 0.5-cm margin. This field is irradiated with 45–50 Gy in 1.8–2 Gy fraction doses [31]. The reason for delineating the whole bladder is that bladder cancer is generally multifocal, and recurs in a multifocal manner [31]. Besides, delineating the microscopic extent of the tumor on a planning CT is difficult. If elective nodal irradiation is to be administered, pelvic LNs are also delineated in CTV1 and receive the same dose. CTV2 for the boost dose is formed with a 0.5-cm margin to the GTV2, and irradiated to a total dose of 60–65 Gy. Another boost technique is to irradiate the whole bladder with an additional 8 Gy and then give a boost dose of 12 Gy to the tumor alone. However, if the site of the tumor is not clear, then the whole bladder is recommended to be treated to the total dose [31].

All anatomical variations such as cystocele and diverticulum should be included in the CTV. If there is involvement of ureteric orifice, distal urethra should be encompassed in the CTV with a 1-cm margin [31]. The prostate is involved in up to 43% of patients with bladder cancer [31]. The risk of urethral involvement, and therefore prostatic involvement, is increased with the existence of carcinoma in-situ in the bladder, multifocal tumors and involvement of the trigone/bladder neck. If any one of these risk factors are present, the whole prostate gland can be included in the CTV1. If there is macroscopic involvement of the prostate and/or urethra, the prostate should be included in both CTV1 and CTV2 [31].

In female patients, the rate of urethral involvement was found 7–46% in cystectomy series [31]. Urethral involvement was shown to be associated with the involvement of bladder neck [31]. Another potential site for microscopic invasion is the anterior vaginal wall in patients with urethral involvement [31]. However, it is difficult to determine microscopic vaginal involvement without cystectomy, and delineating the vagina is not routinely recommended. If there is anterior vaginal wall involvement on imaging or clinical examination, then the vagina should be included in CTV1 together with the proximal urethra.

CTV delineation including pelvic lymph nodes in a muscle-invasive bladder cancer patient treated with bladder preserving multimodal approach IGRT is depicted in Fig. 6.2.

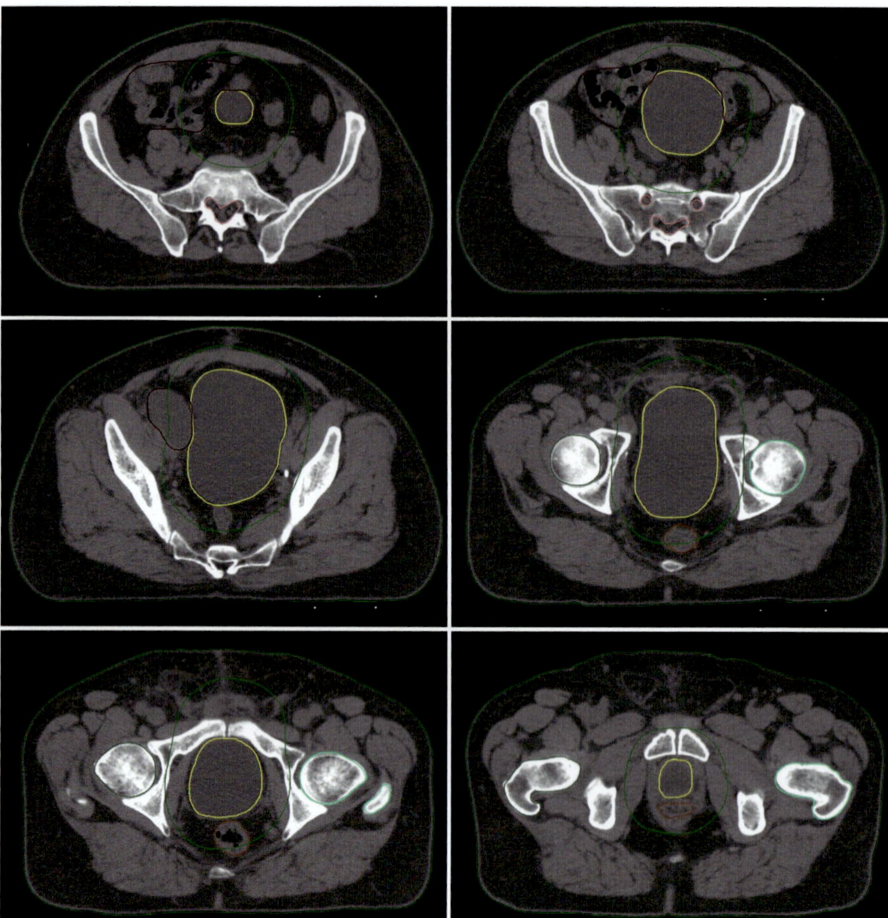

Fig. 6.2 CTV delineation for a muscle-invasive bladder cancer patient treated with definitive IGRT

6.1.3.2 Role of Elective Nodal Irradiation

There are conflicting data on elective nodal irradiation in the treatment of bladder cancer [31]. The rate of LN involvement is approximately 25% according to radical cystectomy series, and this finding helps to indicate the need for extensive LN dissection (LND) and adjuvant chemotherapy [31]. The number of dissected LNs is directly correlated with the outcome of patients, independent of the N stage. Based on these findings, elective nodal irradiation may provide a survival benefit in patients that did not undergo LND whether they are involved or not, with the expense of additional toxicity [31]. Although there is no randomized trial favoring the inclusion of the pelvic nodes in the radiation volume, elective nodal irradiation aims at eradication of micrometastatic disease in the pelvis. However, this approach results in irradiation of a large target volume, encompassing significant amounts of the small bowel and rectum. This can lead to greater gastrointestinal toxicity and potentially limit treatment intensification [32]. The question of whether to include lymph nodes or not in CTV has never been the issue of any randomized trial. Centers that irradiate the bladder alone do not report either increased pelvic failure rates or reduced survival, although direct comparisons are difficult [33]. Retrospective studies comparing patients receiving irradiation to the locoregional lymph nodes with patients treated with small fields to the bladder only showed a significantly worse treatment outcome on irradiation of the nodes [34].

However, the bias of treating the more advanced cases with locoregional nodes may be the reason for these inferior results [35]. However, reviewing the extended pelvic lymphadenectomy data in bladder cancer showed that several prospective and retrospective studies proved that the extent of lymphadenectomy and the number of dissected nodes determine the survival rates, even in node-negative patients [36]. This may reflect the importance of eradication of the disease in the lymph nodes, even in its microscopic form, in bladder cancer end results. With the advancement in radiotherapeutic techniques, it is expected that radiation can improve the tumor control probability and reduce normal tissue complication probability in such patients.

However, pelvic failure and survival rates are not decreased with irradiation of the bladder alone when used together with chemotherapy. The BC20001 study reported a low rate of nodal relapse both in patients that received RT alone (7%) and in patients that received chemoradiotherapy (5%). In a randomized trial that compares 45 Gy of whole pelvic RT including elective nodal irradiation and 20 Gy boost dose with bladder-only irradiation of 65 Gy, no difference was found in the rates of pelvic nodal relapse and overall survival in patients with complete response. Therefore, it may be reasonable to electively irradiate the pelvic lymphatic regions in patients that cannot receive concurrent chemotherapy [31].

6.1.3.3 Planning Target Volume

The whole bladder is usually defined as PTV with a 1.5-cm margin to the uninvolved outer bladder wall and the extravesical extent of the tumor with a 2-cm margin [31]. In other instances, the PTV is formed with a 2-cm margin to the CTV in order to adequately cover all errors based on setup and organ motion. It was shown that the bladder wall can move beyond 1.5 cm at least once during a course of treatment in over 60% of patients, and the GTV can move outside the PTV on at least one course of treatment in over 20% of patients [31]. Daily image-guided therapy can be administered, or insertion of fiducial markers in the bladder wall around the tumor bed may be another solution. The use of these techniques can decrease the margins <1.5 cm [37]. However, besides the movement of the bladder, the change of its shape is also challenging. Therefore, the margins for the PTV do not seem to be reduced at any time soon. The recommended margins for the PTV are 1–1.5 cm in all directions, and 2–2.5 cm in the superior direction when using conventional RT. The inferior margin can be reduced to 1 cm if the prostate or urethra has been included. One should also consider which walls of the bladder are involved by the cancer and the relative mobility of this particular portion of the bladder [31].

6.1.3.4 Simulation, Target Volume and Fields

Tumor location is essential for determining the target volume. For this purpose, operative notes during cystoscopy and histology reports should be available and cross-sectional imaging is mandatory [31]. Standard supine position is the treatment position of choice. Computed tomography simulation is the gold standard for treatment planning, for adequate coverage of whole bladder [37]. Intravesical contrast (30–70 mL) may also be administered via a catheter, with or without additional air (15–30 mL). It is necessary to make sure that the use of contrast does not result in considerable difference of the bladder volume in planning and during daily treatment delivery [38].

All simulations performed with empty bladder in supine position. This makes more reproducible and predictable positioning of bladder. 3D-CT simulation is essential for treatment. Patients underwent 3-mm slice thickness CT from mid L4 to the lower edge of lesser trochanters. Intravenous contrast could be used in suspicious cases, not as clinical routine [31].

Treatment of urinary bladder cancer involves two phases of RT (Figs. 6.3 and 6.4). Bladder and prostate with or without pelvic lymph nodes, are target volumes in the first phase. The second phase boosts the bladder alone. Pelvic lymph nodes consist of obturator, internal and external iliac lymphatics. As there might be occult stromal invasion, prostatic urethra and first 2 cm of proximal urethra needs to be covered in men and women, respectively. The top border of the field starts at the level of the bifurcation of the common iliac vessels and does not include entire pelvis [31].

6.1.3.5 Doses and RT Schedules

There are two main RT schedules in the treatment of urinary bladder cancer [31].

1. CTV1 is treated up to 46 Gy and a boost of 65–66 Gy delivered to CTV2 in once daily 1.8–2 Gy fractions, 5 days per week [26, 39].
2. Twice-daily concomitant boost is used and CTV1 is treated up to 45 Gy in 1.8 Gy fractions and CTV2 is boosted to 67.5 Gy in 1.5 Gy fractions. Typically, 40–45 Gy is delivered to the pelvic lymph nodes and entire bladder while whole bladder boosts additional 20–24 Gy.

The major difference between these schedules is that the first regimen allows assessment of early treatment response following the delivery of first phase. Repeat cystoscopy/biopsy after 3-weeks of treatment break may distinguish the non-responder patients and lead them to immediate radical cystectomy [31].

Day to day variations in bladder size, shape and position is the major technical difficulty in urinary bladder cancer RT. These variations may results inadequate dose homogeneity while increasing the dose to surrounding normal tissues. Also, the need of larger treatment margins might result in the irradiation of significant volumes of small bowel and rectum [31]. Use of fiducial markers may allow decrease in PTV expansion. Daily image guided therapy is the only way to reduce the margins significantly. Also, if the daily treatment is centered on the bladder rather than referenced to bony anatomy, smaller margins could be feasible [31].

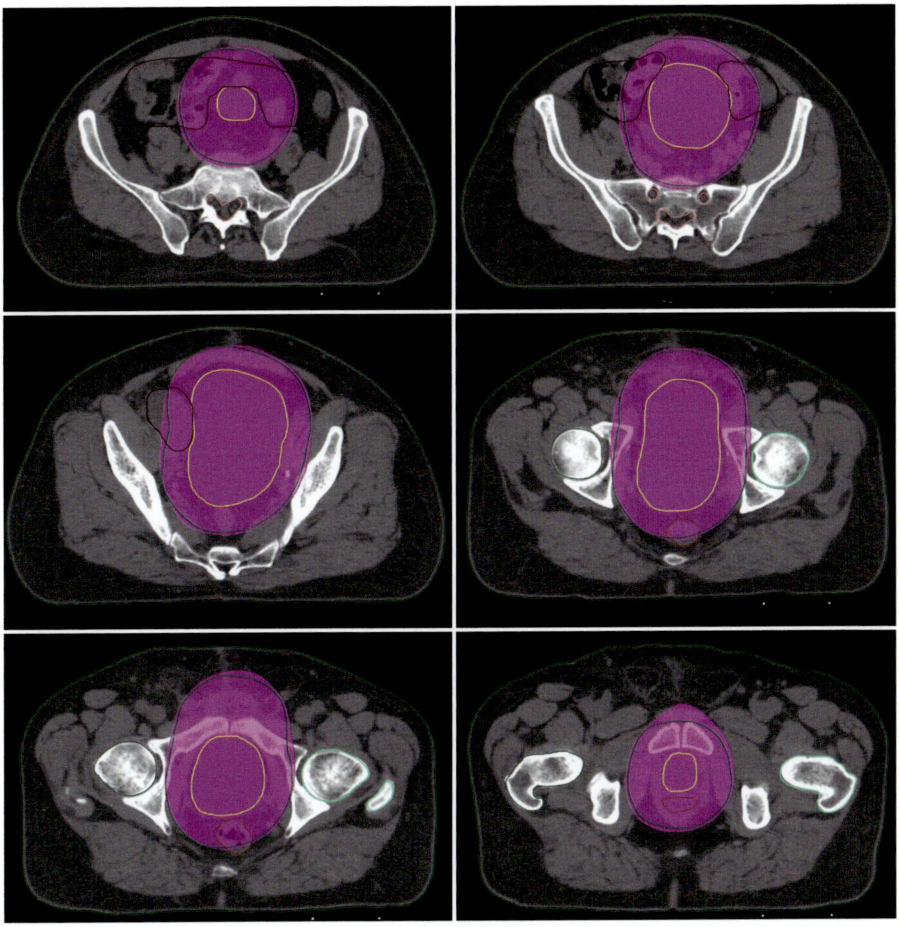

Fig. 6.3 Treatment of urinary bladder cancer: first phases of RT without elective. Pelvic lymph node radiotherapy

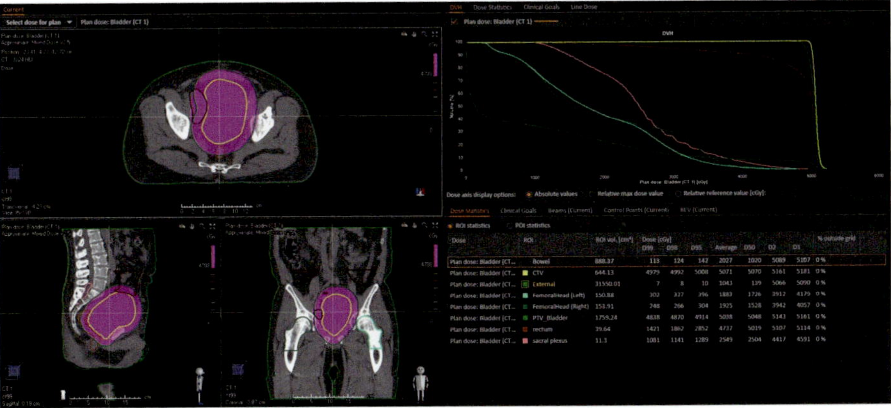

Fig. 6.4 Dose volume histogram for the first phase of radiotherapy

Estimated bladder tolerance in partial bladder irradiation is 80 Gy if one third of the bladder is spared. Partial bladder irradiation does allow for the delivery of a higher dose to the tumor than whole bladder radiation without increase in morbidity [32].

6.2 Prostate Cancer

Overview

Prostate cancer (PC) is the most common tumor in males. Treatment alternatives for localized prostate cancer include radical prostatectomy and radiotherapy (RT), which is delivered either as external beam radiation therapy (EBRT) or brachytherapy (BRT). Radiotherapy of PC has been evolved since last decades with the innovation in technology. More precise radiotherapy (RT) techniques provide sharper dose gradients while sparing organs at risk (OAR). It is also essential that set-up margins could be reduced with image guidance. Hence, precisely defining targets and considering organ movement is gaining much more importance. As a consequence of sharper dose gradients and image guidance, dose escalation became possible. There is a positive correlation between RT dose and biochemical progression free survival (BPFS), with dose-escalated conventionally fractionated up to 76–80 Gy in 2 Gy fractions, which is a biologically equivalent dose (BED1.5) of 180–200 Gy, assuming an α/β of 1.5. A recent meta-analysis clearly demonstrated an increased disease control with a BED1.5 to 200 Gy, with no additional clinical benefit with doses above 200 Gy. It is essential to delineate target volumes properly, to deliver RT with high-technology devices, to immobilize patient and track prostate during RT in order to deliver higher doses to prostate without increasing surrounding organs at risk.

Key Words: Prostate cancer; Radiotherapy

6.2.1 Case Presentation

6.2.1.1 Case 1

He was a 62-year-old male presents with lower urinary tract symptoms, and prostate-specific antigen (PSA) of 7.7 ng/mL. His whole blood count, kidney and liver function tests were normal. His physical examination and were normal. A nodule on prostate gland was palpated in his digital rectal examination. His past medical history was normal. He was referred to urology for transrectal ultrasound (TRUS) of prostate and US-guided needle biopsy. US revealed 45 g prostate with mixed echogenecity. Transrectal biopsy confirmed a diagnosis of clinically localized prostate cancer (cT2, Gleason score 7 (4 + 3), 4/12 cores affected). Prostate MRI of patient revelaed hypointense cancer area in the left posterior peripheral zone with no SV and capsule invasion (Fig. 6.5). AJCC 2017 staging of patient was T2aN0M0 (Table 6.3).

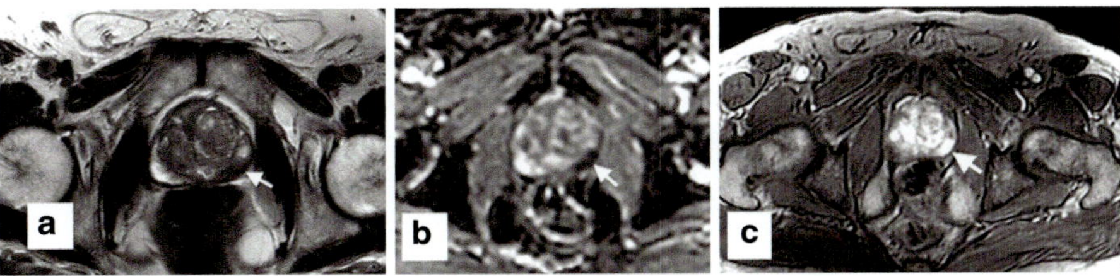

Fig. 6.5 MRI of patient. (**a**) Axial T2-W image demonstrated hypointense cancer area (arrow) in the left posterior peripheral zone. (**b**) ADC map shows signal loss (arrow) in the cancer region. (**c**) DCE-MRI at early phase reveals avid enhancement (arrow) of the lesion

Table 6.3 Prostate cancer TNM staging AJCC UICC 2017

Primary tumor (T)	
Clinical T (cT)	
T category	T criteria
TX	Primary tumor cannot be assessed
T0	No evidence of primary tumor
T1	Clinically inapparent tumor that is not palpable
T1a	Tumor incidental histologic finding in 5% or less of tissue resected
T1b	Tumor incidental histologic finding in more than 5% of tissue resected
T1c	Tumor identified by needle biopsy found in one or both sides, but not palpable
T2	Tumor is palpable and confined within prostate
T2a	Tumor involves one-half of one side or less
T2b	Tumor involves more than one-half of one side but not both sides
T2c	Tumor involves both sides
T3	Extraprostatic tumor that is not fixed or does not invade adjacent structures
T3a	Extraprostatic extension (unilateral or bilateral)
T3b	Tumor invades seminal vesicle(s)
T4	Tumor is fixed or invades adjacent structures other than seminal vesicles such as external sphincter, rectum, bladder, levator muscles, and/or pelvic wall
Pathological T (pT)	
T category	T criteria
T2	Organ confined
T3	Extraprostatic extension
T3a	Extraprostatic extension (unilateral or bilateral) or microscopic invasion of bladder neck
T3b	Tumor invades seminal vesicle(s)
T4	Tumor is fixed or invades adjacent structures other than seminal vesicles such as external sphincter, rectum, bladder, levator muscles, and/or pelvic wall

Note: There is no pathological T1 classification
Note: Positive surgical margin should be indicated by an R1 descriptor, indicating residual microscopic disease

(continued)

Table 6.3 (continued)

Regional lymph nodes (N)	
N category	N criteria
NX	Regional nodes were not assessed
N0	No positive regional nodes
N1	Metastases in regional node(s)

Distant metastasis (M)	
M category	M criteria
M0	No distant metastasis
M1	Distant metastasis
M1a	Nonregional lymph node(s)
M1b	Bone(s)
M1c	Other site(s) with or without bone disease

Note: When more than one site of metastasis is present, the most advanced category is used. M1c is most advanced.

Prostate-specific antigen (PSA)

PSA values are used to assign this category.

PSA values

<10

≥10 < 20

<20

≥20

Any value

Histologic grade group (G)

Recently, the Gleason system has been compressed into so-called Grade Groups

Grade group	Gleason score	Gleason pattern
1	≤6	≤3 + 3
2	7	3 + 4
3	7	4 + 3
4	8	4 + 4, 3 + 5, 5 + 3
5	9 or 10	4 + 5, 5 + 4, or 5 + 5

Used with permission of the American College of Surgeons, Chicago, Illinois. The original and primary source for this information is the AJCC Cancer Staging Manual, Eighth Edition (2017) published by Springer International Publishing

6.2.1.2 Case 2

He was a 66-years-old male applied to clinics with prostate-specific antigen (PSA) level of 26 ng/mL detached during prostate cancer screening. He has past medical history of BPH. His family history includes his father, who was dead with metastatic prostate cancer. He was referred to urology for transrectal ultrasound (TRUS) of prostate and US-guided needle biopsy. His whole blood count, kidney and liver function tests were normal. His physical examination was normal. Digital rectal examination revealed nodularity on the left peripheral zone. US revealed 50 g prostate with capsular invasion on the left peripheral zone of the prostate. Transrectal biopsy confirmed a diagnosis of clinically localized prostate cancer (cT3a, Gleason score 8 (4 + 4), 4/12 cores affected). Contrast-enhanced pelvic computed tomography (CT) revealed no pathological pelvic lymph nodes. Technetium-99 radionuclide bone scan did not show any bone metastases. MRI imaging showed increased uptake at the left peripheral zone of the prostate with capsular invasion (Fig. 6.6). **AJCC 2017 staging of patient was T3aN0M0 (Tables 6.3 and 6.4).**

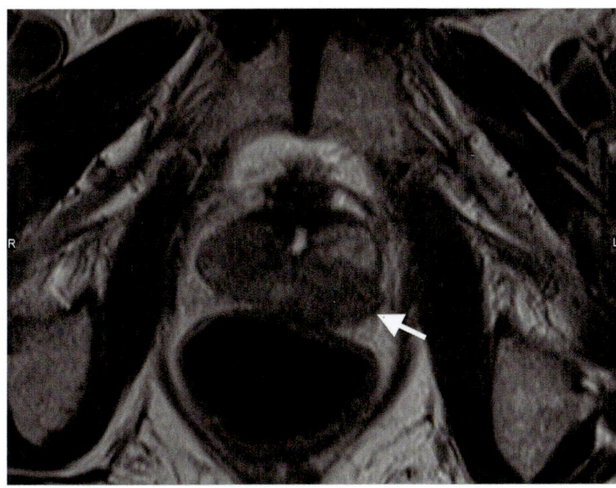

Fig. 6.6 Axial T2-W image demonstrates hypointense mass in right posterolateral peripheral prostate gland. Interruption of prostate capsule in tumoral region suggests capsule invasion (arrow)

Table 6.4 Prostate cancer TNM prognostic stage groups AJCC UICC 2017

When T is...	And N is...	And M is...	And PSA is...	And Grade Group is...	Then the stage group is...
cT1a-c, cT2a	N0	M0	<10	1	I
pT2	N0	M0	<10	1	I
cT1a-c, cT2a, pT2	N0	M0	≥10 <20	1	IIA
cT2b-c	N0	M0	<20	1	IIA
T1-2	N0	M0	<20	2	IIB
T1-2	N0	M0	<20	3	IIC
T1-2	N0	M0	<20	4	IIC
T1-2	N0	M0	≥20	1–4	IIIA
T3-4	N0	M0	Any	1–4	IIIB
Any T	N0	M0	Any	5	IIIC
Any T	N1	M0	Any	Any	IVA
Any T	Any N	M1	Any	Any	IVB

TNM tumor, node, metastasis, *AJCC* American Joint Committee on Cancer, *UICC* Union for International Cancer Control, *PSA* prostate-specific antigen

Note: When either PSA or Grade Group is not available, grouping should be determined by T category and/or either PSA or Grade Group as available

Used with permission of the American College of Surgeons, Chicago, Illinois. The original and primary source for this information is the AJCC Cancer Staging Manual, Eighth Edition (2017) published by Springer International Publishing

6.2.2 Evidence Based Treatment Recommendations

6.2.2.1 Radiotherapy Dose Escalation

Dose escalation for prostate cancer causes improved biochemical control and reduced distant metastasis [40]. However, local failure still occurs in one-third of patients after 78 Gy ERT, and the original IPL is the most frequent location of relapse [41]. Therefore, selectively boosting radiation to these lesions to a very high dose has been hypothesized to be a more effective method to improve the therapeutic ratio than a homogeneous, but more modest, dose escalation to the entire prostate [42]. Randomized trials have shown a gain in BPFS using dose escalation for PC [40, 43]. However, isolated local failure is still reported in nearly one-third of patients, even with higher RT doses [40]. Local recurrence is of clinical importance because a relationship has been suggested between local control, distant metastasis and survival [44]. Also, it has been demonstrated that local failure mainly originates at IPL. This could be result of intrinsic resistance of radio-resistance tumor clones [41]. So, delivering higher doses to IPL using SIB technique may potentially increase local control and treatment outcomes. The SIB technique can be safely performed by static IMRT, VMAT or HT. With VMAT plan and HT plan, a homogenous dose distribution is observed in target volumes with better sparing the surrounding organs.

There are several studies investigating SIB boost to IPL/whole gland in treatment of PC [45–49] (Table 6.5). A boost to the IPL has been found to be effective and safe [50]. The reported BRFS and DFS rates were 78–92% and 90–100% respectively [51]. Although SIB to IPL is not standard approach, several ongoing studies will evaluate whether this approach is effective in local tumor control or not.

6.2.2.2 Hypofractionation/Stereotactic Body Radiotherapy

Larger fraction per treatment is hypothesized with better radiobiological effect in the treatment of PC [52]. In addition to that, the potentially low alpha/beta ratio of PC is hypothesized as the rationale of hypofractionation and SBRT [53–55]. In moderate hypofractionation 2.2–4 Gy per fraction is generally delivered with linear accelerators while doses above 5 Gy is used in SBRT. SBRT uses more intensive immobilization and tracking systems to safely deliver high doses of radiation compared to IMRT.

SBRT and hypofractionation studies generally investigated low risk and intermediate risk patients. Because high-risk disease requires more comprehensive approach due to risk of regional spread, SBRT is generally used as boost in such patients. Also, greater likelihood of local recurrence and resistance of conventional RT dose makes high-risk patients a candidate for dose escalation with larger RT fraction [56].

Summaries of hypofractionation and SBRT studies are depicted in Table 6.6. Briefly, SBRT and hypofractionated RT could be used as monotherapy, whole gland boost therapy or focal boost of IPL. There are various RT schemes for monotherapy

Table 6.5 Published studies demonstrating the feasibility of simultaneous integrated boost intra-prostatic lesion during prostate radiotherapy

Study	Patient no.	RT technique/dose	Toxicity
De Meerleer [101]	15	Step-shoot IMRT Prostate + 7–10 mm 74 Gy IPL + 0 mm 80 Gy	Acute GI Gr II 3/15 Acute GU Gr III 1/15 Acute GU Gr II 6/15
Fonteyne et al. [45]	118 (boost) 112 (no boost)	Step-shoot IMRT Prostate + 8 mm 78 Gy IPL + 4 mm 80 Gy	No increase in toxicity with SIB plan
Miralbell [102]	50	Prostate 64–64.4 Gy Hipofractionated boost 5–8 Gy	Late GI Gr II 10% Late GI Gr III 10% Late GU Gr II 12%
Ippolito [103]	40	Step-shoot IMRT Prostate + 10 mm 72 Gy IPL + 5 mm 80 Gy	Late GI Gr II 5% Late GI Gr III 2.5% Late GU Gr II 5%
Pinkawa [104]	Total 67 SIB 46	Step-shoot IMRT Prostate + 6 mm 75.6 Gy IPL + 0 mm 80 Gy	No increase in toxicity with SIB plan
Aluwini [105]	50 14 IPL (+)	Prostate + 3 mm 38 Gy/4 fx (day) IPL 44 Gy/4 fx	Late GI Gr II 3% Late GU Gr II 10% Late GU Gr III 6%
Onal [106]	173	Dynamic IMRT/VMAT Prostate + 5–8 mm 78 Gy IPL + 4 mm 86 Gy	Late GI Gr II 4% Late GU Gr II 3%

of PC but the optimal fractionation has not been determined. Most of the studies investigated the BPFS, quality of life (QoL) and toxicity. In general, hypofractionation or SBRT are well tolerated with acceptable results without any serious increase in toxicity.

6.2.2.3 Hormonal Therapy in Locally Advanced Disease

ADT was shown to improve OS and PFS in patients with locally advanced disease [57–63]. Table 6.7 represents the results of ADT combined with RT.

ADT was shown to be the most cost-effective therapy if started at the time that the patient developed symptomatic metastases [64] Thus ADT should be started immediately in case of symptomatic metastases in order to palliate symptoms and prevent complications, however, controversy still exists regarding asymptomatic metastatic patients because of the lack of high-quality studies.

6.2.2.4 Role of Elective Nodal Irradiation in Prostate Cancer

For a staging lymphadenectomy to be adequate, the TNM classification recommends at least eight LNs to be resected in order to stage a patient as pN0, but there is no exact requirement. Elective nodal irradiation is not required in a patient with pN0 tumor because of the increased rate of toxicity and the lack of a prospective study that shows the benefit of this treatment. Similarly, elective nodal irradiation has no rationale in patients with cN0 disease [65].

Table 6.6 Published studies of stereotactic radiotherapy and hypofractionation in prostate cancer treatment

Study	N	Design	Risk group	Fractionation	Therapy	Follow-up	Outcome	Toxicity
Arcangeli [107]	168	Randomized	HR	Conv. vs. 3.1 Gy × 20 fr	Monotherapy	70 months	5y BPFS 79–85% No difference	Late Grd 2 ≥ 11–17% No difference
Pollack et a1. [55]	303	Randomized	HR	Conv. vs. 2.7 Gy × 26 fr	Monotherapy	68 months	5y BPFS 81–85% No difference	Late Grd 2 ≥ 13–23% No difference
Hoffman [108]	204	Randomized Phase III	LR, IR, HR	Conv. vs. 2.4 Gy × 30 fr	Monotherapy	57 months	–	Late Grd 2 ≥ 5.1–16.5%
Norkus [109]	124	Randomized	HR	Conv. vs. 3.15 Gy × 20 fr	Monotherapy		–	Acute tx No difference
Wilkins (CHHiP trial) [110]	2054	Randomized Phase III	LR, IR, HR	Conv vs. 3 Gy × 19–20 fr	Monotherapy	50 months	No difference	No difference
Aluvini (HYPRO trial) [111]		Randomized Phase III	IR, HR	Conv. vs. 3.4 Gy × 19 fr	Monotherapy			Hypofractionation is more toxic
King [112]	1100	Prospective Phase II	LR, IR, HR	7 Gy × 5 fr 8 Gy × 5 fr	Monotherapy		5y BPFS 81%	

Table 6.7 Randomized studies of radiotherapy and androgen blockade in patients with high-risk prostate cancer

Study	N	Arms	Results
RTOG 85-31 [60]	977	RT vs. RT + LHRHa (continuous)	Combined arm is better in all end points
RTOG 86-10 [61]	456	RT vs. RT + 4 month CAB	No significant difference in OS GS 2–6 patients have better OS
RTOG 92-02 [62]	1554	RT + 4 month LHRHa vs. RT + 2 year LHRHa	Long term arm is better in all end points except OS GS 8–10 patients have better OS with long term LHRHa
EORTC 22863 [63]	415	RT vs. RT + 3 year LHRHa	Combined arm is better in all end points

RT radiotherapy, *LHRH* Luteinizing hormone releasing hormone agonist, *CAB* complete androgen blockade, *GS* Gleason score, *OS* overall survival

There are three prospective randomized trials questioning the role of elective nodal irradiation in prostate cancer. The first study was Radiation Therapy Oncology Group (RTOG) 77-06 trial which resulted in no benefit from prostatic bed and nodal irradiation compared to prostatic bed irradiation only [66]. However, patients that had undergone lymphadenectomy had significantly better outcomes than the patients that did not.

The second trial was the first report of RTOG 9413 which found that whole pelvis RT (WHRT) with short-term neoadjuvant hormonotherapy (HT) increased the rate of progression-free survival (PFS) in 1275 prostate cancer patients without positive LNs but with a risk of LN involvement >15% [67]. However, this study was criticized because of the bias in the duration of HT in different groups. Eventually, in the update of this study, WHRT had no significant benefit over prostate-only RT (PORT) in addition to an increased rate of late gastrointestinal toxicity [68].

The third study was the Groupe d'étude des tumeurs urogénitales (GETUG)-01 trial which similarly found no benefit of pelvic irradiation even in patients with a higher risk of LN involvement [69]. In 2016, the update of this study was published with a median follow-up of 11.4 years [70]. The 10-year overall survival (OS) and event-free survival (EFS) rates were similar in patients that did and did not undergo pelvic irradiation.

In the light of these data, elective nodal irradiation in patients without nodal involvement is not recommended. However, Murthy et al. analyzed the incidental dose received by the pelvic LNs and found and interesting result [71]. When they compared the dose from 2-dimensional conventional RT (2D CRT), 3-dimensional conformal RT (3D CRT) and intensity-modulated RT (IMRT), they found that the obturator nodes received 44 Gy, 29 Gy, and 22 Gy from 2D CRT, 3D CRT, and IMRT, respectively, and each was significantly different from the others. On the other hand, the dose to other lymphatic regions was low and not clinically relevant. The authors concluded that in patients that will undergo IMRT, elective pelvic irradiation can be considered.

6.2.2.5 Target Volume Delineation

In recent years, the use of intensity-modulated RT (IMRT) and image-guided RT (IGRT) have increased worldwide. These techniques are highly conformal and the target should be more precise. Fiducial markers should be inserted into the prostate via transrectal ultrasound guidance before IGRT administration. In the study of the Mayo Clinic, the inter- and intra-fractional prostate movements were found a mean 2.5 mm (up to 9.1 mm) at the superior-inferior, 3.7 mm (up to 16.3 mm) at the anterior-posterior, and 1.9 mm (up to 15.2 mm) at the right-left planes [72]. Without localization of the fiducials the clinical target volume (CTV) received 95% of the prescribed dose with 5.1, 7.3, and 5 mm margins on the superoinferior, anteroposterior and lateral aspects. The respective margins were decreased to 2.7, 2.9, and 2.8 mm with fiducial visualization. Bony structures should not be trusted while delineating the prostate because the movement of these structures is between 2.8 and 4.4 mm while the prostate can move between 5.6 and 4.4 mm. Crook et al. found a displacement of gold markers of 0.1–0.5 cm in the lateral, and 0.5–1 cm in the inferior aspect of the prostate gland [73]. The displacement in the posterior was >1 cm in 30% of the patients. Zelefsky et al. reported the mean motion of the prostate 1.2, 0.6, and 0.5 cm in the anteroposterior, lateral, and superoinferior directions [74]. They also recommended adding wider margins for the planning target volume (PTV) in patients with large rectal and bladder volumes in order to adequately cover the CTV.

After the fiducials are located, approximately 1 week should be awaited for the planning computerized tomography (CT). That is because of the time for fibrosis to happen around the fiducials so that they cannot move and the target would not change during simulation and between fractions. Intravenous contrast injection is not necessary for the CT simulation unless the pelvic LNs would be irradiated. However, the patient should undergo planning CT with a urinary catheter in order to empty the urinary bladder. The catheter can also be used in every treatment fraction, or patients with good cooperation can be told to undergo treatment after voiding the bladder. The patient is then immobilized with a knee-fix and feet-fix in the supine position in which the prostate gland moves less compared to the prone position. This position also helps to remove the small intestines out of the treatment field [75]. The arms should be on the chest in order to keep them away from the treatment area. To define the isocenter, three radiopaque pellet markers are placed; one at the anterior midline and two at right and left lateral points, respectively, on the skin. The CT scan is then acquired in ≤5 mm (ideally ≤3 mm, particularly for stereotactic body RT [SBRT] planning) slices from the superior level of the iliac bones to the inferior of minor trochanters of the femurs or the perineum [76, 77]. The gross tumor volume (GTV), CTV, PTV and organs at risk (OAR) should be delineated separately in each slice based on the recommendations in International Commission on Radiation Units and Measurements (ICRU) reports 50 and 62 [78, 79].

6.2.2.6 Gross Tumor Volume (GTV)

The GTV is the primary tumor in the prostate gland and extraprostatic tissue, if existent. However, delineating a GTV in prostate cancer is not practical because the total dose is prescribed to the CTV and generally no boost dose to the GTV is applied. On the other hand, institutions using simultaneous integrated boost to malignant nodule determined via MR fusion should delineate entire nodule as boost volume or GTV.

6.2.2.7 Clinical Target Volume (CTV)

The prostatic apex is the structure which is the guide for the delineation of the target because of the fact that it can be visualized easily on CT. However, because the apex is not covered with a capsule, the level of the GUD may vary causing a difficulty in discriminating the prostate from the GUD. In this case, magnetic resonance imaging (MRI) can be helpful on which the GUD can also be easily detected. Roach et al. observed a 32% increase in prostate volume when defined by non-contrast CT scan compared to contrast CT and MRI scans [80]. This discrepancy is mainly the result of misinterpretation of the posterior, apical and posteroinferoapical aspects of the prostate as well as the neurovascular bundles. MRI was found significantly superior in defining the apex and base of the prostate, neurovascular bundle and anterior wall of the rectum while delineating based on fused CT and MRI images [81]. Rasch et al. reported that the volumes of the prostate and SVs were 40% larger when determined on CT compared to MRI [50]. The most apparent difference was at the base of the SVs and prostatic apex which concluded in an additional 8-mm and 6-mm delineation, respectively. MRI also has a higher resolution for soft tissues which more clearly defines the organ-confined disease, SV involvement, and capsular and extracapsular extension. Based on these data CT and MRI should be used together while delineating the prostate.

The CTV is defined as the whole prostate gland and bilateral SVs. Prostate cancer is typically multifocal. It was reported that only 17–24% of prostate cancers arise from a solitary focus [82, 83]. The capsule of the gland is invaded in 8–57% of the patients with prostate cancer [84, 85]. Therefore, whole prostate gland and its capsule should be delineated in all patients independent of the clinical stage and risk group. However, the extent of the delineation of the SVs depend on the risk group. In low-risk and intermediate-risk disease, the delineation of proximal SVs is sufficient, whereas in high-risk disease whole bilateral SVs should be contoured.

There is a wide range of variability among radiation oncologists for prostate-contouring. It is crucial to master in prostate and pelvic anatomy for delineating the target and OARs correctly. In 2009, McLaughlin et al. published a study on the common contouring errors while delineating the apex, mid gland, and base of the prostate on CT images [86]. They reported that the GUD, rectum, and anterior fascia are overestimated at the level of the prostatic apex. The overestimation continued in the anterior and lateral fasciae at the mid gland, and the bladder and anterior fascia at the base. The reason for common errors was claimed to be the transition zone hypertrophy and bladder neck variability at the superior base, and the variability in the relationship between the prostate and SVs at the posterior base. They recommended to inspect the lateral view of prostate contours and to improve recognition of certain anatomic structures on CT images, concluding that most errors can be improved without the direct help of MRI.

The delineation the SVs can also be challenging. The risk of involvement of SVs is 15–20% in intermediate- and high-risk prostate cancer [87]. The median length of SV involvement was found 1 cm, whereas the rate of ≥2-cm involvement decreased to <4% even in high-risk disease [88]. Therefore, the CTV should encompass at least the proximal SVs. However, the definition of proximal SV varies according to different guidelines. The European Organization for Research and Treatment of Cancer (EORTC) recommends adding the proximal 2-cm SV into the CTV in high-risk and the proximal 1-cm in intermediate-risk disease [89]. In the ongoing Radiation Therapy Oncology Group (RTOG) 0815 trial, the proximal 1-cm of SV is recommended to be delineated in both intermediate- and high-risk patients. Qi et al. compared these two recommendations and found that both recommendations failed to encompass the SV under risk, and a 1.4-cm and 2.2 cm SV should be contoured in intermediate- and high-risk patients, respectively, in order to adequately include the proximal SVs [90].

CTV delineation for prostate cancer patient (Sect. 6.2.1.1) treated with definitive SBRT is depicted in Fig. 6.7.

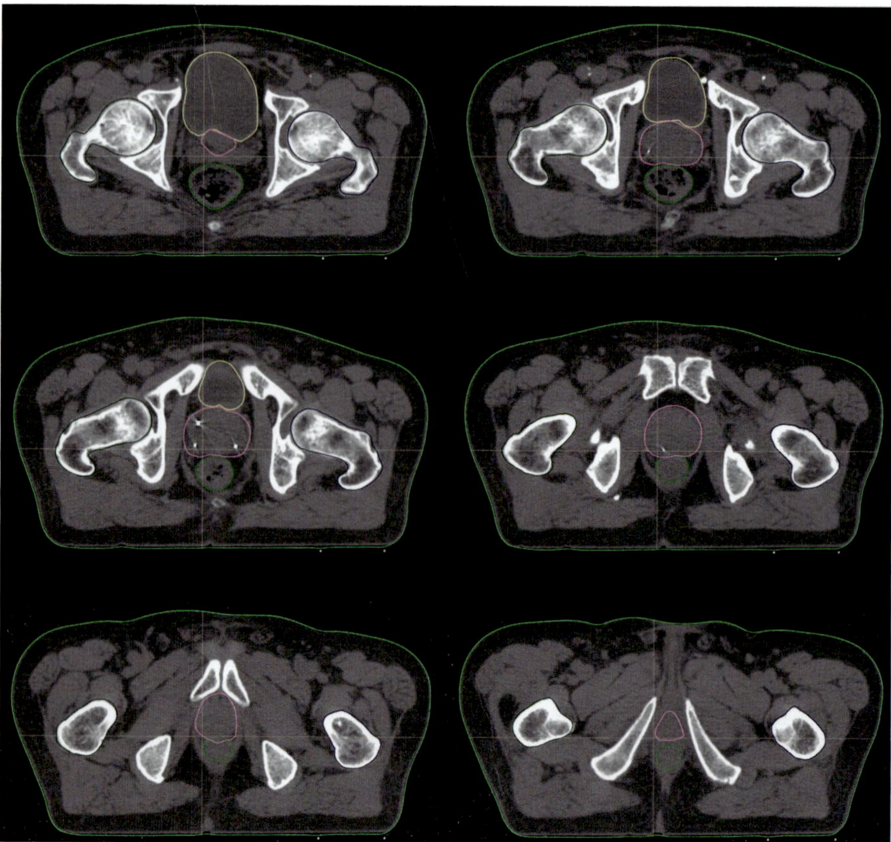

Fig. 6.7 CTV delineation for a prostate cancer patient treated with definitive IGRT

6.2.2.8 Planning Target Volume (PTV)

There are various recommendations for the constitution of the PTV. Memorial Sloan Kettering Cancer Center (MSKCC) proposes a 1-cm margin to the CTV to form the PTV in all directions but to diminish it to 0.6 cm at the posterior [91]. Fox Chase Cancer Center recommends an 8-mm margin in all directions which should be minimized to 5 mm posteriorly [92]. In SBRT and other IGRT techniques, some centers recommend a 0.6 cm margin in all directions, whereas in MSKCC 0.5 mm is recommended in all but 0.3 mm in the posterior direction [92]. In addition, the central 1-cm diameter portion of the prostate encompassing the prostatic urethra is defined for dosimetric consideration and evaluation during high-dose IMRT planning.

CTV delineation for prostate cancer patient (Sect. 6.2.1.2) treated with definitive VMAT is depicted in Fig. 6.8.

6.2.2.9 Target Volume Determination in Adjuvant or Salvage Radiotherapy

In the EORTC-22911 trial, 5-year progression-free survival (PFS) and locoregional control rates were significantly higher in patients with positive SM, extracapsular

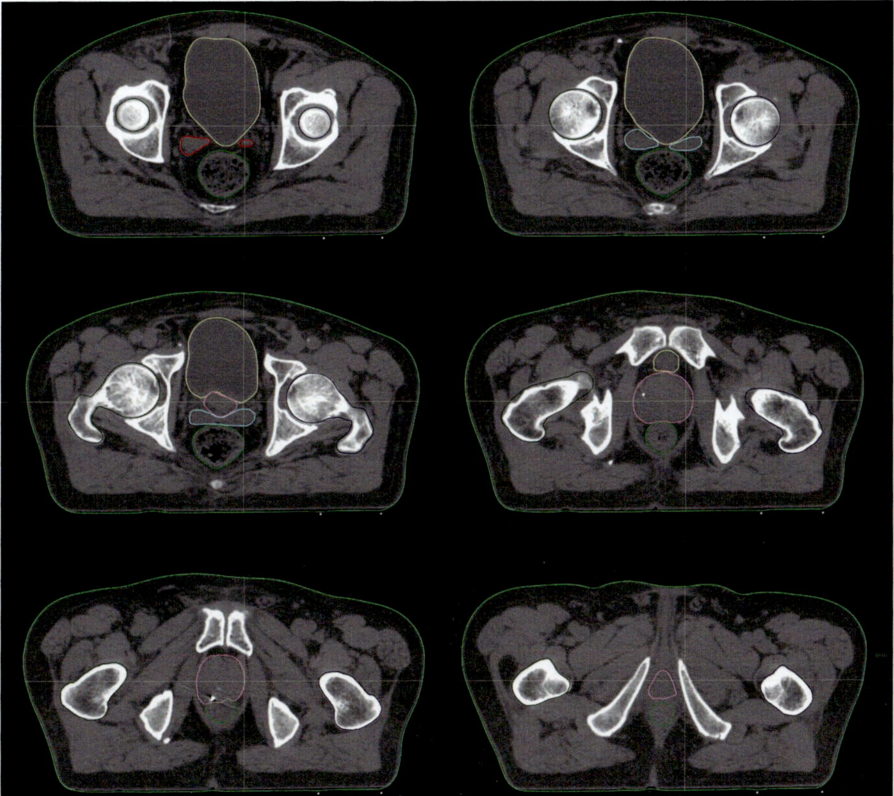

Fig. 6.8 CTV delineation for a prostate cancer patient treated with definitive VMAT

extension (ECE) and SV involvement after radical prostatectomy (RP) [93]. However, in the subgroup analysis of this study, the only group that benefited from adjuvant RT was the patients with positive surgical margins (SM) [94]. In the South Western Oncology Group (SWOG)-8794 trial, patients with pT3 tumors and/or positive SM had significantly better outcomes with adjuvant RT [95]. Similarly, a German study reported better results with adjuvant RT in patients with T3 tumors and positive SM [96]. According to Grossfeld et al., 24% of patients with clinically organ-confined disease are found to have locally advanced disease and/or lymph node (LN) positivity after RP [97]. Based on the previous studies, adjuvant RT to the prostate is indicated in patients with T3–4 tumor and positive SM. In the presence of LN positivity and ECE, lymphatic irradiation should also be performed. The following contouring recommendations can also be used for patients that will undergo salvage RT for biochemical failure after RP.

No GTV is present in the adjuvant setting. Four guidelines have been published for the delineation of CTV in postoperative prostate cancer. The first guideline was reported by the EORTC in 2007 [98]. They stated that the most risky areas for recurrence were the vesicourethral anastomosis (VUA) in the central, the bladder neck at the superior, the vicinity of the outer rectal wall and most posterior portion of the bladder neck at the posterior, the prostatic apex at the caudal, the neurovascular bundles at the lateral, and the anastomosis and the urethral axis at the anterior aspects, respectively. After delineating these structures, they recommend a 5-mm margin in all directions excluding the rectal wall, an additional 5-mm margin in the posterolateral aspect in patients with ECE except the rectal wall (as this is where the recurrence mostly occurs), and an additional 5-mm margin in the direction of positive SM. The base of the SV should be included in all patients. If the SVs are involved, they recommend contouring their original location and/or the remnants without an additional margin and irradiating them with a lower dose.

In the second guideline published in 2007 by Princess Margaret Hospital; the inferior border of the CTV was recommended to be 8-mm below the VUA or superior to the penile bulb, whichever is most superior [99]. The superior border was just above the most superior surgical clip, if present, or 5 mm above the inferior border of the vas deferens, anterior border was posterior to the symphysis pubis caudally and posterior 1.5 cm of the urinary bladder cranially, posterior border was anterior to the rectal wall and levator ani muscle caudally and the mesorectal fascia cranially, and lateral border was the medial border of the levator ani and obturator internus muscles caudally and the sacrorectogenitopubic fascia cranially. In case of salvage RT, 1-cm margin was added to the gross disease and surgical clips for the CTV.

The Australian and New Zealand Radiation Oncology Genito-Urinary Group published another guideline in 2008 [100]. They recommend the inferior border of the CTV 5–6 mm below the VUA including all surgical clips. The VUA is just below the last slice with urine or one slice above the penile bulb. The anterior border is the posterior aspect of the symphysis pubis cranially and encompasses the posterior 1.5 cm of the bladder caudally, posterior border is the posterior rectal wall caudally and the anterior mesorectal fascia cranially, lateral border is the medial border of the levator ani or obturator internus muscle, and the superior border should include whole SV bed and the distal portion of the vas deferens. For the PTV, they recommend a 1-cm margin but claim that this can be lowered to 0.5 cm according to the rectal dose.

In 2010, RTOG published the last consensus guideline [77]. They recommend that the CTV should begin from the level of the cut end of the vas deferens and end at >8–12 mm inferior to the VUA. In case the vas deferens is retracted postoperatively, the superior end can start 3–4 cm above the top of symphysis pubis. In addition, the inferior border may be extended if the apical SM is positive. The VUA can be visualized in one slice below the most inferior urine-containing image in the retropubic region on a CT scan, and can be more clearly seen as a hypertensive signal on T2 images of MRI. The VUA can be better visualized if the urinary bladder is full, and the sagittal images can help the identification of the VUA. If the VUA cannot be visualized, the inferior border of the CTV can extend to the last slice above the penile bulb. If pathologically involved, both SV remnants should be included in the CTV. Other borders for the CTV vary according to its location in the pelvis. Above the superior edge of the symphysis pubis; the anterior border of the CTV encompasses the posterior 1–2 cm of the bladder wall, the posterior border is the mesorectal fascia, and lateral borders extend to the sacrorectogenitopubic fascia but may extend to obturator internus muscles if there is extraprostatic disease at the base of the gland. Below the superior edge of the symphysis pubis; the anterior border is the posterior edge of the pubic bone, the posterior border is the anterior rectal wall (the CTV may need to be curved at the level of the VUA), and lateral borders are medial to the levator ani and obturator internus muscles. The RTOG recommends including all surgical clips in the prostate and SV bed into the CTV. However, the clips above the level of SV can be excluded because they are generally left by the surgeon to control the bleeding, not to mark the sites of the disease.

6.2.3 Radiotherapy Delivery Approaches

With advancements in imaging, more focal 3-dimensional treatment plans were developed to target the prostate and seminal vesicles only. Further advances in radiation delivery techniques such as IMRT and volumetric modulated arc therapy (VMAT) led to greater sparing of adjacent normal tissue to reduce toxicity. Techniques such as VMAT and IMRT are able to generate conformal isodoses, which significantly reduce the OAR doses and normal tissue toxicity [31]. Although IMRT is a commonly used method to treat prostate cancer, the potential downsides of IMRT include increased RT delivery time, resulting in a greater integral body dose, which might increase the risk of secondary cancer development [31].

VMAT is an innovative form of IMRT optimization that allows the radiation dose to be efficiently delivered using a dynamic modulated arc. The VMAT simultaneously coordinates gantry rotation, multi-leaf collimator (MLC) motion and dose rate modulation, and facilitating highly conformal treatment with better normal tissue sparing [31]. Compared with IMRT, the potential advantages of VMAT include a large reduction in monitor units (MU) required to deliver a given fraction size and a concomitant reduction in treatment time. Helical tomotherapy (HT) is an arc-based application of IMRT that uses a fan-beam of radiation in conjunction with binary MLC. The gantry rotates at a constant speed, while the binary MLC leaves open 51 times per rotation and close entirely between projections. This rotational treatment modality can establish target dose conformity and OAR dose reduction (Figs. 6.9, 6.10, 6.11, and 6.12).

Image guidance is essential for delivering the high radiation doses to prostate accurately. The prostate is a mobile organ influenced by bladder and rectal filling. The position of these structures as defined on the planning CT can vary during and between fractions. Delivery of highly conformal treatments with steep dose gradients demands confidence in localization of the target because motion can lead to geographic miss, under-dosing of the tumor and/or unwanted over-dosing of organs at risk. Dedicated CBCT equipment can acquire 3D CT image in real-time in the treatment position just before treatment. Resolution is not of diagnostic quality, but enables visualization of soft tissues (prostate, bladder and rectum) so that table shifts can be made if needed.

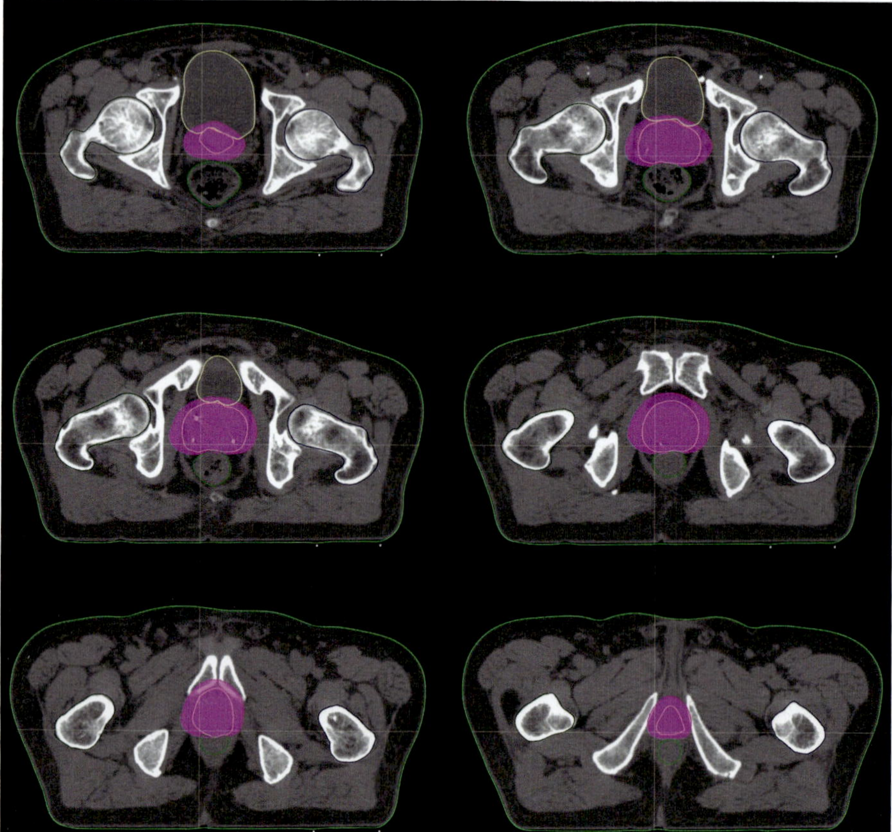

Fig. 6.9 Treatment plan of Case 1. Representative axial computed tomography slices showing 95% of prescribed dose distributions for 6 MV, FFF energy VMAT plans

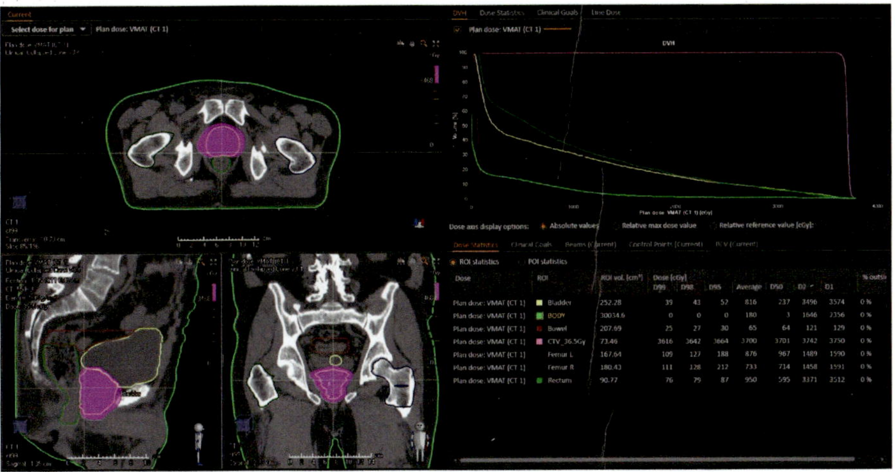

Fig. 6.10 DVH of Case 1

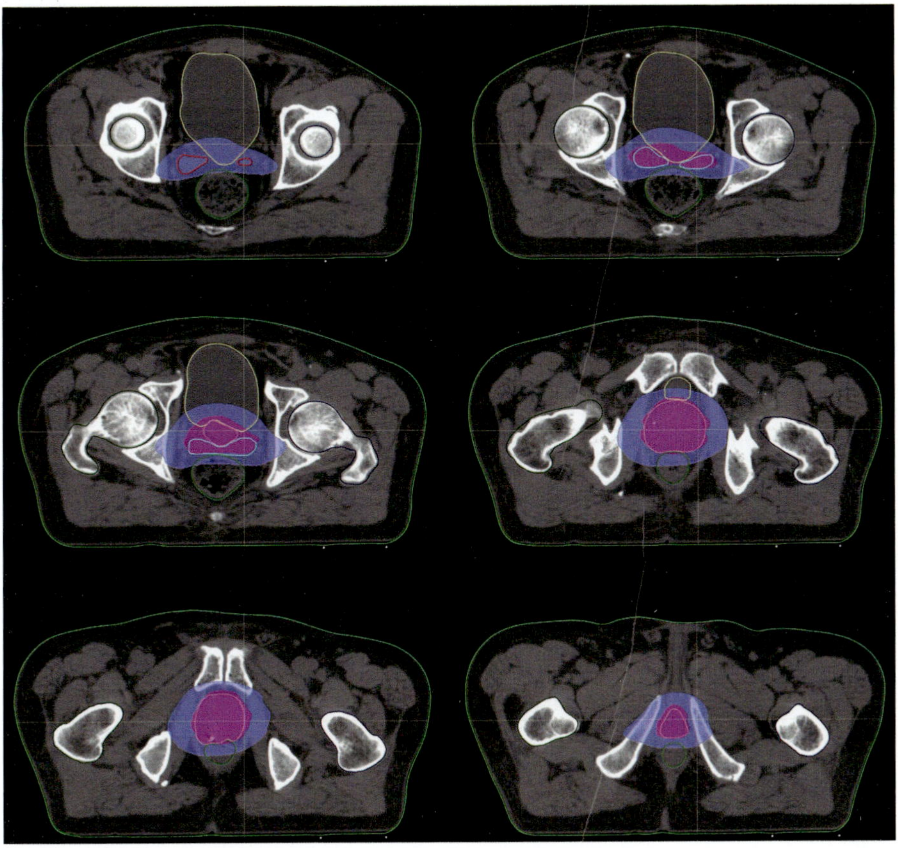

Fig. 6.11 Treatment plan of Case 2. Representative axial computed tomography slices showing 95% of prescribed dose distributions for 6 MV, FFF energy VMAT plans

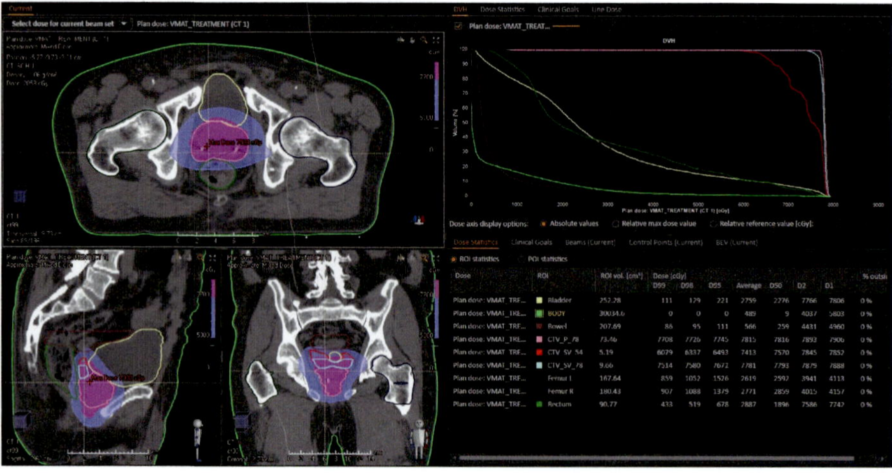

Fig. 6.12 DVH of Case 2

CBCT can be used in conjunction with fiducial seeds. However, the implantation of fiducial markers is an invasive procedure with the potential for discomfort, bleeding and infection. Furthermore, fiducial markers provide little information on deformation of the target, localization of the seminal vesicles, or alteration in the neighboring normal tissue, and may cause deformation of the prostate gland after implantation. Although fiducial marker implantation for image-guided RT in prostate cancer allows the localization of the prostate during treatment, this application may cause some complications and dosimetric uncertainties. Therefore, alternative noninvasive methods of CBCT should be considered for IGRT of prostate cancer patients [31].

Radiofrequency tracking or implanted markers such as fiducial can be used for delivering SBRT. Prostate movement can be minimized with careful bladder and rectal/small bowel preparation [31]. If standard cone beam computerized tomography (CBCT) is used instead of tracking systems, it is recommended to perform before and after treatment. Rectal protection is the one of the major issues in PC SBRT. Care should be taken to ensure the rectum receives less than the prescribed radiation dose. The use of an inflatable rectal balloon for rectal distension or rectoprostatic injectable hydrogel can be used for organ motion. Another issue about PC SBRT is homogeneity. Ideally care should be taken with maximal dose inhomogeneity of <107% of the prescription dose within the prostate to prevent ureteral complications. Caution and care must be taken for appropriate education, immobilization and RT delivery.

6.2.3.1 Robotic Radiosurgery with CyberKnife at Hacettepe University

Patient Selection

We recommend robotic SBRT (rSBRT) with CyberKnife® in low-intermediate risk patients (PSA < 20 ng/mL, Gleason score <8, T1-T2N0M0) (Fig. 6.13). If a patient has a very large prostate volume (>50 cm³), it might be worthwhile to consider having the patient undergo hormonal therapy for volume reduction rSBRT.

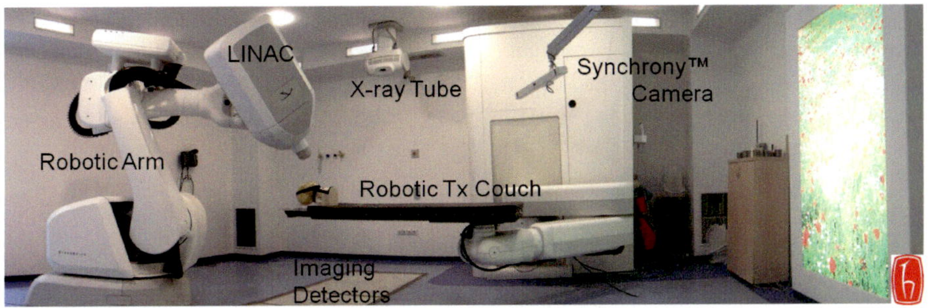

Fig. 6.13 Robotic stereotactic body radiotherapy unit (Courtesy of Hacettepe University)

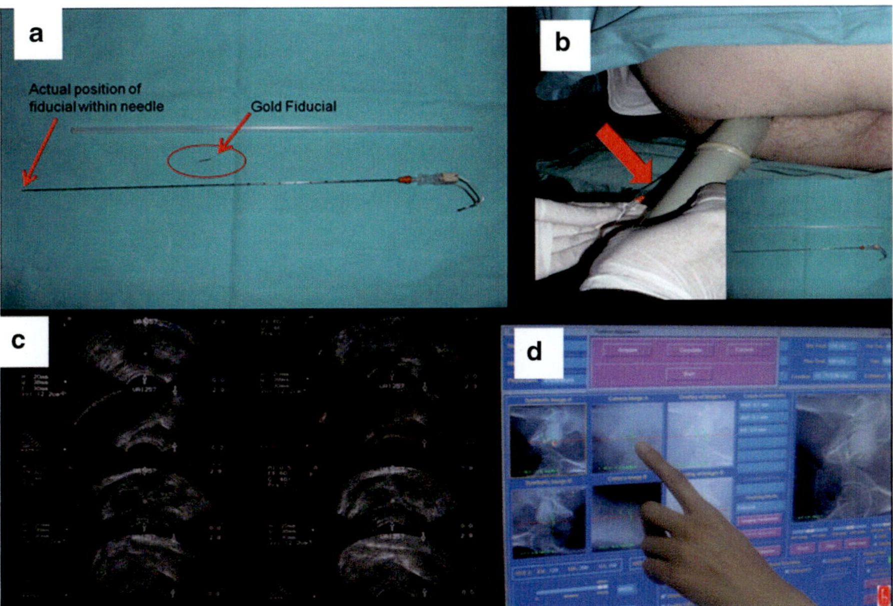

Fig. 6.14 (**a**) Golden fiducials for CyberKnife, (**b**) transrectal fiducial placement for rSBRT, (**c**) locations for the fiducial placement within prostate gland, (**d**) daily kV Imaging of Gold Fiducials for rSBRT: verification of fiducial locations prior to CyberKnife

We do not recommend rSBRT in patients with collagen vascular disease and inflammatory bowel disease. We can treat patients with metal in the pelvis, which consists of artificial hips since the delivery of multiple small beamlets can find an appropriate alternative pathways.

Fiducial Placement

Once the patient is a candidate for rSBRT, the patient is scheduled for his fiducial placement and simulation. We used specific four golden fiducials manufactured to be used with CyberKnife® (Fig. 6.14). Prophylactic antibiotic and urinary antiseptics are given prior to procedure.

At our institution, the fiducials are inserted transrectally under ultrasound guidance by the urologist under local anesthesia (Fig. 6.14). We also try to place the fiducials in certain regions of prostate gland due to the fact that all fiducials should be in certain geometry accordingly with the imaging X-ray tubes (Fig. 6.14). Once the fiducials have been placed, there should be 7–10 days before the simulation is done.

Image Guidance

Daily image-guided radiation therapy (IGRT) is achieved using real time daily kV imaging with fiducials.

Simulation

For the simulation, we place the patient in a supine position and place a 14 Gauge Foley catheter into bladder to visualize prostatic urethra. We then inflate its balloon with 6 cc of water. Once the Foley is placed, a non-contrast planning CT with <1 mm slice thickness is performed of the entire pelvis.

Contouring

At our institution, the CTV for definitive prostate cancer patients is as per the following: prostate only for low-risk; prostate proximal seminal vesicles (SV) for intermediate-risk. Proximal is defined as the proximal 1 cm of the SV.

Dosing

The standard dose is 36.5 Gy in 7.3 Gy daily fractions either in consecutive (Monday to friday) or every other day regimen (2 weeks regimen).

Plan Evaluation

Our rSBRT treatment plan acceptance criteria are summarized as following (Fig. 6.15);

PTV
- PTV prescribed dose: 7.3 Gy in 5 fraction with a total dose of 36.5 Gy
- Inhomogeneities. 110–130% high dose region within CTV if possible within GTV.
- Maximum dose <45.5 Gy
- 95% volume of PTV should receive 36.25 Gy
- Minimum PTV dose 34.4 Gy

Rectum
- V33.5 Gy < 1 cm^3
- Minor variation: V33.5 Gy $\geq$ 1 cm^3 but <3 cm^3
- Major variation: V33.5 Gy $\geq$ 3 cm^3
- Max dose (0.03 cm^3) $\leq$ 38.06 Gy
- <3 cm^3 volume may receive 34.4 Gy.
- V32.6 Gy $\leq$ 90% rectum
- V29 Gy $\leq$ 80% rectum
- V18.125 Gy $\leq$ 50% rectum

Bladder
- V35 Gy < 5 cm^3
- Minor variation: V35 Gy $\geq$ 5 cm^3 but <10 cm^3
- Major variation: V35 Gy $\geq$ 10 cm^3
- Max point dose (0.03 cm^3) $\leq$ 38.06 Gy
- V32.625 Gy $\leq$ 90% bladder
- V18.125 Gy $\leq$ 50% bladder

Urethra
- V45.5 Gy < 10%
- Minor variation: V45.5 Gy $\geq$ 10% but <20%
- Major variation: V45.5 Gy $\geq$ 20%
- Max. Doz < 38.78 Gy

Penile Bulb
- V27.5 Gy $\leq$ 50%
- Minor variation: V27.5 Gy $\geq$ 50% but <70%
- Major variation: V27.5 Gy $\geq$ 70%
- Max. Dose does not exceed the prescribed dose
- V20 Gy < 3 cc

Femur
- V20 Gy < 10 cm^3

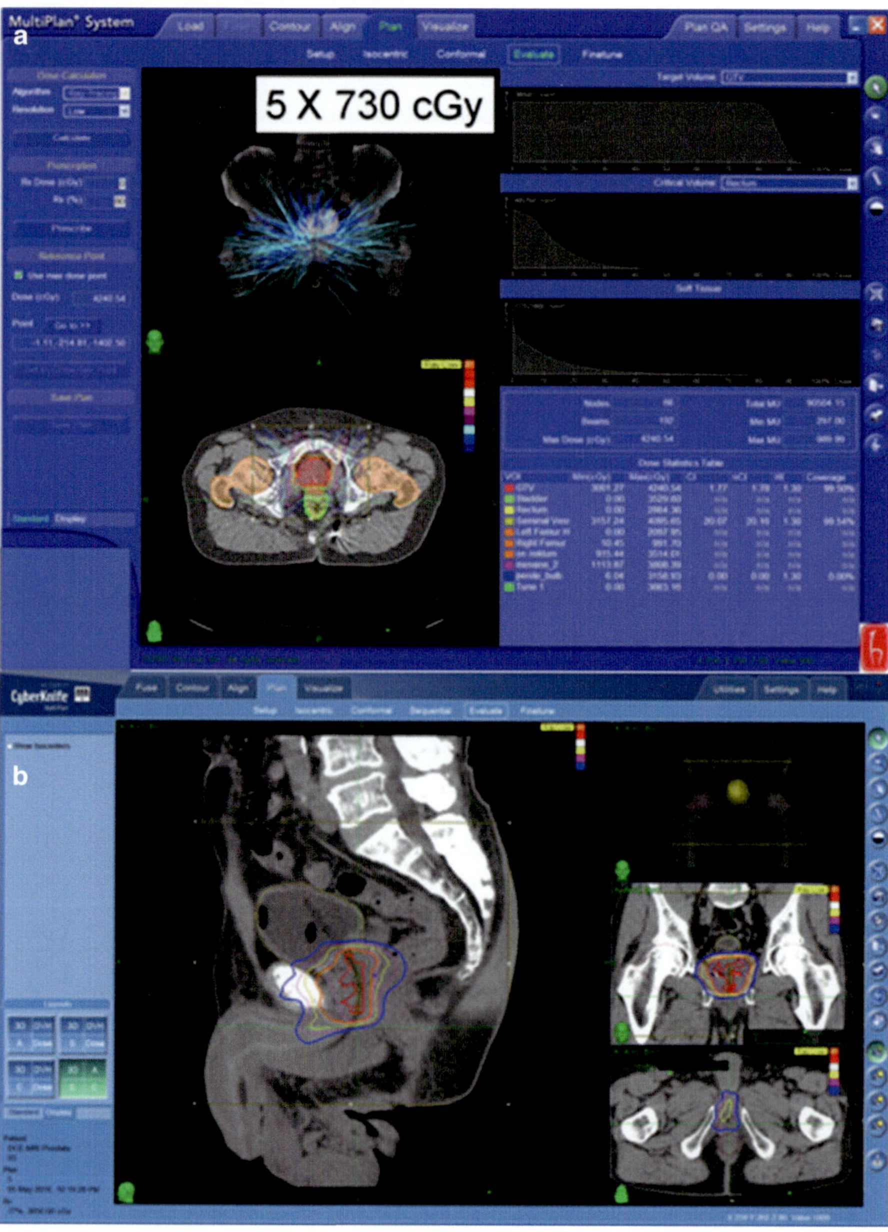

Fig. 6.15 (**a**) Treatment plan of a patient receving rSBRT with every other day protocol. (**b**) 14 G Foley catheter visualized within the prostatic urethra. Sample plan is showing hot points within urethra that is not acceptable

References

1. Gakis G, Efstathiou J, Lerner SP, Cookson MS, Keegan KA, Guru KA, et al. ICUD-EAU international consultation on bladder cancer 2012: radical cystectomy and bladder preservation for muscle-invasive urothelial carcinoma of the bladder. Eur Urol. 2013;63(1):45–57. https://doi.org/10.1016/j.eururo.2012.08.009.

2. Grossman HB, Natale RB, Tangen CM, Speights VO, Vogelzang NJ, Trump DL, et al. Neoadjuvant chemotherapy plus cystectomy compared with cystectomy alone for locally advanced bladder cancer. N Engl J Med. 2003;349(9):859–66. https://doi.org/10.1056/NEJMoa022148.

3. Chahal R, Sundaram SK, Iddenden R, Forman DF, Weston PM, Harrison SC. A study of the morbidity, mortality and long-term survival following radical cystectomy and radical radiotherapy in the treatment of invasive bladder cancer in Yorkshire. Eur Urol. 2003;43(3):246–57.

4. Kotwal S, Choudhury A, Johnston C, Paul AB, Whelan P, Kiltie AE. Similar treatment outcomes for radical cystectomy and radical radiotherapy in invasive bladder cancer treated at a United Kingdom specialist treatment center. Int J Radiat Oncol Biol Phys. 2008;70(2):456–63. https://doi.org/10.1016/j.ijrobp.2007.06.030.

5. Munro NP, Sundaram SK, Weston PM, Fairley L, Harrison SC, Forman D, et al. A 10-year retrospective review of a nonrandomized cohort of 458 patients undergoing radical radiotherapy or cystectomy in Yorkshire, UK. Int J Radiat Oncol Biol Phys. 2010;77(1):119–24. https://doi.org/10.1016/j.ijrobp.2009.04.050.

6. Hussain SA, Stocken DD, Peake DR, Glaholm JG, Zarkar A, Wallace DM, et al. Long-term results of a phase II study of synchronous chemoradiotherapy in advanced muscle invasive bladder cancer. Br J Cancer. 2004;90(11):2106–11. https://doi.org/10.1038/sj.bjc.6601852.

7. Rene NJ, Cury FB, Souhami L. Conservative treatment of invasive bladder cancer. Curr Oncol. 2009;16(4):36–47.

8. Langsenlehner T, Doller C, Quehenberger F, Stranzl-Lawatsch H, Langsenlehner U, Pummer K, et al. Treatment results of radiation therapy for muscle-invasive bladder cancer. Strahlenther Onkol. 2010;186(4):203–9. https://doi.org/10.1007/s00066-010-2053-1.

9. Hall RR, Newling DW, Ramsden PD, Richards B, Robinson MR, Smith PH. Treatment of invasive bladder cancer by local resection and high dose methotrexate. Br J Urol. 1984;56(6):668–72.

10. Herr HW, Bajorin DF, Scher HI. Neoadjuvant chemotherapy and bladder-sparing surgery for invasive bladder cancer: ten-year outcome. J Clin Oncol. 1998;16(4):1298–301. https://doi.org/10.1200/jco.1998.16.4.1298.

11. Prout GR Jr, Shipley WU, Kaufman DS, Heney NM, Griffin PP, Althausen AF, et al. Preliminary results in invasive bladder cancer with transurethral resection, neoadjuvant chemotherapy and combined pelvic irradiation plus cisplatin chemotherapy. J Urol. 1990;144(5):1128–34. discussion 34–6.

12. Coppin CM, Gospodarowicz MK, James K, Tannock IF, Zee B, Carson J, et al. Improved local control of invasive bladder cancer by concurrent cisplatin and preoperative or definitive radiation. The National Cancer Institute of Canada Clinical Trials Group. J Clin Oncol. 1996;14(11):2901–7. https://doi.org/10.1200/jco.1996.14.11.2901.

13. Chung PW, Bristow RG, Milosevic MF, Yi QL, Jewett MA, Warde PR, et al. Long-term outcome of radiation-based conservation therapy for invasive bladder cancer. Urol Oncol. 2007;25(4):303–9. https://doi.org/10.1016/j.urolonc.2006.09.015.

14. Shipley WU, Winter KA, Kaufman DS, Lee WR, Heney NM, Tester WR, et al. Phase III trial of neoadjuvant chemotherapy in patients with invasive bladder cancer treated with selective bladder preservation by combined radiation therapy and chemotherapy: initial results of Radiation Therapy Oncology Group 89-03. J Clin Oncol. 1998;16(11):3576–83. https://doi.org/10.1200/jco.1998.16.11.3576.

15. Rodel C, Weiss C, Sauer R. Trimodality treatment and selective organ preservation for bladder cancer. J Clin Oncol. 2006;24(35):5536–44. https://doi.org/10.1200/JCO.2006.07.6729.

16. Sangar VK, McBain CA, Lyons J, Ramani VA, Logue JP, Wylie JP, et al. Phase I study of conformal radiotherapy with concurrent gemcitabine in locally advanced bladder cancer. Int J Radiat Oncol Biol Phys. 2005;61(2):420–5. https://doi.org/10.1016/j.ijrobp.2004.05.074.

17. Housset M, Maulard C, Chretien Y, Dufour B, Delanian S, Huart J, et al. Combined radiation and chemotherapy for invasive transitional-cell carcinoma of the bladder: a prospective study. J Clin Oncol. 1993;11(11):2150–7. https://doi.org/10.1200/jco.1993.11.11.2150.

18. James ND, Hussain SA, Hall E, Jenkins P, Tremlett J, Rawlings C, et al. Radiotherapy with or without chemotherapy in muscle-invasive bladder cancer. N Engl J Med. 2012;366(16):1477–88. https://doi.org/10.1056/NEJMoa1106106.

19. Tunio MA, Hashmi A, Qayyum A, Mohsin R, Zaeem A. Whole-pelvis or bladder-only chemo-radiation for lymph node-negative invasive bladder cancer: single-institution experience. Int J Radiat Oncol Biol Phys. 2012;82(3):e457–62. https://doi.org/10.1016/j.ijrobp.2011.05.051.

20. Peyromaure M, Slama J, Beuzeboc P, Ponvert D, Debre B, Zerbib M. Concurrent chemo-radiotherapy for clinical stage T2 bladder cancer: report of a single institution. Urology. 2004;63(1):73–7.

21. Kragelj B, Zaletel-Kragelj L, Sedmak B, Cufer T, Cervek J. Phase II study of radioche-motherapy with vinblastine in invasive bladder cancer. Radiother Oncol. 2005;75(1):44–7. https://doi.org/10.1016/j.radonc.2005.01.007.

22. Aboziada MA, Hamza HM, Abdlrahem AM. Initial results of bladder preserving approach by chemo-radiotherapy in patients with muscle invading transitional cell carcinoma. J Egypt Natl Canc Inst. 2009;21(2):167–74.

23. Choudhury A, Cowan R. Bladder preservation multimodality therapy as an alternative to rad-ical cystectomy for treatment of muscle invasive bladder cancer. BJU Int. 2011;108(9):E313. https://doi.org/10.1111/j.1464-410X.2011.10672_3.x.

24. Choudhury A, Swindell R, Logue JP, Elliott PA, Livsey JE, Wise M, et al. Phase II study of conformal hypofractionated radiotherapy with concurrent gemcitabine in muscle-invasive bladder cancer. J Clin Oncol. 2011;29(6):733–8. https://doi.org/10.1200/JCO.2010.31.5721.

25. Kaufman D, Raghavan D, Carducci M, Levine EG, Murphy B, Aisner J, et al. Phase II trial of gemcitabine plus cisplatin in patients with metastatic urothelial cancer. J Clin Oncol. 2000;18(9):1921–7. https://doi.org/10.1200/jco.2000.18.9.1921.

26. Efstathiou JA, Spiegel DY, Shipley WU, Heney NM, Kaufman DS, Niemierko A, et al. Long-term outcomes of selective bladder preservation by combined-modality therapy for invasive bladder cancer: the MGH experience. Eur Urol. 2012;61(4):705–11. https://doi.org/10.1016/j.eururo.2011.11.010.

27. Rodel C, Grabenbauer GG, Kuhn R, Papadopoulos T, Dunst J, Meyer M, et al. Combined-modality treatment and selective organ preservation in invasive bladder cancer: long-term results. J Clin Oncol. 2002;20(14):3061–71.

28. Tester W, Porter A, Asbell S, Coughlin C, Heaney J, Krall J, et al. Combined modality pro-gram with possible organ preservation for invasive bladder carcinoma: results of RTOG pro-tocol 85-12. Int J Radiat Oncol Biol Phys. 1993;25(5):783–90.

29. Kaufman DS, Winter KA, Shipley WU, Heney NM, Wallace HJ 3rd, Toonkel LM, et al. Phase I-II RTOG study (99-06) of patients with muscle-invasive bladder cancer undergo-ing transurethral surgery, paclitaxel, cisplatin, and twice-daily radiotherapy followed by selective bladder preservation or radical cystectomy and adjuvant chemotherapy. Urology. 2009;73(4):833–7. https://doi.org/10.1016/j.urology.2008.09.036.

30. Ploussard G, Daneshmand S, Efstathiou JA, Herr HW, James ND, Rodel CM, et al. Critical analysis of bladder sparing with trimodal therapy in muscle-invasive bladder cancer: a sys-tematic review. Eur Urol. 2014;66(1):120–37. https://doi.org/10.1016/j.eururo.2014.02.038.

31. Ozyigit G, Selek U. Principles and practice of urooncology: radiotherapy, Surgery, and Systemic Therapy. 1st ed. Cham: Springer; 2017.

32. Cowan RA, McBain CA, Ryder WD, Wylie JP, Logue JP, Turner SL, et al. Radiotherapy for muscle-invasive carcinoma of the bladder: results of a randomized trial comparing conven-tional whole bladder with dose-escalated partial bladder radiotherapy. Int J Radiat Oncol Biol Phys. 2004;59(1):197–207. https://doi.org/10.1016/j.ijrobp.2003.10.018.

33. Fokdal L, Hoyer M, von der Maase H. Treatment outcome and prognostic variables for local control and survival in patients receiving radical radiotherapy for urinary bladder cancer. Acta Oncol. 2004;43(8):749–57. https://doi.org/10.1080/02841860410018629.

34. Davidson SE, Symonds RP, Snee MP, Upadhyay S, Habeshaw T, Robertson AG. Assessment of factors influencing the outcome of radiotherapy for bladder cancer. Br J Urol. 1990;66(3):288–93.

35. Fokdal L, Hoyer M, von der Maase H. Radical radiotherapy for urinary bladder cancer: treatment outcomes. Expert Rev Anticancer Ther. 2006;6(2):269–79. https://doi.org/10.1586/14737140.6.2.269.

36. Leissner J, Ghoneim MA, Abol-Enein H, Thuroff JW, Franzaring L, Fisch M, et al. Extended radical lymphadenectomy in patients with urothelial bladder cancer: results of a prospective multicenter study. J Urol. 2004;171(1):139–44. https://doi.org/10.1097/01.ju.0000102302.26806.fb.

37. Rothwell RI, Ash DV, Jones WG. Radiation treatment planning for bladder cancer: a comparison of cystogram localisation with computed tomography. Clin Radiol. 1983;34(1):103–11.

38. Muren LP, Smaaland R, Dahl O. Organ motion, set-up variation and treatment margins in radical radiotherapy of urinary bladder cancer. Radiother Oncol. 2003;69(3):291–304.

39. Turner SL, Swindell R, Bowl N, Marrs J, Brookes B, Read G, et al. Bladder movement during radiation therapy for bladder cancer: implications for treatment planning. Int J Radiat Oncol Biol Phys. 1997;39(2):355–60.

40. Zietman AL, DeSilvio ML, Slater JD, Rossi CJ Jr, Miller DW, Adams JA, et al. Comparison of conventional-dose vs high-dose conformal radiation therapy in clinically localized adenocarcinoma of the prostate: a randomized controlled trial. JAMA. 2005;294(10):1233–9. https://doi.org/10.1001/jama.294.10.1233.

41. Cellini N, Morganti AG, Mattiucci GC, Valentini V, Leone M, Luzi S, et al. Analysis of intraprostatic failures in patients treated with hormonal therapy and radiotherapy: implications for conformal therapy planning. Int J Radiat Oncol Biol Phys. 2002;53(3):595–9.

42. Geier M, Astner ST, Duma MN, Jacob V, Nieder C, Putzhammer J, et al. Dose-escalated simultaneous integrated-boost treatment of prostate cancer patients via helical tomotherapy. Strahlenther Onkol. 2012;188(5):410–6. https://doi.org/10.1007/s00066-012-0081-8.

43. Viani GA, Stefano EJ, Afonso SL. Higher-than-conventional radiation doses in localized prostate cancer treatment: a meta-analysis of randomized, controlled trials. Int J Radiat Oncol Biol Phys. 2009;74(5):1405–18. https://doi.org/10.1016/j.ijrobp.2008.10.091.

44. Kuban DA, Tucker SL, Dong L, Starkschall G, Huang EH, Cheung MR, et al. Long-term results of the M. D. Anderson randomized dose-escalation trial for prostate cancer. Int J Radiat Oncol Biol Phys. 2008;70(1):67–74. https://doi.org/10.1016/j.ijrobp.2007.06.054.

45. Fonteyne V, Villeirs G, Speleers B, De Neve W, De Wagter C, Lumen N, et al. Intensity-modulated radiotherapy as primary therapy for prostate cancer: report on acute toxicity after dose escalation with simultaneous integrated boost to intraprostatic lesion. Int J Radiat Oncol Biol Phys. 2008;72(3):799–807. https://doi.org/10.1016/j.ijrobp.2008.01.040.

46. Ishii K, Ogino R, Okada W, Nakahara R, Kawamorita R, Nakajima T. A dosimetric comparison of RapidArc and IMRT with hypofractionated simultaneous integrated boost to the prostate for treatment of prostate cancer. Br J Radiol. 2013;86(1030):20130199. https://doi.org/10.1259/bjr.20130199.

47. Onal C, Sonmez S, Erbay G, Guler OC, Arslan G. Simultaneous integrated boost to intraprostatic lesions using different energy levels of intensity-modulated radiotherapy and volumetric-arc therapy. Br J Radiol. 2014;87(1034):20130617. https://doi.org/10.1259/bjr.20130617.

48. Ost P, Speleers B, De Meerleer G, De Neve W, Fonteyne V, Villeirs G, et al. Volumetric arc therapy and intensity-modulated radiotherapy for primary prostate radiotherapy with simultaneous integrated boost to intraprostatic lesion with 6 and 18 MV: a planning comparison study. Int J Radiat Oncol Biol Phys. 2011;79(3):920–6. https://doi.org/10.1016/j.ijrobp.2010.04.025.

49. Pinkawa M, Attieh C, Piroth MD, Holy R, Nussen S, Klotz J, et al. Dose-escalation using intensity-modulated radiotherapy for prostate cancer--evaluation of the dose distribution with

and without 18F-choline PET-CT detected simultaneous integrated boost. Radiother Oncol. 2009;93(2):213–9. https://doi.org/10.1016/j.radonc.2009.07.014.

50. von Eyben FE, Kiljunen T, Kangasmaki A, Kairemo K, von Eyben R, Joensuu T. Radiotherapy boost for the dominant intraprostatic cancer lesion-a systematic review and meta-analysis. Clin Genitourin Cancer. 2016;14(3):189–97. https://doi.org/10.1016/j.clgc.2015.12.005.

51. Lips IM, van der Heide UA, Haustermans K, van Lin EN, Pos F, Franken SP, et al. Single blind randomized phase III trial to investigate the benefit of a focal lesion ablative microboost in prostate cancer (FLAME-trial): study protocol for a randomized controlled trial. Trials. 2011;12:255. https://doi.org/10.1186/1745-6215-12-255.

52. Fowler JF, Ritter MA, Chappell RJ, Brenner DJ. What hypofractionated protocols should be tested for prostate cancer? Int J Radiat Oncol Biol Phys. 2003;56(4):1093–104.

53. Lee WR. Extreme hypofractionation for prostate cancer. Expert Rev Anticancer Ther. 2009;9(1):61–5. https://doi.org/10.1586/14737140.9.1.61.

54. Magnuson WJ, Mahal A, Yu JB. Emerging technologies and techniques in radiation therapy. Semin Radiat Oncol. 2017;27(1):34–42. https://doi.org/10.1016/j.semradonc.2016.08.004.

55. Pollack A, Walker G, Horwitz EM, Price R, Feigenberg S, Konski AA, et al. Randomized trial of hypofractionated external-beam radiotherapy for prostate cancer. J Clin Oncol. 2013;31(31):3860–8. https://doi.org/10.1200/JCO.2013.51.1972.

56. Zumsteg ZS, Spratt DE, Romesser PB, Pei X, Zhang Z, Kollmeier M, et al. Anatomical patterns of recurrence following biochemical relapse in the dose escalation era of external beam radiotherapy for prostate cancer. J Urol. 2015;194(6):1624–30. https://doi.org/10.1016/j.juro.2015.06.100.

57. Ozyigit G. The role of radiotherapy in the management of prostate cancer. Turkiye Klinikleri J Med Oncol-Special Topics. 2015;8(3):23–30.

58. Ozdemir Y, Akyol F, Ozyigit G, Hurmuz P, Onal C, Selek U, Karabulut E. Three dimensional conformal radiotherapy and androgen deprivation therapy in patients with clinically localized prostate cancer; Hacettepe University experience. Int J Hematol Oncol. 2015;25(2):107–17.

59. Ozyigit G, Akyol F, Onal C, Sari S, Gurdalli S, Yapici B. Combined Hormonotherapy and Definitive Radiation Therapy in Localized Prostate Adenocarcinoma. Turk Hematoloji-Onkoloji Dergisi. 2003;13(4):177–89.

60. Lawton CA, Winter K, Grignon D, Pilepich MV. Androgen suppression plus radiation versus radiation alone for patients with stage D1/pathologic node-positive adenocarcinoma of the prostate: updated results based on national prospective randomized trial radiation therapy oncology group 85-31. J Clin Oncol. 2005;23(4):800–7.

61. Roach M 3rd, Bae K, Speight J, Wolkov HB, Rubin P, Lee RJ, et al. Short-term neoadjuvant androgen deprivation therapy and external-beam radiotherapy for locally advanced prostate cancer: long-term results of RTOG 8610. J Clin Oncol. 2008;26(4):585–91.

62. Horwitz EM, Bae K, Hanks GE, Porter A, Grignon DJ, Brereton HD, et al. Ten-year follow-up of radiation therapy oncology group protocol 92-02: a phase III trial of the duration of elective androgen deprivation in locally advanced prostate cancer. J Clin Oncol. 2008;26(15):2497–504.

63. Bolla M, Van Tienhoven G, Warde P, Dubois JB, Mirimanoff RO, Storme G, et al. External irradiation with or without long-term androgen suppression for prostate cancer with high metastatic risk: 10-year results of an EORTC randomised study. Lancet Oncol. 2010;11(11):1066–73.

64. Bayoumi AM, Brown AD, Garber AM. Cost-effectiveness of androgen suppression therapies in advanced prostate cancer. J Natl Cancer Inst. 2000;92:1731–9.

65. Dirix P, Haustermans K, Junius S, Withers R, Oyen R, Van Poppel H. The role of whole pelvic radiotherapy in locally advanced prostate cancer. Radiother Oncol. 2006;79(1):1–14.

66. Asbell SO, Martz KL, Shin KH, Sause WT, Doggett RL, Perez CA, et al. Impact of surgical staging in evaluating the radiotherapeutic outcome in RTOG #77-06, a phase III study for T1BN0M0 (A2) and T2N0M0 (B) prostate carcinoma. Int J Radiat Oncol Biol Phys. 1998;40(4):769–82.

67. Roach M 3rd, DeSilvio M, Lawton C, Uhl V, Machtay M, Seider MJ, et al. Phase III trial comparing whole-pelvic versus prostate-only radiotherapy and neoadjuvant versus adjuvant

combined androgen suppression: Radiation Therapy Oncology Group 9413. J Clin Oncol. 2003;21(10):1904–11.

68. Roach M, Yan Y, Lawton CA, Hsu IJ, Lustig RA, Jones CU, et al. Radiation Therapy Oncology Group (RTOG) 9413: randomized trial comparing whole pelvic radiotherapy (WPRT) to prostate only (PORT) and neoadjuvant hormone therapy (NHT) to adjuvant hormone therapy (AHT). J Clin Oncol. 2012;30(5_suppl):96.

69. Pommier P, Chabaud S, Lagrange JL, Richaud P, Lesaunier F, Le Prise E, et al. Is there a role for pelvic irradiation in localized prostate adenocarcinoma? Preliminary results of GETUG-01. J Clin Oncol. 2007;25(34):5366–73.

70. Pommier P, Chabaud S, Lagrange JL, Richaud P, Le Prise E, Wagner JP, et al. Is there a role for pelvic irradiation in localized prostate adenocarcinoma? Update of the long-term survival results of the GETUG-01 randomized study. Int J Radiat Oncol Biol Phys. 2016;96(4):759–69.

71. Murthy V, Lewis S, Sawant M, Paul SN, Mahantshetty U, Shrivastava SK. Incidental dose to pelvic nodal regions in prostate-only radiotherapy. Technol Cancer Res Treat. 2017;16(2):211–7.

72. Schallenkamp JM, Herman MG, Kruse JJ, Pisansky TM. Prostate position relative to pelvic bony anatomy based on intraprostatic gold markers and electronic portal imaging. Int J Radiat Oncol Biol Phys. 2005;63(3):800–11.

73. Crook JM, Raymond Y, Salhani D, Yang H, Esche B. Prostate motion during standard radiotherapy as assessed by fiducial markers. Radiother Oncol. 1995;37(1):35–42.

74. Zelefsky MJ, Crean D, Mageras GS, Lyass O, Happersett L, Ling CC, et al. Quantification and predictors of prostate position variability in 50 patients evaluated with multiple CT scans during conformal radiotherapy. Radiother Oncol. 1999;50(2):225–34.

75. Malone S, Crook JM, Kendal WS, Szanto J. Respiratory-induced prostate motion: quantification and characterization. Int J Radiat Oncol Biol Phys. 2000;48(1):105–9.

76. Benedict SH, Yenice KM, Followill D, Galvin JM, Hinson W, Kavanagh B, et al. Stereotactic body radiation therapy: the report of AAPM Task Group 101. Med Phys. 2010;37(8):4078–101.

77. Michalski JM, Lawton C, El Naqa I, Ritter M, O'Meara E, Seider MJ, et al. Development of RTOG consensus guidelines for the definition of the clinical target volume for postoperative conformal radiation therapy for prostate cancer. Int J Radiat Oncol Biol Phys. 2010;76(2):361–8.

78. Measurements. ICoRUa. ICRU report 50: prescribing, recording and reporting photon beam therapy. Bethesda, MD: Measurements. ICoRUa; 1993.

79. Measurements. ICoRUa. ICRU report 62: prescribing, recording and reporting photon beam therapy (supplement to ICRU report 50). Bethesda, MD: Measurements. ICoRUa; 1999.

80. Roach M 3rd, Faillace-Akazawa P, Malfatti C, Holland J, Hricak H. Prostate volumes defined by magnetic resonance imaging and computerized tomographic scans for three-dimensional conformal radiotherapy. Int J Radiat Oncol Biol Phys. 1996;35(5):1011–8.

81. Kagawa K, Lee WR, Schultheiss TE, Hunt MA, Shaer AH, Hanks GE. Initial clinical assessment of CT-MRI image fusion software in localization of the prostate for 3D conformal radiation therapy. Int J Radiat Oncol Biol Phys. 1997;38(2):319–25.

82. Rasch C, Barillot I, Remeijer P, Touw A, van Herk M, Lebesque JV. Definition of the prostate in CT and MRI: a multi-observer study. Int J Radiat Oncol Biol Phys. 1999;43(1):57–66.

83. Jewett HJ. The present status of radical prostatectomy for stages A and B prostatic cancer. Urol Clin North Am. 1975;2(1):105–24.

84. Wise AM, Stamey TA, McNeal JE, Clayton JL. Morphologic and clinical significance of multifocal prostate cancers in radical prostatectomy specimens. Urology. 2002;60(2):264–9.

85. Catalona WJ, Richie JP, Ahmann FR, Hudson MA, Scardino PT, Flanigan RC, et al. Comparison of digital rectal examination and serum prostate specific antigen in the early detection of prostate cancer: results of a multicenter clinical trial of 6,630 men. J Urol. 1994;151(5):1283–90.

86. McLaughlin PW, Evans C, Feng M, Narayana V. Radiographic and anatomic basis for prostate contouring errors and methods to improve prostate contouring accuracy. Int J Radiat Oncol Biol Phys. 2010;76(2):369–78.

87. Eifler JB, Feng Z, Lin BM, Partin MT, Humphreys EB, Han M, et al. An updated prostate cancer staging nomogram (Partin tables) based on cases from 2006 to 2011. BJU Int. 2013;111(1):22–9.
88. Kestin L, Goldstein N, Vicini F, Yan D, Korman H, Martinez A. Treatment of prostate cancer with radiotherapy: should the entire seminal vesicles be included in the clinical target volume? Int J Radiat Oncol Biol Phys. 2002;54(3):686–97.
89. Boehmer D, Maingon P, Poortmans P, Baron MH, Miralbell R, Remouchamps V, et al. Guidelines for primary radiotherapy of patients with prostate cancer. Radiother Oncol. 2006;79(3):259–69.
90. Qi X, Gao XS, Asaumi J, Zhang M, Li HZ, Ma MW, et al. Optimal contouring of seminal vesicle for definitive radiotherapy of localized prostate cancer: comparison between EORTC prostate cancer radiotherapy guideline, RTOG0815 protocol and actual anatomy. Radiat Oncol. 2014;9:288.
91. Buyyounouski MK, He P, Jr RA, Feigenberg SJ, Pollack A, Prostate IMRT. In: Bortfeld TS-UR, De Neve W, Wazer DE, editors. Image-guided IMRT. Berlin: Springer; 2006. p. 391–410.
92. Desai NZM. Prostate Adenocarcinoma. In: Lee NY, et al., editors. Target volume delineation and field setup, a practical guide for conformal and intensity-modulated radiation therapy. Berlin: Springer; 2013. p. 213–26.
93. Bolla M, van Poppel H, Collette L, van Cangh P, Vekemans K, Da Pozzo L, et al. Postoperative radiotherapy after radical prostatectomy: a randomised controlled trial (EORTC trial 22911). Lancet. 2005;366(9485):572–8.
94. Van der Kwast TH, Bolla M, Van Poppel H, Van Cangh P, Vekemans K, Da Pozzo L, et al. Identification of patients with prostate cancer who benefit from immediate postoperative radiotherapy: EORTC 22911. J Clin Oncol. 2007;25(27):4178–86.
95. Swanson GPTI, Tangen C. Phase III randomized study of adjuvant radiation therapy versus observation in patients with patohologic T3 prostate cancer (SWOG 8794). Int J Radiat Oncol Biol Phys. 2005;63(Suppl 1):S1.
96. Wiegel T, Bottke D, Willich N, et al. Phase III results of adjuvant radiotherapy (RT) versus 'wait and see' (WS) in patients with pT3 prostate cancer following radical prostatectomy (RP) (ARO 96-02/AUO AP 09/95). J Clin Oncol (Meeting Abstracts). 2005;23(16_suppl):4513.
97. Grossfeld GD, Chang JJ, Broering JM, Li YP, Lubeck DP, Flanders SC, et al. Under staging and under grading in a contemporary series of patients undergoing radical prostatectomy: results from the cancer of the prostate strategic urologic research endeavor database. J Urol. 2001;165(3):851–6.
98. Poortmans P, Bossi A, Vandeputte K, Bosset M, Miralbell R, Maingon P, et al. Guidelines for target volume definition in post-operative radiotherapy for prostate cancer, on behalf of the EORTC Radiation Oncology Group. Radiother Oncol. 2007;84(2):121–7.
99. Wiltshire KL, Brock KK, Haider MA, Zwahlen D, Kong V, Chan E, et al. Anatomic boundaries of the clinical target volume (prostate bed) after radical prostatectomy. Int J Radiat Oncol Biol Phys. 2007;69(4):1090–9.
100. Sidhom MA, Kneebone AB, Lehman M, Wiltshire KL, Millar JL, Mukherjee RK, et al. Post-prostatectomy radiation therapy: consensus guidelines of the Australian and New Zealand Radiation Oncology Genito-Urinary Group. Radiother Oncol. 2008;88(1):10–9.
101. De Meerleer G, Villeirs G, Bral S, Paelinck L, De Gersem W, Dekuyper P, De Neve W. The magnetic resonance detected intraprostatic lesion in prostate cancer: planning and delivery of intensity-modulated radiotherapy. Radiother Oncol. 2005;75(3):325–33.
102. Miralbell R, Mollà M, Rouzaud M, Hidalgo A, Toscas JI, Lozano J, Sanz S, Ares C, Jorcano S, Linero D, Escudé L. Hypofractionated boost to the dominant tumor region with intensity modulated stereotactic radiotherapy for prostate cancer: a sequential dose escalation pilot study. Int J Radiat Oncol Biol Phys. 2010;78(1):50–7.
103. Ippolito E, Mantini G, Morganti AG, Mazzeo E, Padula GDA, Digesù C, Cilla S, Frascino V, Luzi S, Massaccesi M, Macchia G, Deodato F, Mattiucci GC, Piermattei A, Cellini N. Intensity-modulated radiotherapy with simultaneous integrated boost to dominant intraprostatic lesion. Am J Clin Oncol. 2012;35(2):158–62.

104. Pinkawa M, Piroth MD, Holy R, Klotz J, Djukic V, Corral NE, Caffaro M, Winz OH, Krohn T, Mottaghy FM, Eble MJ. Dose-escalation using intensity-modulated radiotherapy for prostate cancer–evaluation of quality of life with and without 18F-choline PET-CT detected simultaneous integrated boost. Radiat Oncol. 2012;7(1):14.
105. Aluwini S, van Rooij P, Hoogeman M, Kirkels W, Kolkman-Deurloo I-K, Bangma C. Stereotactic body radiotherapy with a focal boost to the MRI-visible tumor as monotherapy for low- and intermediate-risk prostate cancer: early results. Radiat Oncol. 2013;8(1):84.
106. Onal C, Sonmez S, Erbay G, Guler OC, Arslan G. Simultaneous integrated boost to intraprostatic lesions using different energy levels of intensity-modulated radiotherapy and volumetric-arc therapy. Br J Radiol. 2014;87(1034):20130617.
107. Arcangeli G, Fowler J, Gomellini S, Arcangeli S, Saracino B, Petrongari MG, Benassi M, Strigari L. Acute and late toxicity in a randomized trial of conventional versus hypofractionated three-dimensional conformal radiotherapy for prostate cancer. Int J Radiat Oncol Biol Phys. 2011;79(4):1013–21.
108. Hoffman KE, Ranh Voong K, Levy LB, Allen PK, Choi S, Schlembach PJ, Lee AK, McGuire SE, Nguyen Q, Pugh TJ, Frank SJ, Kudchadker RJ, Du W, Kuban DA. Randomized trial of hypofractionated, dose-escalated, intensity-modulated radiation therapy (IMRT) versus conventionally fractionated IMRT for localized prostate cancer. J Clin Oncol. 2018;36(29):2943–9.
109. Norkus D, Karklelyte A, Engels B, Versmessen H, Griskevicius R, De Ridder M, Storme G, Aleknavicius E, Janulionis E, Valuckas K. A randomized hypofractionation dose escalation trial for high risk prostate cancer patients: interim analysis of acute toxicity and quality of life in 124 patients. Radiat Oncol. 2013;8(1):206.
110. Wilkins A, Mossop H, Syndikus I, Khoo V, Bloomfield D, Parker C, Logue J, Scrase C, Patterson H, Birtle A, Staffurth J, Malik Z, Panades M, Eswar C, Graham J, Russell M, Kirkbride P, O'Sullivan JM, Gao A, Cruickshank C, Griffin C, Dearnaley D, Hall E. Hypofractionated radiotherapy versus conventionally fractionated radiotherapy for patients with intermediate-risk localised prostate cancer: 2-year patient-reported outcomes of the randomised, non-inferiority, phase 3 CHHiP trial. Lancet Oncol. 2015;16(16):1605–16.
111. Aluwini S, Pos F, Schimmel E, Krol S, van der Toorn PP, de Jager H, Alemayehu WG, Heemsbergen W, Heijmen B, Incrocci L. Hypofractionated versus conventionally fractionated radiotherapy for patients with prostate cancer (HYPRO): late toxicity results from a randomised, non-inferiority, phase 3 trial. Lancet Oncol. 2016;17(4):464–74.
112. King CR, Freeman D, Kaplan I, Fuller D, Bolzicco G, Collins S, Meier R, Wang J, Kupelian P, Steinberg M, Katz A. Stereotactic body radiotherapy for localized prostate cancer: pooled analysis from a multi-institutional consortium of prospective phase II trials. Radiother Oncol. 2013;109(2):217–21.

Gynecological Cancers 7

Melis Gultekin, Sezin Yuce Sari, Gozde Yazici,
Pervin Hurmuz, Ferah Yildiz, and Gokhan Ozyigit

7.1 Cervical Cancer

Overview

Epidemiology: Worldwide, cervical cancer is the third-most common gynecologic cancer in women. The incidence and mortality rate of cervical cancer has dramatically declined due to cervical cancer screening and prevention programs in developed countries. However, it is still the leading cause of cancer related death in developing countries.

Pathological and biological features: Over 90% of patients with cervical cancer have related to human papillomavirus (HPV) infection. Most cervical cancers are squamous cell carcinoma (SCC). Less than 10% of tumors have adenocarcinoma histology, which has been rising steadily. Stage, tumor size, and lymph node status are the major prognostic factors influencing treatment outcomes.

Definitive therapy: In cervical cancer, treatment decisions are usually depends on the disease extent at the time of initial presentation and staging evaluation. Cisplatin-based concurrent chemotherapy and radiotherapy (CRT) is the standard treatment for locally advanced cervical cancers. It is also an option for patients with medically inoperable early stage disease or who refuse surgery. Brachytherapy (BRT) is an integral component of definitive treatment.

M. Gultekin (✉) · S. Y. Sari · G. Yazici · P. Hurmuz · G. Ozyigit · F. Yildiz
Department of Radiation Oncology, Faculty of Medicine, Hacettepe University,
Ankara, Turkey
e-mail: melisgultekin@hacettepe.edu.tr

© Springer Nature Switzerland AG 2019
G. Ozyigit, U. Selek (eds.), *Radiation Oncology*,
https://doi.org/10.1007/978-3-319-97145-2_7

Adjuvant therapy: Surgery is often preferred treatment modality for early stage cervical cancer. Postoperative radiotherapy (RT) with or without cisplatin-based concurrent chemotherapy is indicated for patients with intermediate risk factors [tumor size >4 cm, deep stromal invasion, lymphovascular space invasion (LVSI)] or high risk factors (positive surgical margin, lymph node metastasis, parametrial involvement).

Keywords: Cervical cancer, radiotherapy

7.1.1 Case Presentation

A 53-year-old female admitted to the hospital with several month history of postmenopausal bleeding. She had medical history of bronchial asthma. She had a previous history of smoking 10 packs/year, but quitted 10 years ago. Her gynecological examination revealed a 5 cm exophytic cervical mass and right parametrial infiltration. A uterine cervical biopsy specimen revealed invasive squamous cell carcinoma (SCC). Pelvic magnetic resonance imaging (MRI) showed $6.0 \times 4.3 \times 7$ cm cervical mass and suspicious bilateral parametrial involvement (Fig. 7.1). Whole body fluorodeoxyglucose (FDG) positron emission tomography/computed tomography (PET/CT) scan demonstrated accumulation of FDG in cervix with SUVmax of 14.8 (Fig. 7.2). No lymph nodes were detected both MRI and PET/CT scan. Whole blood count, and kidney and liver function tests were normal. She was staged as FIGO IIB cervical SCC (Table 7.1).

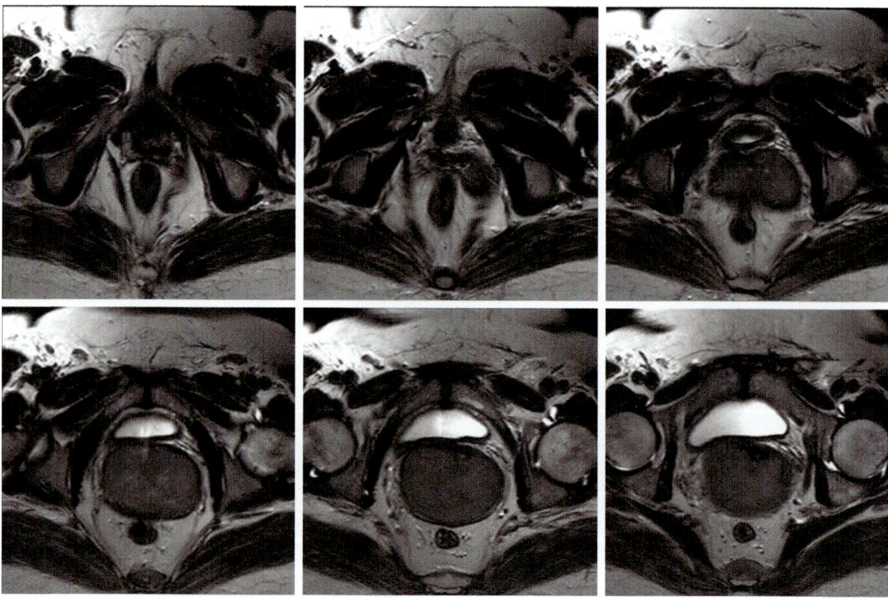

Fig. 7.1 T2-weighted axial MRI images of patient at diagnosis

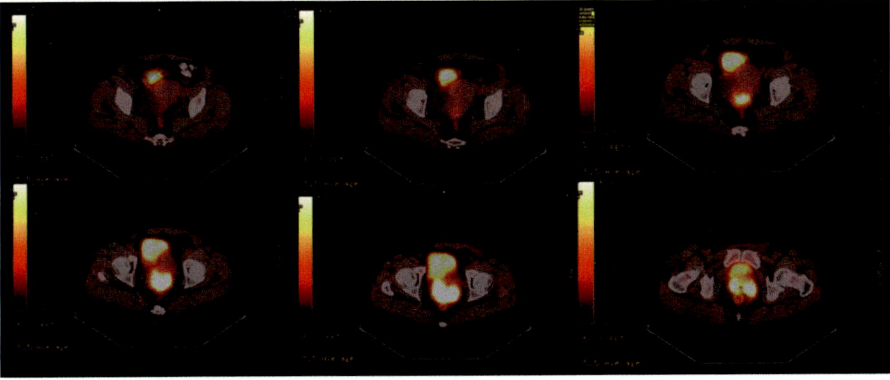

Fig. 7.2 Accumulation of FDG in uterine cervix at diagnosis (SUV max = 14.8)

Table 7.1 Staging of cervical cancer based on FIGO (2009) and AJCC TNM classification (8th edition)

FIGO/TNM Staging		
Primary Tumor (T)		
FIGO	TNM	
TX		Primary tumor cannot be assessed
T0		No evidence of primary tumor
Tis*		Carcinoma in situ (preinvasive carcinoma)
I	T1	Cervical carcinoma confined to uterus (extension to corpus should be disregarded)
IA	T1a**	Invasive carcinoma diagnosed only by microscopy. Stromal invasion with a maximum depth of 5.0 mm measured from the base of the epithelium and a horizontal spread of 7.0 mm or less. Vascular space involvement, venous or lymphatic, does not affect classification
IA1	T1a1	Measured stromal invasion 3.0 mm or less in depth and 7.0 mm or less in horizontal spread
IA2	T1a2	Measured stromal invasion more than 3.0 mm and not more than 5.0 mm with a horizontal spread 7.0 mm or less
IB	T1b	Clinically visible lesion confined to the cervix or microscopic lesion greater than T1a/IA2
IB1	T1b1	Clinically visible lesion 4.0 cm or less in greatest dimension
IB2	T1b2	Clinically visible lesion more than 4.0 cm in greatest dimension
II	T2	Cervical carcinoma invades beyond uterus but not to pelvic wall or to lower third of vagina
IIA	T2a	Tumor without parametrial invasion
IIA1	T2a1	Clinically visible lesion 4.0 cm or less in greatest dimension
IIA2	T2a2	Clinically visible lesion more than 4.0 cm in greatest dimension
IIB	T2b	Tumor with parametrial invasion
III	T3	Tumor extends to pelvic wall and/or involves lower third of vagina, and/or causes hydronephrosis or nonfunctioning kidney
IIIA	T3a	Tumor involves lower third of vagina, no extension to pelvic wall
IIIB	T3b	Tumor extends to pelvic wall and/or causes hydronephrosis or nonfunctioning kidney
IVA	T4	Tumor invades mucosa of bladder or rectum, and/or extends beyond true pelvis (bullous edema is not sufficient to classify a tumor as T4)
*FIGO no longer includes Stage 0 (Tis).		
**All macroscopically visible lesions—even with superficial invasion—are T1b/IB.		

(continued)

Table 7.1 (continued)

Regional Lymph Nodes (N)			
FIGO	TNM		
	NX	Regional lymph nodes cannot be assessed	
	N0	No regional lymph node metastasis	
IIIB	N1	Regional lymph node metastasis	
Distant Metastasis (M)			
FIGO	TNM		
	M0	No distant metastasis	
IVB	M1	Distant metastasis (including peritoneal spread, involvement of	
		supraclavicular, mediastinal, or paraaortic lymph nodes, lung,	
liver, or bone			
Stage Grouping			
Stage 0ᵃ	Tis	N0	M0
Stage Iᵇ T1	N0	M0	
Stage IA	T1a	N0	M0
Stage IA1	T1a1	N0	M0
Stage IA2	T1a2	N0	M0
Stage IB	T1b	N0	M0
Stage IB1	T1b1	N0	M0
Stage IB2	T1b2	N0	M0
Stage II	T2	N0	M0
Stage IIA	T2a	N0	M0
Stage IIA1	T2a1	N0	M0
Stage IIA2	T2a2	N0	M0
Stage IIB	T2b	N0	M0
Stage III	T3	N0	M0
Stage IIIA	T3a	N0	M0
Stage IIIB	T3b	AnyN	M0
	T1-3	N	M0
Stage IVA	T4	AnyN	M0
Stage IVB	AnyT	AnyN	M1

TNM T (tumor) N (regional lymph nodes) M (distant metastasis)

FIGO International Federation of Gynecology and Obstetrics

Used with permission of the American Joint Committee on Cancer (AJCC), Chicago, Illinois. The original source for this material is the AJCC Cancer Staging Manual, Eight Edition (2017) published by Springer Science Business Media LLC, www.springer.com

ᵃFIGO no longer includes Stage 0 (Tis)

ᵇAll macroscopically visible lesions—even with superficial invasion—are T1b/IB

7.1.2 Evidence Based Treatment Recommendations

Cervical cancer is staged clinically based on the International Federation of Gynecology and Obstetrics (FIGO) staging system which includes detailed physical examination and histologic evaluation of a cervical biopsy [1]. These tumors should also be staged according to the American Joint Committee on Cancer (AJCC) Tumor, Node, Metastasis (TNM) classification (8th edition, 2017) [2]. A complete blood count, liver and renal function tests, and urinalysis should be performed. Tumor size and vaginal or parametrial involvement should be evaluated with pelvic examination. Additionally, groin and supraclavicular lymph nodes are palpated to determine the presence of distant metastases. Some patients need pelvic examination under general anesthesia to assess parametrial or pelvic sidewall extension. Punch biopsy, endocervical curettage, colposcopy with directed biopsy and diagnostic conization can be used for tissue diagnosis. FIGO allows a hysteroscopy, cystoscopy, proctoscopy, intravenous pyelogram (IVP), chest x-ray, and radiograph of the skeleton to be used for clinical staging.

Imaging studies can be used for the determination of tumor size or parametrial invasion, as well as metastases to lymph nodes. Although these techniques do not alter the FIGO stage, it impacts treatment decision and RT volumes [3, 4]. MRI helps to assess tumor size and local spread (e.g. parametrial invasion, rectum or bladder involvement) especially for women who are candidates for surgery. PET/CT is also being used in the initial work-up of cervical cancer to detect lymph node metastases which provides information to design RT fields and/or rule out metastasis. The main limitation of PET/CT is a higher false-negative rate for detecting para-aortic lymph node metastases in locally advanced cervical cancer [5, 6].

In cervical cancer, treatment decisions are usually depends on the FIGO stage at diagnosis. For women with early-stage disease, surgery is often the preferred treatment. RT plays a significant role in the management of cervical cancer. It can be used as an adjuvant treatment after surgery in early stage disease or as definitive treatment for locally advanced disease. Locally advanced disease requires combined modality treatment that includes RT and concomitant chemotherapy with or without a subsequent hysterectomy.

7.1.2.1 Early Stage

The definition of early stage cervical cancer includes FIGO stage IA, IB1, or IIA1 disease which was limited to the cervix. Fertility-sparing surgery, modified radical hysterectomy or primary RT with or without chemotherapy can be used depends on the patient and tumor characteristics. Evaluation of the lymph nodes by lymph node dissection or imaging studies is an integral part of the treatment planning in cervical cancer. Sentinel lymph node biopsy is currently considered as investigational [7, 8].

Patients with microinvasive disease (FIGO stage IA1, no LVSI) have a low risk of lymph node metastasis (<1%) and conization or extrafascial (simple, class I) hysterectomy alone is a treatment option for these patients [9]. Extrafascial hysterectomy involves removal of the cervix, uterus, and a small vaginal cuff. If patients have LVSI, lymph nodes should be evaluated with bilateral pelvic lymph node dissection (BPLND).

For patients with FIGO stage IA2 through IB1 (<2 cm) cervical cancer, modified radical hysterectomy (class II) with BPLND is recommended [10, 11]. Surgery provides an opportunity for lower long-term morbidity than primary RT. [12] Modified radical hysterectomy involves removal of the cervix, uterus, upper one-fourth of the vagina, and parametria. Hysterectomy may be performed via laparotomy, conventional laparoscopy, or robotic-assisted laparoscopy. If pretreatment imaging shows para-aortic nodal involvement or if pelvic lymph nodes are suspicious for metastasis, para-aortic lymph node sampling should be done according to frozen section analysis. In premenopausal women, ovaries may be preserved in squamous cell histology which had low rates of ovarian metastases [13]. However, bilateral salpingectomy should be done.

Radical hysterectomy (class III) with BPLND (±para-aortic lymph node sampling) is the preferred treatment approach for patients with a tumor that is confined to the cervix, uterus, or upper third of the vagina (FIGO stage IB1 and IIA1) that is nonbulky (≤4 cm). Radical hysterectomy involves removal of more extensive vaginal and parametrial tissues as well as entire uterosacral and vesicouterine ligaments.

Patients with medically inoperable early stage cervical cancer or who refuse surgery are usually treated with primary RT [pelvic external beam radiotherapy (EBRT) and BRT]. There are no data regarding whether CRT improves treatment outcomes.

In the setting of early stage disease treated with hysterectomy, RT or CRT should be recommended for patients who have poor prognostic factors at final pathology report. Prognostic factors are classified into two groups: Intermediate risk factors and high risk factors. The intermediate risk factors (Sedlis criteria) include tumor size (>4 cm), deep cervical stromal invasion and the presence of LVSI, and patients with any two of these factors should be considered for adjuvant RT [14]. The presence of intermediate risk factors associated with a 30% risk of death and postoperative RT decreased the rate of recurrence [14, 15]. Progression-free survival (PFS) and overall survival (OS) may also improve with the addition of RT. Rogers et al. showed in a 2012 meta-analysis that compared to observation, postoperative RT improved disease control in 397 patients with early stage cervical cancer [16]. There are no high quality data regarding the benefit of CRT in these patients. Although limited data suggest that CRT may reduce the risk of recurrence, it is not known whether this will translate into an OS benefit [17]. Additional risk factors include histologic type (e.g., adenocarcinoma) and grade. Ryu et al. defined the intermediate risk group as a "four-factor model" which was include tumor size ≥3 cm, deep stromal invasion of the outer third of the cervix, LVSI, and adenocarcinoma or adenosquamous carcinoma histology [18]. Among these factors, presence of any two factors may be useful for predicting recurrence after radical hysterectomy.

The high risk factors (Peters criteria) include pathologically lymph node metastasis, positive surgical margins and parametrial involvement and patients with any of these factors should be considered for adjuvant single–agent platinum based CRT with or without BRT [17, 19, 20]. The presence of high-risk factors associated with a 40% risk of recurrence and 50% risk of death following surgery alone [19–21]. In the Gynecologic Oncology Group (GOG) 109 study, the superiority of CRT was demonstrated [19, 20]. In this study, 268 patients with high risk factors were randomized to CRT (4 cycles of cisplatin 70 mg/m^2 on day 1, plus FU 1000 mg/m^2 per day by continuous infusion for four days, every three weeks) versus RT alone (49.3 Gy in 29 fractions to a standard pelvic field) after hysterectomy. With a median follow-up of 42 months, 4-year PFS (80% vs. 63%, p = 0.003) and OS (81% vs. 71%, p = 0.007) were superior with CRT compared to RT alone. However, grade 3–4 toxicity was more frequent in the CRT arm. The role of CRT versus RT alone in node negative high risk disease is controversial.

7.1.2.2 Locally Advanced Stage

Primary surgery is not recommended in locally advanced cervical cancer (bulky FIGO stage IB2, IIA2, IIB, III and IVA disease) due to it is not likely to be curative and these patients usually require adjuvant RT or CRT, which is associated with higher rates of morbidity [19, 22, 23]. Definitive concurrent CRT (EBRT plus BRT), using cisplatin-based chemotherapy, is the standard approach. According to the 5 randomized phase III studies and a metaanalysis, concurrent CRT reduces the risk of death by 30–50% compared to RT alone, which translated into 10% absolute improvement in survival [19, 24–31]. However, there is a significant increase in the risk of acute and long-term toxicity [32, 33].

Concurrent cisplatin alone or cisplatin plus 5-fluorouracil (5-FU) can be used with pelvic EBRT [34, 35]. However, single-agent weekly cisplatin (40 mg/m^2) is the most commonly used agent due to its favorable toxicity profile [34]. Combination therapies of cisplatin with other agents did not show any additional benefit compared to cisplatin alone [36, 37]. If patients have renal insufficiency, concurrent carboplatin or gemcitabine can be administered instead of cisplatin [32]. There is no clear evidence of benefit beside additional toxicity risk to administer adjuvant chemotherapy following CRT thus it is still investigational [38, 39].

Patients with locally advanced cervical cancer should undergo a PET/CT prior to CRT for accurate determination of disease extent and RT fields. It is valuable modality for evaluating lymph node metastases. Although lymph node metastases does not change the FIGO clinical stage, it impacts modification of RT planning in up to 43% of patients [40, 41]. The decision to pursue lymphadenectomy or CT-guided biopsy based on PET/CT findings depends on the clinician's decision [42]. Gold et al. assessed the value of para-aortic lymph node sampling (compared with radiographic determination) in 555 patients who participated in GOG trials (GOG 85, GOG 120, and GOG 165) retrospectively and concluded that it had a positive impact on prognosis [42]. Lymph node dissection can be performed either transperitoneal or extraperitoneal approach. The latter has fewer side effects [43–46]. For women with para-aortic lymph node metastases, primary CRT with extended-field RT (pelvic and para-aortic field) is recommended. However, it is associated with a high rate of acute and late toxicity [47–50]. Prophylactic para-aortic RT may improve treatment outcomes, but it causes severe toxicity [51, 52].

In the setting of initially bulky tumor (>7 cm), lower uterine segment involvement, or a high residual tumor volume after CRT, simple hysterectomy following CRT may be performed to improve pelvic control [53–55]. Complementary hysterectomy may also play a role, especially in patients whose uterine anatomy is not suitable to deliver BRT dose appropriately. However, it is no impact on OS and significantly increased toxicity [55]. In a randomized trial, Morice et al. evaluated the role of hysterectomy after CRT who had a complete response in patients with stage IB2 to II cervical cancer [53]. At 3 years there was no difference in event-free survival (72% vs. 89%) or OS (86% vs. 97%). A recent Cochrane review also did not demonstrate a benefit of complementary hysterectomy [56].

Although neoadjuvant chemotherapy followed by surgery has been used in areas where RT is not available, neoadjuvant chemotherapy prior to definitive hysterectomy does not offer an OS advantage relative to primary CRT either early stage or locally advanced stage cervical cancer. However, it may reduce the need for adjuvant RT by decreasing tumor size and response to neoadjuvant chemotherapy can be used as a prognostic indicator [57–59]. Gupta et al. recently demonstrated in a phase III randomized trial that neoadjuvant chemotherapy (3 cycles of paclitaxel and carboplatin once every three weeks) followed by surgery was associated with inferior 5-year DFS (69.3% vs. 76.7%, p = 0.038) compared to CRT in 633 patients with stage IB2, IIA, or IIB squamous cell cervical cancer [60]. However, 5-year OS was similar between the two groups (75.4% vs. 74.7%, p = 0.87). On the other hand, CRT arm had more increased long-term toxicity compared to neoadjuvant chemotherapy plus surgery arm. Selected phase III randomized controlled trials in cervical cancer are summarized in Table 7.2.

7.1.2.3 Metastatic Disease

Patients with metastatic disease (stage IVB) are often treated with combination cisplatin-based chemotherapy. Palliative RT may also be given with palliative intent in symptomatic patients.

7.1.3 Treatment Recommendations

Recommended algorithm for the treatment of early and locally advanced stage cervical cancer is summarized in Fig. 7.3.

7.1.4 Treatment Planning

7.1.4.1 Simulation

In premenopausal women, surgical ovarian transposition should be considered prior to initiation of RT or CRT to preserve ovarian function [61].

Patients are usually CT simulated in the supine position, arms above chest with immobilization devices (Fig. 7.4). They also simulated in the prone position using a "belly board" which displace small bowel from the treatment field and reduce toxicity.

Prior to simulation, patients undergo a standard bladder and bowel preparation. Rectum should be empty (≤3.5 cm) during CT simulation and daily treatment.

In postoperative cases, to identify the vaginal apex on the CT scan, radiopaque vaginal marker may be inserted into the vaginal apex.

Two CT data sets obtained at simulation for intensity modulated RT (IMRT): (1) with full bladder (2) with empty bladder. These images then should be fused to account for organ motion. During RT, the patient must be treated with the bladder full.

Table 7.2 Selected phase III randomized controlled trials in cervical cancer

Reference	Characteristics	Treatment	FU (mo)	Clinical outcome	Toxicity
Landoni [10]	343 pts Stage IB-IIA Lymphangiography RH + pelvic LND	Primary RT vs. RH (± Adjuvant RT) EBRT (1.8–2 Gy, 40–53 Gy) + LDR BRT Point A: 70–90 Gy If PA LN+: PA RT 45 Gy + (5–10 Gy) boost Adjuvant RT (64%): IB1 54%, IB2 84% If ≥pT2b, LN+, margin+, <3 mm uninvolved cervical stroma Pelvis 50.4 Gy, ±PA 45 Gy	87	No difference in OS (83% for both groups) No difference in DFS (74% for both groups) No difference in recurrence (26% vs. 25%) Prognostic factors: Tumor size, LN status, and adenocarcinoma histology Early stage IB, IIA pts have similar DFS and OS treated with surgery or RT alone Combined surgery and adjuvant RT increased toxicity	Higher rates of urologic complications with combined surgery and RT Severe grade 2–3: 12% vs. 28% (p = 0.0004)
Sedlis [14] (GOG 92/ RTOG 87-06)	277 pts Stage IB RH and pelvic LND LN (−), margin (−), ≥2 risk factors: >1/3 stromal invasion, LVSI+, ≥4 cm	Adjuvant RT vs. Observation EBRT: Pelvis 1.8–2 Gy/46–50.4 Gy No BRT	60	LR: 13% vs. 19% DM: 2% vs. 7% 36% less mortality in the RT group	Grade 3–4: 7% vs. 2%
Rotman [15] (update of GOG 92)			120	RT arm: 46% reduction in risk of recurrence (p = 0.007) 42% reduction in risk of progression or death (p = 0.009) 30% improvement in OS (p = 0.074) AdenoCa/Adenosquamous recurrence rate: 8.8% vs. 44% (p = 0.019) Adjuvant RT reduced local and distant recurrences, and improved PFS	Grade 3–4: 6.6% vs. 2.1% (p = 0.083)

(continued)

Table 7.2 (continued)

Reference	Characteristics	Treatment	FU (mo)	Clinical outcome	Toxicity
Peters [19] (GOG 109/ SWOG 8797)	243 pts Stage IA2, IB, IIA: LN+ and/or margin+ and/or prm+ RH and pelvic LND	Adjuvant RT vs. Adjuvant CRT EBRT: Pelvis 1.7 Gy/49.3 Gy If CI LN+: EFRT 1.5 Gy/45 Gy Chemo: Bolus cisplatin (70 mg/m^2)/96-h infusion 5-FU (4 g/m^2/day) every 3 weeks, 4 cycles	42	4-year PFS: 63% vs. 80% (p = 0.003) 4-year OS: 71% vs. 81% (p = 0.007) CRT: LR decreased by 50% and DM by 30% Adjuvant CRT increased OS in pts with high risk, early stage disease (>2 cm, ≥2 LN+)	Grade 3–4: 3% vs. 61%
Keys [55] (GOG 71)	256 pts Bulky (≥4 cm) stage IB	RT vs. RT + Adjuvant Hysterectomy RT: EBRT + BRT	115	No difference in OS (61% vs. 64%, p = 0.26) No difference in PFS (53% vs. 62%, p = 0.09) Higher LR without surgery (27% vs. 14%, p = 0.08) No benefit of extrafascial hysterectomy	Grade 3–4: 10% for both groups
Rotman [51, 52] (RTOG 79-20)	367 pts Stage IIB, bulky IB and IIA (≥4 cm) Clinically or pathologically PA LN (−)	Pelvic RT vs. EFRT EBRT: Pelvis 1.6–1.8 Gy/40–50 Gy, PA 1.6–1.8 Gy/44–45 Gy BRT: 30-40 Gy to point A		10-year OS: 44% vs. 55%, p = 0.02 10-year DFS: 40% vs. 42% No difference in LRC (65% vs. 69%, p = 0.44) No difference in DM (25–30%) Improved OS with EFRT	Grade 4–5: 4% vs. 8%, p = 0.06
Morris [25] (RTOG 90-01)	403 pts Stage IB, IIA (≥5 cm or LN+), IIB-IVA PA LN (−)	Pelvic RT + Concurrent Cisplatin/5-FU vs. EFRT EBRT: 45 Gy LDR BRT: Point A dose 85 Gy	43	5-year OS: 73% vs. 58%, p = 0.004 5-year DFS: %67 vs. 40%, p < 0.001 5-year LRR: 19% vs. 35%, p < 0.001 5-year DM: 14% vs. 33%, p < 0.001 Stage III-IVA: No difference in OS or DFS	

Study		Treatment		Results	Toxicity
Eifel [30] (update of RTOG 90-01)			55	8-year OS: 67% vs. 41%, p ˂ 0.0001 8-year DFS: 61% vs. 46% CRT: Risk of recurrence or death reduced by 51%, LRR risk reduced by %58 Stage III-IVA: Better DFS ($p = 0.05$) and OS ($p = 0.07$)	Late grade 3–4: 13% vs. 12%
Rose [27, 39] (GOG 120)	526 pts Stage IIB-IVA PA LN (−)	RT + Cisplatin (1) vs. RT + HU (2) vs. RT + Cisplatin/5-FU + HU (3) EBRT: Pelvis 1.7 Gy/40.8–51 Gy LDR BRT (point A dose 81 Gy) (1) Weekly Cisplatin 40 mg/m^2/week, 6 cycles (2) Oral HU 3 g/m^2 biweekly, 6 cycles (3) Cisplatin 50 mg/m^2 on d1, 29; 5-FU 4 g/m^2 at 96-h infusion days 1, 29; oral HU 2 g/m^2 twice weekly, 6 cycles	106	10-year PFS: 46% vs. 26% vs. 43% 10-year OS: 53% vs. 34% vs. 53% 10-year LR: 22% vs. 34% vs. 21% Stage IIB-III: Better PFS ($p < 0.005$) and OS ($p < 0.025$) Cisplatin groups: Higher PFS, OS and LC	Late grade 3–4 GI/urologic 4.7% vs. 2.6% vs. 0.9%
Keys [24] (GOG 123)	369 pts Stage IB2 LN (−)	RT + Hysterectomy vs. RT + Concurrent cisplatin + Hysterectomy EBRT: Pelvis 1.8–2 Gy/45 Gy LDR BRT: Point A dose 75 Gy Cisplatin: 40 mg/m^2/week, 6 cycles Extrafascial hysterectomy: 3–6 weeks following RT	36	RR of progression 0.51 favoring CRT (p˂0.001) RR of death 0.54 favoring CRT ($p = 0.008$)	Grade 3–4 hematologic: 2% vs. 21% Grade 3–4 GI: 5% vs. 14%
Stehman [31] (update of GOG 123)			101	6-year PFS: 60% vs. 71% 6-year OS: 64% vs. 78% Concurrent CRT improved PFS and OS	Late: No difference

(continued)

Table 7.2 (continued)

Reference	Characteristics	Treatment	FU (mo)	Clinical outcome	Toxicity
Whitney [26]	368 pts Stage IIB-IVA PA LN (−)	RT plus HU vs. RT plus 5-FU and cisplatin EBRT: whole pelvic RT	104	PFS: Improved with 5-FU/Cisplatin (21% risk reduction) OS: Improved with 5-FU/Cisplatin (26% risk reduction)	Severe or life-threatening leukopenia: 24% vs. 4%
Duenas Gonzales [38]	515 pts Stage IIB-IVA KPS ≥70	CRT (1) vs. CRT followed by adjuvant chemo (2) (1) Concurrent cisplatin (40 mg/m^2/week) and RT (2) Concurrent gemcitabine (125 mg/m^2/week) plus cisplatin (40 mg/m^2/week) and RT followed by adjuvant gemcitabine (1 g/m^2 on d1, 8), and cisplatin (50 mg/m^2 on d1), every 3 weeks EBRT: 1.8 Gy/50.4 Gy BRT: 30–35 Gy in 96 h	46.9	3-year PFS: 65% vs. 74.4%, p = 0.029 LR: 16.4 vs. 11.2, p = 0.097 DM: 16.4 vs. 8.1, p = 0.005 Gemcitabine plus cisplatin CRT followed by adjuvant gemcitabine and cisplatin improved survival outcomes	Grade 3–4: 46.3% vs. 86.5, p < 0.001
Ryu [18] (KGOG)	2158 pts Stage IB-IIA RH Intermediate risk factors	Development group vs. Validation group To predict recurrence, multivariate models were developed using the development group	64.2	Histology, tumor size, DSI, and LVSI were significantly associated with recurrence "Four-factor model" was defined any two of the four intermediate-risk factors (tumor size ≥3 cm, DSI of the outer third of the cervix, LVSI, and adenocarcinoma or adenosquamous Ca) showed the best performance for predicting recurrence	

Wang [36] (AGOG)	74 pts Stage III-IVA or stage I-II, LN+	CRT with cisplatin vs. CRT with cisplatin plus gemcitabine Cisplatin 40 mg/m²/week Gemcitabine 125 mg/m²/week		3-year PFS: 65.1% vs. 71.0%, p = 0.71 3-year OS: 74.1% vs. 85.9%, p = 0.89 No benefit of adding gemcitabine	Grade 2–4 hematologic: Increased with the addition of gemcitabine
Thakur [37]	81 pts Stage IIA-IIIB	CRT with cisplatin (1) vs. CRT with cisplatin plus paclitaxel (2) (1) Cisplatin 40 mg/m²/week, 5 weeks (2) Cisplatin 30 mg/m²/week and paclitaxel 50 mg/m²/week, 5 weeks EBRT: 2 Gy/50 Gy followed by BRT or EBRT boost	29	CR: 75.6% vs. 84%, p = 0.4095 DFS: 64.3% vs. 79.5%, p = 0.07 OS: 78.6% vs. 87.2%, p = 0.27	Grade 2 hematologic: 12.2% vs. 35% Grade 3 GI: 7.4% vs. 20% Grade 4 GI: 2.4% vs. 12.5%
Gupta [60]	635 pts Stage IB2, IIA, IIB	Neoadjuvant chemo followed by surgery vs. CRT Neoadjuvant chemo: Paclitaxel and carboplatin, every 3 weeks, 3 cycles If indicated, adjuvant RT/CRT CRT: Concurrent cisplatin 40 mg/m²/week	58.5	5-year DFS: 69.3% vs. 76.7%, p = 0.38 5-year OS: 75.4% vs. 74.7%, p = 0.87 Cisplatin-based CRT improved DFS	Late (>24 mo) Rectal: 2.2% vs. 3.5%, p = 0.474 Bladder: 1.6% vs. 3.5%, p = 0.204 Vaginal: 12.0% vs. 25.6%, p ᐸ 0.001

Abbreviations: *FU* follow-up, *mo* months, *pts* patients, *RH* radical hysterectomy, *LND* lymph node dissection, *RT* radiotherapy, *EBRT* external beam radiotherapy, *Gy* gray, *LDR* low dose rate, *BRT* brachytherapy, *PA* para-aortic, *LN* lymph node, *p* pathologic, *T* tumor, *OS* overall survival, *DFS* disease-free survival, *GOG* Gynecologic Oncology Group, *RTOG* Radiation Therapy Oncology Group, *LVSI* lymphovascular space invasion, *LR* local recurrence, *DM* distant metastasis, *Ca* carcinoma, *PFS* progression-free survival, *SWOG* Southwest Oncology Group, *prm* parametrium, *CRT* chemoradiotherapy, *CI* common iliac, *EFRT* extended field radiotherapy, *chemo* chemotherapy, *5-FU* 5-fluorouracil, *LRC* loco-regional control, *LRR* loco-regional recurrence, *HU* hydroxyurea, *d* day, *GI* gastrointestinal, *RR* Relative risk, *KPS* Karnofsky performance status, *KGOG* Korean Gynecologic Oncology Group, *DSI* deep stromal invasion, *AGOG* Asian Gynecologic Oncology Group, *CR* complete response

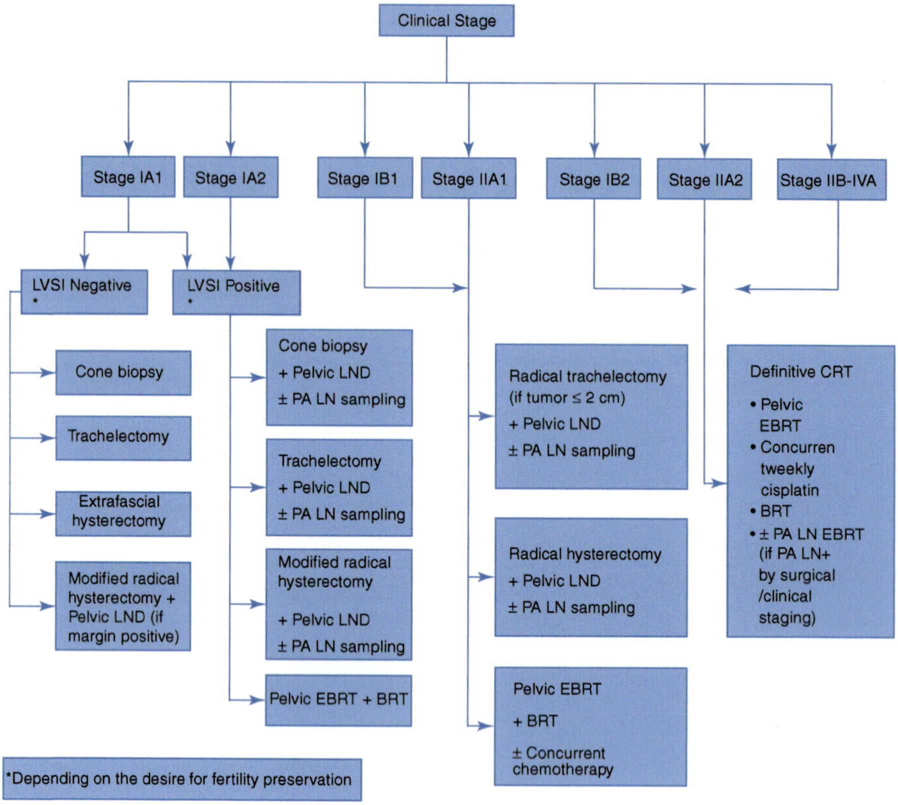

Fig. 7.3 Recommended treatment algorithm for cervical cancer

Fig. 7.4 Immobilization and simulation procedure of the patient

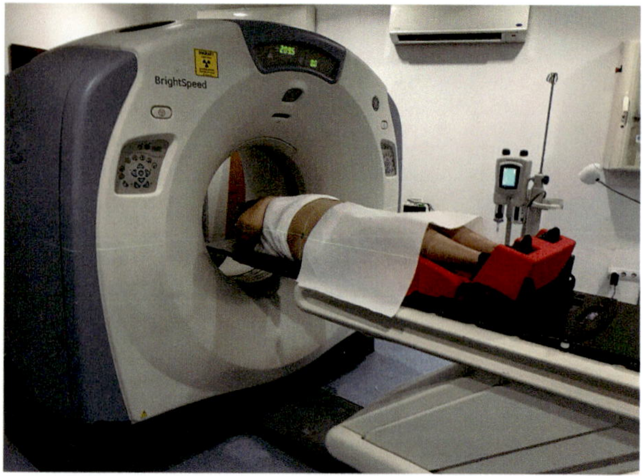

The small bowel may be opacified using oral contrast, rectal marker may be used to define the rectum, and rectum opacified with barium or CT-compatible contrasts as needed.

If patient had gross disease, an inferior margin of the tumor may be marked with a radiopaque wire during simulation.

Intravenous (IV) contrast may be helpful to localize pelvic vascular structures for contouring.

7.1.4.2 Contouring

Traditionally, a four-field "box" (anteroposterior/posteroanterior (AP/PA) and opposed lateral) technique is used. With conventional 2-dimensional (2D) RT, RT field borders are determined by anatomical landmarks, often skeletal anatomy. The superior field border is placed at the L4-L5 interspace. For lymph node negative postoperative cases superior field edge can be reduced to L5-S1 interspace. The distal field border is placed at the bottom of the obturator foramen or 3–4 cm below the lowest extent of disease. Lateral borders are placed at least a 1.5 cm lateral to the pelvic brim. The lateral portal superior and inferior borders remain the same as for AP/PA fields. Posterior border is placed at least at the S2-S3 interspace and the anterior border placed in front of the symphysis pubis. Extended field pelvic and para-aortic RT (EFRT) technique is mainly used for patients with evidence of para-aortic lymph node metastases. The lower border is the same as in the superior pelvic field border. Upper border is extended usually to the T12-L1 interspace or to the level of the renal vessels.

7.1.4.3 External Beam Radiotherapy

In postoperative patients, adjuvant pelvic (±para-aortic) EBRT with or without concurrent chemotherapy indicated based on the risk factors to eradicate potentially harboring occult disease.

In patients with intact cervix, standard treatment approach include concurrent pelvic (±para-aortic) EBRT and chemotherapy then BRT. These patients should not be treated routinely with IMRT or stereotactic body radiotherapy (SBRT) boost instead of BRT.

Weekly 40 mg/m^2 cisplatin is most commonly used and well tolerated agent with EBRT.

The EBRT field determined by the surgical or radiological lymph node status. If para-aortic lymph nodes negative, only pelvic EBRT is given.

Treatment plans can be developed using 3-dimensional conformal RT (3DCRT) or IMRT techniques based on CT images. Nowadays, IMRT has been standard treatment option for the post-operative cases [62]. It allows greater organs at risk (OARs) sparing thus reduce hematologic, gastrointestinal and urinary toxicity especially in the post-hysterectomy setting and in treating the para-aortic region [63]. IMRT may also allow escalation of the gross lymph node dose [64].

IMRT plan is usually created using 5–7 coplanar fields and 6 MV photon beams. It is feasible if careful attention to target volume definitions, reproducibility of treatment and quality assurance. For proper delivery of IMRT routine daily online image guidance (i.e., cone-beam CT) is essential.

Small et al. reported on consensus guidelines for delineation of clinical target volume (CTV) for pelvic IMRT in postoperative treatment of endometrial and cervical cancer to standardize target volume definition [62].

Gross target volume (GTV) (if present), CTV, planning target volume (PTV), and OARs should be defined in conformal RT, especially for IMRT.

For definitive treatment, CTV should include the GTV, cervix, uterus, upper 1/2 vagina (upper 2/3 vagina if upper vagina involved or entire vagina if extensive vaginal involvement), bilateral parametria (including bilateral ovaries), and all locoregionally draining pelvic lymphatics, which include common iliac, external iliac, internal iliac, obturator, and presacral nodes. If para-aortic lymph nodes involved, in addition to the pelvic lymph nodes, the pericaval, interaortacaval, and para-aortic lymph nodes should be contoured. Bilateral inguinofemoral lymph nodes should be included in the RT field if tumors extend to the distal third of the vagina.

For postoperative cases, CTV should include the pelvic lymph nodes, including obturator, presacral, external, internal, and lower common iliac groups (nodal CTV), and upper 1/3 vagina and parametrial/paravaginal tissues (vaginal CTV) [62]. If para-aortic lymph nodes involved, the pericaval, interaortacaval, and para-aortic lymph nodes should also be contoured. Nodal CTV should start from 7 mm below the L4-L5 interspace to the level of the superior aspect of the femoral heads for external iliac and at the level of S3 for the presacral lymph nodes. A nodal CTV is defined as the iliac vessels plus an additional circumferential margin of 7 mm (excluding bowel, muscles and bone). It also should cover contiguous gross or suspicious lymph nodes, lymphoceles, and surgical clips. An additional margin of 7 mm is added in all directions to create nodal PTV. Vaginal CTV should include the gross disease (if present), vaginal cuff and 3 cm below the vaginal marker and parametrial/paravaginal tissues from the vaginal cuff to the medial edge of the internal obturator muscle or ischial ramus on each side. The inferior margin of the vaginal CTV is often at the 1 cm above the inferior extent of the obturator foramen. The rectum, bladder, bone, and muscle should be excluded from the vaginal CTV. To account for vaginal mobility due to bladder filling changes, vaginal CTV is countered using a full-bladder CT scan fused to an empty-bladder CT scan. Then integrated target volume (ITV) created by full bladder plus empty bladder vaginal CTVs (for IMRT planning). A 7 mm margin around ITV in all directions is used to define vaginal PTV.

Small bowel, rectum, bladder and bilateral femoral heads should be defined as OARs in all patients with full bladder CT. If EFRT has been used, bilateral kidneys and spinal cord should also be delineated.

Use of the IGRT system allows reduction of the PTV margin and obviates the need for an ITV, with the daily control of bladder and rectal filling.

IMRT in treating locally advanced cervical cancer remains controversial. Lim et al. reported on consensus guidelines for delineation of clinical target volume (CTV) for pelvic IMRT for the definitive treatment of cervical cancer [65]. MRI immediately before or at the time of simulation is strongly recommended to minimize discrepancies in organ positioning. ITV is created as in postoperative cases. Margin of 7 mm around the nodal CTV and 1.5–2 cm around the primary CTV is added in all directions to create PTVs. Daily soft tissue image-guided RT (IGRT) is recommended to reduce geographical miss.

Case Contouring: Delineation of target volumes for EBRT of the case is shown in Fig. 7.5.

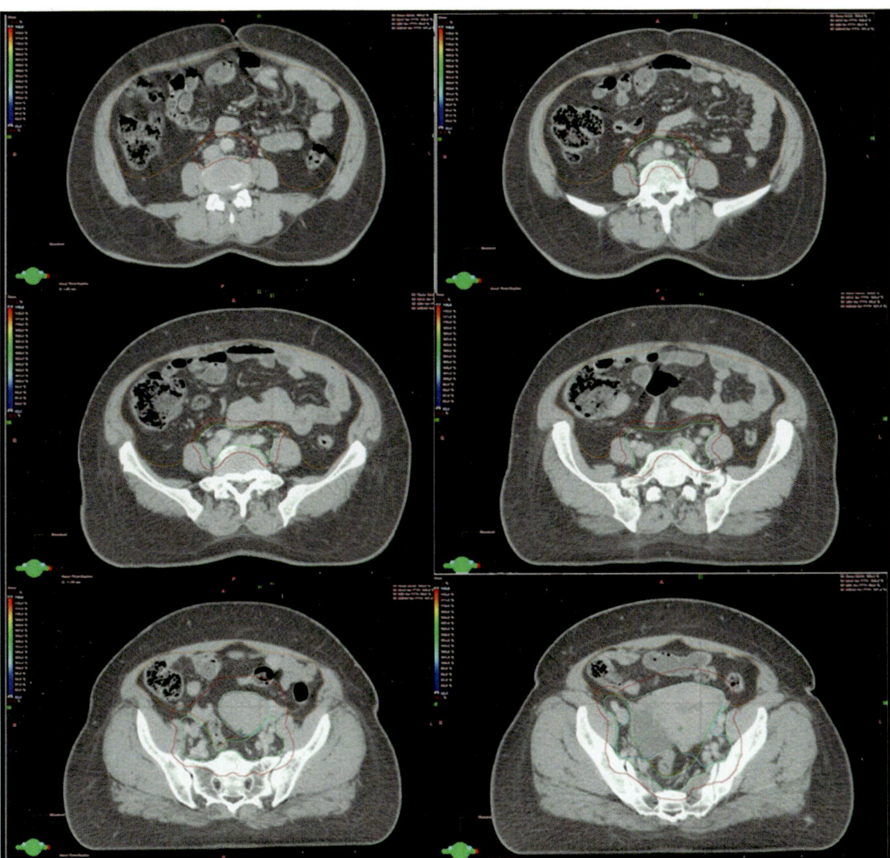

Fig. 7.5 Delineation of target volumes for EBRT of the FIGO stage IIB cervical SCC patient. Red: PTV, green: CTV lymphatic, cyan: CTV primary, orange: bowel, blue: rectum, yellow: bladder, pink: right femur, brown: left femur, light green: body

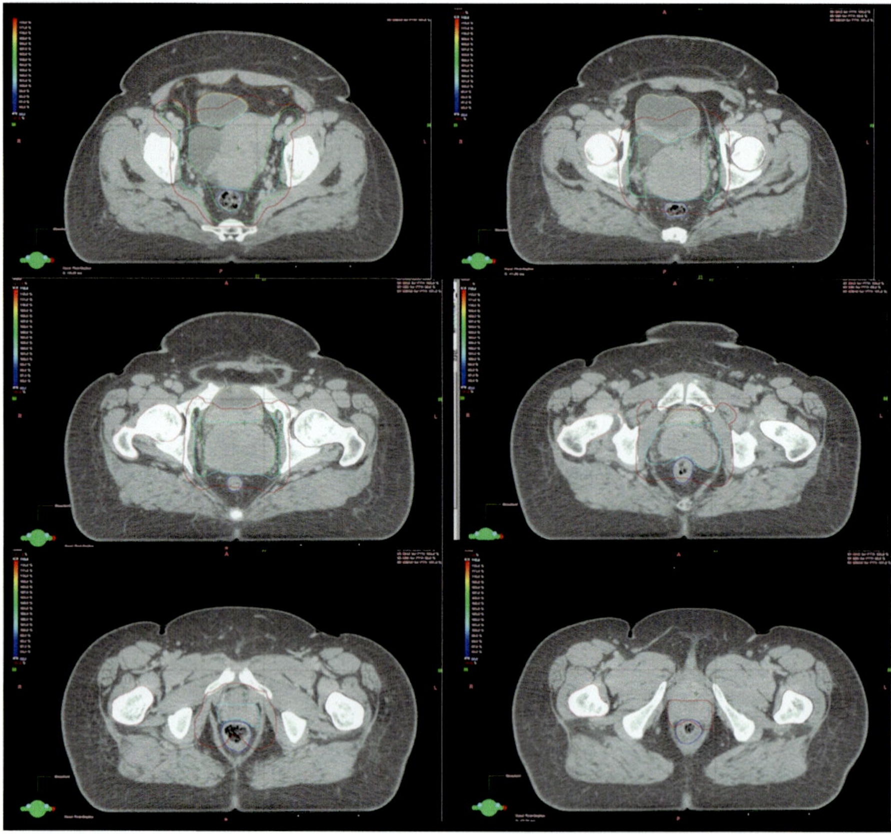

Fig. 7.5 (continued)

7.1.4.4 Brachytherapy

BRT is the local application of RT to the cervix and paracervical tissues. The rapid dose fall-off allows delivery of a very high dose to the cervix while sparing OARs.

A BRT boost is an essential component of treatment to improve local control and OS in definitive treatment of locally advanced cervical cancer [66].

BRT can be delivered with either a low dose rate (LDR), pulse dose rate (PDR), or high dose rate (HDR) system that have similar outcomes and toxicity rates [67–69]. Currently, HDR BRT has been most commonly used form of BRT.

BRT can be performed using an intracavitary, interstitial or hybrid systems in patients with an intact cervix. Depending on the patient and tumor anatomy as well as clinician preference, BRT may be delivered using CT or MRI compatible vaginal ovoids, ring, or cylinder combined with the intrauterine tandem.

Stage IA tumors may be treated with BRT alone.

For patients with positive or close vaginal surgical margins after hysterectomy, BRT may be used as a boost to EBRT.

BRT is usually initiated after completion of EBRT to minimize the amount of residual disease and improve BRT geometry due to tumor shrinkage increasing the distance between the tumor and the OARs.

EBRT and BRT should not be administered on the same day.

Chemotherapy is not recommended during BRT due to the potential for increased toxicity.

The traditional dose prescription system is based on orthogonal radiographs (2D imaging), in which total dose prescribed to point A. It is defined as a point 2 cm above and 2 cm lateral to where the tandem intersects the line connecting the top of the ovoids, which represents the paracervical tissues. Additionally, point B (5 cm lateral to the tandem), bladder and rectal points are defined and doses are calculated according to the International Commission on Radiation Units and Measurements (ICRU) 38 recommendations [70]. However, this system does not take into account tumor volume or surrounding OARs.

Today, 3D image-guided adaptive BRT (IGABT) is considered as standard procedure, which allows individualization of treatment with more precise dose delivery to the tumor while sparing OARs [71–73]. Several observational studies and one prospective study showed that IGABT significantly improved disease control, OS, and morbidity compared to conventional BRT [74–78].

IGABT process involves the following steps: IV conscious sedation or general anesthesia, examination under anesthesia and applicator placement, CT- or MRI-imaging with the applicator in place, contouring of target volumes and OARs, applicator reconstruction, treatment planning, optimization and plan evaluation.

Repetitive gynecological examination is mandatory with documentation in 3D clinical drawings at diagnosis and at the time of BRT to assess tumor extent accurately.

CT and/or MRI can be used for IGABT planning. Although MRI is the gold standard imaging modality with its superior soft tissue contrast and visualization, CT scans are widely available and could be used more frequently for logistic reasons. However, CT-based contours significantly larger than MRI-based contour especially in patients with parametrial extension [79]. The guidelines using CT scans for IGABT already have been published [79–81].

MRI is strongly recommended to assess primary and residual tumor size and geometry at the beginning of the EBRT and immediately before BRT.

Accurate delineation of the tumor and OARs is critical for precise treatment planning. For this purpose, Groupe Europeen Curietherapy-European Society for Therapeutic Radiation Oncology (GEC-ESTRO) published a guideline for MRI-based BRT contouring [73]. The delineation process is based on clinical examination at diagnosis and at BRT and on MRI images taken at diagnosis and at BRT with applicator in place.

GTV: Macroscopic tumor (if present) at time of BRT, high signal intensity mass(es) (FSE, T2) in cervix/corpus, parametria, vagina, bladder and rectum.

High Risk-CTV (HRCTV): High tumor load at time of BRT including GTV, whole cervix, and presumed extracervical tumor extension, grey zones in parametria, uterine corpus, vagina, or rectum, and bladder.

Intermediate Risk-CTV (IRCTV): Microscopic tumor load at time of BRT which encompasses HR-CTV with a safety margin of 5–15 mm according to tumor size and regression and the initial tumor extension at diagnosis.

OARs: Bladder, rectum, sigmoid, and vagina.

Case Contouring: Delineation of target volumes for BRT of the case is shown in Fig. 7.6.

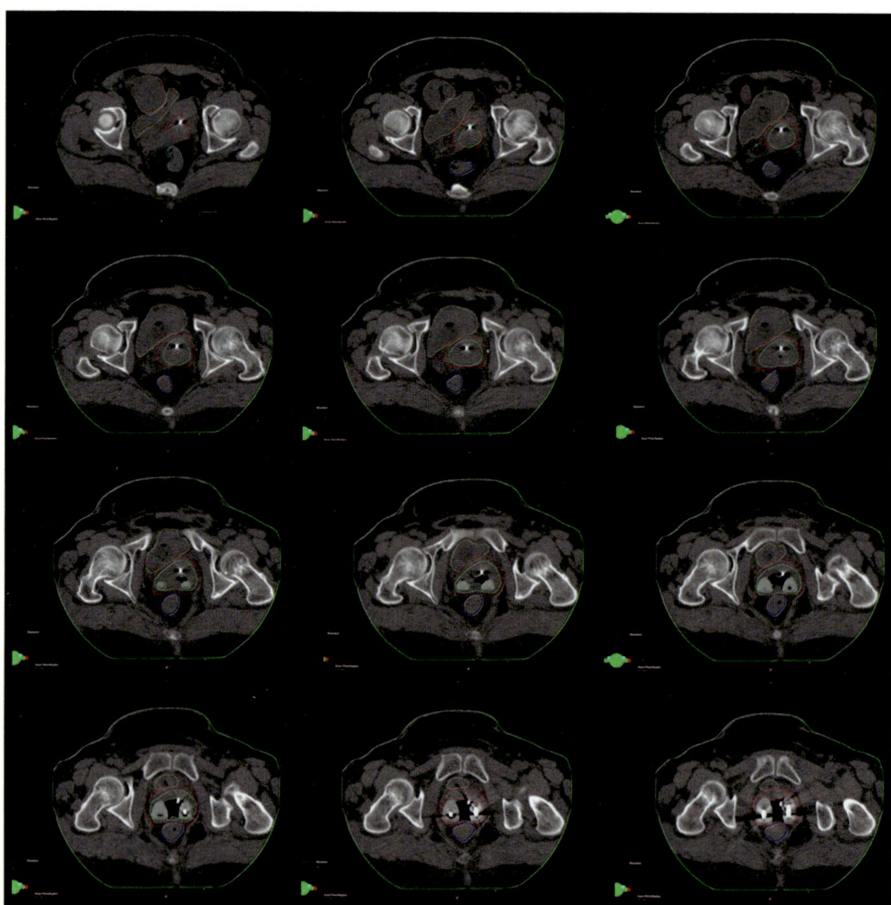

Fig. 7.6 Delineation of target volumes for BRT of the FIGO stage IIB cervical SCC patient. Red: IRCTV, green: HRCTV, blue: rectum, yellow: bladder, sigmoid: cyan, pink: bowel

7.1.4.5 Prescription Dose and Dose Constraints for Critical Structures

Case plan: The patient with FIGO Stage IIB cervical cancer presented here was treated with definitive pelvic EBRT (50.4 Gy in 1.8 Gy/fraction) and concurrent weekly (40 mg/m^2, 6 weeks) cisplatin chemotherapy followed by BRT. EBRT applied with forward-planning IMRT technique. After completion of the EBRT, MRI imaging is performed to assess treatment response and it was showed that $1.7 \times 2 \times 3.2$ cm residual mass in the cervix (Fig. 7.7). CT-based intracavitary BRT

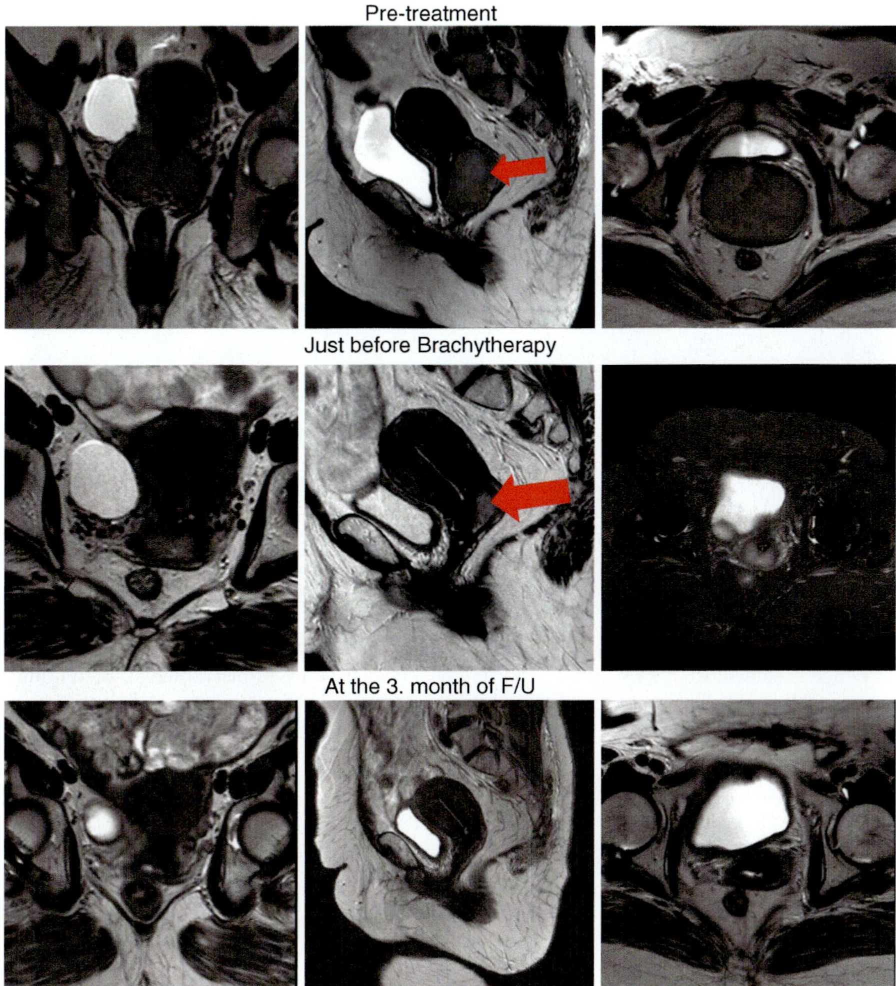

Fig. 7.7 FIGO stage IIB patient with 6.0x4.3x7 cm cervical mass and right parametrial involvement at diagnosis; partial remission after CRT; complete remission at 3-month follow-up. T2-weighted MRI findings of lesion At diagnosis ($6 \times 4.3 \times 7$ cm), just before BRT ($1.7 \times 2 \times 3.2$ cm), and at 3-month follow-up (no lesion) (3)

was applied to patient in 4×7 Gy fraction. The total EQD2: HRCTV D90 = 90 Gy, IRCTV D98 = 65 Gy, Rectum D2cc = 75 Gy, Bowel D2cc = 70 Gy, Bladder D2cc = 85 Gy. At the 3rd-month of follow-up, complete response was observed. Treatment planning details are seen in Figs. 7.8, 7.9, 7.10, and 7.11.

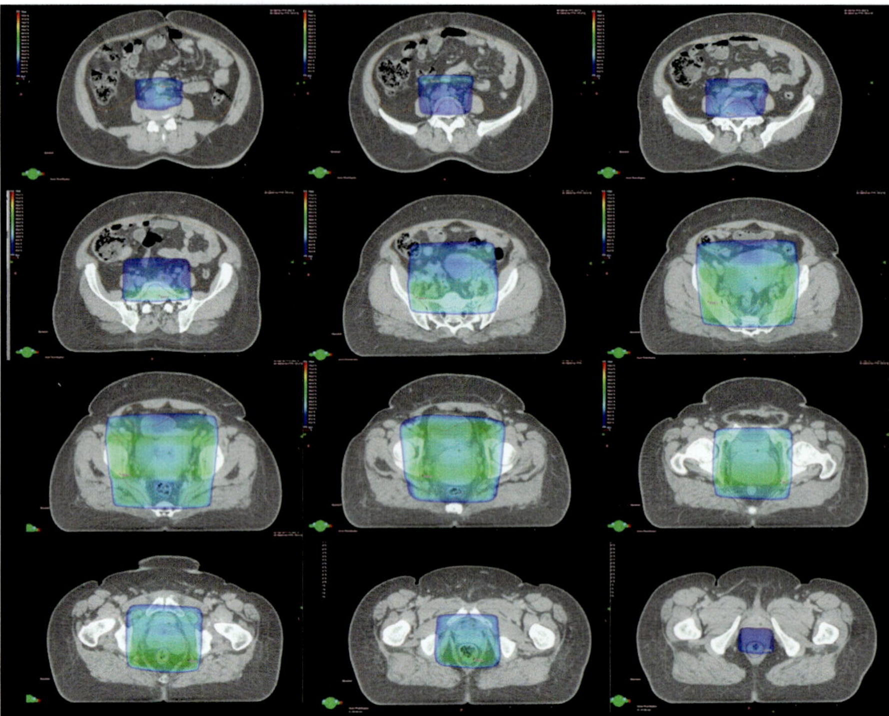

Fig. 7.8 Forward-planning IMRT in the definitive setting of FIGO stage IIB disease. 95% isodose coverage is shown. Red: PTV, green: CTV lymphatic, cyan: CTV primary, orange: bowel, blue: rectum, yellow: bladder, pink: right femur, brown: left femur, light green: body

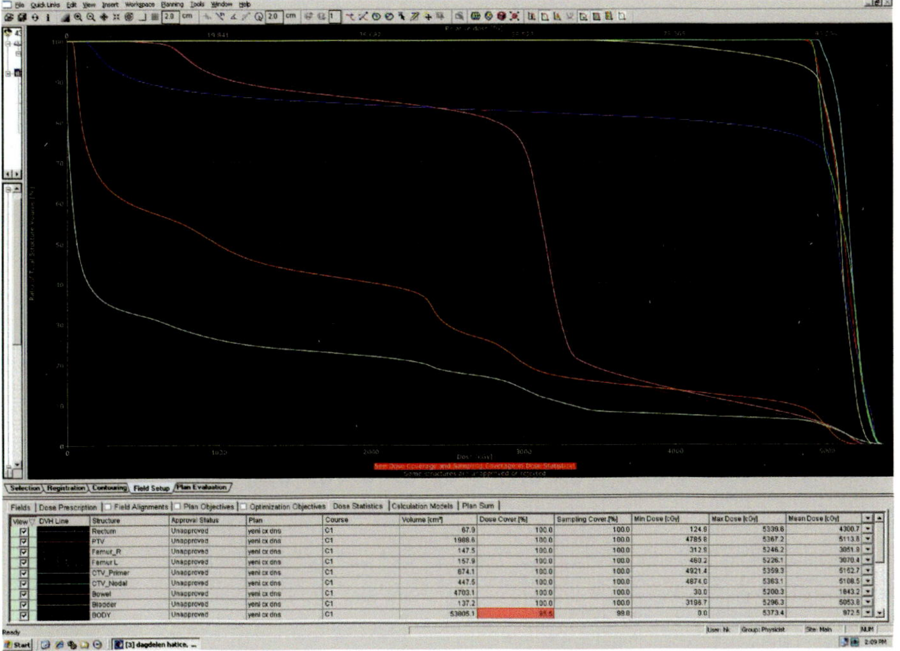

Fig. 7.8 (continued)

7.1.4.6 EBRT Dose

- Whole pelvic RT: 45–50 Gy in 25 once-daily fractions of 1.8–2.0 Gy.
- Microscopic nodal disease: 45–50 Gy in 25 once-daily fractions of 1.8–2.0 Gy.
- Gross nodal disease: An additional 10–20 Gy boost may be administered to reduced volume with highly conformal RT. Bowel, spinal cord, and renal dose limits should not exceed tolerance limits.
- It is recommended that completing the entire RT course (EBRT plus BRT) within 6–8 weeks [82, 83].
- Treatment plans must be done on the full-bladder CT scan.
- Treatment plans should be designed to minimize dose to OARs.
- The treatment plan should be evaluated in each patient using dose volume histogram (DVH) analyses of the PTV and OARs. Prescription goals for the PTV and OARs constraints are needed to be achieved.
- Total prescribed dose should be covered to at least 95% of the PTV. The minimum and maximum dose constraints for the PTV should be within 5% of prescription dose.

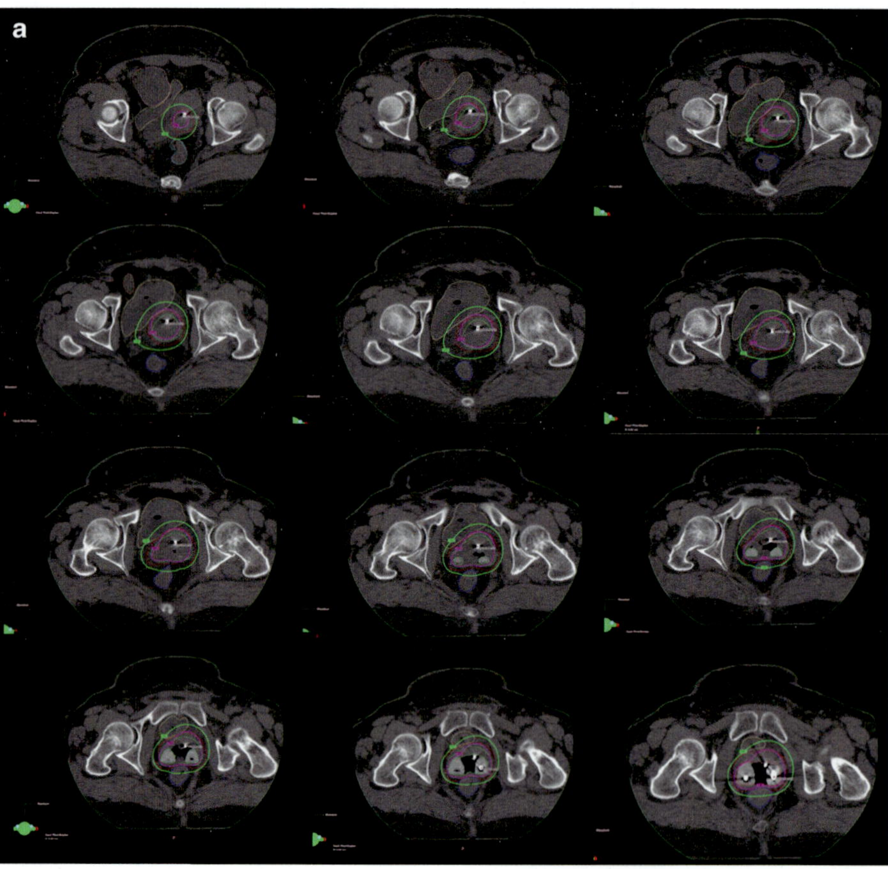

Fig. 7.9 CT-based BRT planning in the definitive setting of FIGO stage IIB disease in first fraction. Tandem applicators and ovoids in place. HRCTV D90: 704 cGy, IRCTV D98: 439 cGy, bladder D2cc: 554 cGy, rectum D2cc: 493 cGy, sigmoid D2cc: 240 cGy. (**a**, **b**) HRCTV and IRCTV well covered within 7 Gy (magenta) and 3.5 Gy (green) isodose volume and (**c**) dose-volume histogram for HRCTV (D90) and rectum (D2cc) are shown. Red: IRCTV, green: HRCTV, blue: rectum, yellow: bladder, sigmoid: cyan, pink: bowel. (**a**) Dose distribution; (**b**) DVHs

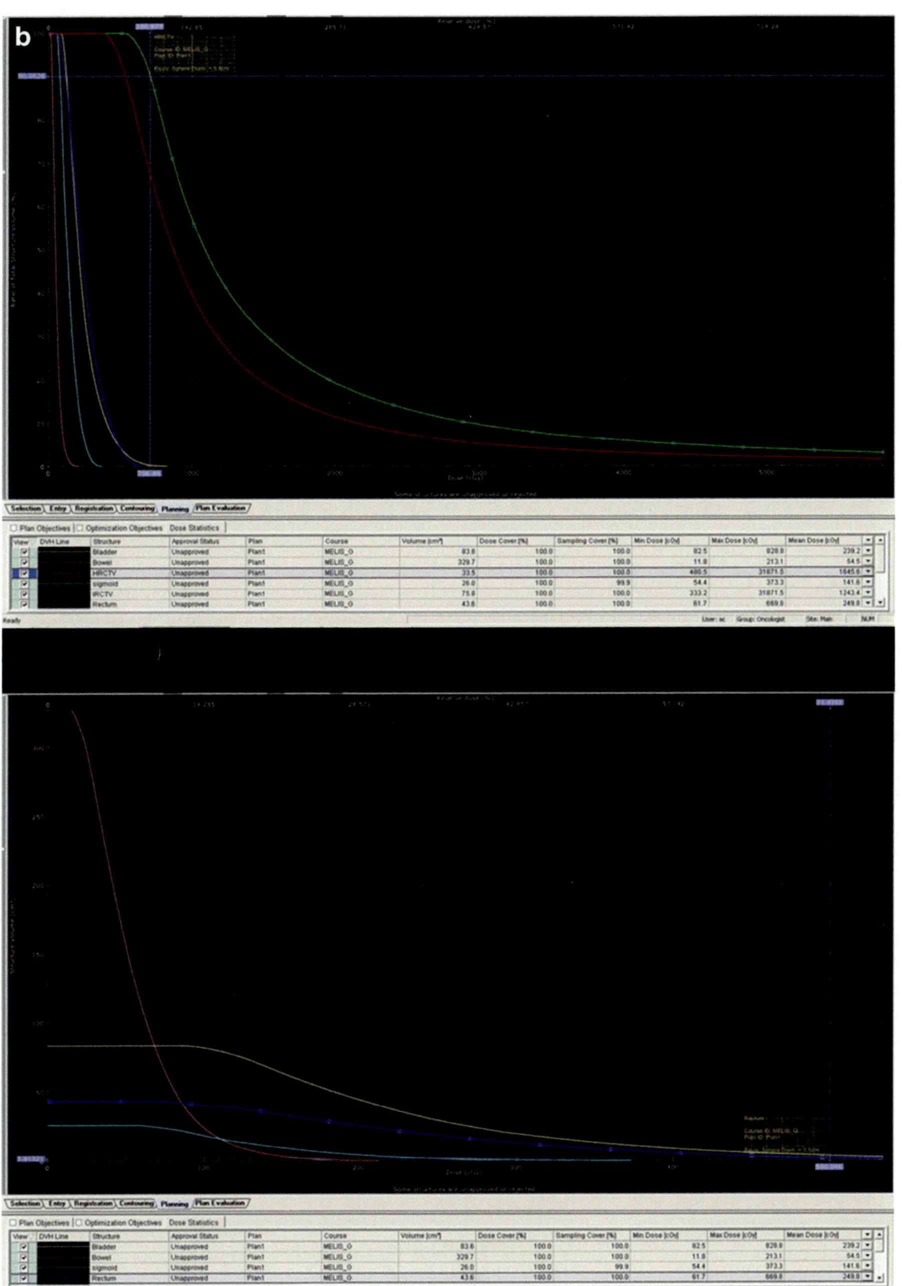

Fig. 7.9 (continued)

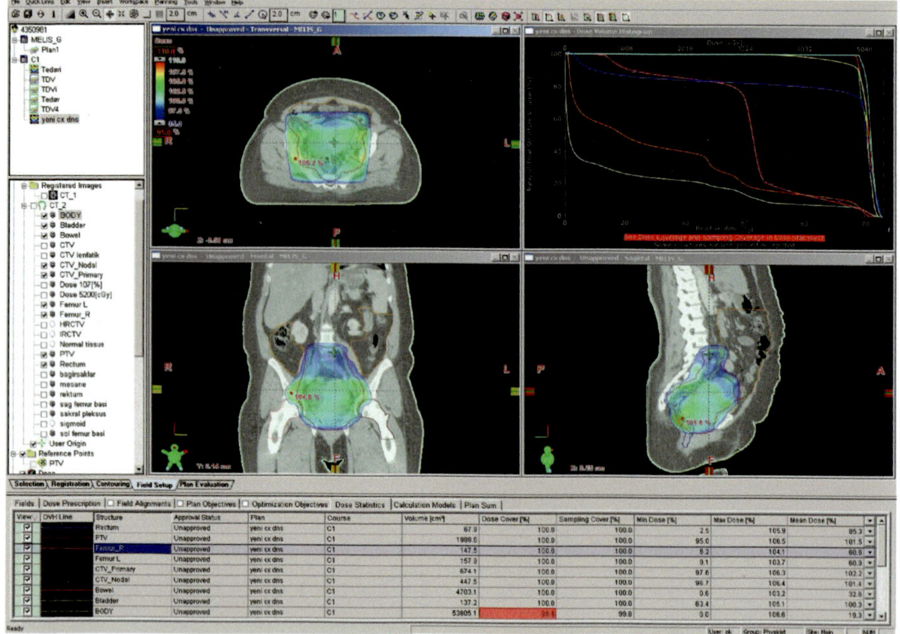

Fig. 7.10 Forward-planning IMRT plan of the patient

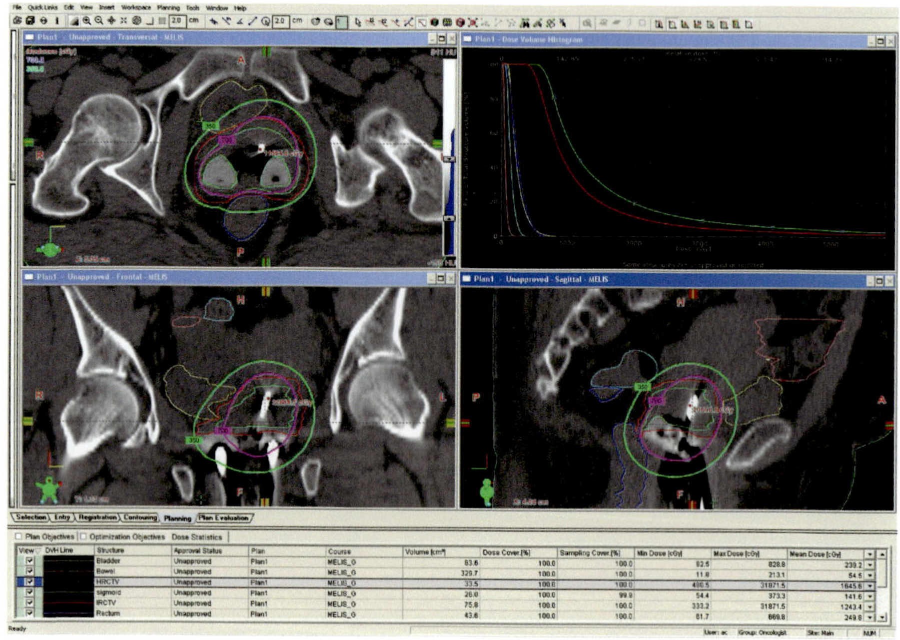

Fig. 7.11 BRT plan of the patient in first fraction

Recommended OARs Doses are Detailed in Below
Small bowel (peritoneal cavity) dose: V45 Gy <195 cm [3], V40 Gy <30%
Bladder dose: V45 Gy <35%
Rectum dose: V30 Gy <60%, V50 Gy <50%
Vaginal surface dose: 100 Gy
Femoral head: V30 Gy <15%, V50 Gy <5%
Bone marrow: Up to 90% receives 10 Gy, up to 37% receives 40 Gy
Kidney dose <18 Gy
Spinal cord dose <45 Gy
Transposed ovaries <8 Gy

7.1.5 BRT Dose

- The prescribed BRT dose depends on the stage and bulk of disease, response to EBRT, and BRT technique [84, 85].
- Different HDR BRT regimens can be used: 5 × 5.5 Gy, 5 × 6 Gy, 4 × 7 Gy, etc.
- Most commonly used LDR BRT regimen is 35–40 Gy in 1–2 insertions.
- For patients with close or positive surgical margin after hysterectomy, a vaginal cylinder or ovoids can be used. Usually, dose is prescribed to the vaginal surface or at 5 mm depth of the upper 3 cm of the vagina (2 × 5.5 Gy at 5 mm, 3 × 6 Gy at vaginal surface, etc.).
- Replanning based on CT- or MRI-imaging with applicator in place is recommended for each fraction. Dose is prescribed to target volumes. For each fraction the following parameters should be recorded: D98 and D90 for GTV, D98 and D90 for HRCTV, D98 for IRCTV, D2cc of bladder, rectum, sigmoid and rectovaginal point. Dose to point A should also be recorded.
- Summation of EBRT and BRT doses must be performed by calculation of a biologically equivalent dose in 2 Gy per fraction (EQD2) using the linear-quadratic model [EQD2 = D × [(d + α/β)/(2 + α/β), α/β = 10 Gy for tumor and α/β = 3 Gy for late responding tissue).
- ICRU 89 recommendations should be followed when planning IGABT [86]. Optimization should be performed with caution to achieve an acceptable dose distribution both HRCTV and OARs. Modifying the dwell positions allows reducing the dose to the OARs and ensuring maximal tumor coverage.

GEC ESTRO Planning Target and OARs Goals [73, 87, 88]
D98 GTV EQD2: >95 Gy
D90 HRCTV EQD2: >90 Gy, <95 Gy
D98 HRCTV EQD2: >75 Gy
D98 IRCTV EQD2: >60 Gy
Point A EQD2: >65 Gy

D2cc rectum ⟨65–75 Gy
D2cc sigmoid ⟨70–75 Gy
D2cc bladder ⟨80–90 Gy
Rectovaginal point EQD2 ⟨65–75 Gy

Interstitial or hybrid BRT systems may be used to treat disease that cannot be adequately covered by intracavitary BRT.

7.1.6 Follow-Up

The optimal surveillance strategy for patients with cervical cancer remains controversial. Following definitive therapy, patients should be seen regularly for careful clinical examination to detect recurrences in early stage that might be amenable to potentially curative salvage therapy [89]. It is suggested that every 3–6 months for the first 2 years, every 6–12 months for years 3–5 and then annually. Surveillance imaging studies should not be routinely performed unless recurrence is suspected. However, PET/CT is often used for prognostic purposes 3–4 months following CRT. Cervicovaginal cytology (Pap smear) is not routinely recommended after RT because it may cause false positivity. However, annual Pap smear should be performed in patients treated with surgery alone [90].

7.2   Endometrial Cancer

Overview
Epidemiology
   Endometrial cancer is the most common gynecologic malignancy in developed countries. It affects predominantly postmenopausal women. It often presents at an early stage due to early warning sign of postmenopausal vaginal bleeding. The main risk factor for endometrial cancer is unopposed estrogen.
   Pathological and biological features
   Endometrioid adenocarcinoma is the most common endometrial cancer which has a favorable prognosis. Other histologic types of endometrial cancer include serous carcinoma, clear cell carcinoma and carcinosarcoma, and they are associated with worse outcomes. Patients with endometrial cancer are initially categorized into risk groups (low-, intermediate- and high-risk) based on risk factors.
   Definitive therapy
   Treatment of endometrial cancer depends on the stage of the disease and patient performance status. Surgery is the main treatment for endometrial cancer. Radiotherapy (RT) plays a significant role in the management of

endometrial cancer both as an adjuvant treatment of surgery or as a definitive treatment for patients with medically inoperable early stage disease or who refuse surgery. RT options include external beam RT (EBRT), brachytherapy (BRT) or both.

Adjuvant therapy

Adjuvant treatment of endometrial cancer following surgery is based on the risk of disease recurrence, which is defined by the stage of disease, histologic subtype, and presence of other prognostic factors (grade, depth of myometrial invasion, lymphovascular space invasion (LVSI), tumor size, patient's age, and lower uterine segment involvement, etc.). Surgery alone is usually adequate treatment for patients with low-risk disease. Patients with intermediate- or high-risk factors may benefit from adjuvant RT, chemotherapy or both.

Keywords: Endometrium cancer, radiotherapy

7.2.1 Case Presentation

7.2.1.1 Case 1

A 66-year-old female admitted to the hospital with a 6-month history of postmenopausal bleeding. She had medical histories of hypertension and diabetes mellitus. She never smoked. Her physical examination revealed no abnormality. Endometrial biopsy revealed grade 1 endometrioid type adenocarcinoma. Chest X-ray, whole blood count, and kidney and liver function tests were normal. She underwent total abdominal hysterectomy (TAH) and bilateral salpingo-oophorectomy (BSO) with pelvic and para-aortic lymph node dissection (LND). Her pathologic evaluation was reported as grade 1, endometrioid type adenocarcinoma with superficial myometrial invasion. The tumor was 3.5 × 2 cm. There was no LVSI, cervical stromal invasion, or adnexal involvement. No metastases were detected in 50 lymph nodes removed. She was classified as International Federation of Gynecology and Obstetrics (FIGO) stage IB, grade 1 intermediate-risk endometrial cancer.

7.2.1.2 Case 2

A 72-year-old female admitted to the hospital with a 12-month history of postmenopausal bleeding. She had a past medical history of controlled diabetes mellitus and hypertension. She never smoked. There were no abnormalities noted on her gynecological examination. Endometrial biopsy revealed grade 1 endometrioid type adenocarcinoma. Chest X-ray, whole blood count, and kidney and liver function tests were normal. She underwent TAH/BSO, pelvic and para-aortic LND and peritoneal washings for cytology. Her pathologic evaluation was reported as grade 1, endometrioid type adenocarcinoma. The largest tumor diameter was 6.5 cm. There was a deep ½ myometrial invasion and LVSI. There was no cervical stromal invasion or adnexal involvement. Peritoneal washing cytology was negative. Out of 30 dissected lymph nodes, 12 were metastatic (5-para-aortic, 7-pelvic). She was classified as FIGO stage IIIC2, grade 1 high-risk endometrial cancer.

7.2.2 Evidence Based Treatment Recommendations

Patients with suspected endometrial cancer should undergo a history and complete pelvic and general physical examination with particular attention to the presence of extrauterine disease [91]. Pelvic or transvaginal sonography is often the first-line imaging study to evaluate other etiologies of abnormal uterine bleeding. Endometrial sampling is the gold standard for the diagnosis and usually performed with an office endometrial biopsy, endometrial curettage (D&C), or hysterectomy specimen. Laboratory tests or imaging studies should be done based on clinical symptoms, physical findings or patient comorbidities to assess disease extent and to decide appropriate treatment (e.g., surgery, chemotherapy, or RT). Measurement of the serum CA 125 level may be useful for predicting extrauterine disease and monitoring clinical response.

After the histopathological diagnosis of endometrial cancer, patients should undergo surgical staging and treatment as appropriate. Staging for endometrial cancer is based on the joint 2017 FIGO/Tumor, Node, Metastasis (TNM) classification system (Table 7.3). Standard surgical staging procedure includes TAH and BSO with pelvic and para-aortic LND [92]. Open, laparoscopic or vaginal approaches can be used for surgery. Minimally invasive surgery is preferred surgical treatment for low- and intermediate-risk patients. Cytoreductive surgery may be required for metastatic implants. FIGO recommends that peritoneal cytology should be collected, but it is not part of the FIGO staging criteria. An omentectomy is usually recommended for patients with serous or clear cell histology.

The extent of surgery (sampling versus LND) for pelvic and paraaortic lymph nodes is controversial [93–96]. At a minimum during surgery, it is recommended to palpate lymph nodes and to remove enlarged or suspicious ones [97]. LND is required for accurate pathologic staging to guide adjuvant treatment recommendations [98]. Two large randomized trials showed no survival benefit of routine LND in low- and intermediate-risk patients, therefore LND is not recommended for these patients [99, 100]. The presence of serous, clear cell, or high-grade histology, myometrial invasion greater than 50%, and large tumor (>2 cm) suggests a benefit for surgical resection of the lymph nodes. The frozen section may help to determine tumor grade and depth of myometrial invasion, however according to the final pathology result a significant portion of low-risk patients shift to high-risk group. The role of sentinel lymph node biopsy for endometrial cancer is not fully established.

Adjuvant treatment of endometrial cancer following surgical staging is based on the risk of disease recurrence, which is defined by the stage of disease, histology of the tumor, and presence of other prognostic factors. These include: grade, depth of myometrial invasion, LVSI, tumor size, patient's age, and lower uterine segment involvement [101]. In high-risk patients (e.g., high grade, deep myometrial invasion) with incomplete surgical staging, computed tomography (CT), magnetic resonance imaging (MRI), or positron emission tomography (PET)/CT is recommended to determine the lymph node status for adjuvant treatment planning [102, 103].

Table 7.3 Staging of endometrial cancer based on FIGO (2009) and AJCC TNM classification (8th edition)

FIGO/TNM Staging			
Primary Tumor (T)			
FIGO	TNM		
TX		Primary tumor cannot be assessed	
T0		No evidence of primary tumor	
Tis*		Carcinoma in situ (preinvasive carcinoma)	
IA	T1a	Tumor limited to endometrium or invades less than one-half of the myometrium	
IB	T1b	Tumor invades one-half or more of the myometrium	
II	T2**	Tumor invades stromal connective tissue of the cervix but does not extend beyond uterus	
IIIA	T3a	Tumor involves serosa and/or adnexa (direct extension or metastasis)	
IIIB	T3b	Vaginal involvement (direct extension or metastasis) or parametrial involvement	
IVA	T4	Tumor invades bladder mucosa and/or bowel mucosa	
(bullous edema is not sufficient to classify a tumor as T4)			
*FIGO staging no longer includes Stage 0 (Tis).			
**Endocervical glandular involvement only should be considered as Stage I and not Stage II.			
Regional Lymph Nodes (N)			
FIGO	TNM		
	NX	Regional lymph nodes cannot be assessed	
	N0	No regional lymph node metastasis	
IIIC1	N1	Regional lymph node metastasis to pelvic lymph nodes	
IIIC2	N2	Regional lymph node metastasis to para-aortic lymph nodes, with or without positive pelvic lymph nodes	
Distant Metastasis (M)			
FIGO	TNM		
M0		No distant metastasis (no pathologic M0; use clinical M to complete stage group)	
IVB	M1	Distant metastasis (includes metastasis to inguinal lymph nodes, intraperitoneal disease, or lung, liver, or bone. It excludes metastasis to para-aortic lymph nodes, vagina, pelvic serosa, or adnexa)	
Stage Grouping			
Stage I	T1	N0	M0
Stage IA	T1a	N0	M0
Stage IB	T1b	N0	M0
Stage II	T2	N0	M0
Stage III	T3	N0	M0
Stage IIIA	T3a	N0	M0
Stage IIIB	T3b	N0	M0
Stage IIIC1	T1,3	N1	M0
Stage IIIC2	T1,3	N2	M0
Stage IVA	T4	AnyN	M0
Stage IVB	AnyT	AnyN	M1

TNM T (tumor) N (regional lymph nodes) M (distant metastasis)

FIGO International Federation of Gynecology and Obstetrics

Used with permission of the American Joint Committee on Cancer (AJCC), Chicago, Illinois. The original source for this material is the AJCC Cancer Staging Manual, Eight Edition (2017) published by Springer Science Business Media LLC, www.springer.com

[a]FIGO staging no longer includes Stage 0 (Tis)

[b]Endocervical glandular involvement only should be considered as stage I and not stage II

7.2.2.1 Low-Risk Endometrial Cancer

Low-risk endometrial cancer is defined as stage I, grade 1 or 2, endometrioid type, ᶜ50% myometrial invasion and LVSI negative disease [104]. The risk of nodal involvement is less than 5%; therefore it is not necessary to perform surgical staging in this patient population. Vaginal BRT may reduce the risk of local recurrence without an improvement in overall survival (OS) [105]. Given the rate of local recurrence is below 5%, adjuvant treatment is not recommended after surgery in low risk endometrial cancer [105–108]. Pelvic RT is associated with an increase the risk of death and a high risk of secondary cancers and treatment-related toxicity [109, 110].

7.2.2.2 Intermediate-Risk Endometrial Cancer

After complete surgical staging, intermediate-risk endometrial cancer is defined as stage I, endometrioid type, grade 1 or 2, ≥50% myometrial invasion and LVSI negative disease [104]. The adjuvant treatment options for women with intermediate-risk disease include observation or vaginal BRT depends on whether or not risk factors are present. The rational for vaginal BRT is to prevent local (vaginal) recurrence.

Several randomized trials have addressed the role of adjuvant pelvic RT in intermediate-risk endometrial cancer and have consistently demonstrated a decrease the risk of locoregional recurrence (from 14% to 4%) without an improvement in OS [108, 111, 112]. All were randomized patients to either pelvic RT or to observation following TAH and BSO. These trials and two meta-analyses demonstrated that pelvic RT although very effective in reducing recurrence, significantly increases the risk of toxicity (predominantly gastrointestinal) [111, 113].

A subset of patients with intermediate-risk endometrial cancer is classified as high-intermediate-risk (HIR) group based on Post-Operative Radiation Therapy in Endometrial Cancer (PORTEC)-1 and Gynecologic Oncology Group (GOG)-99 trial results [108, 112]. The most suitable adjuvant treatment in these patients is pelvic RT to decrease locoregional recurrence. In GOG 99 trial, factors associated with an increased recurrence rate were increasing age, the presence of deep myometrial invasion, grade 2 or 3 histology, or the presence of LVSI [108]. HIR group is defined as follows: (a) ≥70 years of age with one risk factor, (b) age 50–69 years with two risk factors, or (c) any age with all three risk factors. In this trial, two-thirds of all recurrences were observed in patients with HIR disease. By contrast, PORTEC-1 trial defines the HIR group as the presence of two of three clinicopathologic factors: >60 years of age, outer half myometrial invasion, and grade 3 histology [112, 114, 115]. In this trial, patients with HIR factors had an increased pelvic recurrence rate following observation [116].

Nout et al. reported the results of PORTEC-2 trial that, among patients with HIR factors who were treated with vaginal BRT had an excellent vaginal control and a more favorable adverse events and quality of life profile compared with pelvic RT. [114] Although for patients treated with pelvic RT, the incidence of pelvic recurrences was 0.5%, compared to 3.8% (p = 0.02) for those treated with vaginal BRT, there was no difference in OS rates. However, after central pathology review, 14% of the cases were considered as low-intermediate risk disease (grade 1–2 tumors with ≥50% myometrial invasion and without LVSI).

According to the ESMO guideline; HIR endometrial cancer is defined as (1) stage I endometrioid, grade 3, <50% myometrial invasion, regardless of LVSI status or (2) stage I endometrioid, grade 1–2, LVSI unequivocally positive, regardless of depth of invasion [104]. There is a growing interest in using combined chemotherapy and RT to decrease the risk of distant recurrence in addition to the locoregional recurrence in patients with endometrial cancer. Although there are several randomized trials addressing the role of adjuvant chemotherapy in advanced stage endometrial cancer, there is no high quality data for HIR patients [117–123].

The results of 2011 meta-analysis have led to the adoption of adjuvant chemotherapy as a component of combined modality treatment following TAH and BSO for endometrial cancer [124]. There was a significant improvement in progression-free survival (PFS) (HR 0.63, 95% CI 0.44–0.89) and a trend for OS (HR 0.68, 95% CI 0.51–1.06), in favor of platinum-based combination chemotherapy. However, patients included in this trial had both early-stage and advanced-stage (large proportion) disease. Therefore, this data is the rationale for the use of chemotherapy in intermediate-risk patients with high risk factors. Most commonly preferred chemotherapy scheme consist of three to four cycles of carboplatin and paclitaxel following vaginal BRT.

A GOG-249 study randomized 601 patients with HIR and high-risk patients to pelvic RT or vaginal BRT followed by three cycles of carboplatin and paclitaxel chemotherapy [125]. Although relapse-free survival (RFS), OS, and vaginal or distant failure were similar between the two groups, vaginal BRT and chemotherapy arm had a significantly higher risk for pelvic and para-aortic nodal recurrences [126]. Vaginal BRT and chemotherapy arm was associated with significantly more acute toxicity without difference in chronic toxicities.

All patients without LND considered as incompletely staged patients. Pelvic RT can be safely applied in these patients instead of complementary LND [116, 127]. In PORTEC-1 study, 715 patients following TAH and BSO without LND were randomized to pelvic RT or observation [112, 115, 116, 128]. With a median follow-up of 13 years, the rate of 15-year OS (52% vs. 60%, respectively, p = 0.14), distant metastases (9% vs. 7%, p = 0.25), and second primary cancers (22% vs. 16%, p = 0.10) was similar between the treatment arms. The 15-year locoregional recurrence rate was significantly improved with pelvic RT (6% vs. 16%, p < 0.0001).

7.2.2.3 High-Risk Endometrial Cancer

High-risk endometrial cancer represents a heterogeneous group of patients which includes stage I grade 3 deeply invasive endometrioid carcinoma; stage II endometrioid carcinoma; stage III endometrioid carcinoma without residual disease; and non-endometrioid carcinoma (serous, clear cell, undifferentiated carcinoma or carcinosarcoma) regardless of stage. Women with high-risk endometrial cancer have an increased risk of pelvic recurrence and distant metastases that causes poor prognosis. Although adjuvant treatment is usually recommended after surgery to improve locoregional control, the effect on OS is unclear [129–137]. In a subgroup of patients who had stage IIIC disease, adjuvant RT may improve OS [117].

Combined RT and chemotherapy is recommended as opposed to either alone in high-risk disease [138]. Pelvic RT is usually indicated to improve locoregional control, whereas adjuvant chemotherapy is used to prevent distant metastases. Although combination of these treatments may increase the treatment related toxicity, it is a reasonable standard of care. Carboplatin and paclitaxel is the preferred combination chemotherapy regimen. However, the optimal sequence of chemotherapy and RT remains unclear [139–142]. RT can be administered in 3 ways: (1) After completion of six cycles of chemotherapy, (2) Between three cycles of chemotherapy before and after RT (Sandwiched method), (3) Concurrently with chemotherapy.

The RTOG 9708 phase II study provides initial support for concurrent chemoradiotherapy (CRT) followed by adjuvant chemotherapy [120]. Forty-six patients with high-risk endometrial cancer were treated with postoperative pelvic RT with concurrent two cycles of cisplatin (50 mg/m^2 on days 1 and 28) followed by four additional courses of cisplatin (50 mg/m^2) and paclitaxel (175 mg/m^2) at 28 days interval. At 4-years, OS rates were 85% for the whole group and 77% for stage III patients. Following this study, recently completed PORTEC-3 and GOG 258 trials were designed to evaluate the role of combined cisplatin-based CRT plus adjuvant chemotherapy compared with either RT alone or chemotherapy alone, respectively, in patients with high-risk and advanced stage endometrial cancer [143]. Based on PORTEC-3 trial, CRT plus adjuvant chemotherapy demonstrated better 5-year failure-free survival (FFS) (69% vs. 58%; HR 0.66, 95% CI 0.45–0.97), but not OS (79% vs. 70%; HR 0.69, 95% CI 0.44–1.09) in patients with stage III disease compared to RT alone. With a median follow-up of 42 months, CRT increased adverse events and reduced health-related quality of life during 2 years, with rapid recovery thereafter [144]. The GOG 258 trial randomized 813 patients with optimally debulked (<2 cm residual disease) stage III to IVA endometrioid or stage I to II serous or clear cell carcinoma and positive cytology to CRT receiving cisplatin and volume-directed RT followed by four cycles of carboplatin and paclitaxel versus chemotherapy alone receiving six cycles of carboplatin and paclitaxel [135]. The preliminary results of this trial at a median follow-up of 47 months showed that the addition of RT reduced the local (vaginal) recurrence rate (3% vs. 7%; HR 0.36, 95% CI 0.16–0.82) and pelvic/para-aortic relapses (10% vs. 21%; 0.43, 95% CI 0.28–0.66) without differences in RFS (HR 0.9, 95% CI 0.74–1.10) or distant recurrence rates (28% vs. 21%; HR 1.36, 95% CI 1.0–1.86) compared to chemotherapy alone. Rates of ≥grade 3 acute toxicities were similar between the CRT and chemotherapy alone arms. Despite these trials questioning the role of CRT in advanced stage disease, the addition of RT may decrease locoregional recurrences.

Stage II tumors have been described as having cervical stromal invasion. These tumors more often associated with grade 3 histology and deep myometrial invasion, and have a high risk of recurrence [106]. No OS difference between radical hysterectomy and simple hysterectomy [145]. Adjuvant pelvic RT plays a significant role in stage II disease after surgery. Although the role of BRT boost after pelvic RT is controversial, it is a clear role in positive vaginal margin [146]. Based on SEER analysis, in patients with stage IIIC endometrial cancer who had direct extension of the primary tumor, the addition of BRT to pelvic RT improved OS [147]. Other studies have found no difference in local recurrence or OS rates, but it was associated with increased risk of toxicity [148–153].

Non-endometrioid cancers (uterine serous and clear cell tumors) represent an infrequent subset of endometrial cancer. Due to its rarity, it has been difficult to make evidence-based treatment recommendations. Adjuvant chemotherapy is often recommended for these patients because of the high rates of distant metastases [154]. In the largest retrospective study, Viswanathan et al. showed that for patients with uterine serous cancers, combined chemotherapy and RT had a survival benefit [155]. Conversely, a subgroup analysis of the NSGO 9501/EORTC 55991 and MaNGO-ILIADE III trials did not show a survival benefit for patients with serous or clear-cell tumors [132]. One retrospective study investigated the role of vaginal BRT alone for stage I serous or clear-cell tumors and showed that it was adequate adjuvant local therapy for patients with stage IA disease [156]. RT may be preferred in clear cell histology due to the poor response to chemotherapy [157].

7.2.2.4 Inoperable Patients

For patients with medically inoperable stage I endometrial carcinoma, primary RT either intrauterine BRT alone or combination of pelvic RT and BRT should be considered [158, 159]. With RT, 2-year local control rates can be achieved over 90%.

For patients with unresectable stage III or IV disease can be treated with chemotherapy alone. Surgical cytoreduction may have a role in retrospective series [160–163]. Palliative pelvic RT should be considered in patients with symptomatic disease. Selected phase III randomized controlled trials and metaanalyses in cervical cancer are summarized in Table 7.4.

7.2.3 Treatment Recommendations

Adjuvant therapy recommendations for the treatment of endometrial cancer according to the risk groups are summarized in Table 7.5.

Table 7.4 Selected phase III randomized controlled trials and metaanalyses in endometrial cancer

Reference	Characteristics	Treatment	FU (mo/y)	Clinical outcome	Toxicity
Low risk					
Sorbe [105]	645 pts Stage IA (FIGO 2009), E-type, Gr 1–2 TAH+BSO+LN sampling+peritoneal cytology	BRT vs. NFT BRT: HDR/LDR, 3–6 frx, 3–8 Gy	68	5-year CSS 98.4% (No difference) 5-year OS 96.1% (No difference) Vaginal recurrence: 1.2% vs. 3.1%, p = 0.114 All located in the upper 2/3 of the vagina	Dysuria, frequency, and incontinence: 2.8% vs. 0.6%

Intermediate risk					
Creutzberg [112] (PORTEC-1) Scholten [128] (update of PORTEC-1) Creutzberg [116] (update of PORTEC-1)	715 pts Stage IA Gr 2–3, IB Gr 1–2 (FIGO 2009) TAH+BSO, no LND Central pathology review	Pelvic EBRT vs. NFT RT: 2 Gy/46 Gy	52 97 13.3 year	5-year LRR: 4% vs. 14%, p < 0.001 (mostly vaginal 73%) 5-year OS: 81% vs. 85%, p = 0.31 Endometrial-Ca-related death: 9% vs. 6%, p = 0.37 10-year LRR: 5% vs. 14%, p < 0.0001 10-year OS: 66% vs. 73%, p = 0.09 Endometrial-Ca-related death: 11% vs. 9%, p = 0.47 High-risk: At least 2 of 3 risk factors ($\geq$60 year, Gr 3, and $\geq$50% MI) High-risk: 10-year LRR 4.6% vs. 23.1% 15-year LRR: 5.8% vs. 15.5%, p < 0.0001 (mostly vaginal, NFT 74%) 15-year OS 52% vs. 60%, p = 0.14 15-year FFS 50% vs. 54%, p = 0.94 HIR group: 15-year OS 41% vs. 48%, p = 0.51, 15-year endometrial Ca-related death 14% vs. 13% 15-year DMs 9.3% vs. 7.1%, p = 0.25 Second primary cancers over 15 year: 22% vs. 16%, p = 0.10	Late: 25% vs. 6%, p < 0.0001

(continued)

Table 7.4 (continued)

Reference	Characteristics	Treatment	FU (mo/y)	Clinical outcome	Toxicity
Keys [108] (GOG 99)	392 pts TAH+BSO+Selective BPPLND+peritoneal cytology Stage IA, IB, or occult II (FIGO 2009) HIR: Gr 2–3, LVSI+, and deep MI; ‛50 year with all risk factors, 50–70 year with any 2 risk factors, >70 with any risk factor	No adjuvant therapy vs. pelvic EBRT RT: 1.8 Gy/50.4 Gy	69	2-year recurrence: 12% vs. 3%, $p = 0.007$ (HIR: 26% vs. 6%) 2-year isolated LR: 7.4% vs. 1.6% 4-year OS: 86% vs. 92%, $p = 0.557$	Serious adverse events 13% RT: more frequent and more severe toxicity ($p < 0.001$)
Kong [113] (metaanalysis)	Stage I	Role of adjuvant RT 7 trials: EBRT vs. no EBRT (or BRT) 1 trial: BRT vs. no treatment		EBRT: Reduced LRR (HR = 0.36) No improvement in OS (HR = 0.99) No improvement in CSS (HR = 0.96) No improvement in DMs (RR = 1.04) Low-risk (Gr 1–2, ‛50% MI): EBRT increased endometrial Ca–related death (RR = 2.64) Intermediate-risk (IC or Gr 3): No difference in OS (HR = 1.05) or CSS (HR = 1.03)	EBRT: increased risk of severe acute and late toxicity, and reduced QOL scores Severe acute Gr 3 or 4: RR = 4.68 Severe late Gr 3 or 4: RR = 2.58

Nout [114] (PORTEC-2)	427 pts Stage I-IIA HIR: 1) >60 year and stage 1B Gr 1 or 2 , or stage 1A Gr 3 (FIGO 2009) TAH+BSO, no routine LND	BRT vs. Pelvic EBRT RT: 2 Gy/46 Gy BRT: HDR (3 frx/21 Gy) or LDR 30 Gy	45	5-year vaginal recurrence: 1.8% vs. 1.6%, p = 0.74 5-year LRR: 5.1% vs. 2.1%, p = 0.17 5-year pelvic recurrence 3.8% vs. 0.5%, p = 0.02 DMs were similar (8.3% vs. 5.7%, p = 0.46) No differences in OS (84.8% vs. 79.6%, p = 0.57) No differences in DFS (82.7% vs. 78.1%, p = 0.74)	Acute Gr 1–2 GI: 12.6% vs. 53.8% Late Gr 3 GI: <1% vs. 2% (requiring surgery for bowel obstruction)
Blake [111] (Metaanalysis)	905 pts MRC ASTEC/NCIC CTG EN.5 Intermediate or high-risk Stage IA, Gr 3; IB, any Gr; S/CC, all stages, any Gr (FIGO 2009)	Adjuvant EBRT vs. NFT Pelvic RT: 40–46 Gy ±BRT (2 frx, 4 Gy HDR or 15 Gy LDR)	58	No difference in OS (HR 1.05) No difference in CSS (HR 1.13) ASTEC/EN.5: 53% BRT, NFT 5-year LR 6·1%	Severe or life threatening acute: 3% vs. <1% Severe or life threatening late: 8% vs. <3%
Johnson [124] (metaanalysis)	5 RCTs Surgery	Adjuvant RT + chemo vs. RT alone Adjuvant chemo vs. RT		OS advantage of adjuvant chemo (RR 0.88) Modern platinum based chemo: RR of death 0.85 HR for OS 0.74, significantly favoring the addition of postoperative platinum based chemo HR for PFS 0.75 Chemo reduces first recurrence outside the pelvis (RR 0.79), 5% absolute risk reduction Pelvic recurrence: Chemo less effective than RT (RR 1.28), may have added value when used with RT (RR 0.48)	

(continued)

Table 7.4 (continued)

Reference	Characteristics	Treatment	FU (mo/y)	Clinical outcome	Toxicity
Sorbe [149]	527 pts Medium-risk: stage I, E-type, one of the risk factors: FIGO Gr 3, deep MI, or DNA aneuploidy TAH+BSO+LN sampling	EBRT + BRT vs. BRT	62	5-year LRR: 1.5% vs. 5%, p = 0.013 5-year OS 89% vs. 90%, p = 0.548 Endometrial-Ca-related death: 3.8% vs. 6.8%, p = 0.118 EBRT+BRT: Pelvic recurrences (exclusively vaginal) reduced by 93%	Gr 3 late: ˂2% All Gr 1–3: 14.5% vs. 2.7%
Aalders [137] (Norwegian trial) Onsrud [110] (update of Norwegian trial)	540 pts Stage I TAH+BSO, no LND	BRT → EBRT vs. BRT alone	3–10 year 20.5 year	Vaginal and pelvic recurrences: 1.9% vs. 6.9%, p < 0.01 DMs %9.9 vs. 5.4% No difference in 5-year OS Gr 3, deep MI: Benefit from additional EBRT No difference in OS (20.50 y vs. 20.48 y, p = 0.186) ˂60 year: Higher mortality rates after EBRT (HR 1.36, 95% CI, 1.06–1.76) ˂60 year: Secondary cancer increased after EBRT (HR 2.02; 95% CI, 1.30–3.15)	Gr 3–4: 2.9% vs. 0%
Randall [126] (GOG 249)	601 pts Stage I E-type HIR (GOG 99 criteria), stage II or stage I-II S/CC Hysterectomy ± LND	Pelvic EBRT ± BRT vs. BRT → Chemo RT: 45 Gy Chemo: Carboplatin and paclitaxel, 3 cycles	53	3-year RFS: 82% for both 3-year OS: 91% vs. 88% Vaginal or distant failure: no difference BRT + chemo: Pelvic/PA recurrences more common	BRT + chemo: Acute toxicity was more common and severe Late: no difference

High-risk

Morrow [134]	Clinically stage I or II (occult) ≥1 risk factors: >50% MI, pelvic/PA LN+, cervical involvement, or adnexal metastases	EBRT → Doxorubicin vs. No doxorubicin		OS or PFS: No difference Recurrence pattern: no difference	No cases of Gr 3 or 4 cardiac toxicity RT: 6.9% small bowel obstruction
Randall [129] (GOG 122)	422 pts Stage III or IV Postoperative residue ≤2 cm All histologies	WAI vs. Doxorubicin and Cisplatin RT: 20 frx/30 Gy + 15 Gy pelvic boost Chemo: Doxorubicin 60 mg/m^2 and cisplatin 50 mg/m^2 every 3 weeks, seven cycles, followed by one cycle of cisplatin	74	Chemo: HR for progression adjusted for stage 0.71, p < 0.01 Chemo: HR for stage-adjusted death 0.68, p < 0.01 Pelvic recurrence 13% vs. 18% Distant recurrence 38% vs. 32% 5-year PFS: 42% vs. 38% 5-year OS: 53% vs. 42%	Greater acute toxicity was seen with chemo Treatment related death: 2% vs. 4%
Maggi [131] (Italian study)	345 pts High-risk: IC Gr 3, II Gr 3 with deep MI or III	Adjuvant chemo vs. EBRT Chemo: Cisplatin (50 mg/m^2), doxorubicin (45 mg/m^2), cyclophosphamide (600 mg/m^2), every 28 days, 5 cycles RT: 45–50 Gy	95.5	No significant HR for death of 0.95, p = 0.77 No significant HR for event of 0.88, p = 0.45 3-, 5- and 7-year OS: 78, 69 and 62% in RT group and 76, 66 and 62% in chemo group 3-, 5- and 7-year PFS: 69, 63 and 56% in RT group and 68, 63 and 60% in chemo group RT delayed LR and chemo delayed metastases	Both treatments were well tolerated

(continued)

Table 7.4 (continued)

Reference	Characteristics	Treatment	FU (mo/y)	Clinical outcome	Toxicity
Susumi [130] (JGOG Study)	385 pts Intermediate- and high-risk Stage IC-IIIC, >50% MI LIR: Stage IC, ＜70 year, Gr 1/2 E-type HIR: Stage IC, >70 year, Gr 3 E-type; stage II or IIIA (+cytology)	Adjuvant pelvic EBRT vs. chemo Chemo: Cyclophosphamide (333 mg/m^2), doxorubicin (40 mg/m^2), cisplatin (50 mg/m^2), every 4 weeks, $\geq$3 cycles RT: $\geq$40 Gy		No differences in 5-year PFS (83.5% vs. 81.8%) No differences in 5-year OS (85.3% vs. 86.7%) LIR: No differences in PFS or OS HIR: Higher PFS (83.8% vs. 66.2%, p = 0.024) and higher OS (89.7% vs. 73.6%, p = 0.006) with chemo	Adverse events: No difference (1.6% vs. 4.7%)
Kuoppala [136] (Finn study)	156 pts High-risk Stage IA-IB Gr 3 (n = 28), stage IC-IIIA Gr 1–3 (n = 128)	RT vs. RT + chemo CT: Cisplatin (50 mg/m^2), epirubicin (60 mg/m^2), cyclophosphamide (500 mg/m^2), 3 cycles RT: 56 Gy	60	5-year OS: 84.7% vs. 82.1%, p = 0.148 Median DFS: 18 mo vs. 25 mo, p = 0.134 Median time to recurrence: 15 mo vs. 20 mo, p = 0.170	Chemo: Acceptable rate of acute toxicity Gr 3–4 nausea <8% Gr 3 infection 6.2% Intestinal complications and surgery: 2.7% vs. 9.5%
Hogberg [132] (NSGO-EC-9501/ EORTC-55991 and MaNGO ILIADE-III)	540 pts TAH+BSO, LND optional No residue Stage-I-III	Adjuvant RT ± chemo ERT: $\geq$44 Gy ± BRT CT (83%): Doxorubicin/epirubicin (50 mg/m^2) and cisplatin (50 mg/m^2) every 4 weeks, 4 cycles		PFS favoring CRT: HR 0.63, p = 0.009 NSGO/EORTC-trial (HR 0.64, p = 0.04) MaNGO-trial: no significant difference (HR 0.61, p = 0.10) Pooled analysis: trend for improved OS (82% vs. 75%, p = 0.07)	

Park [138] (metaanalysis)	High-risk 3 observational studies and 3 RCT	Adjuvant chemo + RT vs. Adjuvant RT		Chemo + RT: survival benefit in advanced stage (OS HR 0.53; PFS HR 0.54) No benefit in early stage (OS HR 0.96; PFS HR 1.00)	
Galaal [133] (metaanalysis)	1269 pts Stage III-IV 4 RCT Primary cytoreductive surgery	Adjuvant chemo vs. RT or CRT		Adjuvant chemo: OS (HR 0.75) and PFS (HR 0.74) were longer Chemo increases survival by approximately 25% in stage III-IV pts	Chemo: More haematological and neurological toxicity and alopecia (RR 5.73) No difference in treatment-related deaths (RR 1.67)
Gao [139] (metaanalysis)	Advanced stage 5 articles	Sandwich method: Chemo-Involved field RT-additional chemo		3-year PFS: 68% (p = 0.77) 3-year OS 75% (p = 0.01)	Pooled analysis of toxicity was not performed (heterogeneity)
Matei [135] (GOG 258)	813 pts Stage III-IVA E-type (≤2 cm residue) or I-II S/ CC and cytology positive Optimal debulking	CRT → Chemo vs. Chemo alone CRT: Cisplatin and RT → Four 21 day cycles Carboplatin + Paclitaxel Chemo: Cisplatin days 1. and 28, 50 mg/m^2; Carboplatin AUC5; Paclitaxel 175 mg/m^2 Chemo alone: Six 21 day cycles Carboplatin + Paclitaxel Pelvic EBRT: 45 Gy ± BRT boost	47	No differences in RFS (HR 0.9) No difference in distant recurrence (28% vs. 21%; HR 1.36) RT reduced vaginal recurrences (3% vs. 7%; HR 0.36) RT reduced pelvic and PA relapses (10% vs. 21%)	>Gr 3: 58% vs. 63%

(continued)

Table 7.4 (continued)

Reference	Characteristics	Treatment	FU (mo/y)	Clinical outcome	Toxicity
de Boer [139] (PORTEC-3)	660 pts High-risk FIGO 2009 stage I, E-type Gr 3 with deep MI or LVSI (or both) Stage II-II E-type Stage I-III S/CC	CRT → Chemo vs. Pelvic EBRT alone CRT: 2 cycles of cisplatin 50 mg/m^2 given during RT Chemo: 4 cycles of Carboplatin (AUC5) + Paclitaxel (175 mg/m^2) Pelvic EBRT: 1.8 Gy/48.6 Gy If cervical involvement: BRT boost (2 × 5 Gy, HDR)	60.2	5-year OS: 81·8% vs. 76·7%, p = 0.11 5-year FFS: 75·5% vs. 68·6%, p = 0.022 Stage I-II 80.8% vs. 76.6%, p = 0.47 Stage III 69.3% vs. 58%, p = 0.031 5-year pelvic recurrence: 4.9% vs. 9.2%, p = 0.026 ≥70 year had the greatest benefit from CRT	Acute ≥Gr 3: 60% vs. 12%, p < 0.0001 ≥Gr 2 sensory neuropathy at 3-year: 8% vs. 1%, p < 0.0001

Abbreviations: *FU* follow-up, *mo* months, *y* years, *pts* patients, *FIGO* International Federation of Gynecology and Obstetrics, *E* endometrioid, *Gr* grade, *TAH* total abdominal hysterectomy, *BSO* bilateral salpingo-oophorectomy, *LN* lymph node, *BRT* brachytherapy, *NFT* no further treatment, *HDR* high dose rate, *LDR* low dose rate, *frx* fraction, *Gy* gray, *CSS* cancer specific survival, *OS* overall survival, *PORTEC* post operative radiation therapy in endometrial carcinoma, *LND* lymph node dissection, *EBRT* external beam radiotherapy, *RT* radiotherapy, *LRR* locoregional recurrence, *Ca* cancer, *MI* myometrial invasion, *FFS* failure-free survival, *HIR* high intermediate risk, *DM* distant metastasis, *GOG* Gynecologic Oncology Group, *BPPLND* bilateral pelvic/para-aortic lymph node dissection, *LVSI* lymphovascular space invasion, *LR* local recurrence, *HR* hazard ratio, *QOL* quality of life, *RR* relative risk, *DFS* disease-free survival, *GI* gastrointestinal, *MRC ASTEC* Medical Research Council A Study in the Treatment of Endometrial Cancer, *NCIC CTGEN.5* National Cancer Institute of Canada Clinical Trials Group EN.5 Trial, *S* serous, *CC* clear cell, *RCT* randomized controlled trial, *chemo* chemotherapy, *DNA* deo, *CI* confidence interval, *RFS* relapse-free survival, *PA* para-aortic, *PFS* progression-free survival, *WAI* whole abdominal irradiation, *JGOG* Japanese Gynecologic Oncology Group, *LIR* low intermediate risk, *NSGO-EC* Nordic Society of Gynaecological Oncology-Endometrial Cancer, *EORTC* European Organisation for Research and Treatment of Cancer, *MaNGO* Gynaecological Oncology Group at the Mario Negri Institute, *CRT* chemoradiotherapy, *AUC* area under curve

Table 7.5 Adjuvant therapy recommendations for the treatment of endometrial cancer according to the risk groups

- **Low-risk**
  - Stage IA Gr 1–2, endometrioid type, no LVSI
  - *No adjuvant treatment is recommended following surgery*
- **Intermediate-risk**
  - Stage IB Gr 1–2, endometrioid type, no LVSI
  - *The adjuvant treatment options include observation or vaginal BRT*
- **High-intermediate (HIR) risk**
  - Stage IA Gr 3, endometrioid type, ±LVSI
  - Stage IA-B Gr 1–2, endometrioid type, LVSI+
  - *If surgical nodal staging performed, vaginal BRT alone is recommended*
  - *If no surgical nodal staging:*
    LVSI (+): Pelvic EBRT
    Gr 3, LVSI (−): vaginal BRT alone
  - *Role of systemic therapy is not clear*
- **High-risk**
  - Stage IB Gr 3, endometrioid type, ±LVSI
  - Stage II, endometrioid type
  - Stage III, endometrioid type, no residual disease
  - Non-endometrioid (serous, clear-cell, undifferentiated carcinoma, or carcinosarcoma), regardless of stage
  - *Combined pelvic EBRT (±para-aortic) and chemotherapy is recommended*
- **Advanced stage or metastatic disease**
  - Stage III, residual disease or stage IVA
  - Stage IVB
  - *Systemic therapy is recommended*

RT may be indicated for primary tumors that are unresectable or symptomatic

7.2.4 Treatment Planning

7.2.4.1 Simulation

- Patients are usually CT simulated in the supine position, arms above chest with immobilization devices (**Fig. 7.12**). They also simulated in the prone position using a "belly board" which displace small bowel from the treatment field and reduce toxicity.
- Prior to simulation, patients undergo a standard bladder and bowel preparation. Rectum should be empty (≤3.5 cm) during CT simulation and daily treatment.
- Two CT data sets obtained at simulation for intensity modulated RT (IMRT): (1) with full bladder (2) with empty bladder. These images then should be fused to account for organ motion. During RT, the patient must be treated with the bladder full.
- Oral contrast may be used to opacify small bowel. A vaginal or rectal marker may be used to define the vaginal cuff and the rectum.
- Intravenous (IV) contrast may be helpful to localize pelvic vascular structures for contouring.

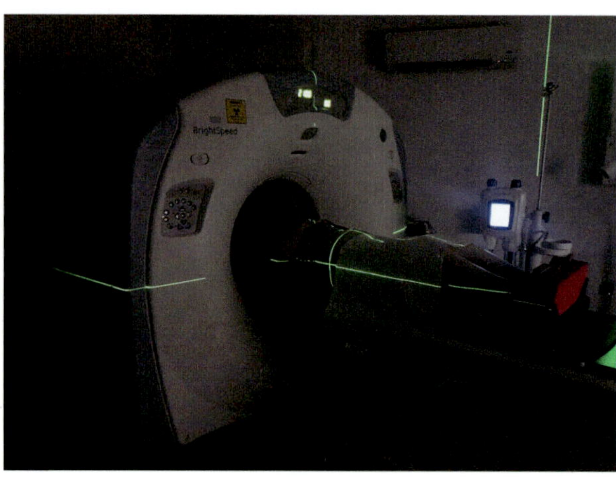

Fig. 7.12 Immobilization and simulation procedures

7.2.4.2 Contouring

External Beam Radiotherapy

- In patients with endometrial cancer, "tumor-directed RT" indicated based on the risk factors. It refers to RT directed at sites of known or suspected to harbor disease and may include EBRT directed to the pelvis with or without the para-aortic region and/or vaginal BRT.
- Traditionally, a four-field "box" (anteroposterior/posteroanterior (AP/PA) and opposed lateral) technique is used. With conventional 2-dimensional (2D) RT, RT field borders are determined by anatomical landmarks, often skeletal anatomy. The superior field border is placed at the L4-L5 interspace. For lymph node negative postoperative cases superior field edge can be reduced to L5-S1 interspace. The distal field border is placed at the bottom of the obturator foramen or at least 3 cm below the vaginal cuff (defined by the vaginal marker). Lateral borders are placed at least a 1.5 cm lateral to the pelvic brim. The lateral portal superior and inferior borders remain the same as for AP/PA fields. Posterior border is placed at least at the S2-S3 interspace and the anterior border placed in front of the symphysis pubis. Custom blocks used to shield small bowel and femoral heads. This technique resulting in substantial irradiation of normal organs such as small bowel, rectum and bone marrow.
- Extended field pelvic and para-aortic RT (EFRT) technique is mainly used for patients with evidence of para-aortic lymph node metastases. The lower border is the same as in the superior pelvic field border. Upper border is extended usually to the T12-L1 interspace or to the level of the renal vessels.
- Treatment plans can be developed using 3-dimensional conformal RT (3DCRT) or IMRT/volumetric-modulated arc therapy (VMAT) techniques based on CT images. Nowadays, IMRT has been standard treatment option for the postoperative cases [62]. It allows greater organs at risk (OARs) sparing thus reduce

hematologic, gastrointestinal and urinary toxicity especially in treating the para-aortic region [164].

- IMRT plan is usually created using 5–7 coplanar fields and 6 MV photon beams. It is feasible if careful attention to target volume definitions, reproducibility of treatment and quality assurance. For proper delivery of IMRT routine daily online image guidance (i.e., cone-beam CT) is essential.

- Small et al. reported on consensus guidelines for delineation of clinical target volume (CTV) for pelvic IMRT in postoperative treatment of endometrial and cervical cancer to standardize target volume definition [62].

- Gross target volume (GTV) (if present), CTV, planning target volume (PTV), and OARs should be defined in conformal RT, especially for IMRT.

- Postoperative pelvic EBRT should target the pelvic lymph nodes, including obturator, external, internal, and lower common iliac groups (nodal CTV), and upper 1/3 vagina and parametrial/paravaginal tissues (vaginal CTV) [62]. If patients have gross cervical involvement presacral lymph nodes should be included. If para-aortic lymph nodes involved, in addition to the pelvic lymph nodes, the pericaval, interaortacaval, and para-aortic lymph nodes should be contoured (refers to as extended field RT).

- Nodal CTV should start from 7 mm below the L4-L5 interspace to the level of the superior aspect of the femoral heads for external iliac and at the level of S3 for the presacral lymph nodes (if gross cervical involvement). A nodal CTV is defined as the iliac vessels plus an additional circumferential margin of 7 mm (excluding bowel, muscles and bone). It also should cover contiguous gross or suspicious lymph nodes, lymphoceles, and surgical clips. An additional margin of 7 mm is added in all directions to create nodal PTV. Vaginal CTV should include the gross disease (if present), vaginal cuff and 3 cm below the vaginal marker and parametrial/paravaginal tissues from the vaginal cuff to the medial edge of the internal obturator muscle or ischial ramus on each side. The inferior margin of the vaginal CTV is often at the 1 cm above the inferior extent of the obturator foramen. The rectum, bladder, bone, and muscle should be excluded from the vaginal CTV. To account for vaginal mobility due to bladder filling changes, vaginal CTV is countered using a full-bladder CT scan fused to an empty-bladder CT scan. Then integrated target volume (ITV) created by full bladder plus empty bladder vaginal CTVs (for IMRT planning). A 7 mm margin around ITV in all directions is used to define vaginal PTV.

- Small bowel, rectum, bladder and bilateral femoral heads should be defined as OARs in all patients with full bladder CT. If EFRT has been used, bilateral kidneys and spinal cord should also be delineated.

- Use of the IGRT system allows reduction of the PTV margin and obviates the need for an ITV, with the daily control of bladder and rectal filling.

Case Contouring: Delineation of target volumes for the case 2 is shown in Fig. 7.13.

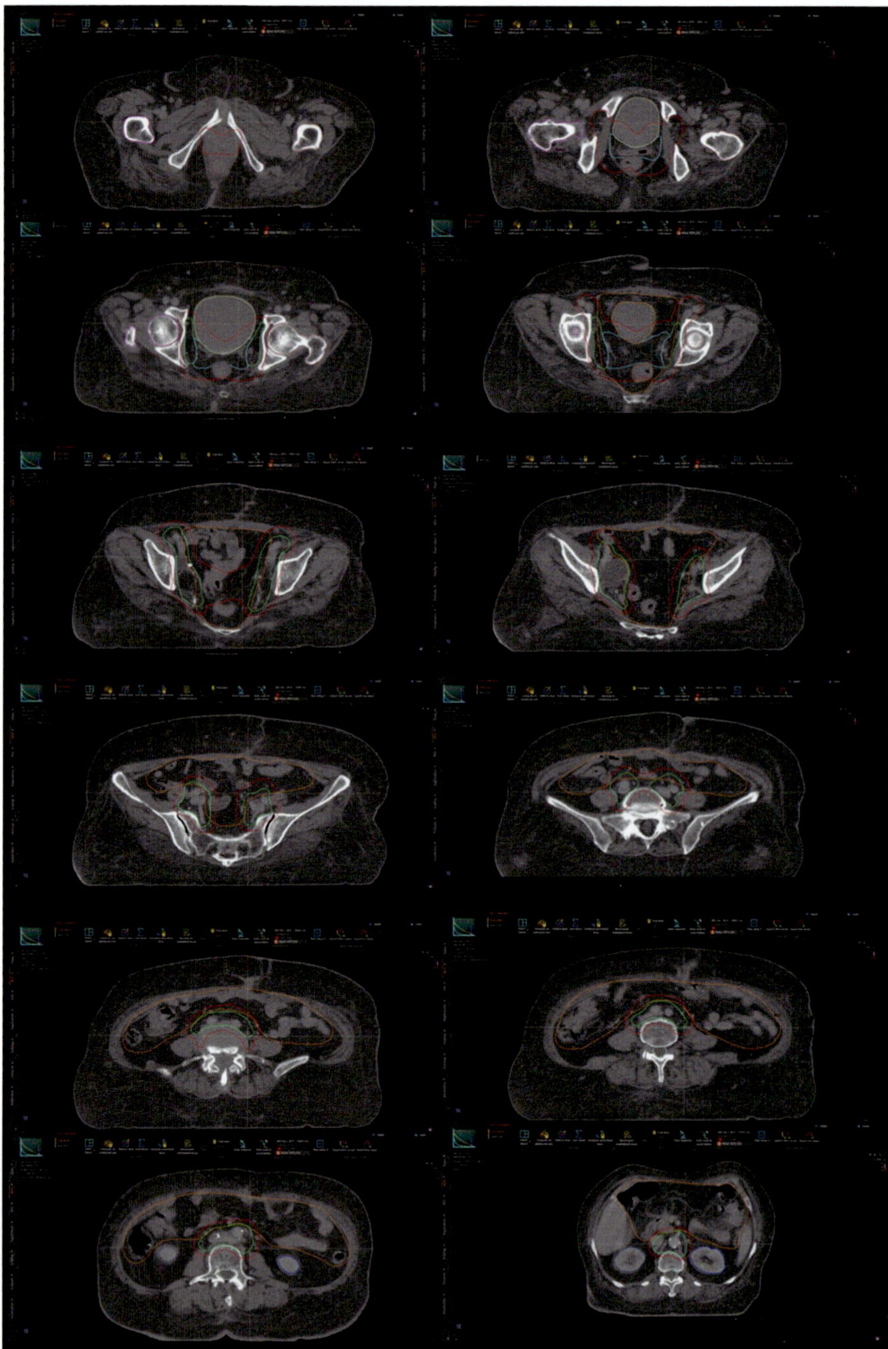

Fig. 7.13 Delineation of target volumes for pelvic and para-aortic EBRT of the patient with FIGO stage IIIC2 endometrial cancer (Case 2). Red: PTV, green: CTV lymphatic, cyan: CTV vagina, brown: rectum, yellow: bladder, orange: bowel, pink: left femur, magenta: right femur, blue: left kidney, dark blue: right kidney, light green: spinal cord

Brachytherapy

- Vaginal BRT allows delivery of a very high dose to the vaginal mucosa while sparing the surrounding OARs.
- Although vaginal BRT is most commonly delivered postoperatively, it can also be used in inoperable patients as a definitive treatment.
- Adjuvant vaginal BRT alone can be used in intermediate-risk endometrial cancer. For patients with positive or close vaginal surgical margins, grade 3 disease, extensive LVSI or cervical stromal invasion after hysterectomy, BRT may be used as a boost to EBRT.
- BRT can be delivered with either a low dose rate (LDR), pulse dose rate (PDR), or high dose rate (HDR) system. Currently, HDR vaginal BRT has been most commonly used on an outpatient basis.
- Vaginal BRT should be delivered 4–6 weeks postoperatively to allow for adequate vaginal cuff healing.
- In 2012, American Brachytherapy Society (ABS) published a consensus guideline for adjuvant vaginal cuff BRT after hysterectomy which is summarized below [165].
- In endometrial cancer patients, most commonly used applicators are vaginal cylinder (single channel/multichannel) or ovoids. Vaginal cylinders ranging from 2.0 to 4 cm lengths and diameters can be used based on the patient anatomy. If possible, the largest diameter applicators should be used. Proper applicator selection is an important part of the vaginal BRT. Ovoids allow treatment of the only upper length of the vagina, whereas entire vagina can be treated with the cylinder.
- Placement of a radio-opaque marker at the vaginal apex to confirm that the applicator is in contact with the vaginal mucosa should be considered. Pretreatment imaging should be used to check the applicator position. CT simulation has been used more commonly to better delineate vaginal cuff and OARs. It can help to confirm that there is no significant air gap and the applicator is in contact with the upper vagina.
- In general, the proximal 3–5 cm of the vagina is treated. When there is serous or clear cell histology, grade 3 disease, or extensive LVSI, the entire length of the vagina should be treated.
- The dose is prescribed to vaginal mucosa or 5 mm depth from the vaginal mucosa.
- The treatment plan only in the first fraction and the same plan used for all fractions are sufficient.
- For patients with medically inoperable endometrial cancer, radiotherapeutic approaches including EBRT and BRT or BRT alone have been used. In 2015, ABS published a consensus statement for BRT for the treatment of medically inoperable endometrial cancer [166]. CT- or MRI-guided BRT is recommended. GTV, CTV and OARs are defined. CTV includes entire uterus, cervix, and upper 1–2 cm of the vagina.

Case Contouring: Delineation of target volumes for BRT of the case 1 is shown in Fig. 7.14.

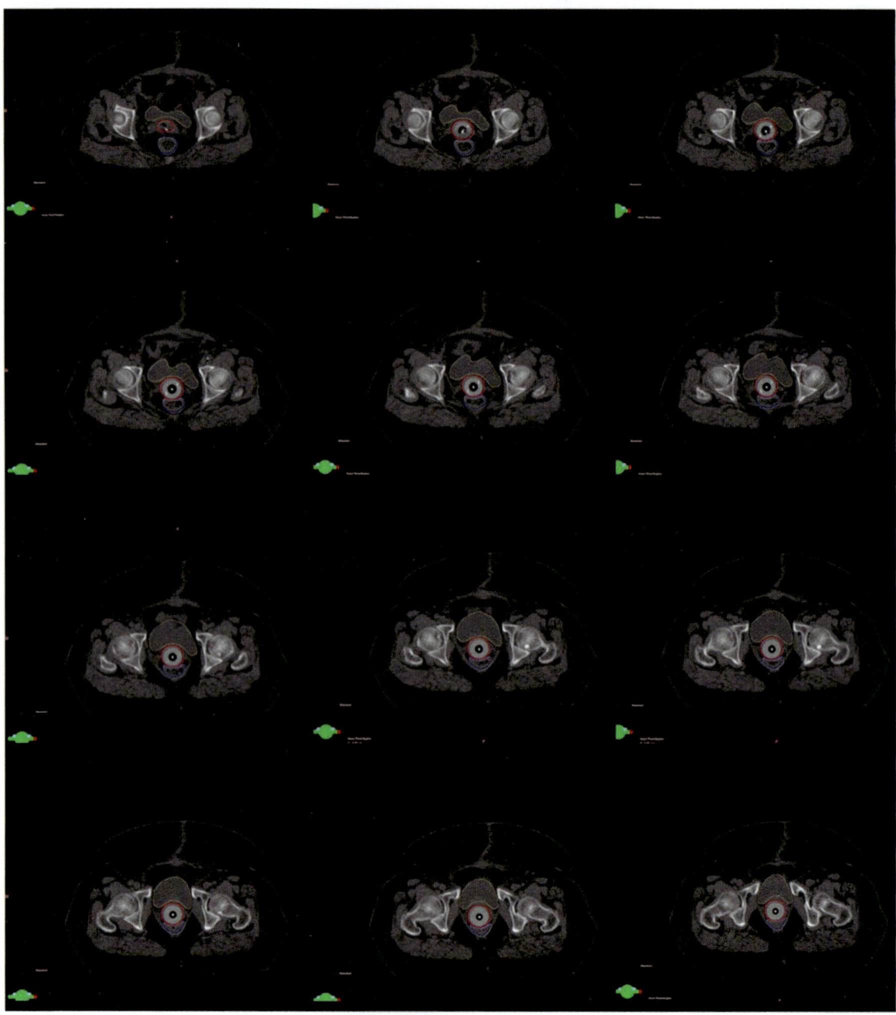

Fig. 7.14 Delineation of target volumes for BRT of the patient with FIGO stage IB, grade 1 endometrial cancer (case 1). Red: CTV, blue: rectum, yellow: bladder

7.2.4.3 Prescription Dose and Dose Constraints for Critical Structures

Case 1 plan: The patient with FIGO Stage IB, grade 1 intermediate-risk endometrial cancer presented here was treated with vaginal cuff BRT alone postoperatively. A 3.5 cm diameter cylinder was used. HDR BRT was given in 5.5 Gy × 5 fraction. Dose is prescribed to 5 mm below the vaginal mucosa. Treatment planning details are seen in Figs. 7.15, 7.16, and 7.17.

Case 2 plan: The patient with FIGO stage IIIC2, grade 1 high-risk endometrial cancer presented here was treated with combined 6 cycles of taxol and carboplatin

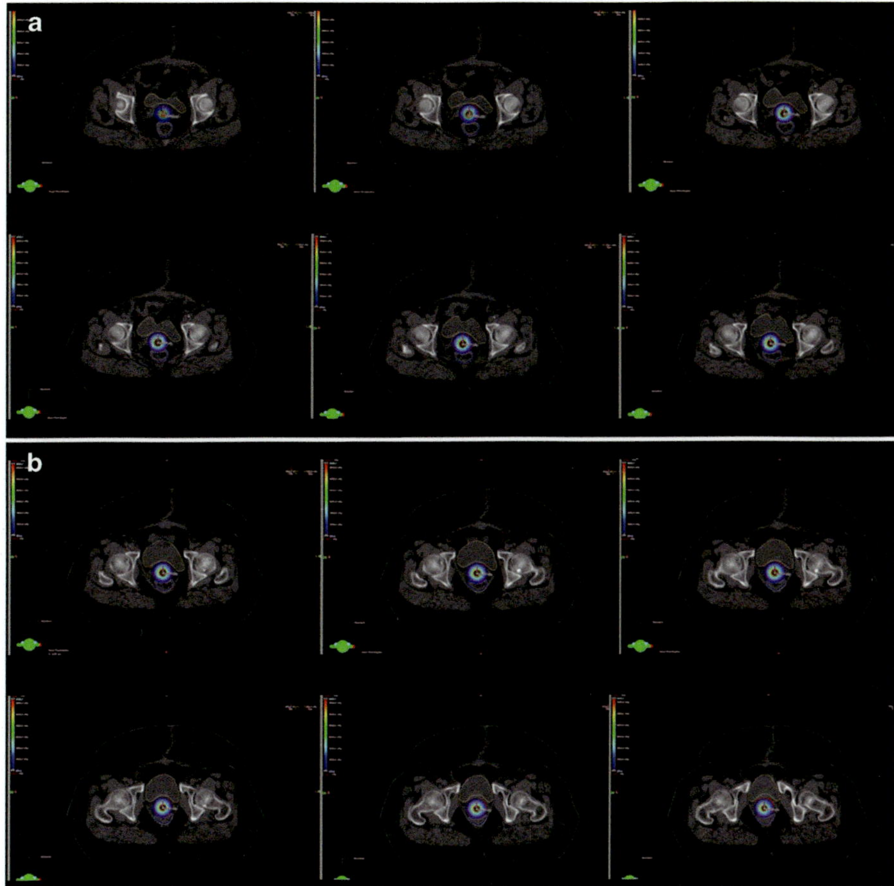

Fig. 7.15 CT-based BRT planning in the postoperative setting of FIGO stage IB, grade 1 endometrial cancer (case 1). The patient was prescribed to receive a dose of 5 × 550 cGy to 5 mm below the vaginal mucosa using HDR BRT alone. (**a**, **b**) 550 cGy isodose volume is shown in blue and (**c**) dose-volume histogram. Red: CTV, blue: rectum, yellow: bladder

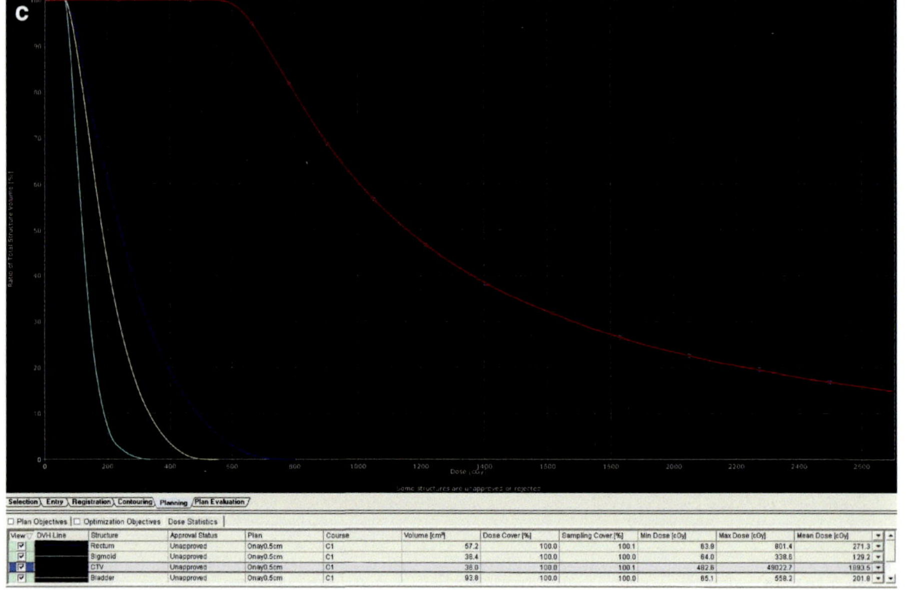

View	DVH Line	Structure	Approval Status	Plan	Course	Volume [cm³]	Dose Cover [%]	Sampling Cover.[%]	Min Dose [cGy]	Max Dose [cGy]	Mean Dose [cGy]
✓		Rectum	Unapproved	Onay0.5cm	C1	57.2	100.0	100.1	63.9	801.4	271.3
✓		Sigmoid	Unapproved	Onay0.5cm	C1	38.4	100.0	100.0	64.0	338.8	129.2
✓		CTV	Unapproved	Onay0.5cm	C1	36.0	100.0	100.1	482.8	49022.7	1893.5
✓		Bladder	Unapproved	Onay0.5cm	C1	93.8	100.0	100.0	85.1	558.2	201.8

Fig. 7.15 (continued)

chemotherapy followed by pelvic and para-aortic EBRT (EFRT). EFRT applied with VMAT technique (50.4 Gy in 1.8 Gy/fraction). Treatment planning details are seen in Figs. 7.16 and 7.18.

7.2.4.4 EBRT Dose

- Generally, a total dose of 45–50.4 Gy should be delivered in 1.8–2.0 Gy per fraction over five to six weeks. If combined EBRT and BRT are planned, EBRT dose should be restricted to 45 Gy.
- Treatment plans must be done on the full-bladder CT scan.
- Treatment plans should be designed to minimize dose to OARs.
- The treatment plan should be evaluated in each patient using dose volume histogram (DVH) analyses of the target volumes and OARs. Prescription goals for the PTV and OARs constraints are needed to be achieved.
- Total prescribed dose should be covered to at least 95% of the PTV. The minimum and maximum dose constraints for the PTV should be within 5% of prescription dose.
- Treatment plans should be designed to minimize dose to critical structures.

a

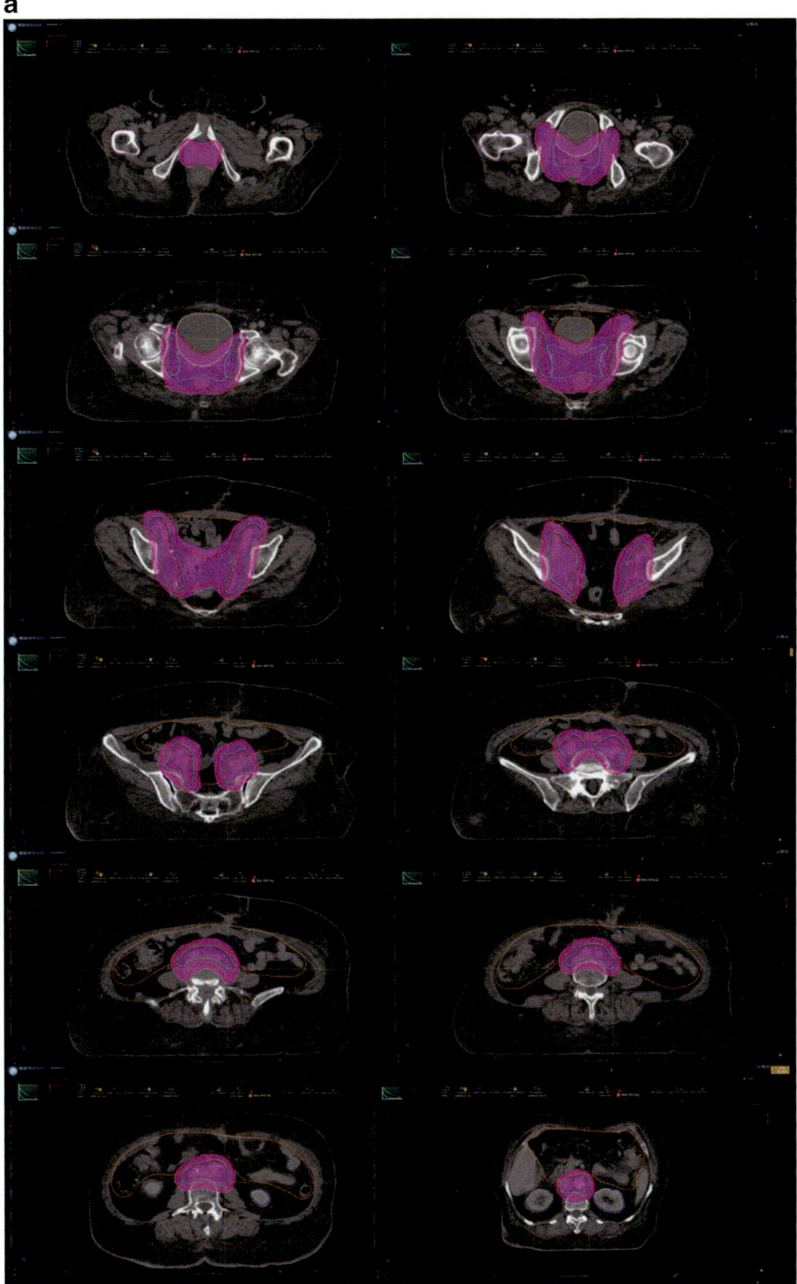

Fig. 7.16 VMAT planning in the postoperative setting of FIGO stage IIIC2 disease. Total dose of 50.4 Gy in 1.8 Gy/fraction was delivered to pelvic and para-aortic region. (**a**, **b**) 95% isodose coverage (pink) and (**c**) dose-volume histogram are shown. Red: PTV, green: CTV lymphatic, cyan: CTV vagina, brown: rectum, yellow: bladder, orange: bowel, pink: left femur, magenta: right femur, blue: left kidney, dark blue: right kidney, light green: spinal cord

b

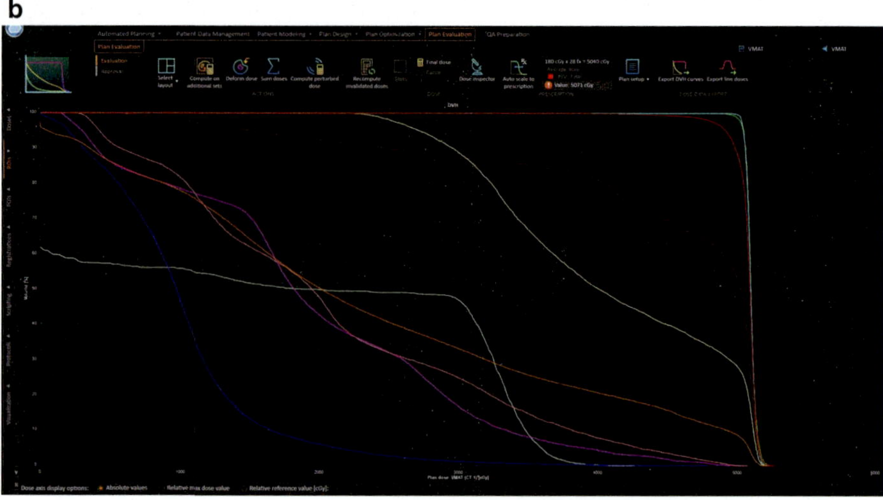

Fig. 7.16 (continued)

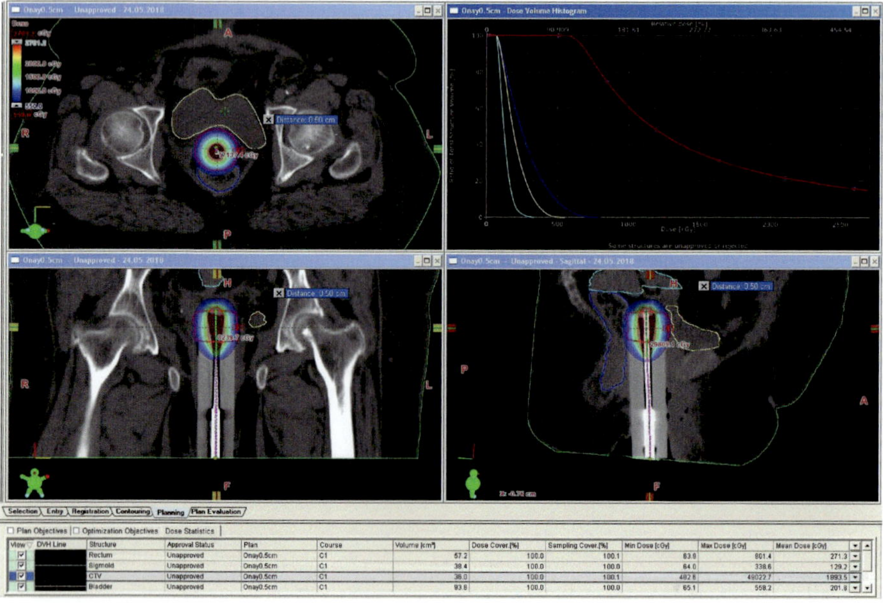

Fig. 7.17 BRT plan of the patient

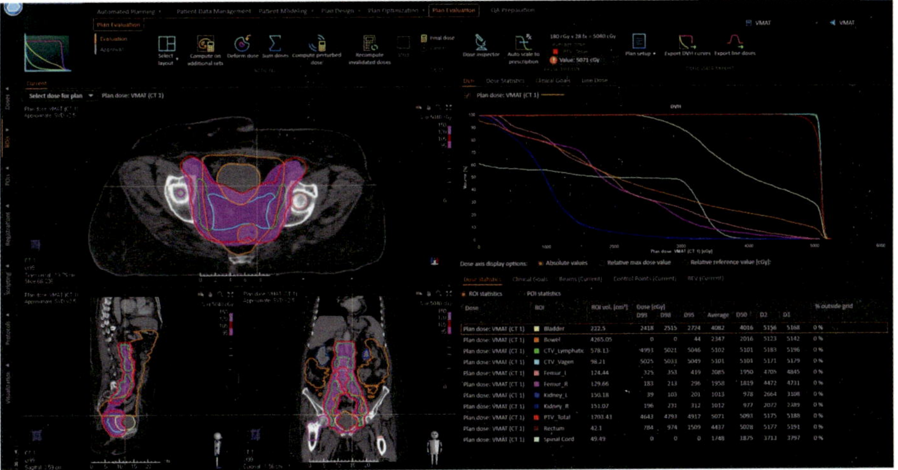

Fig. 7.18 VMAT plan of the patient

Recommended OARs Doses are Detailed in Below
- Small bowel (peritoneal cavity) dose: V45 Gy <195 cc, V40 Gy <30%
- Bladder dose: V45 Gy <35%
- Rectum dose: V30 Gy <60%, V50 Gy <50%
- Vaginal surface dose: 100 Gy
- Femoral head: V30 Gy <15%, V50 Gy <5%
- Bone marrow: Up to 90% receives 10 Gy, up to 37% receives 40 Gy
- Kidney dose <18 Gy
- Spinal cord dose <45 Gy

7.2.4.5 BRT Dose
The prescribed BRT dose depends on the dose specification point, length of vagina treated, BRT technique and whether EBRT is given [165].

Postoperatively Various Fractionation Schedules can be Used But Most Commonly Used Schedules are
Vaginal BRT alone:
5 × 6 Gy or 6 × 4 Gy prescribed to the vaginal mucosa
3 × 7 Gy, 5 × 5 Gy prescribed to 5 mm below the vaginal mucosa
EBRT and BRT:
45 Gy EBRT + 3 × 6 Gy prescribed to the vaginal mucosa or 3 × 5 Gy prescribed to 5 mm below the vaginal mucosa
50.4 Gy EBRT + 2 × 6 Gy prescribed to the vaginal mucosa or 2 × 5 Gy prescribed to 5 mm below the vaginal mucosa
There is no need to calculate bladder and rectum doses in patients treated with BRT alone because of the relatively low dose to OARs [165].

For Medically Inoperable Patients [166]
BRT alone:
  Stage I, grade 1–2, minimal myometrial invasion:
  GTV D90 80–90 Gy, CTV D90 48–62.5 Gy
  6 × 6 Gy/6 × 6.4 Gy/5 × 7.3 Gy/4 × 8.5 Gy/9–10 × 5 Gy
  EBRT and BRT:
  Stage I, grade 1–2, deep myometrial invasion or stage II or stage III:
  GTV D90 80–90 Gy, CTV D90 65–75 Gy
  45 Gy EBRT plus 3 × 6.5 Gy/3 × 6.3 Gy/4 × 5.2 Gy/5 × 5 Gy/2 × 8.5 Gy
BRT
  50 Gy EBRT plus 6 × 3.75 Gy BRT
  Recommended OARs doses are:
  D2cc rectum ‹70–75 Gy
  D2cc sigmoid ‹70–75 Gy
  D2cc bladder ‹80–100 Gy

7.2.5 Follow-up Recommendations

The optimal surveillance strategy for patients with endometrial cancer involves gynecological examination and monitoring for symptoms. Following therapy, patients should be seen every 3–6 months for the first 2 years, every 6–12 months for years 3–5 and then annually. Surveillance imaging studies, serum CA 125 and cervicovaginal cytology (PAP smear) should not be routinely performed unless clinically indicated.

7.3 Vulvar Cancer

Overview
Epidemiology
  Vulvar cancer is the fourth most common gynecologic malignancy. It has a bimodal age distribution, both young and elderly patients can be affected. It is usually diagnosed at an early stage and prognosis is good.
  Pathological and biological features
  Over 80% of vulvar cancers are squamous cell carcinoma (SCC). Risk factors for vulvar cancer include human papillomavirus (HPV) infection, vulvar intraepithelial neoplasia (VIN), cigarette smoking, lichen sclerosus, and immunodeficiency syndromes. Major prognostic factors are stage, tumor size, surgical margin status, and lymph node metastasis.
  Definitive therapy
  In vulvar SCC, treatment decisions are depends on the disease extent at the time of initial presentation and patient performance status. Cisplatin-based

concurrent chemotherapy and radiotherapy (CRT) is the standard treatment for locally advanced vulvar cancer. It is also an option for patients with medically inoperable early stage disease or who refuse surgery.

Adjuvant therapy

For most medically fit patients without evidence of distant metastasis, the standard approach to treatment is surgery. Postoperative radiotherapy (RT) with or without cisplatin-based concurrent chemotherapy is indicated for high risk patients.

Keywords: Vulvar cancer, radiotherapy

7.3.1 Case Presentation

A 85-year-old female admitted to the hospital with several month history of pruritis and mass on her vulva. She had a past medical history of controlled diabetes mellitus and hypertension. Her physical examination revealed a 3 × 3 cm lesion in the left labium minus which was located 2 cm away from the urethra. There were no palpable lymph nodes. Chest X-ray, whole blood count, and kidney and liver function tests were normal. In the pelvic magnetic resonance imaging (MRI), nonspecific contrast enhancement was observed in the distal periurethral region without a vulvar mass. No lymph nodes were detected. The incisional biopsy from vulvar lesion revealed SCC. She underwent left radical hemivulvectomy and bilateral inguinofemoral lymph node (IFLN) dissection. The pathologic evaluation was reported as well differentiated SCC. The largest diameter of the tumor was 3 cm. The depth of stromal invasion by carcinoma was 0.6 cm. The distance from urethral surgical margin was 0.7 cm. All other surgical margins were negative for invasive carcinoma. There was no lymphovascular space invasion (LVSI). Out of 20 dissected lymph nodes, 2 were metastatic in left side. Size of metastases was 5 mm and no extracapsular extension present. Lichen sclerosis was present in the remaining vulva. According to 8th edition AJCC/UICC staging system, she was staged as T1bN2bM0 (Stage IIIB) vulvar cancer (Table 7.6).

7.3.2 Evidence Based Treatment Recommendations

A complete clinical history and physical examination, complete blood count, liver and renal function tests, and chest X-ray should be performed. Tumor size, depth of invasion and local extent are assessed by physical examination and vulvar biopsy. Vulvar cancer staged according to the American Joint Committee on Cancer (AJCC) and the International Federation of Gynecology and Obstetrics (FIGO) staging systems using hybrid surgical and clinical/pathologic evaluation. Staging should include complete surgical resection of the primary tumor and IFLN dissection (unilateral/bilateral) with a separate incision or sentinel lymph node biopsy (SLNB) in selected patients. Pelvic MRI may be used to assist surgery and/or RT planning.

Table 7.6 Staging of vulvar cancer based on FIGO (2009) and AJCC TNM classification (8th edition)

FIGO/TNM Staging			
Primary Tumor (T)			
FIGO	TNM		
TX		Primary tumor cannot be assessed	
T0		No evidence of primary tumor	
Tis*		Carcinoma in situ (preinvasive carcinoma)	
IA	T1a**	Lesions ≤2 cm in size, confined to the vulva or perineum and with stromal invasion ≤1 mm	
IB	T1b	Lesions >2 cm in size or any size with stromal invasion >1 mm, confined to the vulva or perineum	
II	T2***	Tumor of any size with extension to adjacent perineal structures (Lower/distal 1/3 urethra, lower/distal 1/3 vagina, anal involvement)	
IVA	T3****	Tumor of any size with extension to any of the following: upper/proximal 2/3 of urethra, upper/proximal 2/3 vagina, bladder mucosa, rectal mucosa, or fixed to pelvic bone	
	*FIGO staging no longer includes Stage 0 (Tis).		
	**The depth of invasion is defined as the measurement of the tumor from the epithelial-stromal junction of the adjacent most superficial dermal papilla to the deepest point of invasion.		
	***FIGO uses the classification T2/T3. This is defined as T2 in TNM.		
	****FIGO uses the classification T4. This is defined as T3 in TNM.		
Regional Lymph Nodes (N)			
FIGO	TNM		
	NX	Regional lymph nodes cannot be assessed	
	N0	No regional lymph node metastasis	
N1		One or two regional lymph nodes with the following features:	
IIIA	N1a	One or two lymph node metastasis each 5 mm or less	
IIIA	N1b	One lymph node metastasis 5 mm or greater	
	N2	Regional lymph node metastasis with the following features:	
IIIB	N2a	Three or more lymph node metastases each less than 5 mm	
IIIB	N2b	Two or more lymph node metastases 5 mm or greater	
IIIB	N2c	Lymph node metastasis with extracapsular spread	
IVA	N3	Fixed or ulcerated regional lymph node metastasis	
An effort should be made to describe the site and laterality of lymph node metastases			
Distant Metastasis (M)			
FIGO	TNM		
M0		No distant metastasis (no pathologic M0; use clinical M to complete stage group)	
IVB	M1	Distant metastasis (including pelvic lymph node metastasis)	
Stage Grouping			
Stage I	T1	N0	M0
Stage IA	T1a	N0	M0
Stage IB	T1b	N0	M0
Stage II	T2	N0	M0
Stage IIIA	T1,2	N1	M0
Stage IIIB	T1,2	N2a,b	M0
Stage IIIC	T1,2	N2c	M0
Stage IVA	T1,2	N3	M0
	T3	AnyN	M0
Stage IVB	AnyT	AnyN	M1

TNM T (tumor) N (regional lymph nodes) M (distant metastasis)

FIGO International Federation of Gynecology and Obstetrics

Used with permission of the American Joint Committee on Cancer (AJCC), Chicago, Illinois. The original source for this material is the AJCC Cancer Staging Manual, Eight Edition (2017) published by Springer Science Business Media LLC, www.springer.com

aFIGO staging no longer includes stage 0 (Tis)

bThe depth of invasion is defined as the measurement of the tumor from the epithelial-stromal junction of the adjacent most superficial dermal papilla to the deepest point of invasion

cFIGO uses the classification T2/T3. This is defined as T2 in TNM

dFIGO uses the classification T4. This is defined as T3 in TNM

Consider whole body positron emission tomography (PET)/computed tomography (CT) or chest/abdominal/pelvic CT for locally advanced disease or if patients with an symptoms suspicious for metastasis [167].

After the vulvar cancer was diagnosed histopathologically, the patient should be evaluated for which patients are candidate for surgery and adjuvant therapy or non-surgical treatment takes into account both the stage of the disease as well as the patient's baseline health status. For most medically fit patients without evidence of metastatic disease, the standard approach to treatment is conservative surgery, with the potential integration of adjuvant RT and/or chemotherapy based on pathology and extent of disease [168].

7.3.2.1 Early Stage (I-II)

After careful clinical evaluation and staging, standard primary treatment for early stage (T1, smaller T2: ≤4 cm) vulvar cancer is wide local excision with a 1–2 cm margin of grossly normal tissue to the deep fascia and IFLN evaluation. Depending on the size and extent of disease (e.g. midline lesions), radical local excision or modified radical vulvectomy may be required. Although there is no phase III ran-domized study, several retrospective studies comparing results of these resection techniques generally reported similar outcomes [169, 170].

For stage IA disease (≤1 mm depth of invasion), wide local excision or radical local resection is recommended. IFLN evaluation is not required due to the risk of lymph node metastasis is <1% [171]. Patients should be observed after surgery. However, for stage IB or higher disease (>1 mm invasion), IFLN evaluation (SLNB or dissection) in addition to primary site surgery is recommended because the risk of IFLN metastases is ≥8% [172]. Patients with well-lateralized lesions located ≥2 cm from the vulvar midline should undergo ipsilateral IFLN evaluation, whereas patients with midline lesions should undergo bilateral IFLN evaluation [170, 173, 174]. A complete IFLN dissection should be performed if no ipsilateral SLNs are detected. Adjuvant therapy may be required based on primary tumor and nodal sur-gical pathology assessment.

A negative ipsilateral groin nodes after lymphadenectomy have <3% risk of con-tralateral metastases [175]. Contralateral lymphadenectomy or RT of the contralat-eral groin is recommended if the groin nodes are involved after unilateral lymphadenectomy [176]. The excision of all grossly enlarged or suspicious lymph nodes and intraoperative assesment for metastases during the unilateral lymphade-nectomy is essential to decide the extent and bilaterality of the lymph node dissection.

There has been an increasing interest in SLNB to reduce the morbidity associ-ated with IFLN dissection while maintaining low groin recurrences in selected stage IB or II vulvar cancer [177–179]. Ideally, patients with unifocal tumor <4 cm, no clinical IFLNs, and no previous history of vulvar surgery are candidates for SLNB [180]. The current standard for patients with a positive SLN is to undergo comple-tion IFLN dissection and/or administration of adjuvant RT to the affected groin. Additionally, the contralateral groin should be evaluated surgically and/or treated with RT.

van der Velden et al. evaluated IFLN dissection or primary groin RT in early stage vulvar cancer in systematic review at 2011 [168]. Although there was less lymphedema and life-threatening cardiovascular complications in the patients who were treated with primary groin RT than in those who underwent IFLN dissection, it was associated with a higher recurrence rate and lower disease-specific survival (DSS). However, this analysis included only one randomized trial which had inadequate RT technique that groin doses were low and marginal misses were observed [181]. Surgical treatment of the groin has been associated with lower groin recurrence rates, therefore, IFLN dissection is performed even if RT is planned (e.g., tumor size >4 cm) [181]. Primary RT may be an alternative treatment option for patients who are not candidates for surgery [182].

7.3.2.2 Adjuvant Therapy to the Primary Site

Data are limited in regards to which patients with early-stage (I or II) vulvar cancer require adjuvant therapy after surgical treatment. If postoperative adjuvant treatment is required, it should be initiated as soon as possible after adequate healing is achieved, preferably within 6–8 weeks. Resection margin status has been postulated as a significant prognostic factor for recurrence in vulvar cancer. In the retrospective series (n = 135) of Heaps et al., local recurrence rates were 0% in patients with ≥ 1 cm surgical margin versus 50% in patients with ≤ 8 mm surgical margin [183]. It is important to perform a re-excision in the setting of a close or positive surgical margin (≤ 8 mm). However, re-excision of tumors close to the urethra, clitoris and anal sphincter can be difficult without significant morbidity and in these situations adjuvant RT can be applied. Also patients with positive surgical margins after re-excision should receive postoperative RT to the primary tumor bed area [184, 185]. Ignatov et al. reported in a retrospective study of 257 patients with vulvar SCC, the 5-year OS rate was 68% for patients receiving RT in comparison with 29% for patients not receiving RT in 65 patients with close or positive surgical margins (p = 0.038) [184]. There is no benefit of adjuvant RT when the surgical margin is negative, but patients with close or positive margins who received RT had similar OS rates as patients with negative surgical margins (68% vs. 66%). In patients with close or positive surgical margins who require RT due to lymph node metastasis, there is no need for re-excision.

In addition to margin status (≤ 8 mm), a number of primary tumor risk factors may influence adjuvant therapy decisions, which include LVSI , tumor size >4 cm, depth of invasion >5 mm, and/or diffuse/spray pattern of invasion [186]. If patients had negative surgical margins and there were no additional risk factors, adjuvant RT is not recommended.

7.3.2.3 Adjuvant Therapy to the Nodes

Lymph node involvement is an important prognostic factor in vulvar cancer. For patients with negative groin lymph nodes, observation can be considered [177, 187]. In the presence of lymph node metastases, adjuvant RT or CRT is recommended according to number and extent of lymph node metastases [188]. If patients had positive SLNB, completion IFLN dissection followed by RT or CRT could be applied.

Adjuvant RT is controversial if there is a single lymph node metastasis without extracapsular spread [189–192]. Using SEER database, Parthasarathy et al. reported on the results of 208 patients with stage III, single LN positive vulvar SCC [191]. In this series 5-year DSS rate significantly improved with the addition of adjuvant RT compared with patients who did not receive RT following inadequate IFLN dissection. For adequate IFLN dissection at least 12 lymph nodes should be removed.

In the randomized GOG 37 trial, pelvic node dissection and pelvic node RT was compared in 114 patients with groin node-positive vulvar cancer after radical vulvectomy and bilateral IFLN dissection [190, 193]. This study was stopped early due to adjuvant RT resulted in improved 2-year survival compared with pelvic node dissection, particularly among patients with clinical nodal involvement (59% vs. 31%) and those with ≥ 2 positive groin nodes (63% vs. 37%). At median 74 months of follow-up, disease related-death was higher in pelvic node dissection group (51% vs. 29%, p = 0.015).

There is no randomized data comparing adjuvant RT to CRT. Preferred approach is adjuvant RT alone in patients with single nodal micrometastasis and CRT in patients with any macrometastatic disease or micrometastatic disease with ≥ 2 lymph node after IFLN dissection. Based upon limited experience, the most commonly used concurrent chemotherapeutic agent is 40 mg/m^2 cisplatin.

Gill et al. reported the outcome of 1797 patients with node positive resected vulvar SCC treated with RT alone or CRT using United States National Cancer Database (NCDB) [194]. This trial showed that CRT was associated with a trend towards a reduction in the risk of death compared with RT alone (HR 0.81, 95% CI 0.65–1.01). Most commonly chemotherapy was started in the first week of RT.

Adjuvant RT is recommended to the bilateral groins and the pelvis for patients with IFLN metastases. It is usually suggested that also treat the vulva in cases of lymph nodes irradiated to reduce vulvar recurrences [195].

7.3.2.4 Locally Advanced Stage (III-IVA)

Locally advanced disease (larger T2 (>4 cm) or T3 tumors) defined as tumors that can not be resected secondary to tumor or lymph node fixation to adjacent structures. As the treatment for vulvar cancer has evolved with the goal of organ preservation, multimodality therapies have become the standard of care, particularly for patients with locally advanced disease [196]. Despite the lack of high-quality data, concurrent CRT approach is recommended to all patients with unresectable, locally advanced vulvar SCC. In the 2011 Cochrane database review there was no statistically significant overall survival (OS) difference between primary surgery and primary or neoadjuvant CRT in locally advanced vulvar SCC (HR 1.09, 95% CI 0.37–3.17) [197]. Han et al. demonstrated that CRT increased 5-year OS rate compared to RT alone in a series of 54 patients with locally advanced disease (54% vs. 10%, p = 0.04) [198]. Most commonly used chemotherapeutic agents are cisplatin (50 mg/m^2), 5-fluorouracil (5-FU)/cisplatin, and 5-FU/mitomycin-C.

Patients with clinically positive groin nodes should undergo a lymph node biopsy to confirm nodal metastases. Based on limited data, the preferred treatment in patients with clinically involved lymph nodes is debulking surgery followed by adjuvant CRT instead of IFLN dissection to prevent morbidity [199, 200]. Alternatively, definitive platinum-based CRT alone can be used [201, 202]. Nooij et al. investigated the risk of groin recurrence and morbidity in patients with lymph node positive vulvar SCC after standard full IFLN dissection versus less radical debulking of clinically involved lymph nodes or removal of sentinel lymph nodes only followed by RT [199]. They found similar groin recurrence rate in all treatment groups (13%, 16% and 25%, p = 0.495). Debulking of clinically involved lymph nodes was related to a significant lower risk of complications especially regarding lymphocysts and lymphedema compared to IFLN dissection. RT treatment portal should include the vulva, both groins, and lower pelvic lymph nodes. Selected patients without clinically or pathologically involved lymph nodes and at very low risk of having nodal involvement may be treated to the vulvar area alone [203].

Preoperative RT or concurrent platinum-based CRT can lead to decrease in tumor size and reduce the extent of surgery [204]. For patients with locally advanced disease, adjuvant therapy decisions should be made based on the response to treatment, which is usually assessed by clinical evaluation and biopsy 6–12 weeks after completion of CRT. Complete response was observed in approximately 60% of patients after CRT [205–214]. The role of surgery after CRT has not been well defined [201, 215]. If patients had clinically and pathologically complete response at the primary site or in the groin, observation has been advocated. If there is a residual mass at the site of the primary tumor or lymph node, surgical resection of the residual disease should be considered in patients with resectable disease who are eligible for surgery [216]. Moore et al. reported the first part of GOG 101 study which was evaluated the role of preoperative CRT in 73 patients with unresectable T3-T4 vulvar SCC [207]. In this study, preoperative CRT reduced the need for radical surgery including pelvic exenteration [207]. Only 2.8% of patients had residual unresectable disease and in 4% of patients urinary and/or gastrointestinal continence was not possible. For unresectable residual disease, it is recommended that additional RT and/or chemotherapy, or best supportive care. In the second part of GOG 101, the same preoperative CRT scheme was used in 46 patients with unresectable N2-N3 vulvar cancer and they showed that 38 patients were able to undergo surgery after neoadjuvant CRT [215]. With a median follow-up of 6.5 years, nodal and local control was achieved in 36 of 37 patients and 29 of 38 patients, respectively. In GOG 205 study, 58 patients with unresectable vulvar cancer were treated with preoperative CRT with a higher RT dose than GOG 101 study and weekly cisplatin [201]. With a median follow-up of 24.8 months, CRT with weekly cisplatin achieved better clinical complete response and pathologic complete response. The selected studies of treatment in vulvar cancer are summarized in Table 7.7.

Table 7.7 Selected studies of treatment in vulvar cancer

Reference	Study design	Characteristics	Treatment	FU (mo)	Clinical outcomes	Toxicity
Homesley [190] (GOG 37)	RCT	114 pts cStage I-IV RV + Bilateral groin LND pLN+	Ipsilateral PLND vs. Bilateral groin and pelvic RT RT: 2 Gy/45–50 Gy No CT planning Midline block to central vulva	–	Closed early due to better results in RT arm Groin recurrence: 23.6% vs. 5.1%, p = 0.02 Pelvic failure: 1.8% vs. 6.8% 2-year OS: 54% vs. 68%, p = 0.03 cN2-3 groin nodes 31% vs. 59%, p = 0.01 ≥2 inguinal LNs 37% vs. 63%, p ‹ 0.0001 No benefit in patients with 1 LN+	No significant difference
Kunos [193] (update of GOG 37)	Retrospective			74	6-year OS: 51% vs. 41%, p = 0.18 6-year RFS: 48% vs. 59% 6-year Ca-related death: 51% vs. 29%, p = 0.015 6-year OS benefit for RT: Clinically suspected or fixed ulcerated groin LNs (p = 0.004) and ≥2 positive groin LNs (p < 0.001) Positive/Resected LNs number >20%: Significantly associated with contralateral LN mts, relapse, and Ca-related death	Chronic lymphedema: 16% vs. 22%, p = 0.47 Cutaneous desquamation: 19% vs. 15%, p = 0.62

(continued)

Table 7.7 (continued)

Reference	Study design	Characteristics	Treatment	FU (mo)	Clinical outcomes	Toxicity
Stehman [187] (GOG 88)	RCT	52 pts cT1-T3, cN0 RV	Bilateral groin RT vs. Bilateral groin LND RT: 2 Gy/50 Gy, prescribed to 3 cm from the skin If pLN+ (20%): RT to bilateral groin and pelvis	6	Closed early: Groin recurrences seen only in RT arm Groin recurrence: 18.5% vs. 0%, p = 0.033 All recurrences were in field OS: 63% vs. 88%, p = 0.035 RT cannot control groin disease but inadequate RT technique was used	Groin RT: shorter hospitalization (p = 0.0001)
Moore [207] (GOG 101)	Phase II	73 pts Unresectable (T3-T4) cStage III-IV	Preoperative CRT followed by resection of residual tumor and bilateral groin LND CRT: Cisplatin/5-FU + split course RT RT: 47.6 Gy	50	47% cCR, 70% of those had pCR 84% of residual disease had negative margins Only 2 pts (2.8%) had residual unresectable disease 3 pts: No preservation of urinary and/or GI continence Preoperative CRT may reduce the need for pelvic exenteration in locally advanced vulvar Ca	Toxicity was acceptable
Montana [215] (GOG 101)	Phase II	46 pts Unresectable LNs (N2-N3)	Preoperative CRT followed by resection of residual tumor and bilateral groin LND CRT: Cisplatin/5-FU + split course RT RT: 47.6 Gy	77	Became resectable in 38/40 pts pN0 in 15/37 pts (41%) Primary tumor had pCR in 20/38 pts (31%) LC of LNs in 36/37 and primary tumor in 29/38	2 pts died

Han [198]	Retrospective	54 pts Locally advanced stage	Primary or adjuvant CRT vs. RT 2 cycles of 5-FU and Mitomycin C or Cisplatin	17	OS, DSS, RFS: Primary CRT is better than primary RT 5-year OS: 54% vs. 10%, p = 0.04 5-year DSS: 62% vs. 14%, p = 0.03 Adjuvant CRT vs. adjuvant RT: No difference	-
Gill [194] (NCDB)	Retrospective	1797 pts Extirpative surgery Stage IIIA-IVA Groin LN+	Adjuvant RT ± Adjuvant chemo 76.6% 1-3LN+ 26.3% received adjuvant chemo Most pts initiated chemo within 1 week of RT	28.3	Median survival (mo): Chemo (+) 44 vs. chemo (−) 29.7, p = 0.001 Adjuvant chemo resulted in a 38% reduction in the risk of death	–
van der Velden [168]	Cochrane review	52 pts 1/12 papers met the selection criteria	Primary groin RT vs. Primary groin surgery	–	RT: Increased groin recurrence (RR 10.21, 95% CI 0.59 to 175.78) and lower DSS (RR 3.70, 95% CI 0.87 to 15.80)	RT: less lymphedema and fewer life-threatening CV complications Primary surgery: Longer hospital stay
Moore [201] (GOG 205)	Phase II	58 pts Unresectable (T3-T4, any N)	RT and weekly cisplatin followed by surgical resection of residual tumor (or biopsy to confirm cCR) RT: 1.8 Gy/57.6 Gy Cisplatin: 40 mg/m^2 Surgery: 6–8 weeks after CRT	24.8	69% completed CRT Primary vulvar tumor: cCR: 64% (37/58), pCR in cCR (29/37): 78%, pCR (29/58) in total 50% RT and weekly cisplatin: High cCR and pCR with acceptable toxicity	Acceptable toxicity

(continued)

Table 7.7 (continued)

Reference	Study design	Characteristics	Treatment	FU (mo)	Clinical outcomes	Toxicity
Viswanathan [222]	Retrospective	205 pts Stage I-IVA	Relationship of margin status and RT dose to recurrence was evaluated Margin status: negative ($\geq$1 cm) (34%), close (<1 cm) (56%), positive (10%)	49	4-year RFS 53%; 4-year OS 73% 4-year rates of freedom from vulvar recurrence (p for trend = 0.005): Negative margins: 82%; close margins: 63%; positive margins: 37% Increased risk of vulvar relapse (Multivariate analysis): Close margins (HR = 3.03, 95% CI 1.46–6.26) Positive margins (HR = 7.02, 95% CI 2.66–18.54) $\geq$56 Gy had a lower risk of relapse than $\leq$50.4 Gy (p < 0.05) Highest risk of vulvar recurrence: Margins $\leq$5 mm (p = 0.002)	–
Shylasree [197]	Cochrane review	141 pts Locally advanced stage 1 RCT and 2 non-randomized studies	Neoadjuvant and Primary CRT vs. Primary surgery or Primary RT	-	No OS difference between neoadjuvant CRT and primary surgery (RR = 1.29, 95% CI 0.87–1.91) No OS difference between primary CRT vs. primary surgery (n = 63, HR = 1.09, 95% CI 0.37–3.17)	No significant difference
Mahner [188]	Retrospective	1249 pts 447 pts (35.8%) LN+ 1 LN+ (38.5%) 2 LN+ (22.8%)	Adjuvant RT (+) vs. (−)	39.4	3-year PFS: 39.6% vs. 25.9%, p = 0.004 3-year OS: 57.7% vs. 51.4%, p = 0.17 Adjuvant RT: Improved outcomes in LN+ pts	–

Nooij [199]	Retrospective	68 pts LN+ vulvar Ca	Groin dissection vs. cLN debulking vs. SND Adjuvant RT (82%) More pts received RT after debulking vs. groin dissection (90% vs. 67%)	20.5	Groin recurrence: 13% vs. 16% vs. 25%, p = 0.495 cLN+: debulking surgery followed by RT is preferred	Morbidity: 53% vs. 13% vs. 13%, p = 0.003 Lymphocysts: 27% vs. 0% vs. 6%, p = 0.032 Lymphedema: 43% vs. 0% vs. 6%, p = 0.002
Ignatov [184]	Retrospective	257 pts	RT (+) vs. RT (−) Negative margin vs. close/positive margin	39.8	5-year OS: Negative margin 66.1% vs. close/positive margin 49.2%, p = 0.005 5-year OS for close/positive margin: RT (+) 67.6% vs. RT (−) 29% Close/positive margins: adjuvant RT reduced mortality risk (HR 0.36, p = 0.038)	–
Chapman [185] (NCDB)	Retrospective	3075 pts Margin positive	Observation (64.7%) vs. Adjuvant RT (35.3%)	36.4	3-year OS: 58.5% vs. 67.4%, p < 0.001 3-year OS for RT dose: 30.0–45.0 Gy: 54.3 45.1–53.9 Gy: 55.7% 54.0–59.9 Gy: 70.1% >60 Gy: 65.3% Adjuvant RT improves OS: Optimal dose range 54.0–59.9 Gy	–

(continued)

Table 7.7 (continued)

Reference	Study design	Characteristics	Treatment	FU (mo)	Clinical outcomes	Toxicity
Rao [223] (NCDB)	Retrospective	1352 pts Unresectable or medically inoperable	Definitive CRT vs. Definitive RT Median RT dose: 59.4 Gy CRT: Younger (p < 0.001) and more advanced stage (p < 0.001)	45.2 vs. 34.4	5-year OS: 49.9% vs. 27.4%, p $<$ 0.001 FIGO stage I: Improved OS with CRT (p = 0.058) CRT: 24% reduction in the risk of death Definitive CRT was associated with higher OS compared to RT alone who did not receive surgery	–

Abbreviations: *FU* follow-up, *mo* months, *RCT* randomized controlled trial, *pts* patients, *c* clinical, *RV* radical vulvectomy, *LND* lymph node dissection, *p* pathologic, *LN* lymph node, *PLND* pelvic lymph node dissection, *RT* radiotherapy, *Gy* gray, *CT* computed tomography, *OS* overall survival, *GOG* Gynecologic Oncology Group, *RFS* relapse free survival, *Ca* cancer, *mts* metastases, *T* tumor, *CRT* chemoradiotherapy, *5-FU* 5-fluorouracil, *CR* complete response, *GI* gastrointestinal, *LC* local control, *DSS* disease specific survival, *NCDB* national cancer database, *chemo* chemotherapy, *RR* relative risk, *CI* confidence interval, *CV* cardiovascular, *CR* complete response, *HR* hazard ratio, *PFS* progression free survival, *SND* sentinel node dissection, *FIGO* International Federation of Gynecology and Obstetrics

7.3.2.5 Metastatic Disease (Any T, Any N, M1 Beyond Pelvis) (IVB)

Patients with metastatic disease usually treated with combined carboplatin and paclitaxel chemotherapy. RT can be used for symptom palliation and best supportive care is other treatment alternative.

7.3.2.6 Treatment Recommendations

Recommended algorithms for the treatment of early and locally advanced stage vulvar cancer are summarized in Figs. 7.19, 7.20, 7.21, and 7.22.

7.3.3   Treatment Planning

7.3.3.1 Simulation

- When patients are simulated, the extent of disease based on physical examination and imaging findings should be considered [217, 218].
- Patient traditionally simulated in the supine, arms on chest and "frog-leg" position which allows sparing of the skin in the upper inner thigh (**Fig. 7.23**).
- If possible treat with specific bladder and rectal filling protocols. Some clinicians prefer to treat patients with full bladder to minimize small bowel toxicity, whereas others recommend treating with empty bladder because of better reproducibility.
- For locally advanced vulvar cancer, integrated target volume (ITV) is defined to account for bladder and rectal volume. If the rectum is distended at simulation (>3.5 cm diameter), it is advocated that re-simulate patient with an empty rectum after further bowel preparation.
- Planning CT scan obtained with intravenous (IV) contrast if available.
- Wires or radio-opaque markers should be placed on the vulvar skin during simulation to define the primary target volume, anus, urethra, clitoris and all surgical scars.

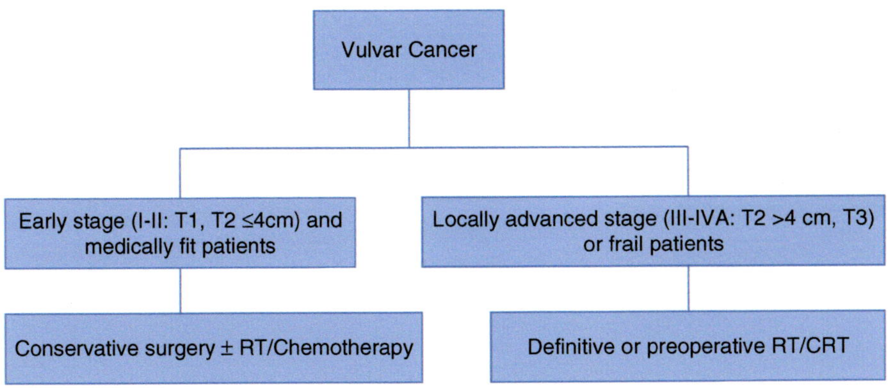

Fig. 7.19 Recommended general treatment algorithm for vulvar cancer

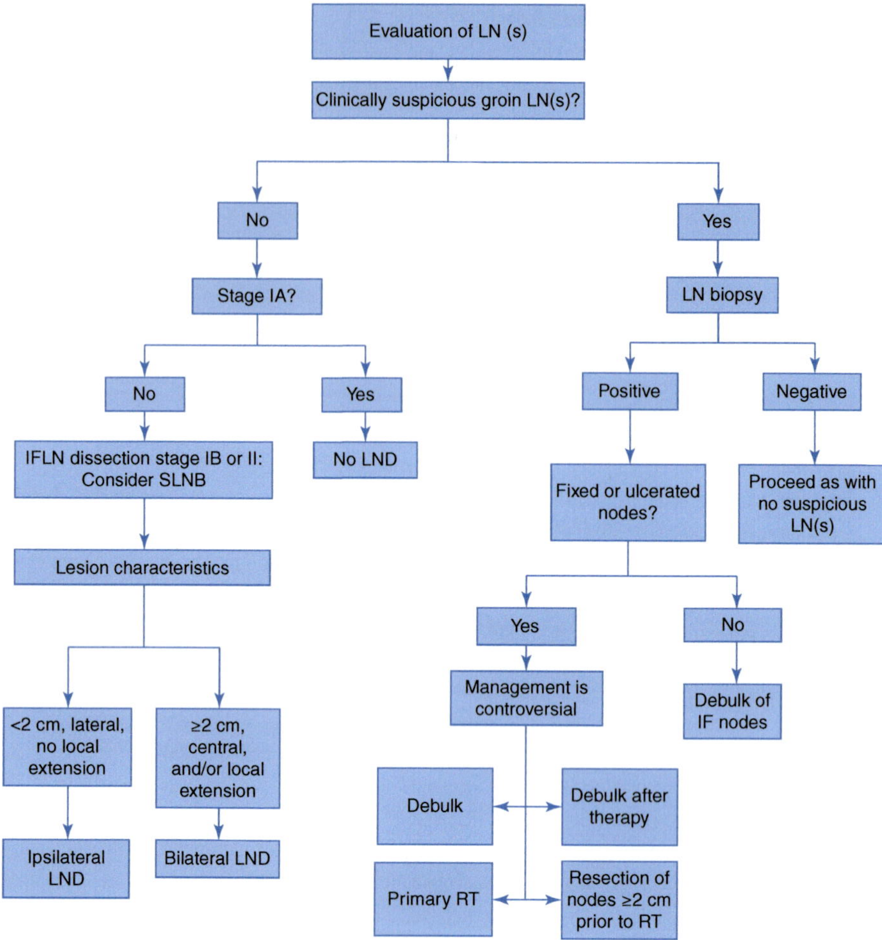

Fig. 7.20 Recommended algorithm for lymph node evaluation in vulvar cancer

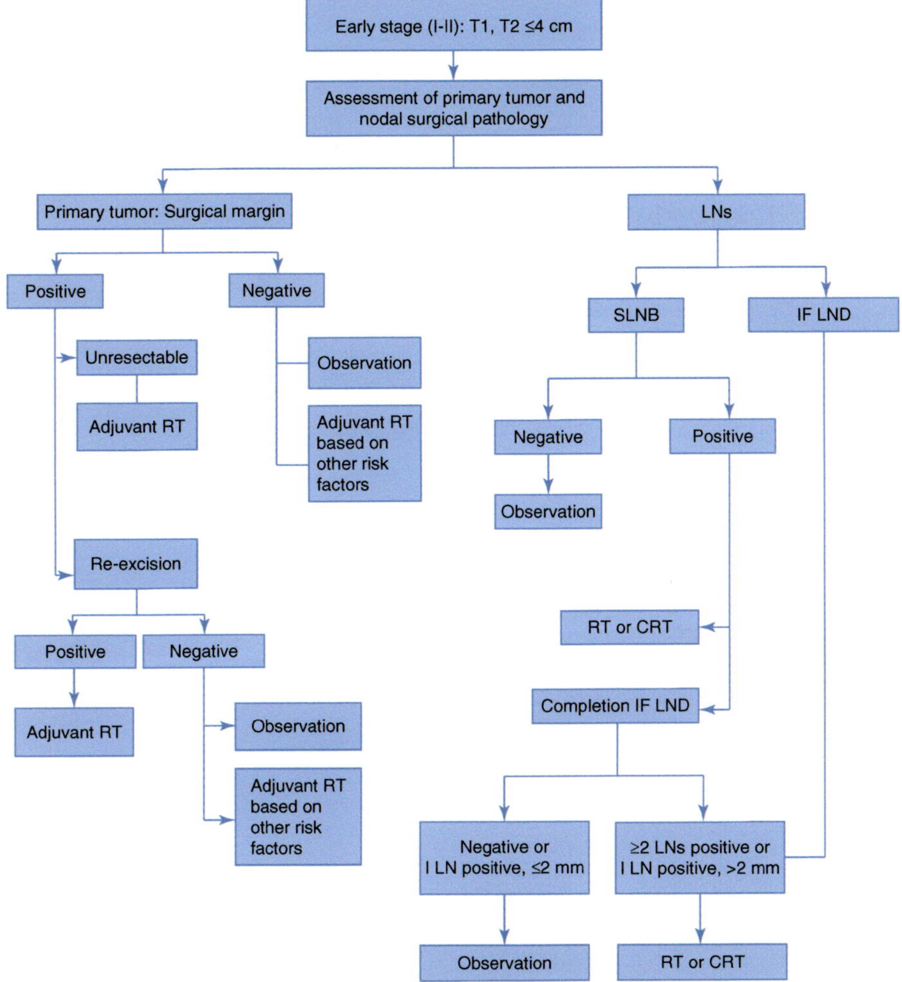

Fig. 7.21 Recommended algorithm for adjuvant therapy in early stage vulvar cancer

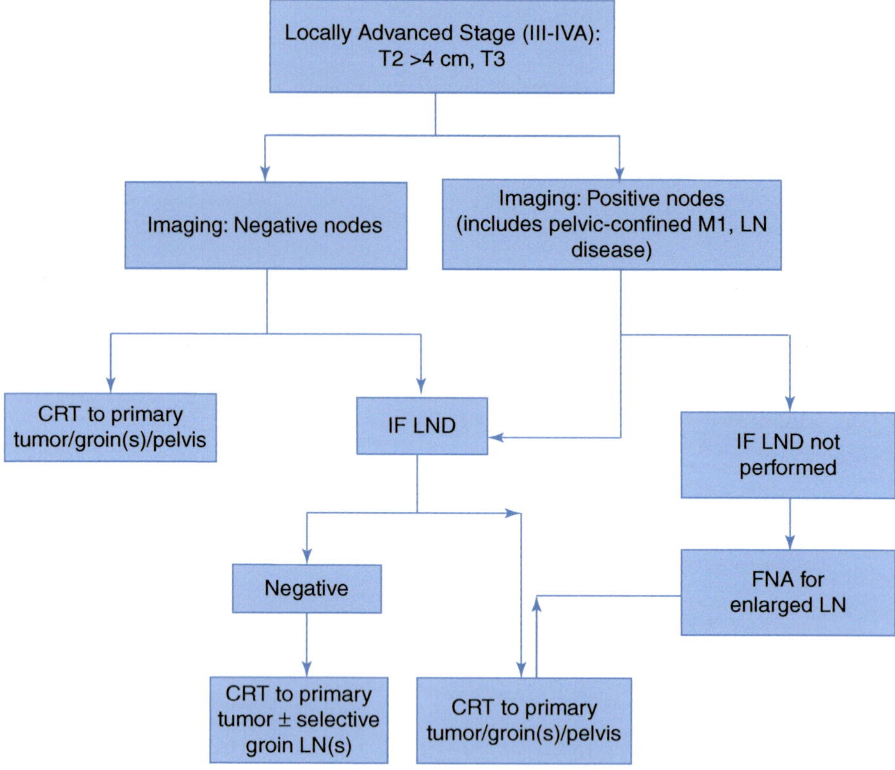

Fig. 7.22 Recommended algorithm for locally advanced stage vulvar cancer

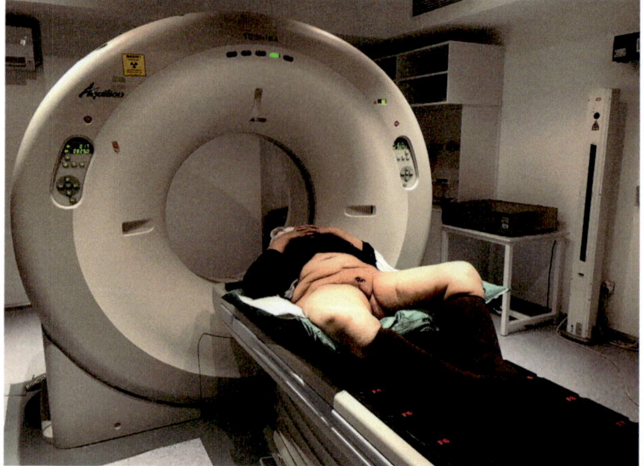

Fig. 7.23 Immobilization and simulation procedures

7.3.3.2 Contouring

- The vulvar and nodal target volumes and critical structures are usually derived from a treatment planning CT.
- RT is applied to known or suspected tumor involvement, which is called "tumor-directed RT".
- CT or MRI planning, with possible image fusion technology, should be used to delineate the primary tumor gross tumor volume (GTV), and the inguinofemoral and iliac lymph nodes.
- Any gross vulvar disease should be contoured as a GTV and include any visible and/or palpable extension beyond the vulva. The vulvar clinical target volume (CTV) encompasses the GTV or tumor bed including the entire vulva, adjacent skin, mucosa, and subcutaneous tissue excluding bony tissue and the soft tissues of the thigh and buttock. If the GTV extends beyond the vulva, an extra 1 cm margin should be encompassed by the CTV.
- If patients have extensive disease with satellite lesions, LVSI, dermal lymphatic invasion, or muscle invasion CTV should be included these lesions with extra margins.
- If there is a vaginal involvement, CTV should also be included GTV plus 3 cm margin. Care must be taken to include the entire vaginal length in the CTV, if there is any uncertainty as to the proximal extent of the vaginal extension or if there is LVSI.
- If there is an involvement of clitoris, urethra, anus, anal canal, or bladder, CTV should also be included GTV plus at least 2 cm of these structures. If disease extends into the mid or proximal urethra, CTV should include the entire urethra and bladder neck.
- If there is a close or positive margins after surgery, these regions should be marked with wire and covered by CTV at least 2 cm margin. Boost dose should also be considered in this region.
- The planning target volume (PTV) includes the CTV or ITV plus a 0.7–1 cm margin to account for positional and setup uncertainties. The treatment 3-dimensional conformal radiotherapy (3DCRT) or intensity modulated radiotherapy (IMRT) and image guidance technique also should be considered to determine margin width.
- There is no adjuvant groin RT indication for patients without pathologic evidence of groin node metastasis.
- For patients with lymph node metastases (unilateral or bilateral) confirmed after bilateral IFLN dissection, treatment should include the inguinofemoral, external iliac, internal iliac, and obturator regions bilaterally [190, 219]. The pelvic nodal CTV consist of a symmetrical 7 mm expansion around corresponding vessels. For groin nodal CTV; anteromedial $\geq$35 mm, anterior $\geq$23 mm, anterolateral $\geq$25 mm, and medial $\geq$22 mm margin on inguinofemoral vessels is optimal. It should extend laterally from the inguinofemoral vessels to the medial border of the sartorius and rectus femoris muscles, posteriorly to the anterior vastus medialis muscle, and medially to the pectineus muscle. Anteriorly the volume should extend to the anterior border of the sartorius muscle. The superior border is at the

level of the where the external iliac artery leaves the bony pelvis to become the femoral artery. The inferior border is 2 cm below the sapheno-femoral junction or the top of the lesser trochanter of the femur [218].

- It is usually suggested that also treat the vulva in cases of lymph nodes irradiated.
- If there is no skin involvement, the groin CTV will not extend outside the skin and should be trimmed to 3 mm below the skin surface. Any tumor involve the skin, the CTV should include the skin with bolus.
- Invasion into the proximal half of the posterior vaginal wall would necessitate coverage of the pre-sacral lymph nodes (from S1 to S3) in the nodal CTV.
- Invasion into the anus or anal canal would necessitate coverage of the perirectal (including mesorectum) and presacral lymph nodes (from S1 to S3).
- Nodal PTV can be defined as the nodal CTV plus symmetrical 7–10 mm expansion.
- For conventional field borders, the superior border is bottom of the sacroiliac joints or L4-L5 for pelvic nodal involvement, the inferior border is at least 2 cm below the most distal part of the vulva, the lateral border extends laterally to the widest point of the pelvic inlet. To adequately cover the IFLNs, the inferior border should be extended to the intertrochanteric line of the femur or 1.5–2 cm distal to the saphenofemoral junction.
- Bowel, bladder, rectum, and bilateral femoral heads defined as critical structures. If patients receive chemotherapy, the pelvic bone marrow should also be defined.

Case Contouring: Delineation of target volumes for the case is shown in Fig. 7.24.

7.3.3.3 Prescription Dose and Dose Constraints for Critical Structures

Case plan: The patient with T1bN2b (Stage IIIB) vulvar cancer presented here was treated with IMRT including vulvar and lymphatic region (bilateral pelvic and groin) postoperatively. RT was given daily, five days per week in 1.8 Gy per fractions to a total 50.4 Gy. Concurrent chemotherapy was not given due to her age and comorbidities. Treatment planning details are seen in Figs. 7.25 and 7.26.

7.3.3.4 Treatment Delivery Techniques

- RT can be applied with 3DCRT or IMRT/Volumetric modulated arc therapy (VMAT) technique. These techniques particularly effective at conforming radiation dose to the target structures while limiting adjacent normal tissue toxicity (e.g. bone marrow, femoral head, small bowel, rectum and bladder).
- Consensus guidelines have been published to better standardize RT use and techniques [220].
- 3DCRT: To encompass more accurately the regional lymph nodes and to reduce the dose to the femoral heads, frequently used technique is a wide anterior-posterior (AP) field that includes the pelvic and groin nodes and a narrow

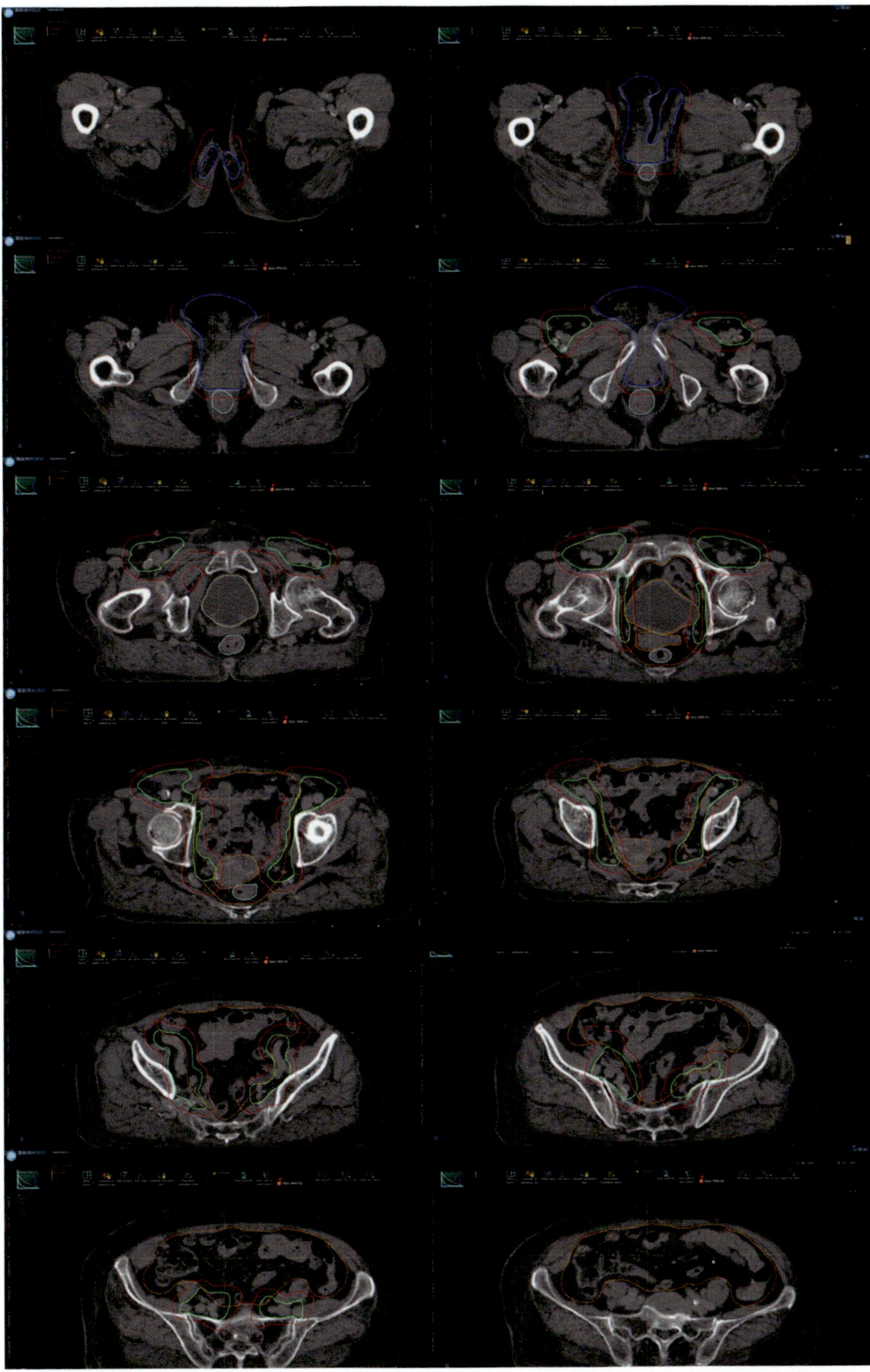

Fig. 7.24 Delineation of treatment volumes for pT1bN2bM0 vulvar SCC patient. Red: PTV, blue: CTV vulva, green: CTV groin, light blue: rectum, yellow: bladder, orange: bowel, pink: right femur, brown: left femur, dark green: body

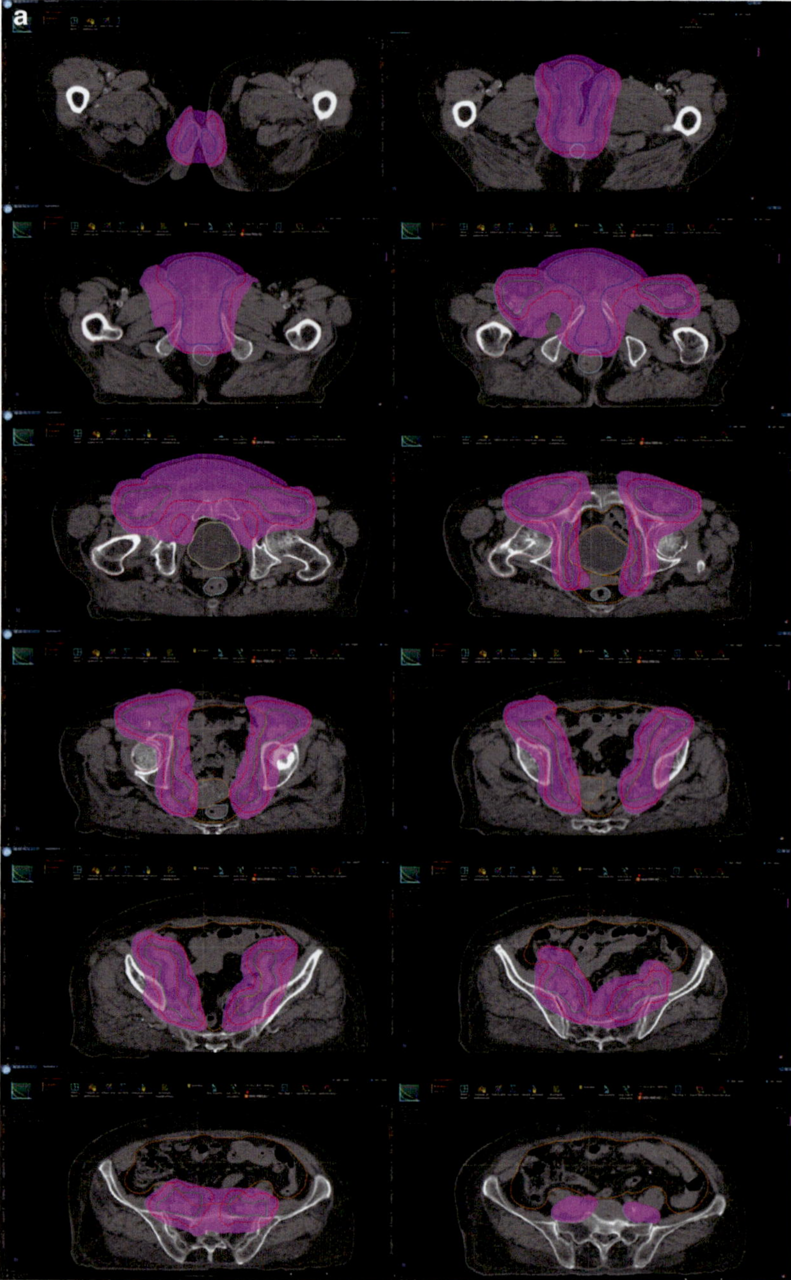

Fig. 7.25 VMAT planning in the postoperative setting of pT1bN2bM0 disease. Total dose of 50.4 Gy in 1.8 Gy/fraction was delivered. (**a**) 95% isodose coverage (pink) and (**b**) dose-volume histogram are shown. Red: PTV, blue: CTV vulva, green: CTV groin, light blue: rectum, yellow: bladder, orange: bowel, pink: right femur, brown: left femur, dark green: body

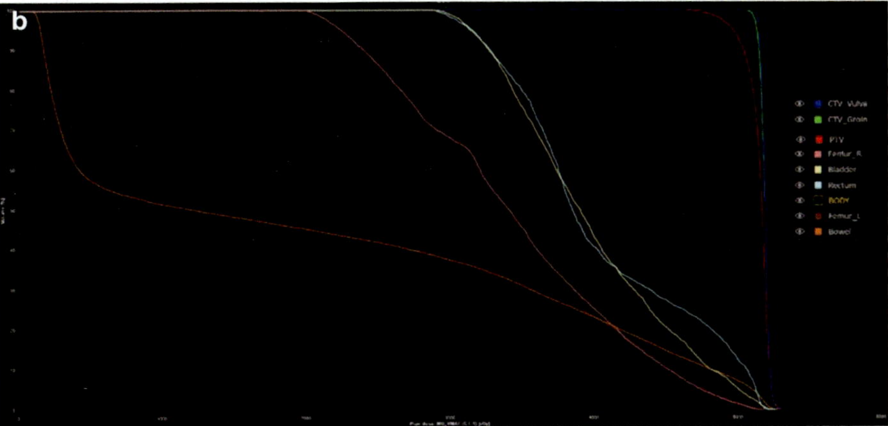

Fig. 7.25 (continued)

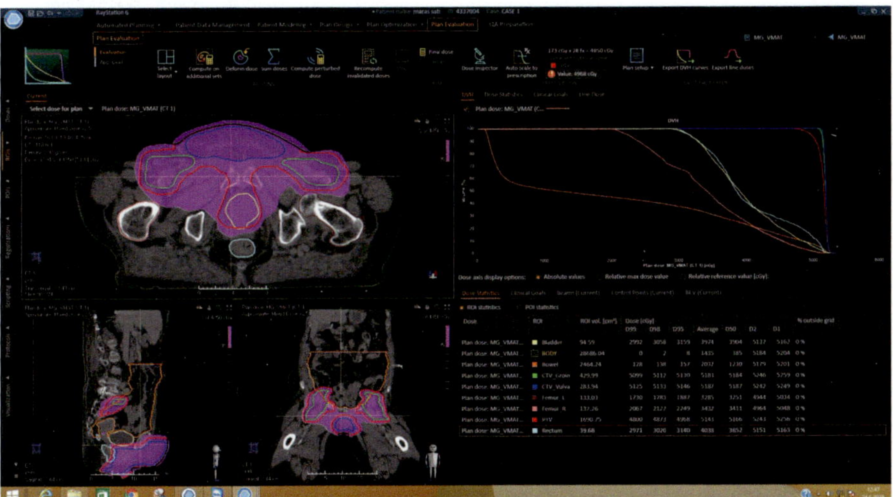

Fig. 7.26 Treatment plan of the patient

posterior-anterior (PA) field (just medial to the femoral necks and heads) covering only the pelvis. A direct anterior electron fields are used to supplement the dose to the inguinal nodes if the depth of the inguinal nodes allow for electron coverage. However, this technique has considerable dosimetric problems due to the overlap of the photon-electron fields at the groin.

- IMRT: This technique has dosimetric advantages over 3DCRT which reduce doses to normal structures, eliminate hot spots and improve dose homogeneity [221]. This treatment is well tolerated with a low incidence of severe toxicity. Bolus over the vulva is not routinely recommended, however it may provide improved dose distribution over the superficial target volume both at the vulva and the groin region. A thermoluminescent dosimeter (TLD) should be placed over the vulva both with and without bolus to confirm skin dose. IMRT should always be performed in image guidance.

7.3.3.5 Dose Recommendations

- RT is given in once daily fractions in 5 days per week. In the postoperative setting, the recommended RT dose is 45–50.4 Gy in 1.8–2.0 Gy per fraction for negative margins, 50–55 Gy for close margins and 54–59.9 Gy for positive margins [185]. Recommended doses are 50 Gy for the cases of microscopic inguinal metastases and up to 60 Gy for multiple lymph node metastases and/or presence of extracapsular extension.
- Viswanathan et al. evaluated in a retrospective study the correlation between RT dose and vulvar recurrence [222]. This study demonstrated that radiation dose $\geq$56 Gy had a lower risk of recurrence than doses $\leq$50.4 Gy.
- Patients with unresectable locally advanced disease have been treated with concurrent weekly cisplatin-based definitive CRT (60–70 Gy) [223]. Alternatively, pre-op CRT (57.6 Gy and weekly 40 mg/m^2 cisplatin) may be considered to improve resectability [201]. If there is an unresectable disease, additional therapy such as concurrent chemotherapy, dose escalation, and brachytherapy may be considered.
- If a patient cannot tolerate chemotherapy, RT alone with dose of 50.4 Gy followed by boost 14.4 Gy to total dose of 64.8 Gy can be used.
- The treatment plan and dose-volume histograms of the target and normal tissue structures should carefully be checked. Target volumes should be adequately covered by prescribed dose homogenously. Hot spots or cold spots should be avoided as well. Additionally, normal tissue dose constraints should be keep in tolerance limits.

> **Normal Tissue Dose Constraints Detailed Below were Based on Previous Radiation Therapy Oncology Group (RTOG) Protocols Using IMRT for Pelvic Tumors**
> Rectum: V45 Gy <60%
>   Bladder: V45–50 Gy <35%
>   Small bowel: V40–45 Gy <30%, 45 Gy <195 cm^3
>   Femoral head: V30 Gy <50%, V40 Gy <35%, and V44 Gy <5%, V50 Gy <5%

> **Another Dose Constraints for IMRT is Presented Below [221]**
> Rectum: V40 Gy $\leq$40%, maximum dose (Dmax) 50 Gy
>   Bladder: V40 Gy $\leq$40%, Dmax 50 Gy
>   Small bowel: V35 Gy $\leq$35%, Dmax 50 Gy
>   Ideally, 95% of the volume of each PTV should receive the prescription dose.
>   The plans were considered acceptable if <5% of the PTV received <100% of the prescribed dose, <10% of the PTV received >110% of the prescribed dose, and <1% of the PTV received >120% of the prescribed dose.

7.3.4 Follow-up Recommendations

The optimal surveillance strategy for patients with vulvar cancer remains controversial. Following therapy, patients should be seen regularly for careful clinical examination of the vulva and groins. It is suggested that every 3–6 months for the first 2 years, every 6–12 months for years 3–5 and then annually. Long-term follow-up is advised patients at high risk of recurrence (i.e., lichen sclerosus) [224]. Surveillance imaging studies should not be routinely performed unless recurrence is suspected. However, PET/CT is often recommended 10–12 weeks following definitive CRT to evaluate treatment response. Cervicovaginal cytology (PAP smear) is not routinely recommended.

References

1. Pecorelli S, Zigliani L, Odicino F. Revised FIGO staging for carcinoma of the cervix. Int J Gynaecol Obstet. 2009;105(2):107–8.
2. Cibula D, Potter R, Planchamp F, et al. The European Society of Gynaecological Oncology/European Society for Radiotherapy and Oncology/European Society of Pathology guidelines for the management of patients with cervical cancer. Radiother Oncol. 2018;28(4):641–55.
3. Grigsby PW, Siegel BA, Dehdashti F. Lymph node staging by positron emission tomography in patients with carcinoma of the cervix. J Clin Oncol. 2001;19(17):3745–9.
4. Scheidler J, Hricak H, Yu KK, Subak L, Segal MR. Radiological evaluation of lymph node metastases in patients with cervical cancer. A meta-analysis. JAMA. 1997;278(13):1096–101.
5. Leblanc E, Gauthier H, Querleu D, et al. Accuracy of 18-fluoro-2-deoxy-D-glucose positron emission tomography in the pretherapeutic detection of occult para-aortic node involvement in patients with a locally advanced cervical carcinoma. Ann Surg Oncol. 2011;18(8):2302–9.
6. Ramirez PT, Jhingran A, Macapinlac HA, et al. Laparoscopic extraperitoneal para-aortic lymphadenectomy in locally advanced cervical cancer: a prospective correlation of surgical findings with positron emission tomography/computed tomography findings. Cancer. 2011;117(9):1928–34.
7. Cormier B, Diaz JP, Shih K, et al. Establishing a sentinel lymph node mapping algorithm for the treatment of early cervical cancer. Gynecol Oncol. 2011;122(2):275–80.
8. Robison K, Holman LL, Moore RG. Update on sentinel lymph node evaluation in gynecologic malignancies. Curr Opin Obstet Gynecol. 2011;23(1):8–12.

9. Mota F. Microinvasive squamous carcinoma of the cervix: treatment modalities. Acta Obstet Gynecol Scand. 2003;82(6):505–9.

10. Landoni F, Maneo A, Colombo A, et al. Randomised study of radical surgery versus radiotherapy for stage Ib-IIa cervical cancer. Lancet. 1997;350(9077):535–40.

11. Bansal N, Herzog TJ, Shaw RE, Burke WM, Deutsch I, Wright JD. Primary therapy for early-stage cervical cancer: radical hysterectomy vs radiation. Am J Obstet Gynecol. 2009;201(5):485.e481–9.

12. Donovan KA, Taliaferro LA, Alvarez EM, Jacobsen PB, Roetzheim RG, Wenham RM. Sexual health in women treated for cervical cancer: characteristics and correlates. Gynecol Oncol. 2007;104(2):428–34.

13. Shimada M, Kigawa J, Nishimura R, et al. Ovarian metastasis in carcinoma of the uterine cervix. Gynecol Oncol. 2006;101(2):234–7.

14. Sedlis A, Bundy BN, Rotman MZ, Lentz SS, Muderspach LI, Zaino RJ. A randomized trial of pelvic radiation therapy versus no further therapy in selected patients with stage IB carcinoma of the cervix after radical hysterectomy and pelvic lymphadenectomy: a Gynecologic Oncology Group study. Gynecol Oncol. 1999;73(2):177–83.

15. Rotman M, Sedlis A, Piedmonte MR, et al. A phase III randomized trial of postoperative pelvic irradiation in Stage IB cervical carcinoma with poor prognostic features: follow-up of a gynecologic oncology group study. Int J Radiat Oncol Biol Phys. 2006;65(1): 169–76.

16. Rogers L, Siu SS, Luesley D, Bryant A, Dickinson HO. Radiotherapy and chemoradiation after surgery for early cervical cancer. Cochrane Database Syst Rev. 2012;5:CD007583.

17. Okazawa M, Mabuchi S, Isohashi F, et al. Impact of the addition of concurrent chemotherapy to pelvic radiotherapy in surgically treated stage IB1-IIB cervical cancer patients with intermediate-risk or high-risk factors: a 13-year experience. Int J Gynecol Cancer. 2013;23(3):567–75.

18. Ryu SY, Kim MH, Nam BH, et al. Intermediate-risk grouping of cervical cancer patients treated with radical hysterectomy: a Korean Gynecologic Oncology Group study. Br J Cancer. 2014;110(2):278–85.

19. Peters WA, Liu PY, Barrett RJ, et al. Concurrent chemotherapy and pelvic radiation therapy compared with pelvic radiation therapy alone as adjuvant therapy after radical surgery in high-risk early-stage cancer of the cervix. J Clin Oncol. 2000;18(8):1606–13.

20. Monk BJ, Wang J, Im S, et al. Rethinking the use of radiation and chemotherapy after radical hysterectomy: a clinical-pathologic analysis of a Gynecologic Oncology Group/Southwest Oncology Group/Radiation Therapy Oncology Group trial. Gynecol Oncol. 2005;96(3):721–8.

21. Feng SY, Zhang YN, Liu JG. Risk factors and prognosis of node-positive cervical carcinoma. Ai Zheng. 2005;24(10):1261–6.

22. Yessaian A, Magistris A, Burger RA, Monk BJ. Radical hysterectomy followed by tailored postoperative therapy in the treatment of stage IB2 cervical cancer: feasibility and indications for adjuvant therapy. Gynecol Oncol. 2004;94(1):61–6.

23. Yamashita H, Okuma K, Kawana K, et al. Comparison between conventional surgery plus postoperative adjuvant radiotherapy and concurrent chemoradiation for FIGO stage IIB cervical carcinoma: a retrospective study. Am J Clin Oncol. 2010;33(6):583–6.

24. Keys HM, Bundy BN, Stehman FB, et al. Cisplatin, radiation, and adjuvant hysterectomy compared with radiation and adjuvant hysterectomy for bulky stage IB cervical carcinoma. N Engl J Med. 1999;340(15):1154–61.

25. Morris M, Eifel PJ, Lu J, et al. Pelvic radiation with concurrent chemotherapy compared with pelvic and para-aortic radiation for high-risk cervical cancer. N Engl J Med. 1999;340(15):1137–43.

26. Whitney CW, Sause W, Bundy BN, et al. Randomized comparison of fluorouracil plus cisplatin versus hydroxyurea as an adjunct to radiation therapy in stage IIB-IVA carcinoma of the cervix with negative para-aortic lymph nodes: a Gynecologic Oncology Group and Southwest Oncology Group study. J Clin Oncol. 1999;17(5):1339–48.

27. Rose PG, Bundy BN, Watkins EB, et al. Concurrent cisplatin-based radiotherapy and chemotherapy for locally advanced cervical cancer. N Engl J Med. 1999;340(15):1144–53.
28. Thomas GM. Improved treatment for cervical cancer--concurrent chemotherapy and radiotherapy. N Engl J Med. 1999;340(15):1198–200.
29. Chemoradiotherapy for Cervical Cancer Meta-analysis C. Reducing uncertainties about the effects of chemoradiotherapy for cervical cancer: individual patient data meta-analysis. Cochrane Database Syst Rev. 2010;1:CD008285.
30. Eifel PJ, Winter K, Morris M, et al. Pelvic irradiation with concurrent chemotherapy versus pelvic and para-aortic irradiation for high-risk cervical cancer: an update of radiation therapy oncology group trial (RTOG) 90-01. J Clin Oncol. 2004;22(5):872–80.
31. Stehman FB, Ali S, Keys HM, et al. Radiation therapy with or without weekly cisplatin for bulky stage 1B cervical carcinoma: follow-up of a Gynecologic Oncology Group trial. Am J Obstet Gynecol. 2007;197(5):503.e501–6.
32. Chemoradiotherapy for Cervical Cancer Meta-Analysis C. Reducing uncertainties about the effects of chemoradiotherapy for cervical cancer: a systematic review and meta-analysis of individual patient data from 18 randomized trials. J Clin Oncol. 2008;26(35):5802–12.
33. King M, McConkey C, Latief TN, Hartley A, Fernando I. Improved survival after concurrent weekly cisplatin and radiotherapy for cervical carcinoma with assessment of acute and late side-effects. Clin Oncol. 2006;18(1):38–45.
34. Monk BJ, Tewari KS, Koh WJ. Multimodality therapy for locally advanced cervical carcinoma: state of the art and future directions. J Clin Oncol. 2007;25(20):2952–65.
35. Kim YS, Shin SS, Nam JH, et al. Prospective randomized comparison of monthly fluorouracil and cisplatin versus weekly cisplatin concurrent with pelvic radiotherapy and high-dose rate brachytherapy for locally advanced cervical cancer. Gynecol Oncol. 2008;108(1):195–200.
36. Wang CC, Chou HH, Yang LY, et al. A randomized trial comparing concurrent chemoradiotherapy with single-agent cisplatin versus cisplatin plus gemcitabine in patients with advanced cervical cancer: An Asian Gynecologic Oncology Group study. Gynecol Oncol. 2015;137(3):462–7.
37. Thakur P, Seam R, Gupta M, Gupta M. Prospective randomized study comparing concomitant chemoradiotherapy using weekly cisplatin & paclitaxel versus weekly cisplatin in locally advanced carcinoma cervix. Ann Transl Med. 2016;4(3):48.
38. Duenas-Gonzalez A, Zarba JJ, Patel F, et al. Phase III, open-label, randomized study comparing concurrent gemcitabine plus cisplatin and radiation followed by adjuvant gemcitabine and cisplatin versus concurrent cisplatin and radiation in patients with stage IIB to IVA carcinoma of the cervix. J Clin Oncol. 2011;29(13):1678–85.
39. Rose PG, Degeest K, McMeekin S, Fusco N. A phase I study of gemcitabine followed by cisplatin concurrent with whole pelvic radiation therapy in locally advanced cervical cancer: a Gynecologic Oncology Group study. Gynecol Oncol. 2007;107(2):274–9.
40. Cosin JA, Fowler JM, Chen MD, Paley PJ, Carson LF, Twiggs LB. Pretreatment surgical staging of patients with cervical carcinoma: the case for lymph node debulking. Cancer. 1998;82(11):2241–8.
41. Goff BA, Muntz HG, Paley PJ, Tamimi HK, Koh WJ, Greer BE. Impact of surgical staging in women with locally advanced cervical cancer. Gynecol Oncol. 1999;74(3):436–42.
42. Gold MA, Tian C, Whitney CW, Rose PG, Lanciano R. Surgical versus radiographic determination of para-aortic lymph node metastases before chemoradiation for locally advanced cervical carcinoma: a Gynecologic Oncology Group study. Cancer. 2008;112(9):1954–63.
43. Zanvettor PH, Filho DF, Neves AR, et al. Laparoscopic surgical staging of locally advanced cervix cancer (IB2 to IVA): initial experience. Gynecol Oncol. 2011;120(3):358–61.
44. Moore KN, Gold MA, McMeekin DS, Walker JL, Rutledge T, Zorn KK. Extraperitoneal para-aortic lymph node evaluation for cervical cancer via pfannenstiel incision: technique and peri-operative outcomes. Gynecol Oncol. 2008;108(3):466–71.
45. Sonoda Y, Leblanc E, Querleu D, et al. Prospective evaluation of surgical staging of advanced cervical cancer via a laparoscopic extraperitoneal approach. Gynecol Oncol. 2003;91(2):326–31.

46. Weiser EB, Bundy BN, Hoskins WJ, et al. Extraperitoneal versus transperitoneal selective paraaortic lymphadenectomy in the pretreatment surgical staging of advanced cervical carcinoma (a Gynecologic Oncology Group study). Gynecol Oncol. 1989;33(3):283–9.
47. Grigsby PW, Lu JD, Mutch DG, Kim RY, Eifel PJ. Twice-daily fractionation of external irradiation with brachytherapy and chemotherapy in carcinoma of the cervix with positive para-aortic lymph nodes: phase II study of the Radiation Therapy Oncology Group 92-10. Int J Radiat Oncol Biol Phys. 1998;41(4):817–22.
48. Varia MA, Bundy BN, Deppe G, et al. Cervical carcinoma metastatic to para-aortic nodes: extended field radiation therapy with concomitant 5-fluorouracil and cisplatin chemotherapy: a Gynecologic Oncology Group study. Int J Radiat Oncol Biol Phys. 1998;42(5):1015–23.
49. Small W Jr, Winter K, Levenback C, et al. Extended-field irradiation and intracavitary brachytherapy combined with cisplatin chemotherapy for cervical cancer with positive para-aortic or high common iliac lymph nodes: results of ARM 1 of RTOG 0116. Int J Radiat Oncol Biol Phys. 2007;68(4):1081–7.
50. Grigsby PW, Heydon K, Mutch DG, Kim RY, Eifel P. Long-term follow-up of RTOG 92-10: cervical cancer with positive para-aortic lymph nodes. Int J Radiat Oncol Biol Phys. 2001;51(4):982–7.
51. Rotman M, Choi K, Guse C, Marcial V, Hornback N, John M. Prophylactic irradiation of the para-aortic lymph node chain in stage IIB and bulky stage IB carcinoma of the cervix, initial treatment results of RTOG 7920. Int J Radiat Oncol Biol Phys. 1990;19(3):513–21.
52. Rotman M, Pajak TF, Choi K, et al. Prophylactic extended-field irradiation of para-aortic lymph nodes in stages IIB and bulky IB and IIA cervical carcinomas. Ten-year treatment results of RTOG 79-20. JAMA. 1995;274(5):387–93.
53. Morice P, Rouanet P, Rey A, et al. Results of the GYNECO 02 study, an FNCLCC phase III trial comparing hysterectomy with no hysterectomy in patients with a (clinical and radiological) complete response after chemoradiation therapy for stage IB2 or II cervical cancer. Oncologist. 2012;17(1):64–71.
54. Darus CJ, Callahan MB, Nguyen QN, et al. Chemoradiation with and without adjuvant extrafascial hysterectomy for IB2 cervical carcinoma. Int J Gynecol Cancer. 2008;18(4):730–5.
55. Keys HM, Bundy BN, Stehman FB, et al. Radiation therapy with and without extrafascial hysterectomy for bulky stage IB cervical carcinoma: a randomized trial of the Gynecologic Oncology Group. Gynecol Oncol. 2003;89(3):343–53.
56. Kokka F, Bryant A, Brockbank E, Powell M, Oram D. Hysterectomy with radiotherapy or chemotherapy or both for women with locally advanced cervical cancer. Cochrane Database Syst Rev. 2015;4:CD010260.
57. Kim HS, Sardi JE, Katsumata N, et al. Efficacy of neoadjuvant chemotherapy in patients with FIGO stage IB1 to IIA cervical cancer: an international collaborative meta-analysis. Eur J Surg Oncol. 2013;39(2):115–24.
58. Landoni F, Sartori E, Maggino T, et al. Is there a role for postoperative treatment in patients with stage Ib2-IIb cervical cancer treated with neo-adjuvant chemotherapy and radical surgery? An Italian multicenter retrospective study. Gynecol Oncol. 2014;132(3):611–7.
59. Ye Q, Yuan HX, Chen HL. Responsiveness of neoadjuvant chemotherapy before surgery predicts favorable prognosis for cervical cancer patients: a meta-analysis. J Cancer Res Clin Oncol. 2013;139(11):1887–98.
60. Gupta S, Maheshwari A, Parab P, et al. Neoadjuvant chemotherapy followed by radical surgery versus concomitant chemotherapy and radiotherapy in patients with stage IB2, IIA, or IIB squamous cervical cancer: a randomized controlled trial. J Clin Oncol. 2018;36:1548–55.
61. Pahisa J, Martinez-Roman S, Martinez-Zamora MA, et al. Laparoscopic ovarian transposition in patients with early cervical cancer. Int J Gynecol Cancer. 2008;18(3):584–9.
62. Small W Jr, Mell LK, Anderson P, et al. Consensus guidelines for delineation of clinical target volume for intensity-modulated pelvic radiotherapy in postoperative treatment of endometrial and cervical cancer. Int J Radiat Oncol Biol Phys. 2008;71(2):428–34.
63. Folkert MR, Shih KK, Abu-Rustum NR, et al. Postoperative pelvic intensity-modulated radiotherapy and concurrent chemotherapy in intermediate- and high-risk cervical cancer. Gynecol Oncol. 2013;128(2):288–93.

64. Du XL, Sheng XG, Jiang T, et al. Intensity-modulated radiation therapy versus para-aortic field radiotherapy to treat para-aortic lymph node metastasis in cervical cancer: prospective study. Croat Med J. 2010;51(3):229–36.

65. Lim K, Small W Jr, Portelance L, et al. Consensus guidelines for delineation of clinical target volume for intensity-modulated pelvic radiotherapy for the definitive treatment of cervix cancer. Int J Radiat Oncol Biol Phys. 2011;79(2):348–55.

66. Han K, Milosevic M, Fyles A, Pintilie M, Viswanathan AN. Trends in the utilization of brachytherapy in cervical cancer in the United States. Int J Radiat Oncol Biol Phys. 2013;87(1):111–9.

67. Parker K, Gallop-Evans E, Hanna L, Adams M. Five years' experience treating locally advanced cervical cancer with concurrent chemoradiotherapy and high-dose-rate brachytherapy: results from a single institution. Int J Radiat Oncol Biol Phys. 2009;74(1):140–6.

68. Hellebust TP, Kristensen GB, Olsen DR. Late effects after radiotherapy for locally advanced cervical cancer: comparison of two brachytherapy schedules and effect of dose delivered weekly. Int J Radiat Oncol Biol Phys. 2010;76(3):713–8.

69. Liu R, Wang X, Tian JH, et al. High dose rate versus low dose rate intracavity brachytherapy for locally advanced uterine cervix cancer. Cochrane Database Syst Rev. 2014;10:CD007563.

70. ICRU. International Commission of Radiation Units and Measurements. Dose and volume specification for reporting intracavitary therapy in gynaecology. ICRU Report 38, Bethesda, MD; 1985.

71. Zwahlen D, Jezioranski J, Chan P, et al. Magnetic resonance imaging-guided intracavitary brachytherapy for cancer of the cervix. Int J Radiat Oncol Biol Phys. 2009;74(4):1157–64.

72. Potter R, Haie-Meder C, Van Limbergen E, et al. Recommendations from gynaecological (GYN) GEC ESTRO working group (II): concepts and terms in 3D image-based treatment planning in cervix cancer brachytherapy-3D dose volume parameters and aspects of 3D image-based anatomy, radiation physics, radiobiology. Radiother Oncol. 2006;78(1):67–77.

73. Haie-Meder C, Potter R, Van Limbergen E, et al. Recommendations from Gynaecological (GYN) GEC-ESTRO Working Group (I): concepts and terms in 3D image based 3D treatment planning in cervix cancer brachytherapy with emphasis on MRI assessment of GTV and CTV. Radiother Oncol. 2005;74(3):235–45.

74. Charra-Brunaud C, Harter V, Delannes M, et al. Impact of 3D image-based PDR brachytherapy on outcome of patients treated for cervix carcinoma in France: results of the French STIC prospective study. Radiother Oncol. 2012;103(3):305–13.

75. Potter R, Dimopoulos J, Georg P, et al. Clinical impact of MRI assisted dose volume adaptation and dose escalation in brachytherapy of locally advanced cervix cancer. Radiother Oncol. 2007;83(2):148–55.

76. Castelnau-Marchand P, Chargari C, Maroun P, et al. Clinical outcomes of definitive chemoradiation followed by intracavitary pulsed-dose rate image-guided adaptive brachytherapy in locally advanced cervical cancer. Gynecol Oncol. 2015;139(2):288–94.

77. Lindegaard JC, Fokdal LU, Nielsen SK, Juul-Christensen J, Tanderup K. MRI-guided adaptive radiotherapy in locally advanced cervical cancer from a Nordic perspective. Acta Oncol. 2013;52(7):1510–9.

78. Rijkmans EC, Nout RA, Rutten IH, et al. Improved survival of patients with cervical cancer treated with image-guided brachytherapy compared with conventional brachytherapy. Gynecol Oncol. 2014;135(2):231–8.

79. Viswanathan AN, Erickson B, Gaffney DK, et al. Comparison and consensus guidelines for delineation of clinical target volume for CT- and MR-based brachytherapy in locally advanced cervical cancer. Int J Radiat Oncol Biol Phys. 2014;90(2):320–8.

80. Viswanathan AN, Dimopoulos J, Kirisits C, Berger D, Potter R. Computed tomography versus magnetic resonance imaging-based contouring in cervical cancer brachytherapy: results of a prospective trial and preliminary guidelines for standardized contours. Int J Radiat Oncol Biol Phys. 2007;68(2):491–8.

81. Ohno T, Wakatsuki M, Toita T, et al. Recommendations for high-risk clinical target volume definition with computed tomography for three-dimensional image-guided brachytherapy in cervical cancer patients. J Radiat Res. 2017;58(3):341–50.

82. Song S, Rudra S, Hasselle MD, et al. The effect of treatment time in locally advanced cervical cancer in the era of concurrent chemoradiotherapy. Cancer. 2013;119(2):325–31.

83. Nugent EK, Case AS, Hoff JT, et al. Chemoradiation in locally advanced cervical carcinoma: an analysis of cisplatin dosing and other clinical prognostic factors. Gynecol Oncol. 2010;116(3):438–41.

84. Nag S, Chao C, Erickson B, et al. The American Brachytherapy Society recommendations for low-dose-rate brachytherapy for carcinoma of the cervix. Int J Radiat Oncol Biol Phys. 2002;52(1):33–48.

85. Viswanathan AN, Beriwal S, De Los Santos JF, et al. American Brachytherapy Society consensus guidelines for locally advanced carcinoma of the cervix. Part II: high-dose-rate brachytherapy. Brachytherapy. 2012;11(1):47–52.

86. International Commission on Radiation Units and Measurements. Prescribing R, and reporting brachytherapy for cancer of the cervix (ICRU report 89), Bethesda, 2016.

87. Potter R, Georg P, Dimopoulos JC, et al. Clinical outcome of protocol based image (MRI) guided adaptive brachytherapy combined with 3D conformal radiotherapy with or without chemotherapy in patients with locally advanced cervical cancer. Radiother Oncol. 2011;100(1):116–23.

88. Potter R, Tanderup K, Kirisits C, et al. The EMBRACE II study: the outcome and prospect of two decades of evolution within the GEC-ESTRO GYN working group and the EMBRACE studies. Clin Transl Radiat Oncol. 2018;9:48–60.

89. Elit L, Fyles AW, Devries MC, Oliver TK, Fung-Kee-Fung M, Gynecology Cancer Disease Site G. Follow-up for women after treatment for cervical cancer: a systematic review. Gynecol Oncol. 2009;114(3):528–35.

90. Salani R, Backes FJ, Fung MF, et al. Posttreatment surveillance and diagnosis of recurrence in women with gynecologic malignancies: Society of Gynecologic Oncologists recommendations. Am J Obstet Gynecol. 2011;204(6):466–78.

91. American College of O, Gynecologists. ACOG practice bulletin, clinical management guidelines for obstetrician-gynecologists, number 65, August 2005: management of endometrial cancer. Obstet Gynecol. 2005;106(2):413–25.

92. Pecorelli S. Revised FIGO staging for carcinoma of the vulva, cervix, and endometrium. Int J Gynaecol Obstet. 2009;105(2):103–4.

93. Aalders JG, Thomas G. Endometrial cancer--revisiting the importance of pelvic and para aortic lymph nodes. Gynecol Oncol. 2007;104(1):222–31.

94. Homesley HD, Kadar N, Barrett RJ, Lentz SS. Selective pelvic and periaortic lymphadenectomy does not increase morbidity in surgical staging of endometrial carcinoma. Am J Obstet Gynecol. 1992;167(5):1225–30.

95. Franchi M, Ghezzi F, Riva C, Miglierina M, Buttarelli M, Bolis P. Postoperative complications after pelvic lymphadenectomy for the surgical staging of endometrial cancer. J Surg Oncol. 2001;78(4):232–7. discussion 237–40

96. Russell AH. Forwards through the rear-view mirror. Gynecol Oncol. 2009;115(1):1–3.

97. Benedet JL. Editorial. Int J Gynaecol Obstet. 2000;70(2):207–8.

98. Frederick PJ, Straughn JM Jr. The role of comprehensive surgical staging in patients with endometrial cancer. Cancer Control. 2009;16(1):23–9.

99. Benedetti Panici P, Basile S, Maneschi F, et al. Systematic pelvic lymphadenectomy vs. no lymphadenectomy in early-stage endometrial carcinoma: randomized clinical trial. J Natl Cancer Inst. 2008;100(23):1707–16.

100. Kitchener H, Swart AM, Qian Q, Amos C, Parmar MK, AS Group. Efficacy of systematic pelvic lymphadenectomy in endometrial cancer (MRC ASTEC trial): a randomised study. Lancet. 2009;373(9658):125–36.

101. Creasman WT, Morrow CP, Bundy BN, Homesley HD, Graham JE, Heller PB. Surgical pathologic spread patterns of endometrial cancer. A Gynecologic Oncology Group study. Cancer. 1987;60(8 Suppl):2035–41.

102. Manfredi R, Mirk P, Maresca G, et al. Local-regional staging of endometrial carcinoma: role of MR imaging in surgical planning. Radiology. 2004;231(2):372–8.

103. Akin O, Mironov S, Pandit-Taskar N, Hann LE. Imaging of uterine cancer. Radiol Clin N Am. 2007;45(1):167–82.
104. Colombo N, Creutzberg C, Amant F, et al. ESMO-ESGO-ESTRO consensus conference on endometrial cancer: diagnosis, treatment and follow-up. Ann Oncol. 2016;27(1):16–41.
105. Sorbe B, Nordstrom B, Maenpaa J, et al. Intravaginal brachytherapy in FIGO stage I low-risk endometrial cancer: a controlled randomized study. Int J Gynecol Cancer. 2009;19(5):873–8.
106. Morrow CP, Bundy BN, Kurman RJ, et al. Relationship between surgical-pathological risk factors and outcome in clinical stage I and II carcinoma of the endometrium: a Gynecologic Oncology Group study. Gynecol Oncol. 1991;40(1):55–65.
107. Eifel PJ, Ross J, Hendrickson M, Cox RS, Kempson R, Martinez A. Adenocarcinoma of the endometrium. Analysis of 256 cases with disease limited to the uterine corpus: treatment comparisons. Cancer. 1983;52(6):1026–31.
108. Keys HM, Roberts JA, Brunetto VL, et al. A phase III trial of surgery with or without adjunctive external pelvic radiation therapy in intermediate risk endometrial adenocarcinoma: a Gynecologic Oncology Group study. Gynecol Oncol. 2004;92(3):744–51.
109. Kong A, Johnson N, Kitchener HC, Lawrie TA. Adjuvant radiotherapy for stage I endometrial cancer. Cochrane Database Syst Rev. 2012;4:CD003916.
110. Onsrud M, Cvancarova M, Hellebust TP, Trope CG, Kristensen GB, Lindemann K. Long-term outcomes after pelvic radiation for early-stage endometrial cancer. J Clin Oncol. 2013;31(31):3951–6.
111. Blake P, Swart AM, Group AES, et al. Adjuvant external beam radiotherapy in the treatment of endometrial cancer (MRC ASTEC and NCIC CTG EN.5 randomised trials): pooled trial results, systematic review, and meta-analysis. Lancet. 2009;373(9658):137–46.
112. Creutzberg CL, van Putten WL, Koper PC, et al. Surgery and postoperative radiotherapy versus surgery alone for patients with stage-1 endometrial carcinoma: multicentre randomised trial. PORTEC Study Group. Post operative radiation therapy in endometrial carcinoma. Lancet. 2000;355(9213):1404–11.
113. Kong A, Johnson N, Kitchener HC, Lawrie TA. Adjuvant radiotherapy for stage I endometrial cancer: an updated Cochrane systematic review and meta-analysis. J Natl Cancer Inst. 2012;104(21):1625–34.
114. Nout RA, Smit VT, Putter H, et al. Vaginal brachytherapy versus pelvic external beam radiotherapy for patients with endometrial cancer of high-intermediate risk (PORTEC-2): an open-label, non-inferiority, randomised trial. Lancet. 2010;375(9717):816–23.
115. Creutzberg CL, van Putten WL, Koper PC, et al. The morbidity of treatment for patients with Stage I endometrial cancer: results from a randomized trial. Int J Radiat Oncol Biol Phys. 2001;51(5):1246–55.
116. Creutzberg CL, Nout RA, Lybeert ML, et al. Fifteen-year radiotherapy outcomes of the randomized PORTEC-1 trial for endometrial carcinoma. Int J Radiat Oncol Biol Phys. 2011;81(4):e631–8.
117. Klopp AH, Jhingran A, Ramondetta L, Lu K, Gershenson DM, Eifel PJ. Node-positive adenocarcinoma of the endometrium: outcome and patterns of recurrence with and without external beam irradiation. Gynecol Oncol. 2009;115(1):6–11.
118. Alvarez Secord A, Havrilesky LJ, Bae-Jump V, et al. The role of multi-modality adjuvant chemotherapy and radiation in women with advanced stage endometrial cancer. Gynecol Oncol. 2007;107(2):285–91.
119. Frigerio L, Mangili G, Aletti G, et al. Concomitant radiotherapy and paclitaxel for high-risk endometrial cancer: first feasibility study. Gynecol Oncol. 2001;81(1):53–7.
120. Greven K, Winter K, Underhill K, Fontenesci J, Cooper J, Burke T. Final analysis of RTOG 9708: adjuvant postoperative irradiation combined with cisplatin/paclitaxel chemotherapy following surgery for patients with high-risk endometrial cancer. Gynecol Oncol. 2006;103(1):155–9.
121. Lupe K, D'Souza DP, Kwon JS, et al. Adjuvant carboplatin and paclitaxel chemotherapy interposed with involved field radiation for advanced endometrial cancer. Gynecol Oncol. 2009;114(1):94–8.

122. Onda T, Yoshikawa H, Mizutani K, et al. Treatment of node-positive endometrial cancer with complete node dissection, chemotherapy and radiation therapy. Br J Cancer. 1997;75(12):1836–41.

123. Lupe K, Kwon J, D'Souza D, et al. Adjuvant paclitaxel and carboplatin chemotherapy with involved field radiation in advanced endometrial cancer: a sequential approach. Int J Radiat Oncol Biol Phys. 2007;67(1):110–6.

124. Johnson N, Bryant A, Miles T, Hogberg T, Cornes P. Adjuvant chemotherapy for endometrial cancer after hysterectomy. Cochrane Database Syst Rev. 2011;10:CD003175.

125. McMeekin DSFV, Aghajanian C, et al. Randomized phase III trial of pelvic radiation therapy (PXRT) versus vaginal cuff brachytherapy followed by paclitaxel/ carboplatin chemotherapy (VCB/C) in patients with high risk (HR), early stage endometrial cancer (EC): a Gynecologic Oncology Group trial. Gynecol Oncol. 2014;134:438.

126. Randall MEFV, McMeekin DS, et al. A phase 3 trial of pelvic radiation therapy versus vaginal cuff brachytherapy followed by paclitaxel/carboplatin chemotherapy in patients with high-risk, early-stage endometrial cancer: a Gynecology Oncology Group study. Int J Radiat Oncol Biol Phys. 2017;99(5):1313.

127. Parthasarathy A, Kapp DS, Cheung MK, Shin JY, Osann K, Chan JK. Adjuvant radiotherapy in incompletely staged IC and II endometrioid uterine cancer. Obstet Gynecol. 2007;110(6):1237–43.

128. Scholten AN, van Putten WL, Beerman H, et al. Postoperative radiotherapy for Stage 1 endometrial carcinoma: long-term outcome of the randomized PORTEC trial with central pathology review. Int J Radiat Oncol Biol Phys. 2005;63(3):834–8.

129. Randall ME, Filiaci VL, Muss H, et al. Randomized phase III trial of whole-abdominal irradiation versus doxorubicin and cisplatin chemotherapy in advanced endometrial carcinoma: a Gynecologic Oncology Group Study. J Clin Oncol. 2006;24(1):36–44.

130. Susumu N, Sagae S, Udagawa Y, et al. Randomized phase III trial of pelvic radiotherapy versus cisplatin-based combined chemotherapy in patients with intermediate- and high-risk endometrial cancer: a Japanese Gynecologic Oncology Group study. Gynecol Oncol. 2008;108(1):226–33.

131. Maggi R, Lissoni A, Spina F, et al. Adjuvant chemotherapy vs radiotherapy in high-risk endometrial carcinoma: results of a randomised trial. Br J Cancer. 2006;95(3):266–71.

132. Hogberg T, Signorelli M, de Oliveira CF, et al. Sequential adjuvant chemotherapy and radiotherapy in endometrial cancer--results from two randomised studies. Eur J Cancer. 2010;46(13):2422–31.

133. Galaal K, Al Moundhri M, Bryant A, Lopes AD, Lawrie TA. Adjuvant chemotherapy for advanced endometrial cancer. Cochrane Database Syst Rev. 2014;5:CD010681.

134. Morrow CP, Bundy BN, Homesley HD, et al. Doxorubicin as an adjuvant following surgery and radiation therapy in patients with high-risk endometrial carcinoma, stage I and occult stage II: a Gynecologic Oncology Group Study. Gynecol Oncol. 1990;36(2):166–71.

135. Matei DFV, Randall M, Steinhoff M, DiSilvestro P, Moxley KM. A randomized phase III trial of cisplatin and tumor volume directed irradiation followed by carboplatin and paclitaxel vs. carboplatin and paclitaxel for optimally debulked, advanced endometrial carcinoma. J Clin Oncol. 2017;35:5505.

136. Kuoppala T, Maenpaa J, Tomas E, et al. Surgically staged high-risk endometrial cancer: randomized study of adjuvant radiotherapy alone vs. sequential chemo-radiotherapy. Gynecol Oncol. 2008;110(2):190–5.

137. Aalders J, Abeler V, Kolstad P, Onsrud M. Postoperative external irradiation and prognostic parameters in stage I endometrial carcinoma: clinical and histopathologic study of 540 patients. Obstet Gynecol. 1980;56(4):419–27.

138. Park HJ, Nam EJ, Kim S, Kim YB, Kim YT. The benefit of adjuvant chemotherapy combined with postoperative radiotherapy for endometrial cancer: a meta-analysis. Eur J Obstet Gynecol Reprod Biol. 2013;170(1):39–44.

139. Secord AA, Havrilesky LJ, O'Malley DM, et al. A multicenter evaluation of sequential multimodality therapy and clinical outcome for the treatment of advanced endometrial cancer. Gynecol Oncol. 2009;114(3):442–7.

140. Abaid LN, Rettenmaier MA, Brown JV, et al. Sequential chemotherapy and radiotherapy as sandwich therapy for the treatment of high risk endometrial cancer. J Gynecol Oncol. 2012;23(1):22–7.
141. Geller MA, Ivy JJ, Ghebre R, et al. A phase II trial of carboplatin and docetaxel followed by radiotherapy given in a "Sandwich" method for stage III, IV, and recurrent endometrial cancer. Gynecol Oncol. 2011;121(1):112–7.
142. Gao H, Zhang Z. Sequential chemotherapy and radiotherapy in the sandwich method for advanced endometrial cancer: a meta-analysis. Medicine (Baltimore). 2015;94(16):e672.
143. de Boer SM, Powell ME, Mileshkin L, et al. Adjuvant chemoradiotherapy versus radiotherapy alone for women with high-risk endometrial cancer (PORTEC-3): final results of an international, open-label, multicentre, randomised, phase 3 trial. Lancet Oncol. 2018;19(3):295–309.
144. de Boer SM, Powell ME, Mileshkin L, et al. Toxicity and quality of life after adjuvant chemoradiotherapy versus radiotherapy alone for women with high-risk endometrial cancer (PORTEC-3): an open-label, multicentre, randomised, phase 3 trial. Lancet Oncol. 2016;17(8):1114–26.
145. Wright JD, Fiorelli J, Kansler AL, et al. Optimizing the management of stage II endometrial cancer: the role of radical hysterectomy and radiation. Am J Obstet Gynecol. 2009;200(4):419. e411–7.
146. Klopp A, Smith BD, Alektiar K, et al. The role of postoperative radiation therapy for endometrial cancer: executive summary of an American Society for Radiation Oncology evidence-based guideline. Pract Radiat Oncol. 2014;4(3):137–44.
147. Rossi PJ, Jani AB, Horowitz IR, Johnstone PA. Adjuvant brachytherapy removes survival disadvantage of local disease extension in stage IIIC endometrial cancer: a SEER registry analysis. Int J Radiat Oncol Biol Phys. 2008;70(1):134–8.
148. Randall ME, Wilder J, Greven K, Raben M. Role of intracavitary cuff boost after adjuvant external irradiation in early endometrial carcinoma. Int J Radiat Oncol Biol Phys. 1990;19(1):49–54.
149. Greven K, Winter K, Underhill K, et al. Preliminary analysis of RTOG 9708: adjuvant postoperative radiotherapy combined with cisplatin/paclitaxel chemotherapy after surgery for patients with high-risk endometrial cancer. Int J Radiat Oncol Biol Phys. 2004;59(1):168–73.
150. Scotti V, Borghesi S, Meattini I, et al. Postoperative radiotherapy in stage I/II endometrial cancer: retrospective analysis of 883 patients treated at the University of Florence. Int J Gynecol Cancer. 2010;20(9):1540–8.
151. Jobsen JJ, Lybeert ML, van der Steen-Banasik EM, et al. Multicenter cohort study on treatment results and risk factors in stage II endometrial carcinoma. Int J Gynecol Cancer. 2008;18(5):1071–8.
152. Crosby MA, Tward JD, Szabo A, Lee CM, Gaffney DK. Does brachytherapy improve survival in addition to external beam radiation therapy in patients with high risk stage I and II endometrial carcinoma? Am J Clin Oncol. 2010;33(4):364–9.
153. Sorbe B, Horvath G, Andersson H, Boman K, Lundgren C, Pettersson B. External pelvic and vaginal irradiation versus vaginal irradiation alone as postoperative therapy in medium-risk endometrial carcinoma--a prospective randomized study. Int J Radiat Oncol Biol Phys. 2012;82(3):1249–55.
154. Hasegawa K, Nagao S, Yasuda M, et al. Gynecologic Cancer InterGroup (GCIG) consensus review for clear cell carcinoma of the uterine corpus and cervix. Int J Gynecol Cancer. 2014;24(9 Suppl 3):S90–5.
155. Viswanathan AN, Macklin EA, Berkowitz R, Matulonis U. The importance of chemotherapy and radiation in uterine papillary serous carcinoma. Gynecol Oncol. 2011;123(3):542–7.
156. Barney BM, Petersen IA, Mariani A, Dowdy SC, Bakkum-Gamez JN, Haddock MG. The role of vaginal brachytherapy in the treatment of surgical stage I papillary serous or clear cell endometrial cancer. Int J Radiat Oncol Biol Phys. 2013;85(1):109–15.
157. Bernardini MQ, Gien LT, Lau S, et al. Treatment related outcomes in high-risk endometrial carcinoma: Canadian high risk endometrial cancer consortium (CHREC). Gynecol Oncol. 2016;141(1):148–54.

158. Podzielinski I, Randall ME, Breheny PJ, et al. Primary radiation therapy for medically inoperable patients with clinical stage I and II endometrial carcinoma. Gynecol Oncol. 2012;124(1):36–41.
159. Fishman DA, Roberts KB, Chambers JT, Kohorn EI, Schwartz PE, Chambers SK. Radiation therapy as exclusive treatment for medically inoperable patients with stage I and II endometrioid carcinoma with endometrium. Gynecol Oncol. 1996;61(2):189–96.
160. Patsavas K, Woessner J, Gielda B, et al. Optimal surgical debulking in uterine papillary serous carcinoma affects survival. Gynecol Oncol. 2011;121(3):581–5.
161. Rauh-Hain JA, Growdon WB, Schorge JO, et al. Prognostic determinants in patients with stage IIIC and IV uterine papillary serous carcinoma. Gynecol Oncol. 2010;119(2):299–304.
162. Shih KK, Yun E, Gardner GJ, Barakat RR, Chi DS, Leitao MM Jr. Surgical cytoreduction in stage IV endometrioid endometrial carcinoma. Gynecol Oncol. 2011;122(3):608–11.
163. Bristow RE, Zerbe MJ, Rosenshein NB, Grumbine FC, Montz FJ. Stage IVB endometrial carcinoma: the role of cytoreductive surgery and determinants of survival. Gynecol Oncol. 2000;78(2):85–91.
164. Beriwal S, Jain SK, Heron DE, et al. Clinical outcome with adjuvant treatment of endometrial carcinoma using intensity-modulated radiation therapy. Gynecol Oncol. 2006;102(2):195–9.
165. Small W Jr, Beriwal S, Demanes DJ, et al. American Brachytherapy Society consensus guidelines for adjuvant vaginal cuff brachytherapy after hysterectomy. Brachytherapy. 2012;11(1):58–67.
166. Schwarz JK, Beriwal S, Esthappan J, et al. Consensus statement for brachytherapy for the treatment of medically inoperable endometrial cancer. Brachytherapy. 2015;14(5):587–99.
167. Viswanathan C, Kirschner K, Truong M, Balachandran A, Devine C, Bhosale P. Multimodality imaging of vulvar cancer: staging, therapeutic response, and complications. AJR Am J Roentgenol. 2013;200(6):1387–400.
168. van der Velden J, Fons G, Lawrie TA. Primary groin irradiation versus primary groin surgery for early vulvar cancer. Cochrane Database Syst Rev. 2011;5:CD002224.
169. DeSimone CP, Van Ness JS, Cooper AL, et al. The treatment of lateral T1 and T2 squamous cell carcinomas of the vulva confined to the labium majus or minus. Gynecol Oncol. 2007;104(2):390–5.
170. Ansink A, van der Velden J. Surgical interventions for early squamous cell carcinoma of the vulva. Cochrane Database Syst Rev. 2000;2:CD002036.
171. Farias-Eisner R, Cirisano FD, Grouse D, et al. Conservative and individualized surgery for early squamous carcinoma of the vulva: the treatment of choice for stage I and II (T1-2N0-1M0) disease. Gynecol Oncol. 1994;53(1):55–8.
172. Hacker NF, Berek JS, Lagasse LD, Nieberg RK, Leuchter RS. Individualization of treatment for stage I squamous cell vulvar carcinoma. Obstet Gynecol. 1984;63(2):155–62.
173. Woelber L, Eulenburg C, Grimm D, et al. The risk of contralateral non-sentinel metastasis in patients with primary vulvar cancer and unilaterally positive sentinel node. Ann Surg Oncol. 2016;23(8):2508–14.
174. Coleman RL, Ali S, Levenback CF, et al. Is bilateral lymphadenectomy for midline squamous carcinoma of the vulva always necessary? An analysis from Gynecologic Oncology Group (GOG) 173. Gynecol Oncol. 2013;128(2):155–9.
175. Gonzalez Bosquet J, Magrina JF, Magtibay PM, et al. Patterns of inguinal groin metastases in squamous cell carcinoma of the vulva. Gynecol Oncol. 2007;105(3):742–6.
176. Burger MP, Hollema H, Emanuels AG, Krans M, Pras E, Bouma J. The importance of the groin node status for the survival of T1 and T2 vulval carcinoma patients. Gynecol Oncol. 1995;57(3):327–34.
177. Van der Zee AG, Oonk MH, De Hullu JA, et al. Sentinel node dissection is safe in the treatment of early-stage vulvar cancer. J Clin Oncol. 2008;26(6):884–9.
178. Levenback CF, Ali S, Coleman RL, et al. Lymphatic mapping and sentinel lymph node biopsy in women with squamous cell carcinoma of the vulva: a gynecologic oncology group study. J Clin Oncol. 2012;30(31):3786–91.

179. Oonk MH, van Hemel BM, Hollema H, et al. Size of sentinel-node metastasis and chances of non-sentinel-node involvement and survival in early stage vulvar cancer: results from GROINSS-V, a multicentre observational study. Lancet Oncol. 2010;11(7):646–52.
180. Covens A, Vella ET, Kennedy EB, Reade CJ, Jimenez W, Le T. Sentinel lymph node biopsy in vulvar cancer: Systematic review, meta-analysis and guideline recommendations. Gynecol Oncol. 2015;137(2):351–61.
181. Stehman FB, Bundy BN, Thomas G, et al. Groin dissection versus groin radiation in carcinoma of the vulva: a Gynecologic Oncology Group study. Int J Radiat Oncol Biol Phys. 1992;24(2):389–96.
182. Hallak S, Ladi L, Sorbe B. Prophylactic inguinal-femoral irradiation as an alternative to primary lymphadenectomy in treatment of vulvar carcinoma. Int J Oncol. 2007;31(5):1077–85.
183. Heaps JM, Fu YS, Montz FJ, Hacker NF, Berek JS. Surgical-pathologic variables predictive of local recurrence in squamous cell carcinoma of the vulva. Gynecol Oncol. 1990;38(3):309–14.
184. Ignatov T, Eggemann H, Burger E, Costa SD, Ignatov A. Adjuvant radiotherapy for vulvar cancer with close or positive surgical margins. J Cancer Res Clin Oncol. 2016;142(2):489–95.
185. Chapman BV, Gill BS, Viswanathan AN, Balasubramani GK, Sukumvanich P, Beriwal S. Adjuvant radiation therapy for margin-positive vulvar squamous cell carcinoma: defining the ideal dose-response using the national cancer data base. Int J Radiat Oncol Biol Phys. 2017;97(1):107–17.
186. Te Grootenhuis NC, Pouwer AW, de Bock GH, et al. Prognostic factors for local recurrence of squamous cell carcinoma of the vulva: a systematic review. Gynecol Oncol. 2018;148(3):622–31.
187. Stehman FB, Bundy BN, Dvoretsky PM, Creasman WT. Early stage I carcinoma of the vulva treated with ipsilateral superficial inguinal lymphadenectomy and modified radical hemivulvectomy: a prospective study of the Gynecologic Oncology Group. Obstet Gynecol. 1992;79(4):490–7.
188. Mahner S, Jueckstock J, Hilpert F, et al. Adjuvant therapy in lymph node-positive vulvar cancer: the AGO-CaRE-1 study. J Natl Cancer Inst. 2015;107(3):dju426.
189. Chan JK, Sugiyama V, Pham H, et al. Margin distance and other clinico-pathologic prognostic factors in vulvar carcinoma: a multivariate analysis. Gynecol Oncol. 2007;104(3):636–41.
190. Homesley HD, Bundy BN, Sedlis A, Adcock L. Radiation therapy versus pelvic node resection for carcinoma of the vulva with positive groin nodes. Obstet Gynecol. 1986;68(6):733–40.
191. Parthasarathy A, Cheung MK, Osann K, et al. The benefit of adjuvant radiation therapy in single-node-positive squamous cell vulvar carcinoma. Gynecol Oncol. 2006;103(3):1095–9.
192. Fons G, Groenen SM, Oonk MH, et al. Adjuvant radiotherapy in patients with vulvar cancer and one intra capsular lymph node metastasis is not beneficial. Gynecol Oncol. 2009;114(2):343–5.
193. Kunos C, Simpkins F, Gibbons H, Tian C, Homesley H. Radiation therapy compared with pelvic node resection for node-positive vulvar cancer: a randomized controlled trial. Obstet Gynecol. 2009;114(3):537–46.
194. Gill BS, Bernard ME, Lin JF, et al. Impact of adjuvant chemotherapy with radiation for node-positive vulvar cancer: A National Cancer Data Base (NCDB) analysis. Gynecol Oncol. 2015;137(3):365–72.
195. Dusenbery KE, Carlson JW, LaPorte RM, et al. Radical vulvectomy with postoperative irradiation for vulvar cancer: therapeutic implications of a central block. Int J Radiat Oncol Biol Phys. 1994;29(5):989–98.
196. Boronow RC. Combined therapy as an alternative to exenteration for locally advanced vulvo-vaginal cancer: rationale and results. Cancer. 1982;49(6):1085–91.
197. Shylasree TS, Bryant A, Howells RE. Chemoradiation for advanced primary vulval cancer. Cochrane Database Syst Rev. 2011;4:CD003752.
198. Han SC, Kim DH, Higgins SA, Carcangiu ML, Kacinski BM. Chemoradiation as primary or adjuvant treatment for locally advanced carcinoma of the vulva. Int J Radiat Oncol Biol Phys. 2000;47(5):1235–44.

199. Nooij LS, Ongkiehong PJ, van Zwet EW, et al. Groin surgery and risk of recurrence in lymph node positive patients with vulvar squamous cell carcinoma. Gynecol Oncol. 2015;139(3):458–64.
200. Hyde SE, Valmadre S, Hacker NF, Schilthuis MS, Grant PT, van der Velden J. Squamous cell carcinoma of the vulva with bulky positive groin nodes-nodal debulking versus full groin dissection prior to radiation therapy. Int J Gynecol Cancer. 2007;17(1):154–8.
201. Moore DH, Ali S, Koh WJ, et al. A phase II trial of radiation therapy and weekly cisplatin chemotherapy for the treatment of locally-advanced squamous cell carcinoma of the vulva: a Gynecologic Oncology Group study. Gynecol Oncol. 2012;124(3):529–33.
202. Stecklein SR, Frumovitz M, Klopp AH, Gunther JR, Eifel PJ. Effectiveness of definitive radiotherapy for squamous cell carcinoma of the vulva with gross inguinal lymphadenopathy. Gynecol Oncol. 2018;148(3):474–9.
203. Reade CJ, Eiriksson LR, Mackay H. Systemic therapy in squamous cell carcinoma of the vulva: current status and future directions. Gynecol Oncol. 2014;132(3):780–9.
204. van Doorn HC, Ansink A, Verhaar-Langereis M, Stalpers L. Neoadjuvant chemoradiation for advanced primary vulvar cancer. Cochrane Database Syst Rev. 2006;3:CD003752.
205. Eifel PJ, Morris M, Burke TW, Levenback C, Gershenson DM. Prolonged continuous infusion cisplatin and 5-fluorouracil with radiation for locally advanced carcinoma of the vulva. Gynecol Oncol. 1995;59(1):51–6.
206. Lupi G, Raspagliesi F, Zucali R, et al. Combined preoperative chemoradiotherapy followed by radical surgery in locally advanced vulvar carcinoma. A pilot study. Cancer. 1996;77(8):1472–8.
207. Moore DH, Thomas GM, Montana GS, Saxer A, Gallup DG, Olt G. Preoperative chemoradiation for advanced vulvar cancer: a phase II study of the Gynecologic Oncology Group. Int J Radiat Oncol Biol Phys. 1998;42(1):79–85.
208. Geisler JP, Manahan KJ, Buller RE. Neoadjuvant chemotherapy in vulvar cancer: avoiding primary exenteration. Gynecol Oncol. 2006;100(1):53–7.
209. Landoni F, Maneo A, Zanetta G, et al. Concurrent preoperative chemotherapy with 5-fluorouracil and mitomycin C and radiotherapy (FUMIR) followed by limited surgery in locally advanced and recurrent vulvar carcinoma. Gynecol Oncol. 1996;61(3):321–7.
210. Berek JS, Heaps JM, Fu YS, Juillard GJ, Hacker NF. Concurrent cisplatin and 5-fluorouracil chemotherapy and radiation therapy for advanced-stage squamous carcinoma of the vulva. Gynecol Oncol. 1991;42(3):197–201.
211. Koh WJ, Wallace HJ, Greer BE, et al. Combined radiotherapy and chemotherapy in the management of local-regionally advanced vulvar cancer. Int J Radiat Oncol Biol Phys. 1993;26(5):809–16.
212. Cunningham MJ, Goyer RP, Gibbons SK, Kredentser DC, Malfetano JH, Keys H. Primary radiation, cisplatin, and 5-fluorouracil for advanced squamous carcinoma of the vulva. Gynecol Oncol. 1997;66(2):258–61.
213. Gerszten K, Selvaraj RN, Kelley J, Faul C. Preoperative chemoradiation for locally advanced carcinoma of the vulva. Gynecol Oncol. 2005;99(3):640–4.
214. Tans L, Ansink AC, van Rooij PH, Kleijnen C, Mens JW. The role of chemo-radiotherapy in the management of locally advanced carcinoma of the vulva: single institutional experience and review of literature. Am J Clin Oncol. 2011;34(1):22–6.
215. Montana GS, Thomas GM, Moore DH, et al. Preoperative chemo-radiation for carcinoma of the vulva with N2/N3 nodes: a Gynecologic Oncology Group study. Int J Radiat Oncol Biol Phys. 2000;48(4):1007–13.
216. Stehman FB, Look KY. Carcinoma of the vulva. Obstet Gynecol. 2006;107(3):719–33.
217. Beriwal S, Shukla G, Shinde A, et al. Preoperative intensity modulated radiation therapy and chemotherapy for locally advanced vulvar carcinoma: analysis of pattern of relapse. Int J Radiat Oncol Biol Phys. 2013;85(5):1269–74.
218. Kim CH, Olson AC, Kim H, Beriwal S. Contouring inguinal and femoral nodes; how much margin is needed around the vessels? Pract Radiat Oncol. 2012;2(4):274–8.

219. Jackson KS, Fankam EF, Das N, et al. Unilateral groin and pelvic irradiation for unilaterally node-positive women with vulval carcinoma. Int J Gynecol Cancer. 2006;16(1):283–7.

220. Gaffney DK, King B, Viswanathan AN, et al. Consensus recommendations for radiation therapy contouring and treatment of vulvar carcinoma. Int J Radiat Oncol Biol Phys. 2016;95(4):1191–200.

221. Beriwal S, Heron DE, Kim H, et al. Intensity-modulated radiotherapy for the treatment of vulvar carcinoma: a comparative dosimetric study with early clinical outcome. Int J Radiat Oncol Biol Phys. 2006;64(5):1395–400.

222. Viswanathan AN, Pinto AP, Schultz D, Berkowitz R, Crum CP. Relationship of margin status and radiation dose to recurrence in post-operative vulvar carcinoma. Gynecol Oncol. 2013;130(3):545–9.

223. Rao YJ, Chin RI, Hui C, et al. Improved survival with definitive chemoradiation compared to definitive radiation alone in squamous cell carcinoma of the vulva: a review of the National Cancer Database. Gynecol Oncol. 2017;146(3):572–9.

224. Oonk MHM, Planchamp F, Baldwin P, et al. European Society of Gynaecological Oncology guidelines for the management of patients with vulvar cancer. Int J Gynecol Cancer. 2017;27(4):832–7.

Sarcoma

8

Sezin Yuce Sari, Gozde Yazici, Melis Gultekin,
Pervin Hurmuz, Murat Gurkaynak, and Gokhan Ozyigit

8.1   Soft Tissue Sarcoma

Overview

Epidemiology: Soft tissue sarcomas (STS) are rare tumors and comprise <1% of all new cancer diagnoses in adults (www.seer.cancer.gov). The etiology is unknown for most STS; however, environmental factors such as radiation and chemical exposures, immunosuppression, lymphedema, viruses, and genetic syndromes (e.g. Li-Fraumeni syndrome, Werner syndrome, neurofibromatosis type 1, Gardner syndrome) can be responsible for some of them [1, 2].

Pathology: Soft tissue sarcomas can arise from any anatomic location and have various histological subtypes. The most common anatomic site is an extremity (60%) (mostly lower), then comes the trunk (15–20%), retroperitoneum (10–15%), and head and neck region (8%) [3]. STS tend to invade longitudinally along musculoaponeurotic planes, and generally do not invade fascial boundaries or bones [4, 5]. As they grow, the surrounding normal tissue is compressed and a pseudocapsule is formed. Microscopic tumor cells can perforate this pesudocapsule and extend beyond it. At the time of diagnosis, involvement of regional lymph nodes (LN) is very rare. However, certain subtypes such as clear cell sarcoma, angiosarcoma, and epithelioid sarcoma have a higher probability of invading LNs [6]. Distant metastasis (DM) at the time of diagnosis can be detected in nearly 25% of patients [3], the lung being the first and the most common site. According to the World Health

S. Y. Sari (✉) · G. Yazici · M. Gultekin · P. Hurmuz · M. Gurkaynak · G. Ozyigit
Department of Radiation Oncology, Faculty of Medicine, Hacettepe University, Ankara, Turkey

© Springer Nature Switzerland AG 2019
G. Ozyigit, U. Selek (eds.), *Radiation Oncology*,
https://doi.org/10.1007/978-3-319-97145-2_8

Organization, STS are divided into four categories as benign, intermediate-locally aggressive, intermediate-rarely metastasizing, and malignant [1]. There are more than 50 histologic subtypes of STS, the most common being liposarcoma, leiomyosarcoma, synovial sarcoma, malignant peripheral nerve sheath tumor, and pleomorphic sarcoma [1]. The most widely used grading systems are the United States National Cancer Institute (NCI) and the French Federation Nationale des Centres de Lutte Contre le Cancer grading systems which grade these tumors as low, intermediate, and high grade according to their scores of tumor differentiation, mitotic count and necrosis between 2 and 8 [7].

Diagnosis: The majority of patients present with a painless mass. Imaging should be performed for both the primary and potential sites of metastasis. The best imaging modality for STS is a magnetic resonance imaging (MRI) scan as it can show the relation between the tumor and adjacent structures as well as the associated edema. For ruling out metastasis, computed tomography (CT) of the chest and/or positron emission tomography (PET)/CT scan is recommended. For the exact diagnosis, an incisional biopsy or CT-guided core biopsy should be performed.

Treatment: The main treatment for STS is surgery. Based on prognostic factors, adjuvant or neoadjuvant radiotherapy (RT) is generally added to surgery with or without chemotherapy. The most important prognostic factor is shown to be the TNM stage. This staging is made based on the tumor size and grade, which are also independent risk factors for tumor recurrence [8–10]. Other prognostic factors include the depth, location and histopathology of the tumor, age, gender, surgical margin status, bone or neurovascular invasion, recurrent disease, and although rare, LN involvement [7–9, 11, 12].

Key Words: Soft tissue sarcoma; Radiotherapy

8.1.1 Case Presentation

A 21-year old woman applied to the hospital with a growing mass in the right lower leg in July 2013. A 5 × 5 cm mass lesion was palpated in the medial side of the right tibia without any sign of inflammation or pathologic LNs. The lab findings and chest x-ray were normal. Superficial ultrasonography revealed a 41 × 32 mm, hypoechoic, clearly-defined solid mass in the right tibia. On MRI, a 31 × 22 × 39 mm, lobulated, clearly-defined mass was identified in the middle 1/3 of the right tibia in the posterior compartment between the superficial and deep muscle layers which was hyperintense on T2- and isointense with the muscle tissue on T1-weighted images, respectively (Fig. 8.1). Tru-cut biopsy revealed a low-grade fibromyxoid sarcoma. In August 2013, marginal resection from the right tibia was performed. The final pathology revealed a 45 × 35 × 30 mm, low-grade fibromyxoid sarcoma with positive surgical margins on several sides. Re-excision was not planned due to

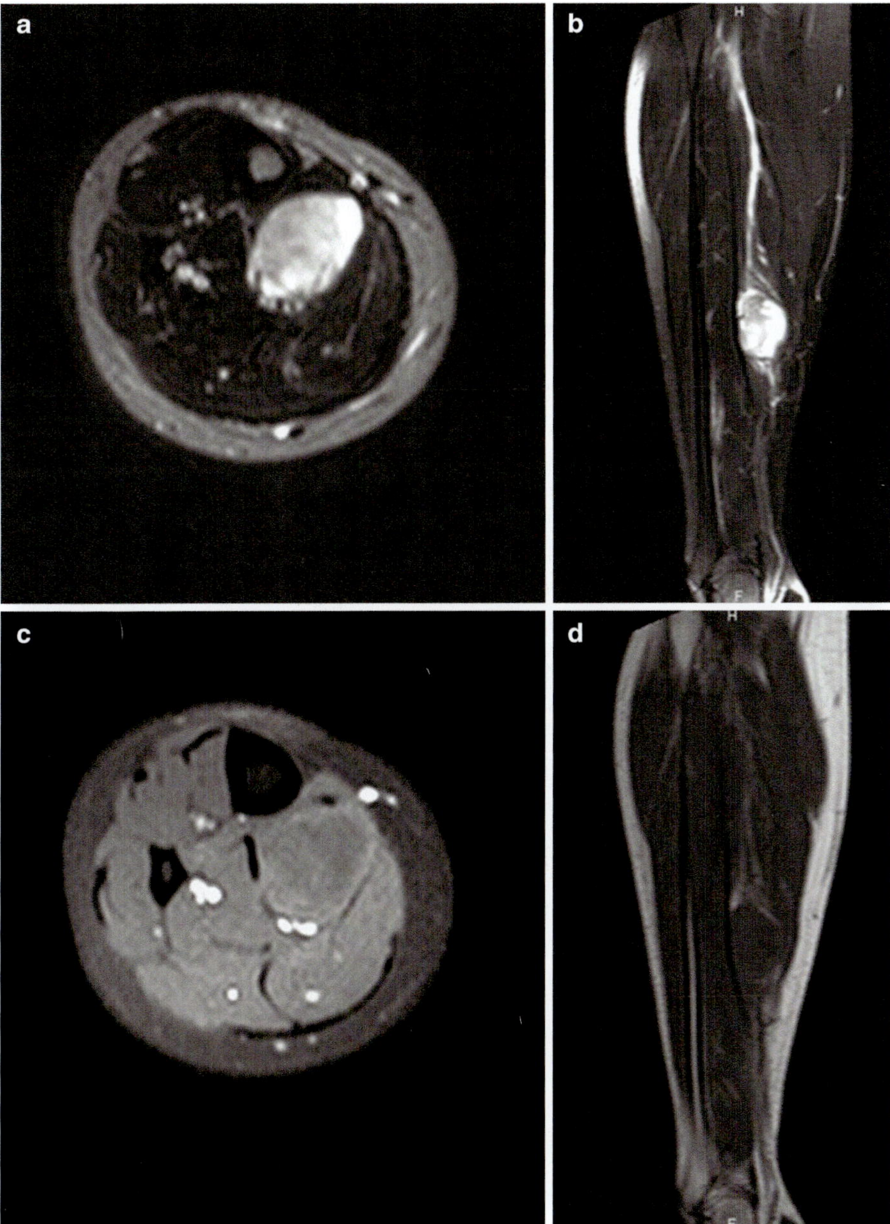

Fig. 8.1 The diagnostic MRI of the case ((**a**) T2-weighted transverse image, (**b**) T2-weighted sagittal image, (**c**) T1-weighted transverse image, (**d**) T1-weighted sagittal image)

the close proximity to local veins and nerves. According to the 8th edition AJCC/ UICC staging system, the patient had stage IA (pT1N0M0) STS (Tables 8.1 and 8.2) (https://www.cancer.org/cancer/soft-tissue-sarcoma/detection-diagnosis-staging/staging.html). Because of the surgical margin positivity, adjuvant RT was indicated.

Table 8.1 Soft tissue sarcomas—TNM staging AJCC UICC, 2017

Primary tumor (T), trunk and extremity sarcomas	
T category	T criteria
TX	Main tumor cannot be assessed
T0	No evidence of a primary tumor
T1	Tumor size is ≤5 cm
T2	Tumor size is 5–10 cm
T3	Tumor size is 10–15 cm
T4	Tumor size is >15 cm
Regional lymph nodes (N), trunk and extremity sarcomas	
N category	N criteria
NX	Regional lymph nodes cannot be assessed
N0	No regional lymph node metastasis
N1	Metastasis in regional lymph nodes
Distant metastasis (M), trunk and extremity sarcomas	
M category	M criteria
M0	No distant metastasis
M1	Distant metastasis
Histologic grade (G), trunk and extremity sarcomas	
G	G definition
GX	Grade cannot be assessed
G1	Total differentiation, mitotica count and necrosis score of 2–3
G2	Total differentiation, mitotica count and necrosis score of 4–5
G3	Total differentiation, mitotica count and necrosis score of 6–8

Used with permission of the American College of Surgeons, Chicago, Illinois. The original and primary source for this information is the AJCC Cancer Staging Manual, Eighth Edition (2017) published by Springer International Publishing

Table 8.2 Pathologic stage groups for trunk and extremity sarcomas—AJCC UICC, 2017

Pathologic stage	T	N	M	Grade
IA	T1	N0	M0	G1, GX
IB	T2–T4	N0	M0	G1, GX
II	T1	N0	M0	G2–3
IIIA	T2	N0	M0	G2–3
IIIB	T3–4	N0	M0	G2–3
IV	Any T	N1	M0	Any G
	Any T	Any N	M1	Any G

Used with permission of the American College of Surgeons, Chicago, Illinois. The original and primary source for this information is the AJCC Cancer Staging Manual, Eighth Edition (2017) published by Springer International Publishing

8.1.2 Evidence Based Treatment Recommendations

The treatment of STS requires a multidisciplinary approach including an experienced radiologist, pathologist, orthopedic surgeon, reconstructive surgeon, medical oncologist, and radiation oncologist. The main goal is to eradicate the tumor with minimal toxicity. Surgical resection is essential for the curative treatment. Surgical procedures include a marginal resection or excisional biopsy, wide resection, and radical resection or amputation. A marginal resection is the removal of the tumor with its pseudocapsule which has up to 90% local recurrence (LR) rate, and is not an appropriate treatment for STS [5]. A wide resection is the en bloc removal of the tumor with some normal tissue which can spare the limb but LR rates can reach up to 25–60% [5]. A radical resection is the removal of all muscles and neurovascular structures within the compartment where the tumor resides with LR rates of 0–18% [5, 13]; however, the loss of limb is the disadvantage of this procedure. Taking all these data into account, wide resection with pre- or postoperative RT is the current standard of care in most patients.

Some single institution series have reported satisfactory results with surgery alone, the LR rate being 0–20% [14–17]. However, these studies are mostly retrospective, and include highly selected patients with small and subcutaneous tumors with wide resection margins. The prospective trial from Pisters et al. [15] reported the results of patients with tumors <5 cm and negative surgical margins after surgery alone. The rate of LR was 8% in total and 5% in patients with subcutaneous tumors. Baldini et al. [14] also reported significantly reduced rates of LR with surgery alone in patients with resection margins ≥1 cm compared to patients with resection margins <1 cm (0% vs. 13% in 10 years). The LR rates after surgery alone are satisfactory in low-grade tumors with a range of 0–5% and the treatment of choice is surgery alone in these tumors [14, 15, 17]. However, if there is positive surgical margins or local recurrence, adjuvant RT is indicated for low-grade STS.

The main purpose of the surgeon should be to attain negative margins as the presence of positive margins increases LR rates even when RT is used [8, 9, 13]. If the first pathology reveals positive margins, re-excision should be performed as the probability of finding a residual disease is 24–63% [18, 19]. When performing re-resection; previous incisions, biopsy tracts, drain sites, and any tissues contaminated by the first surgery are also needed to be removed en bloc along with tumor-bed margins. However, if this wide of surgery would lead to loss of function or would require the removal of a body part such as a nerve or a bone, a planned positive margin is acceptable.

There are 3 randomized trials that show the role of RT combined with conservative surgery in the treatment of STS, and 1 randomized trial that compares adjuvant and neoadjuvant RT (Table 8.3).

As a result, adjuvant external beam RT (EBRT) decreases the rate of LR in high- and, particularly, low-grade tumors in patients that underwent conservative surgery. However, adjuvant brachytherapy (BRT) is not recommended for low-grade tumors

Table 8.3 Randomized trials with combined surgery and radiotherapy

Trial	N of patients	Tumor location	Treatment arms	RT dose (Gy)	LC (%)	5y-OS (%)	5y-DFS (%)
Rosenberg et al. [13]	43	Extremity	HG tumors: Amputation +adj CHT[a] CS + adj CHT[a] + EBRT	60–70	100 85 (p = 0.06)	88 83 (NS)	78 71 (NS)
Pisters et al. [20]	164	Extremity, trunk	HG tumors: CS CS + adj BRT LG tumors: CS CS + adj BRT	42–45 42–45	70 91 (p = 0.0025) 74 64 (NS)	In all: 81 84 (NS)	In all: 76 83 (NS)
Yang et al. [21]	141	Extremity	HG tumors: CS + adj CHT[b] CS + adj CHT[b] + EBRT LG tumors: CS CS + adj EBRT	63 63	100 80 (p = 0.003) 96 67 (p = 0.016)	74[c] 75[c] (NS) 92[c] 92[c] (NS)	– –
O' Sullivan et al. [22]	190	Extremity	Neoadj RT + CS CS + adj RT	50 66	93 92 (NS)	73 67 (NS)	58 59 (NS)

Abbreviations: *N* number, *EBRT* external beam radiotherapy, *LC* local control, *OS* overall survival, *DFS* disease-free survival, *adj* adjuvant, *CHT* chemotherapy, *CS* conservative surgery, *neoadj* neoadjuvant, *NS* not significant, *BRT* brachytherapy, *HG* high-grade, *LG* low-grade
[a]Doxorubicin, cyclophosphamide, methotrexate
[b]Doxorubicin, cyclophosphamide
[c]10-year

as it has no impact on local control (LC) or survival. It is also known that in the presence of positive surgical margins, LR rates are higher in high-grade tumors treated with adjuvant BRT [23]. Therefore, adjuvant BRT can only be administered in patients with high-grade tumors with negative margins after conservative surgery [24]. In case of positive margins, EBRT should be performed either alone or in combination with BRT in high-grade tumors. The rate of LR after conservative surgery and adjuvant RT in high-grade tumors is <15% in more recent series [19, 22, 25–27]. In low-grade tumors, wide excision alone seems adequate, and the rate of LR is <20% if the surgical margins are negative [28]. In case of positive margins or locally recurrent disease in low-grade tumors, adjuvant EBRT is indicated after wide excision.

EBRT can be administered either before or after surgery, and the timing is still a controversial issue between radiation oncologists and surgeons. The LC rates are similar with each approach, and the randomized trial by O'Sullivan et al. [22] reported LC rates of 93% and 92% for the pre- and postoperative approach, respectively, without a significant difference in survival rates in the updated 7-year results. The main difference between these approaches is the toxicity profile. The authors reported the rate of wound complications 17% vs. 35% in post- and preoperative setting, respectively (p = 0.01). It has been shown that preoperative RT leads to an increased rate of acute wound complications with a range of 25–46% in other studies [29, 30]. However, it should not be forgotten that although wound complications increased in the early postoperative period with preoperative RT, the adverse effects were mostly reversible, and the statistically significant difference vanished 1 year after resection. On the contrary, postoperative RT resulted in increased rates of serious late and mostly irreversible toxicities such as subcutaneous fibrosis, joint stiffness, edema, and bone fractures [31, 32]. A systematic review and meta-analysis that compared the results of pre- and postoperative RT included 5 studies with 1098 patients [33]. They reported that the risk of LR was lower in patients that received preoperative RT with an odds ratio of 0.61 without statistical significance. The mean survival rate was 76% (62–88%) and 67% (41–83%) in the pre- and postoperative group, respectively.

There are certain advantages and disadvantages of each approach. In the preoperative RT setting, the RT field is smaller and the total dose is lower, both which reduce the rate of late toxicity. Owing to the lower dose of RT which is associated with good oxygenation of the tumor leading to increased efficacy of RT, the treatment time and cost are reduced, as well as the risk of second malignancies. Preoperative RT can also render unresectable tumors resectable, and tumor seeding of the operative bed or systemic circulation is prevented. On the other hand, the risk of wound complications is higher in the early period; however, they are generally treatable and reversible. Another disadvantage of preoperative RT is that the prior treatment leads to a potentially less informative pathology specimen. The advantages of postoperative RT are the complete pathological review, and lower risk of wound complications. However, the RT field is large due to uncertain tumor location and the need to include all drain and incision sites, the dose is higher due to hypoxic environment related to surgery, and these both lead to increased rates of long-term toxicity which are mostly irreversible. In conclusion, when these pros and cons of each approach are taken into account, preoperative RT seems the most appropriate treatment for STS.

Intensity modulated RT (IMRT) provides a more homogeneous dose distribution while better preserving the organs at risk. Alektiar et al. [34] reported 5-year LC rate of 94% with IMRT even in patients with positive or close (<1 mm) surgical margins. Folkert et al. [35] compared conventional EBRT and IMRT, and found the 5-year rate of LR 15% and 7.6%, respectively, although the number of patients with positive and close margins was higher in the IMRT group. When compared to BRT, significantly better LC rates were achieved with IMRT (5y-LC rate: 19% vs. 8%), and again more patients with positive and close margins and larger tumors were included in the IMRT group [36]. O'Sullivan et al. [37] reported the results of 59 patients with lower-extremity STS whom they treated with image-guided (IG)-IMRT, and the 5-year LC rate was found 88.2%. The results of Radiation therapy Oncology Group (RTOG)-0630 phase II trial using preoperative IGRT in extremity

STS revealed the rate of LC 93% [38]. To sum up, although not being the standard treatment yet, modern RT techniques can provide satisfactory LC rate while decreasing the rate of RT-related morbidity and can be preferred in selected patients.

The role of adjuvant chemotherapy in the treatment of STS is unclear, and studies have reported conflicting results. In a meta-analysis, adjuvant chemotherapy resulted in a longer LR-free interval and distant recurrence-free interval with better overall survival (OS) rates, although not statistically significant [39]. An updated second meta-analysis found a limited benefit of adjuvant chemotherapy with optimal doses of doxorubicin and ifosfamide [40]. The largest randomized trial, on the other hand, reported no benefit of adjuvant chemotherapy, leading to the thought that improvements in surgery and modern RT techniques may have dimmed the role of adjuvant chemotherapy [41].

The role of neoadjuvant chemotherapy has been studied in several trials. A randomized controlled trial showed no benefit of neoadjuvant chemotherapy over surgery alone in patients with resectable high-risk primary and recurrent STS [42]. The phase II study of RTOG 9514 reported 3-year OS, disease-free survival (DFS) and DM-free survival (DMFS) rates of 75%, 57%, and 65%, respectively; however, 83% of the patients suffered grade 4 toxicity [43]. In the updated phase II study of Delaney et al. [44], neoadjuvant chemotherapy resulted in a significant survival benefit without severe complications.

In summary, the role of either adjuvant or neoadjuvant chemotherapy is not clear in the treatment of STS. It may be administered in the context of patient-based data.

8.1.3 Treatment Recommendations

Treatment recommendations for STS according to the National Comprehensive Cancer Network (NCCN) guidelines are summarized in Table 8.4 (https://www.nccn.org/professionals/physician_gls/pdf/sarcoma.pdf).

8.1.4 Target Volume Determination and Delineation Guidelines

8.1.4.1 Simulation

Appropriate positioning of the patient is important in RT planning. The patient should be in a reproducible position, and the extremity be positioned as far away from the body and the opposite extremity as possible. For the upper extremity, the arm should be in the abduction position with the arm supinated or pronated based on the tumor location. If the patient would be more comfortable the arm can be extended above the head while the patient is in prone position, which is called the 'swimmer position'. For the lower extremity, the patient can be positioned either supinely or pronely based on the tumor location (i.e. on the anterior or the posterior

Table 8.4 NCCN guideline version 2.2018 (extremity/superficial trunk)

Stage	Recommended treatment			
IA, IB	Surgery	Negative margins/ intact fascial plane	– Observe	
		Positive margins/ no intact fascial plane	– Re-resection OR – Observe (stage IA) OR – RT	
II (resectable with functional outcomes)	Surgery	Negative margins/ intact fascial plane	– Observe	
		Positive margins/ no intact fascial plane	– RT	
	Preoperative RT		– Surgery	
IIIA (resectable with functional outcomes)	Surgery	RT OR RT + adjuvant CXT		
	Preoperative RT/ CRT	Surgery	– Consider RT boost ± adjuvant CXT	
	Preoperative CXT	Surgery	– RT OR – RT + adjuvant CXT	
II, IIA (unresectable/ resectable without functional outcomes)	RT OR CRT OR CXT OR Regional limb therapy	Resectable with functional outcomes	Surgery	– RT OR – CRT OR – (if previous RT+) consider RT boost ± adjuvant CXT
		Unresectable/ resectable without functional outcomes	– Definitive RT OR – CXT OR – Palliative surgery OR – Observe (if asymptomatic) OR – Best supportive care OR – Amputation	

IV	Single organ metastasis and limited tumor bulk	– Treat like resectable stage II, III and consider these:
		  – Metastasectomy ± CXT ± RT
		  – Ablation procedures (i.e. RFA, cryotherapy)
		  – Embolization procedures
		  – SBRT
		  – Observe		

	Isolated regional disease or LN	– Regional LN dissection ± RT ± CXT – Metastasectomy ± CXT ± RT – SBRT – Isolated limb perfusion/infusion ± surgery		
	Disseminated disease	– CXT – RT/SBRT – Surgery – Observe (if asymptomatic) – Supportive care – Ablation procedures (i.e. RFA, cryotherapy) – Embolization procedures		

Abbreviations: *RT* radiotherapy, *CXT* chemotherapy, *CRT* chemoradiotherapy, *RFA* radiofrequency ablation, *SBRT* stereotactic body radiotherapy, *LN* lymph node

of the leg). If the tumor is in the proximal thigh the 'frog-leg position' can be used to optimally spare the perineum and inguinal regions, as well as the contralateral leg. Another way to stabilize the patient is the decubitus position for lower extremity tumors in the true anterior or posterior compartments. The treated leg is placed directly on the table and the untreated leg is flexed at the knee and placed either posterior or anterior to the treated leg, and the legs are separated as much as possible.

8.1.4.2 Contouring

Radiotherapy for STS can be administered either pre- or postoperatively. In the preoperative setting, the gross target volume (GTV) is the tumor detected in physical examination and on imaging studies. The RTOG Sarcoma Working Group reported a consensus for appropriate target volumes for preoperative RT [45]. Fusion of a diagnostic MRI and planning CT is strongly recommended, and the optimal sequence for MRI is the T1 post-contrast series. For the clinical target volume (CTV) longitudinal margins of as large as 5 cm and 2-cm radial margins were used. However, in recent years, attempts to minimize the margins have been raised, and in the RTOG report, the CTV is formed by adding 3-cm margins longitudinally and 1.5-cm margins radially to the GTV, respectively. If these margins extend beyond the compartment or an intact fascia or bone which are natural barriers, these margins can be truncated. With these margins, the peritumoral edema on T2 MRI will often be included in the CTV. Whether to include the whole edema is at the discretion of the radiation oncologist. It has been shown that microscopic tumor cells can be located 1–4 cm beyond the tumor; however, this does not correlate with the location or extent of peritumoral edema on MRI [46]. Therefore, it is reasonable to try to include the edema in the CTV if this would not require a significant increase in the treatment field. The planning target volume (PTV) is not specified in the RTOG report, but it is traditionally formed by adding 5–10 mm to the CTV. By using these margins, excellent LC rates up to 93% were achieved in various studies [22, 26, 27].

In the postoperative setting, there is no gross tumor, and therefore there is no GTV. However, it can be helpful to draw a virtual GTV in the location where the gross tumor was preoperatively. The CTV should include the whole surgical bed together with the incision and drain sites and metallic clips, and an additional 2–4 cm longitudinal and 1.5–2 cm radial margins should be added to form the final CTV. The PTV is formed by adding 5–10 mm margins to the CTV. With these margins, the historical 2–5 cm margins to the surgical bed is achieved. Typically, these fields are reduced after a certain dose, with diminishing all margins to 2 cm. This is the current standard of care in the postoperative setting, and excellent LC rates are achieved by using these margins [22, 26, 34].

If BRT is to be applied as monotherapy, the CTV should include the operative bed; however, there is no consensus on the margins. In a randomized trial from the Memorial Sloan Kettering Cancer Center, margins of 1.5–2 cm were used beyond the tumor bed [20].

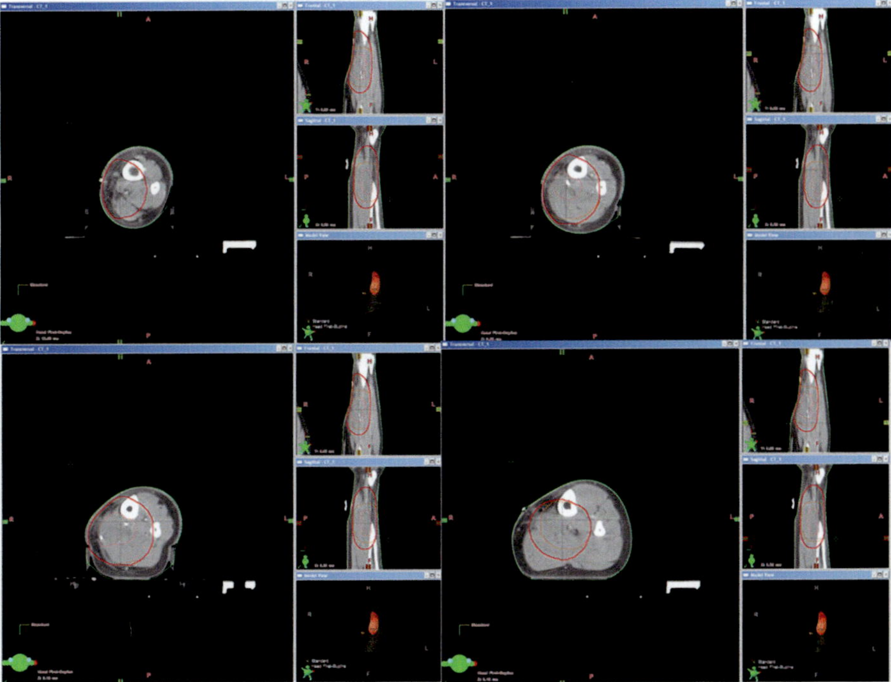

Fig. 8.2 The first phase contouring of the case (pink = GTV, red = CTV1, orange = CTV2)

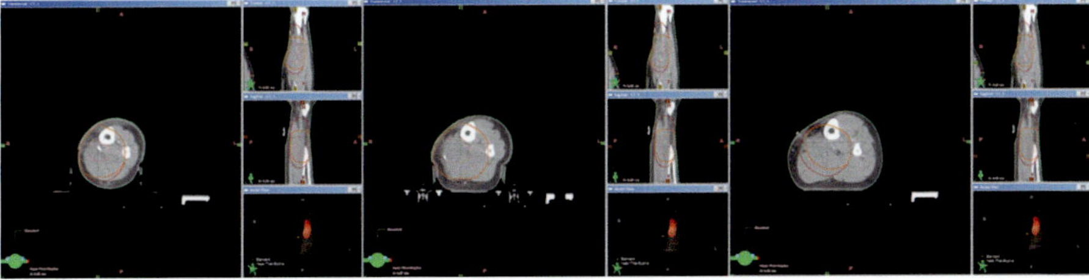

Fig. 8.3 The boost phase contouring of the case (pink = GTV, red = CTV1, orange = CTV2)

8.1.4.3 Case Contouring

In the case presented here, we administered 50 Gy to the postoperative bed with 3-cm margins longitudinally and 2-cm margins radially (Fig. 8.2). In the second phase, we administered a boost dose of 14 Gy to the tumor bed with 2-cm margins in all directions (Fig. 8.3).

8.1.5   Treatment Planning

8.1.5.1 Prescription Dose

In the preoperative setting, the standard dose for EBRT is 50 Gy delivered in 2-Gy fractions [9, 29]. In case of positive surgical margins in a patient that was irradiated

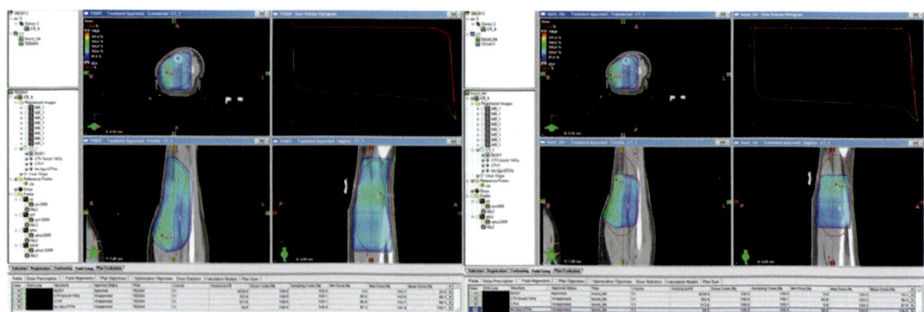

Fig. 8.4 The first and boost phase plans of the case

preoperatively, a boost dose of 16–20 Gy can be applied. However, the efficacy of a boost dose has not been studied, and there is a concern that increased doses can also increase the rate of toxicity [47, 48].

The best timing for postoperative RT is 4–6 weeks after surgery which is a time for allowing the wound to fully heal. In the postoperative setting, the total dose varies based on the surgical margin status. As the oxygenation of the tumor bed is negatively affected after surgery, a higher total dose is required to achieve a similar LC with preoperatively-irradiated tumors. As stated in the 'Contouring' section, 50 Gy is prescribed to the wide-margined CTV and then the margins are diminished. A total dose of 60–66 Gy is adequate if the surgical margins are negative or close. If there is a positive surgical margin, a total dose of 66–68 Gy is recommended [9, 25]. In our center, we administer 60 Gy in case of negative and 64–66 Gy in case of close (<5 mm) or microscopic surgical margins, whereas 70 Gy is applied in case of a gross residual tumor. The dose-volume histogram of the case is shown in Fig. 8.4.

When BRT is used as monotherapy, American Brachytherapy Society (ABS) recommends 4–50 Gy, 30–54 Gy, and 45–50 Gy for low dose rate (LDR), high dose rate (HDR), and pulse dose rate (PDR)-BRT, respectively [49]. When combined with EBRT, the recommended doses are 15–25 Gy, 15–20 Gy, and 15–25 Gy for respective dose rates.

8.1.6 Follow-Up (F/U) Recommendations

Patients with STS should be carefully followed up for both LR and DM. The MRI of the relevant extremity and a chest x-ray should be performed every 3–6 months in the first 2–3 years, and annually thereafter. Patients that underwent surgery should also be evaluated for rehabilitation and it should be continued until maximal function is achieved (https://www.nccn.org/professionals/physician_gls/pdf/sarcoma.pdf).

8.2   Retroperitoneal Sarcoma

Overview

Epidemiology: Primary retroperitoneal sarcomas (RPS) constitute approximately 15% of all soft tissue sarcomas [50]. The age at diagnosis of RPS makes a peak during the sixth decade of life. Risk factors for the development of RPS are not clearly understood yet.

Pathology: There are various histopathologic types of RPS. The most common subtype is liposarcoma, followed by leiomyosarcoma.

Diagnosis: Most patients with RPS are asymptomatic until the tumor grows into a giant mass. When symptomatic, these tumors cause nonspecific abdominal pain, anorexia, and weight loss. For initial diagnosis, a magnetic resonance imaging (MRI) scan of the abdomen and pelvis is required as well as a computed tomography (CT) scan of the chest to rule out lung and liver lesions which are the most common sites of metastasis. Core biopsy with image guidance is the preferred diagnostic procedure.

Treatment: The treatment of choice is surgery for RPS, and although not adequate alone, it has been shown to improve the outcomes. The most important prognostic factors for RPS are the extent of resection, tumor volume, grade, and histopathology. Based on these prognostic factors, most RPS require radiotherapy (RT) that can be administered in the pre- or postoperative setting which have their own advantages and disadvantages.

Key Words: Retroperitoneal sarcoma; Radiotherapy

8.2.1   Case Presentation

A 68-year old woman applied to the hospital with pain in the left flank region in February 2018. Abdominal CT revealed a neoplastic mass of 90 × 80 mm in the left flank, infiltrating the abdominal wall muscles. The fat plan between the mass lesion and anterior pararenal fascia could not be visualized (Fig. 8.5). Because of a metallic implant, an MRI could not be performed on the patient. On thorax CT, no lung metastasis was detected. A tru-cut biopsy was performed and a malignant mesenchymal tumor was diagnosed. The Ki-67 proliferation index was 10%, and dedifferentiated liposarcoma was the most probable diagnose owing to morphologic findings and tumor location. According to 8th edition AJCC/UICC staging system, the patient was diagnosed as stage IIIA (cT2N0M0, grade 3) RPS (Tables 8.5 and 8.6) (https://www.cancer.org/cancer/soft-tissue-sarcoma/detection-diagnosis-staging/staging.html). Neoadjuvant RT followed by surgical resection was planned.

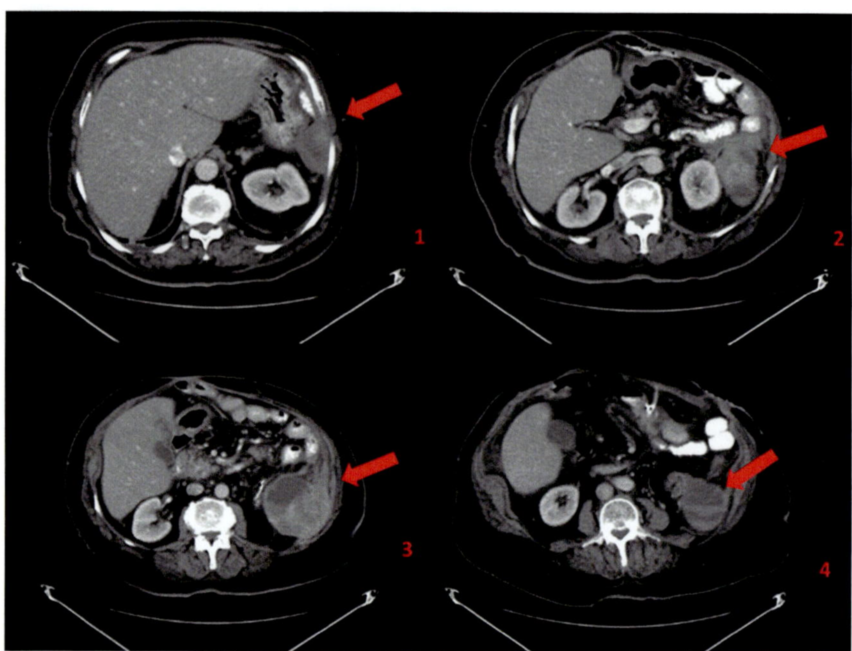

Fig. 8.5 The diagnostic CT images of the case

Table 8.5 Retroperitoneal sarcomas—TNM staging AJCC UICC, 2017

Primary tumor (T), retroperitoneal sarcomas	
T category	T criteria
TX	Main tumor cannot be assessed
T0	No evidence of a primary tumor
T1	Tumor size is ≤5 cm
T2	Tumor size is 5–10 cm
T3	Tumor size is 10–15 cm
T4	Tumor size is >15 cm
Regional lymph nodes (N), retroperitoneal sarcomas	
N category	N criteria
NX	Regional lymph nodes cannot be assessed
N0	No regional lymph node metastasis
N1	Metastasis in regional lymph nodes
Distant metastasis (M), retroperitoneal sarcomas	
M category	M criteria
M0	No distant metastasis
M1	Distant metastasis
Histologic grade (G), retroperitoneal sarcomas	
G	G definition
GX	Grade cannot be assessed
G1	Total differentiation, mitotica count and necrosis score of 2–3
G2	Total differentiation, mitotica count and necrosis score of 4–5
G3	Total differentiation, mitotica count and necrosis score of 6–8

Used with permission of the American College of Surgeons, Chicago, Illinois. The original and primary source for this information is the AJCC Cancer Staging Manual, Eighth Edition (2017) published by Springer International Publishing

Table 8.6 Pathologic stage groups for retroperitoneal sarcomas—AJCC UICC, 2017

Pathologic stage	T	N	M	Grade
IA	T1	N0	M0	G1, GX
IB	T2–T4	N0	M0	G1, GX
II	T1	N0	M0	G2–3
IIIA	T2	N0	M0	G2–3
IIIB	T3–4	N0	M0	G2–3
	Any T	N1	M0	Any G
IV	Any T	Any N	M1	Any G

Used with permission of the American College of Surgeons, Chicago, Illinois. The original and primary source for this information is the AJCC Cancer Staging Manual, Eighth Edition (2017) published by Springer International Publishing

8.2.2 Evidence Based Treatment Recommendations

One of the most challenging issues in the management of RPS is that the patients often present with a large mass owing to delayed symptoms due to the anatomic location. The primary treatment for RPS is surgery, and gross total resection is the treatment of choice. It has been shown that an aggressive surgery increases the survival of patients with RPS [28, 51, 52]. However, it is not always possible due to tumor location and its close proximity with vital organs [53]. The total resectability rate of RPS was reported 65–85% [54–56].

The resection margin status defines the extent of surgical resection; R0 resection means the total resection of the tumor with microscopically negative margins, whereas R1 resection leaves microscopically positive margins, and R2 resection leaves a gross tumor residual behind. The rates of local control (LC) and survival increase with at least an R1 resection [55]. However, even an R0 resection alone do not lead to satisfactory results; the local recurrence (LR) and 5-year overall survival (OS) rate ranges between 33 and 77% and 35–63%, respectively [54, 55, 57]. It has clearly been shown that the primary cause of death in patients with RPS is LR which is responsible for the death of 75% of these patients [54, 55, 58]. Although LC rates are not satisfactory with surgery alone, the only curative treatment modality for RPS is complete surgical resection [59]. Five-year OS rates in patients with non-metastatic and completely resected RPS range between 49% and 70%, whereas LR rates can reach up to 82% in 10 years [54, 55, 57]. Hassan et al. [56] reported a median survival of 103 months for completely resected RPS compared to 18 months in patients that underwent an incomplete resection. Besides, in another study the 5-year OS was 62% and 26% in patients with and without complete resection, respectively [55]. Therefore, it is crucial the control the local disease with an additional treatment method.

There are no randomized controlled studies comparing surgery alone to surgery with neoadjuvant or adjuvant RT in the treatment of RPS. The American College of Surgeons Oncology Group (ACOSOG) Z9031 trial was opened in 2004 to compare neoadjuvant RT and surgery to surgery alone in patients with RP sarcoma; however,

Table 8.7 Retrospective studies comparing surgery with and without adjuvant radiotherapy

Study	N of patients	Follow-up	RT dose (Gy)	LC rate (with vs. without RT)	p value
Stoeckle et al. [54]	165	47 months	Median 50	5-y: 55% vs 23%	0.002
Catton et al. [57]	104	6.3 years	Median 40	LRF interval: 103 months vs. 30 months	0.06
Ferrario and Karakousis [60]	130	41 months	NS	62% vs. 47%	0.16

Abbreviations: *N* number, *RT* radiotherapy, *LC* local control, *LRF* local recurrence-free, *NS* not specified

was closed prematurely due to poor accrual. The European Organization for the Treatment of Cancer (EORTC) 62092-22092, a phase III trial is now closed to patient entry that aims to compare surgery alone to neoadjuvant RT and surgery, and the results are pending. However, some retrospective studies have reported increased rates of LC with adjuvant RT without a significant effect on OS [54, 57, 60] (Table 8.7).

Radiotherapy can be applied either in the adjuvant or neoadjuvant setting, and these two approaches have both their advantages and disadvantages [61]. In adjuvant RT, the field is larger because the whole surgical bed together with the incision and drain sites and surgical clips should be included. Besides, as the oxygenation of the tissues in the field is impaired due to surgery, a higher dose has to be applied for biological efficacy. In neoadjuvant RT, the field is smaller and a lower dose can be applied. Only the tumor is included in the RT field and the organs at risk (e.g. the bowels) can be spared easily, and the risk of intraoperative seeding is reduced. The main disadvantage of preoperative RT is that it increases the rate of wound complications after surgery; however, these complications are mostly curable and reversible. It also leads to a limited histologic sampling and delays definitive surgery. On the other hand, postoperative RT leads to more serious late complications that can be irreversible. Preoperative RT can also be preferred for unresectable tumors to make them amenable to surgery.

8.2.3 Treatment Recommendations

Treatment recommendations for RPS according to the National Comprehensive Cancer Network (NCCN) guidelines are summarized in Table 8.8.

Baldini et al. [61] published the treatment guidelines for RPS in 2015. In this report, they recommend preoperative RT over postoperative RT based on the advantages and disadvantages of both modalities. For a patient to be a candidate for preoperative RT followed by surgery, the following should be present: there should be no symptoms that necessitate urgent surgery, the tumor should be resectable with negative margins, the tumor should be localized and unifocal for the administration of RT (or at most 2 tumors close to each other), and the prescription dose of 50.4 Gy could be administered without unacceptable toxicity. The authors also recommend

Table 8.8 NCCN guidelines version 2.2018

Status	Treatment recommendations			
Resectable disease	Biopsy performed	– Surgery ± IORT **OR** – Preoperative RT/ CHT followed by surgery ± IORT	Adjuvant treatment: – R0 resection: Observe – R1 resection: Consider boost dose (10–16 Gy) if previous RT+ – R2 resection: Consider re-resection	
	Biopsy not performed/ non-diagnostic	– Surgery ± IORT		
Unresectable disease/stage IV	Biopsy	Attempt down-staging	– CXT **OR** – CRT **OR** – RT	If resectable, follow recommendations for resectable disease If unresectable or progressive, follow no down-staging recommendations
		No down-staging	Palliative care: – CXT – RT – Surgery for symptom control – Supportive care – Observe if asymptomatic	

Abbreviations: *IORT* intraoperative radiotherapy, *RT* radiotherapy, *CHT* chemotherapy, *CRT* chemoradiotherapy

the radiation oncologist and surgeon argue about the treatment before it is initiated. In cases where the RPS invades or abuts one kidney which would result in radical nephrectomy, the function of the contralateral kidney must be measured prior to RT and it should be maximally spared during RT. Similarly, if the RPS invades or abuts the liver, the need for partial liver resection should be kept in mind. Liver functions should be evaluated prior to RT, and the sections of the liver to be resected should be spared from high dose.

8.2.4 Target Volume Determination and Delineation Guidelines

8.2.4.1 Simulation

For the CT planning, the patient should be in a reproducible supine position. As the abdomen is the target region, the arms should be over the head either by the patient holding arms up or by using a t-bar or a wing board. Using an intravenous contrast can identify the target volume more clearly. Oral contrast can also help the visualization of the gastrointestinal tract better [61]. The slice thickness of the planning CT is recommended to be ≤3-mm. As the tumor and organs at risk in the upper abdomen can move up to 9 mm with respiration, 4-dimensional (4D) CT scan is strongly recommended for tumors above the level of the iliac crest, if possible [61–63]. In case tumor motion of >1 cm is detected, a form of respiratory control (gating, abdominal compression, breath-hold) is recommended to be used.

8.2.4.2 Contouring

A fusion with a diagnostic MRI and/or positron emission tomography (PET)/CT is recommended while contouring. The ACOSOG Z9031 trial defined the preoperative gross tumor volume (GTV) as the gross tumor that can be visualized in the imaging studies, clinical target volume (CTV) as the tissues adjacent to the GTV that are not visualized by imaging studies but have a potential for microscopic disease and should be given a margin of at least 1.5 cm, and the planning target volume (PTV) with an additional margin to the CTV for setup errors and patient/organ movements. The PTV margin should be at least 0.5 cm to the CTV. However, Langen and Jones [64] showed that the intrafraction motion of the kidneys can be 11–19 mm and the pancreas 18–22 mm, respectively, during normal breathing. Therefore, using cone-beam CT imaging, active breathing control, or respiratory gating can help to decrease the margin for the PTV.

The panel for the treatment guidelines for RPS recommends to delineate an iGTV for tumors above the iliac crest by using 4D motion [61]. The authors choose to add an internal target volume (ITV) which the iGTV accounts for the internal margin, and they recommend adding a 1.5-cm margin for the CTV. The ITV should not include the anatomical barriers such as uninvolved bone, kidney, or liver, but may expand into bowel and air cavity 5 mm, and should be cropped 3–5 mm from the involved skin surface. If the ipsilateral kidney is to be resected after RT, there is no need to exclude it from the ITV. In case the tumor lies within the inguinal canal, the inferior margin is recommended to be 3 cm. The ITV does not need to cover the prior biopsy tract. For tumors below the iliac crest GTV and CTV are the terms to be used rather than iGTV and ITV when 4D motion assessment is not used [61]. The CTV is again formed by adding 1.5-cm margins to the GTV. However, if 4D motion is not used for upper abdominal tumors, the panel recommends adding 2–2.5 cm margins longitudinally and 1.5–2 cm margins radially to the GTV to form the CTV. The PTV is created by adding a 5-mm margin to the ITV or CTV if 4D motion assessment is or is not used, respectively. However, the panel recommends adding 9–12 mm margins for the PTV if image-guided RT (IGRT) is not to be administered due to tumor and organ motions.

For postoperative RT, there may be no GTV after complete resection but it may be helpful to delineate a virtual GTV using preoperative imaging studies in order to define the CTV better. The CTV should include this virtual GTV (and the residual disease if present) and the whole surgical bed with incision and drain sites and surgical clips. Then a longitudinal margin of 3–4 cm and radial margins of 2 cm should be added, limited by the anatomical boundaries. After a dose of 45–50 Gy to this CTV, a boost dose of 5.4–9 Gy should be added based on resection margins with a smaller margin of 2 cm at all directions.

8.2.4.3 Case Contouring

The tumor was contoured on the planning CT with a fusion of the diagnostic CT. As preoperative RT was planned, the CTV was formed by adding 4 cm longitudinally and 2 cm radially. However, due to the anatomical barriers at the superior and inferior, the longitudinal margins were also decreased to 2 cm (Fig. 8.6). 50 Gy was prescribed to this volume.

8.2.4.4 Prescription Dose and Dose Constraints for Critical Structures

Dose Recommendations: There is not an optimal dose for adjuvant RT in the treatment of RPS. In the study of Fein et al. [65], adjuvant RT doses of >55 Gy significantly decreased the rate of LR when compared to doses of <55 Gy (25% vs. 38%, respectively). Sindelar et al. [66] reported a locoregional control rate of 60% after 20 Gy intraoperative RT (IORT) and adjuvant 35–40 Gy external beam RT (EBRT) compared to 20% after adjuvant 50–55 Gy EBRT alone. Similarly, the rate of LC rate in Alektiar et al.'s study [67] was 66% in patients that underwent 12–15 Gy IORT and adjuvant 45–50.4 Gy EBRT, whereas it was 50% in patients that underwent IORT alone. Based on these results, an EBRT dose of ≥55 to 60 Gy seems adequate for the adjuvant treatment of RPS.

For neoadjuvant RT, Jones et al. [68] reported 19.6% LR and 88% 2-year OS rates in patients that underwent a median 45 Gy EBRT prior to resection and adjuvant brachytherapy (BRT). Gieschen et al. [69] treated patients with neoadjuvant 45–50 Gy EBRT followed by surgery and IORT (10 Gy after complete resection, 12.5–15 Gy after microscopic residue and 15–20 Gy after macroscopic residue). In patients with a complete resection, the LC rate increased from 61% to 83% without statistical significance. Petersen et al. [70] reported the results of patients with primary and recurrent RPS or pelvic sarcomas that underwent neoadjuvant EBRT,

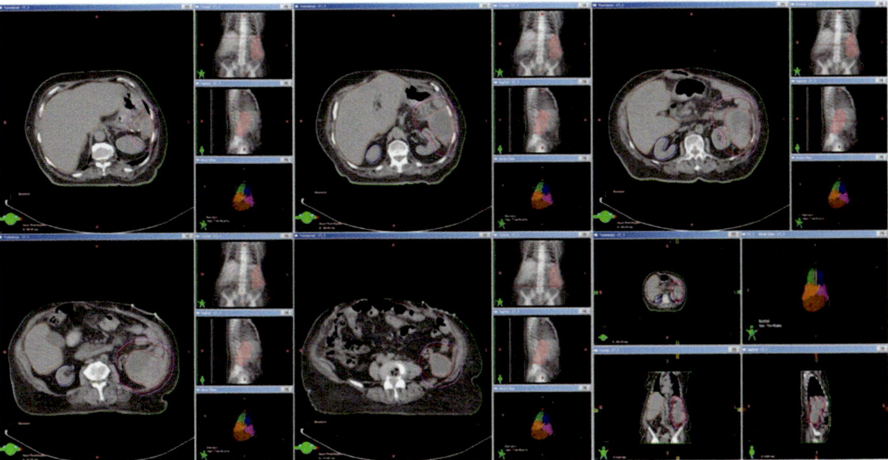

Fig. 8.6 Contouring of the case (pink = GTV, red = CTV, magenta = PTV)

adjuvant EBRT, or both with a median dose of 47.6 Gy together with IORT with a median dose of 15 Gy. The 5-year rate of LC was found 100%, 60%, and 41% in patients with complete resection, microscopic residue, and gross residue, respectively. The 5-year OS rate was 37% in patients with gross residual disease and 52% in others. The recommended doses for preoperative RT is 50–50.4 Gy in 1.8–2-Gy fraction doses [61]. Surgery can be performed 4–6 weeks following the completion of RT [61].

In our center, preoperative RT dose is 50 Gy in 2-Gy fractions. In the postoperative setting, first we administer 50 Gy to the first CTV with larger margins, then the margins are decreased and a boost dose 10 Gy, 14–16 Gy and 20 Gy is applied in patients with complete resection, microscopic residual disease and gross tumor, respectively. 95% of the PTV should receive >95%, of the prescription dose, and 99–100% of the CTV should receive >95% of the prescription dose. Intensity modulated RT (IMRT) should be preferred as the treatment technique for RPS [61]. The RT plan of the case is shown in Fig. 8.7.

Dose Constraints for Critical Structures: The organs at risk at the retroperitoneal area include the kidneys, liver, bowel, rectum, stomach, duodenum, spinal cord, testicles, ovaries, perineum, urinary bladder, and the femoral head. These structures are needed to be delineated if they are within 2 cm of the PTV. As the spinal cord and bowel are serial organs, the whole organ is not necessarily contoured, but the area including 2 cm superior and inferior to the PTV. It is not recommended to subtract the organs at risk from the PTV in order to calculate the doses accurately. The recommended dose constraints for critical structures are shown in Table 8.9.

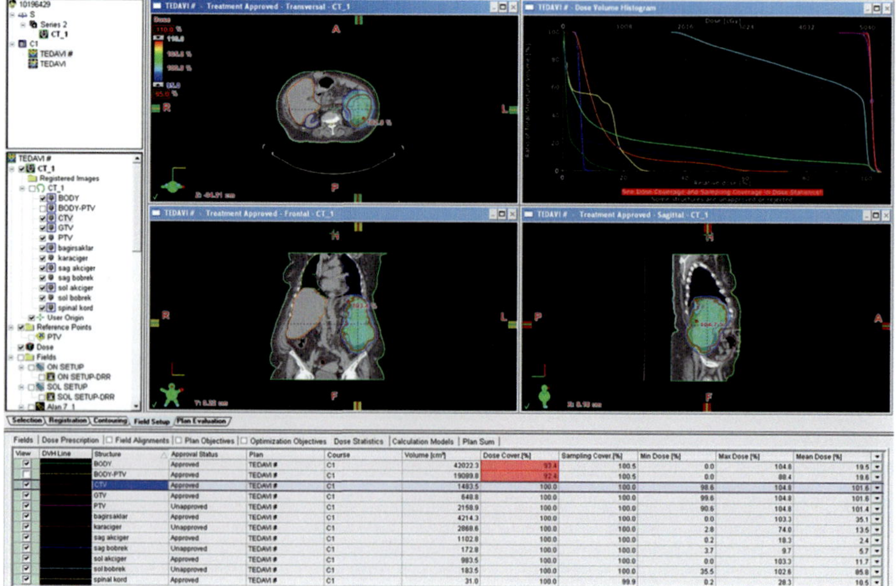

Fig. 8.7 Treatment plan of the case

Table 8.9 Dose constraints for critical structures [61]

Critical structure	Dose constraints
Kidneys	Mean dose <15 Gy and V18 < 50%
	If one kidney to be resected; V18 of the remaining kidney <15%
Liver	Mean dose <26 Gy
Bowel	If contoured together as 'bowel bag'; V15 < 830 cm^3 and V45 < 195 cm^3
	If contoured individually;
	– Small bowel V15 < 120 cc and V55 < 20 cm^3
	– Large bowel V60 < 20 cm^3
Rectum	V50 < 50%
Stomach and duodenum	V45 ≤ 100%, V50 < 50%, and maximum dose 56 Gy
Spinal cord	Maximum dose 50 Gy
Testicles	As low as possible;
	V3 < 50% for fertility and maximum dose <18 Gy
	Consider cryopreservation in young men
Ovaries	Maximum dose <3 Gy for fertility
	Consider cryopreservation in young women
Perineum	If possible; V30 < 50%
Urinary bladder	If necessary; V50 ≤ 100%
Femoral head	If possible; maximum dose <50 Gy, V40 < 64%, and mean dose <37 Gy

8.2.5 Follow-Up (F/U) Recommendations

Patients with RPS should be followed up with an abdominopelvic MRI and chest x-ray every 3–6 months in the first 2–3 years, every 6 months in year 4, and annually thereafter (https://www.cancer.org/cancer/soft-tissue-sarcoma/detection-diagnosis-staging/staging.html).

8.3 Ewing's Sarcoma

Overview

Epidemiology: Ewing's sarcoma (ES), atypical ES, and primitive neuroectodermal tumor (PNET) of the bone constitute Ewing's sarcoma family of tumors (ESFT). Ewing's sarcoma is the second most common primary tumor of bone in childhood, and seen in 2.8 cases per million children per year. Median age is 14 years. Most lesions occur in the pelvis, followed by the lower extremity, the trunk, and upper extremity. The etiology of ESFT is unknown.

Pathology: ESFT are composed of small, round blue cells. They are characterized by a reciprocal translocation involving breakpoints on the EWSR1 gene on chromosome 22q12A. The majority of ESFT has the translocations tl1:22(q24:q12) or t21;22(q22;q12). Besides, there is expression of the c-myc proto-oncogene, without expression of n-myc. Approximately ¾ of patients with ES present with localized disease at the time of diagnosis. However, the majority of the patients have not-yet-identifiable micrometastases at that time, the most common sites being the lung and bones.

Diagnosis: Patients commonly present with localized pain, swelling, and a palpable mass. Systemic symptoms such as fever, malaise, and weakness may also be present. On plain x-rays, bone tumors are observed as a moth-eaten lesion with osteolytic and osteoblastic areas. An 'onion skin' appearance can be seen due to the subperiosteal reactive new bone. On the computed tomography (CT) scan, bone destruction can be seen better, whereas a magnetic resonance imaging (MRI) scan can show the presence of invasion to the adjacent soft tissues or bone marrow. Besides, for accurate staging of the disease, a chest x-ray or CT scan, a bone scan, and a bone marrow biopsy should also be performed. A positron emission tomography (PET)/CT can detect bone and lymph node metastases more sensitively. Biopsy is recommended to be performed at the same institution where the surgery will be performed. The biopsy specimen should be taken from the soft-tissue component. As the cytogenetics is important, a large sample should be achieved. The contamination of uninvolved areas and vital structures, and hematoma development should be avoided. No staging system is present for Ewing's sarcoma; patients are classified as having either localized or metastatic disease.

Treatment: The treatment consists of both local and systemic therapy. It starts with chemotherapy (CHT) of multiple agents, and followed by a definitive therapy; surgery ± radiotherapy (RT), and of adjuvant CHT. Treatment of metastatic sites should also be considered as it increases survival rates. With this multimodality approach, the 5-year survival rate is 70%.

Key Words: Ewing's sarcoma; Radiotherapy

8.3.1 Case Presentation

A 6-year-old boy was brought to the emergency room by his parents with left hip pain in May 2015. The x-ray of the pelvis revealed serious destruction in the medullary spongiosus structure of the left iliac wing, and irregular and ill-defined sclerosis and osteolytic areas in the vicinity of the left sacroiliac joint (Fig. 8.8). On bilateral sacroiliac joint MRI, a 60 × 58 × 78 mm soft tissue mass infiltrating the left iliac muscle, causing expansion and cortical irregularity in the iliac bone with a suspicion of invasion to the minimus and medius gluteus muscles was observed (Fig. 8.9 and Fig. 8.10). The tru-cut biopsy from the left iliac wing revealed a small round cell neoplasm, and the fluorescent in-situ hybridization (FISH) supporting the presence of EWSR gene, ES was diagnosed. Thorax CT revealed a parenchymal nodule in the left lung (Fig. 8.11). On PET/CT, a 62 × 47-mm mass lying from the left iliac

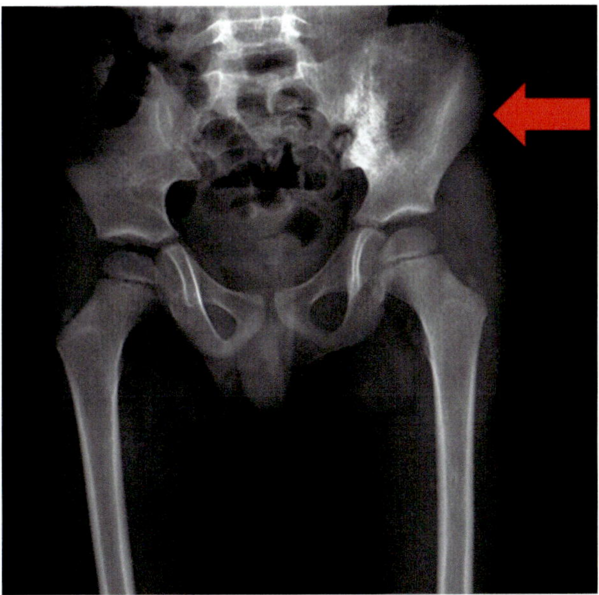

Fig. 8.8 Plain radiograph of the case at presentation

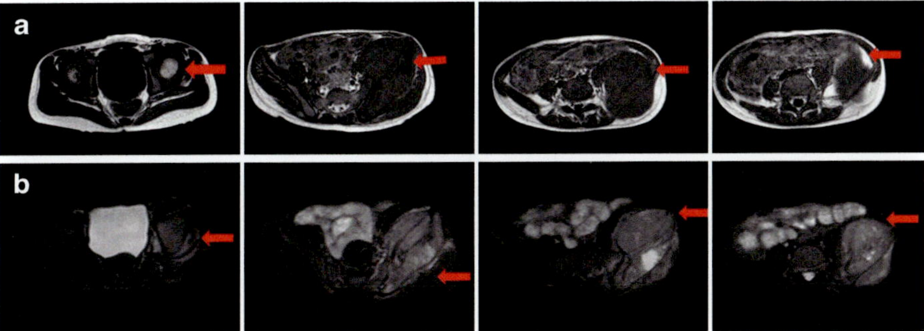

Fig. 8.9 The diagnostic MRI scan of the case ((**a**) T1-weighted transverse images, (**b**) T2-spare transverse images)

bone to the left acetabulum with a soft tissue component which destructs the bones and includes necrotic areas was detected with a SUVmax value of 6.4 (Fig. 8.12). In addition, a 6 × 5-mm subpleural nodule in the left lung with a SUVmax value of 1.5 was also observed (Fig. 8.13).

The patient then received the Euro-EWING 99 protocol, and partial response in both the primary tumor and pulmonary nodule was observed in August 2015. On sacroiliac joint MRI, the tumor was decreased to 2/3 of its initial volume (Fig. 8.14). On PET/CT, the SUVmax of the primary lesion decreased to 2.8 (Fig. 8.15), and no fluouro-deoxy-glucose (FDG) involvement was detected in the lung nodule.

Fig. 8.10 The diagnostic MRI scan of the case (T2-spare coronal image)

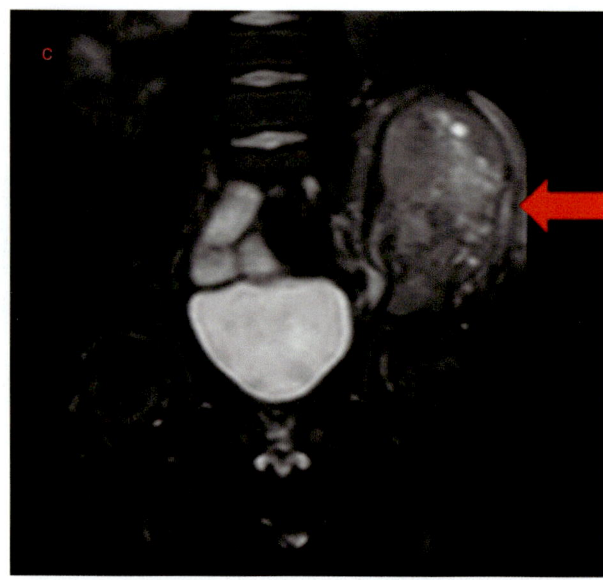

Fig. 8.11 Thorax CT at diagnosis

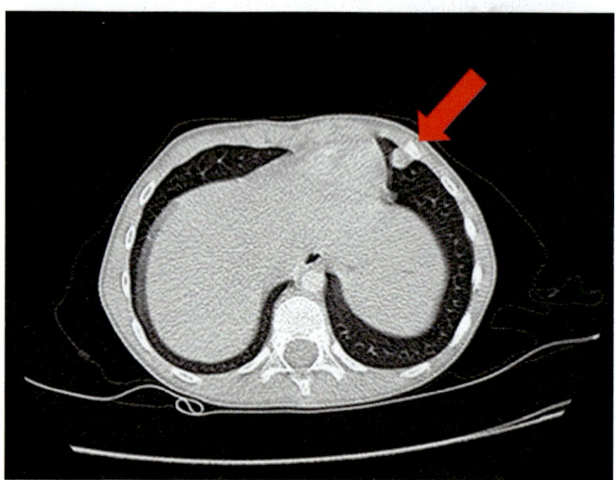

Chemotherapy was continued. In October 2015, although the primary lesion and the lung nodule decreased in size on sacroiliac joint MRI and thorax CT, sclerosis in the primary lesion was increased and the FDG-involved area was widened on PET/CT and progression was thought (Fig. 8.16). After the decision of the tumor board with specialists of Pediatric Oncology, Pediatric Surgery, Radiation Oncology, Radiology and Nuclear Medicine, surgery was decided. In November 2015, the patient underwent internal hemipelvectomy and pelvic fixation. The final pathology revealed ES with vascular invasion. The tumor had invaded the bony cortex and soft tissues. Resection margins were negative but the response to CHT was minimal. The CHT protocol was changed in the tumor board, and RT was planned to both the primary tumor bed and lungs.

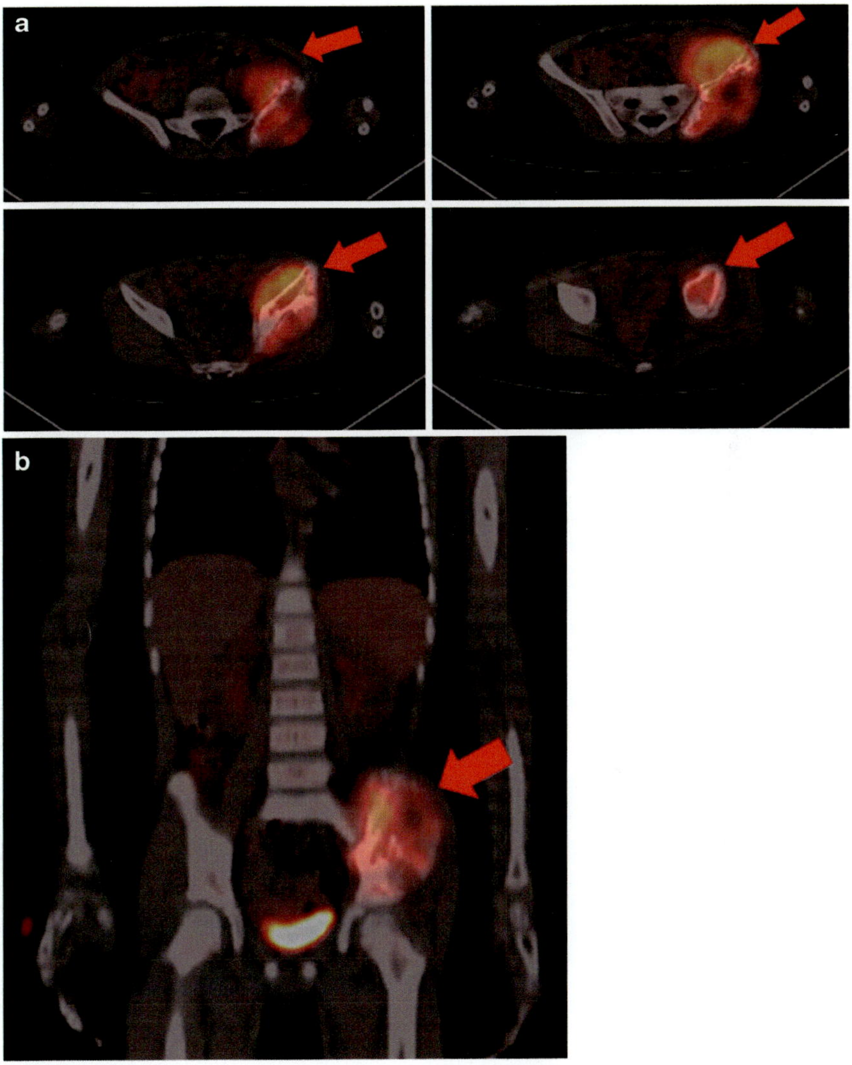

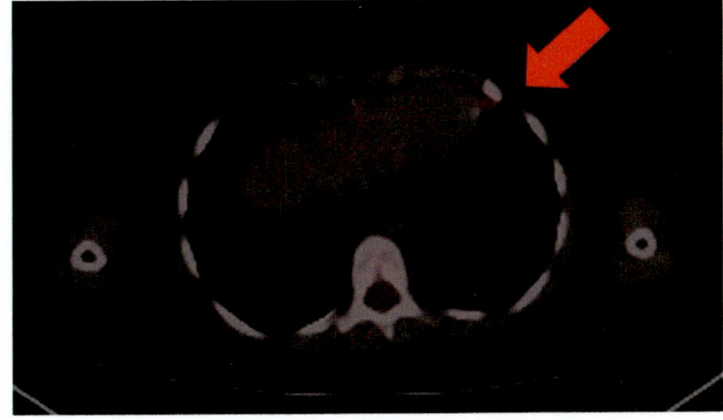

Fig. 8.12 PET/CT images of the primary tumor ((**a**) transverse images, (**b**) Coronal image)

Fig. 8.13 PET/CT image
of the solitary pulmonary
nodule

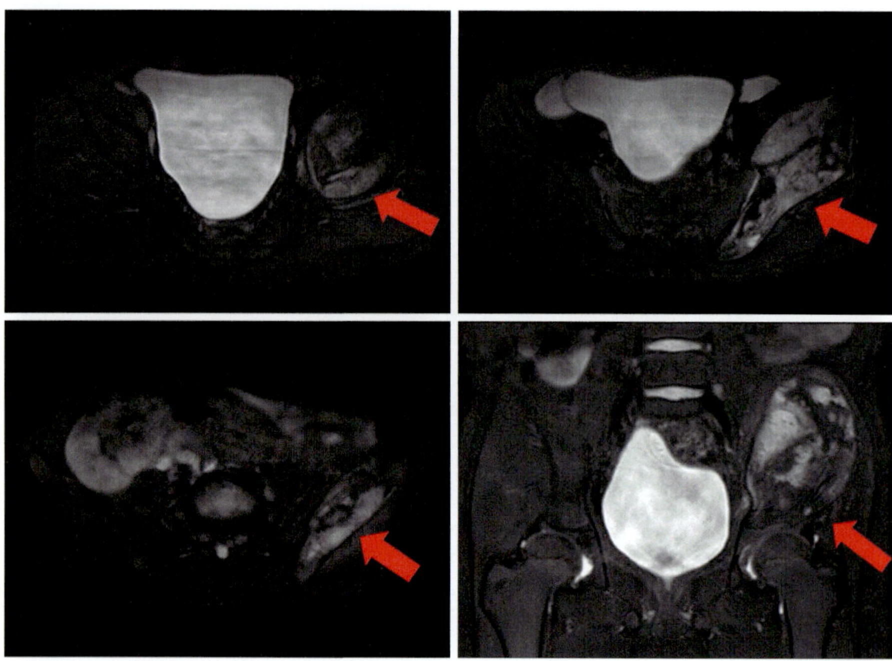

Fig. 8.14 Transverse and coronal T2-weighted MR images of the case after initial chemotherapy

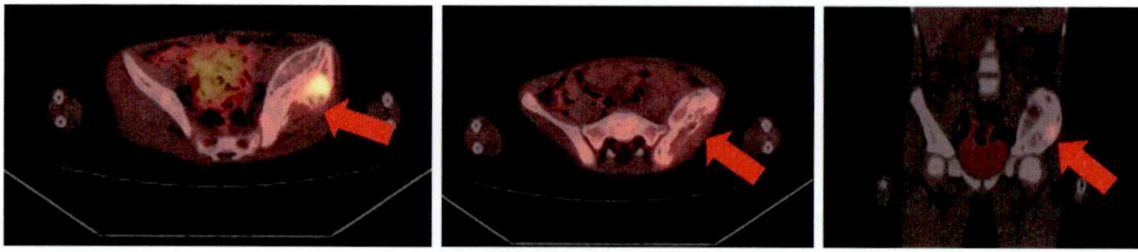

Fig. 8.15 Transverse and coronal images of the PET/CT scan after initial chemotherapy

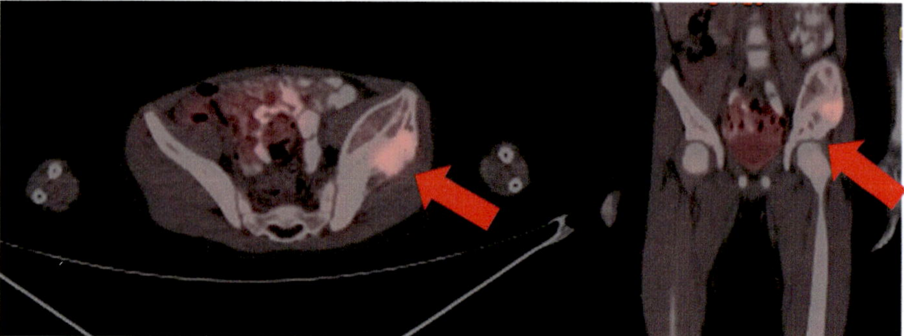

Fig. 8.16 Transverse and coronal images of the PET/CT scan after the completion of induction chemotherapy

8.3.2 Evidence Based Treatment Recommendations

The treatment of ES starts with induction CHT of multiple agents. Induction CHT helps the clinician to evaluate the effectiveness of the regimen, leads to a degree of bone healing which diminishes the risk of pathologic fractures, shrinks the tumor so that the volume to be resected and irradiated gets smaller, and increases the probability of achieving negative surgical margins. Response rates up to 90% have been reported, and the rate is directly correlated with the survival of the patient [71–73]. Following induction CHT, local therapy is essential as cure cannot be achieved with systemic therapy alone. Local therapy can be surgery, RT, or both. Retrospective analyses of randomized studies reported better local control (LC) with surgery; however, there may be a selection bias of patients with favorable characteristics that underwent surgery [74–76]. The risk of secondary malignancy with RT results in surgery being the first local treatment of choice. However, RT is recommended for tumors that cannot be resected without significant morbidity, as ES is known to be radiosensitive and RT is a curative option in these patients. Table 8.10 shows the results of major randomized trials.

Table 8.10 The results of major randomized trials for the treatment of Ewing sarcoma

Study	N of patients	Treatment	5-year EFS (%)
IESS-I [77]	342	VAC	24
(1973–1978)		VACD	44
		VAC + WLI	40
IESS-II [78]	214	VACD-HD	68
(1978–1982)		VACD-MD	48
CCG/POG I (INT-0091) [79]	200	VACD	54
(1988–1993)	198	VACD + IE	69
	120	VACD ± IE (metastatic)	22
CCG/POG INTERGROUP II	247	VCD + IE-48 weeks	70
[80] (1995–1998)	231	VCD + IE-30 weeks	72
COG-AEWS 0031 [81]	247	VCD + IE	65
	231	VCD + IE	73
CESS 81 [82]	93	VACD	80 (<100 mL) (3 years)
(1981–1985)			31 (≥100 mL) (3 years)
CESS 86 [83]	301	VACD (SR)	52 (10 years)
(1986–1991)		VAID (HR)	51 (10 years)
ICESS 92 [84]	155	VAID/VACD (SR)	68/67
(1992–1999)	492	VAID/EVAID (HR)	44/52
UKCCSG-ET1 [85]	120	VACD	41
(1978–1986)			
UKCCSG-ET2 [86]	201	VAID	62
(1987–1993)			

(continued)

Table 8.10 (continued)

Study	N of patients	Treatment	5-year EFS (%)
MSKCC-T2 [87] (1970–1978)	20	VACD (adjuvant)	75
MSKCC-P6 [88] (1990–1995)	36	HD-CVD + IE	77 (2 years)
MSKCC-P6 [89] (1991–2001)	68	HD-CVD + IE	81 (4 years) (localized) 12 (4 years) (metastatic)
St. Jude ES-79 [90] (1978–1986)	52	VACD	82 (<8 cm) (3 years) 64 (≥8 cm) (3 years)
St. Jude ES-87 [91] (1987–1991)	26	IE	Clinical response in 96%
St. Jude EW-92 [92] (1992–1996)	34	VCD-IE	78 (3 years)
REN-3 [93] (1991–1997)	157	VDC + VIA + IE	71
SFOP EW-88 [94] (1988–1991)	141	VD + VD/VA	58
SFOP EW-93 [95] (1993–1999)	116	VD + VD/VA (SR)	70
	46	VD + VD/VA + IE (IR)	54
	48	VD + VD/VA + IE + HD (HR)	48
SSG IX [96] (1990–1999)	88	VID + PID	58 (DMFS)
Euro-EWING 99 [97] (1999–2005)	281	VIDE + VAI + HD	27 (3 years)

Abbreviations: *N* number, *EFS* event-free survival, *WLI* whole lung irradiation, *IESS* Intergroup Ewing's Sarcoma Study, *CCG* Children's Cancer Group, *POG* Pediatric Oncology Group, *INT* intergroup, *COG* Children's Oncology Group, *CESS* Cooperative Ewing's Sarcoma Study, *EICESS* European Intergroup Cooperative Ewing Sarcoma Study, *UKCCSG ET* United Kingdom Children's Cancer Study Group Ewing Tumor, *MSKCC* Memorial Sloan Kettering Cancer Center, *SFOP* French Society of Pediatric Oncology, *SSG* Scandinavian Sarcoma Group, *V* vincristine, *A* actinomycin-D, *C* cyclophosphamide, *D* doxorubicin, *HD* high-dose, *MD* moderate-dose, *I* ifosfamide, *E* etoposide, *P* cisplatin, *SR* standard-risk, *HR* high-risk, *R* intermediate-risk, *DMFS* distant metastasis-free survival

For patients that will undergo surgery, limb-sparing techniques are preferred over amputation. Tumors located in the scapula, clavicle, ribs, proximal fibula, and wing of the ilium can easily be resected. However, amputation may be an option for younger patients with lesions of the fibula, tibia, and foot. After surgery, RT is indicated in most patients. To start with, adjuvant RT should be applied following debulking procedures that are not oncologic resections as they do not provide adequate LC. After a complete oncologic resection, in which the whole compartment of the muscle tissue is resected, the rate of local failure (LF) was reported 4%, compared to 25% and 50% for wide resection (tumor is resected with the surrounding reactive zone) and marginal resection (tumor is resected without its surrounding reactive zone), respectively [98]. Children's Oncology Group (COG) trials recommend adjuvant RT if the resection margins are close (<1 cm for bone, <5 mm for muscle, and <2 mm along a fascial plane). The rate of LC was excellent with surgery alone in the Cooperative Ewing's Sarcoma Study (CESS) and European Intergroup Cooperative Ewing Sarcoma Study (EICESS) trials [99]. However, the rate of LF was reported 12% in patients with a poor histologic response (soft tissue component reduction of <50%) to induction CHT and underwent wide resection, and it was decreased to 6% with adjuvant RT [75]. On the other hand, Bacci et al. [100] did not show any benefit of adjuvant RT in patients that underwent wide or marginal resection with LF rates of 6% and 7% with and without adjuvant RT, respectively. With these data in hand, adjuvant RT is indicated in patients with a poor histologic response to induction CHT and positive/close resection margins following surgery.

Neoadjuvant RT following induction CHT is an option for patients with a poor response [101, 102]. This was studied in the EICESS-92 trial in patients who were thought to leave the operation room with positive/close resection margins, with an aim of sterilizing the compartment to be resected and reducing the risk of dissemination during surgery [75]. This effort resulted in a LC rate of 95% without any benefit on systemic disease control. However, it should be kept in mind that postoperative infection risk may increase with neoadjuvant RT.

Patients who are not candidates for surgery undergo definitive RT. These patients usually present with large tumors that are amenable to surgery without significant morbidity. In the EICESS trials, the LF rate was found 26% in patients that underwent RT only compared to 10% and 4% in patients that underwent surgery only and surgery + RT, respectively [75, 76]. Bacci et al. [100] also reported higher LF rates with RT alone compared to surgery alone and surgery + RT (19% vs. 9% vs. 11%). The important point in this trial is that RT did not decrease LC for tumors in central parts of the body where the surgery is also not successful to control the disease. The COG INT-0091 trial was retrospectively analyzed for the LC of pelvic tumors only, and the LF rate was 22% in both surgery and RT arms [103]. However, although not statistically significant, patients that received both local therapies had better outcomes. Therefore, definitive RT is indicated when a gross residual tumor is suspected to be left with surgery. If an oncologic resection will not be able to be performed, debulking surgery is an unnecessary procedure because it results in increased rate of morbidity without any benefit on LC [75, 76, 100].

Nearly 75% of patients with ES present with localized disease but the majority of them have unidentifiable micrometastases at the time of diagnosis. The prognosis of these patients is poor despite aggressive multiagent CHT. The Euro-EWING 99 protocol included 6 cycles of VIDE (vincristine, ifosfamide, doxorubicin, etoposide) CHT followed by one cycle of VID and local therapy prior to high-dose busulfan and melphalan followed by stem cell rescue, and resulted in 3-year overall survival (OS) and event-free survival (EFS) rates of 34% and 27%, respectively [97]. Patients with lung metastasis constitute a more favorable group. In the CESS and EICESS trials, patients that received whole-lung irradiation (WLI) had higher EFS rates compared to patients who did not (5-year EFS rate was 40% vs. 19%) [104]. As a result, definitive treatment of all metastatic sites improves the outcomes in patients with metastatic ES. If definitive RT does not seem feasible for some sites, palliative RT is recommended.

8.3.3 Treatment Recommendations

Treatment recommendations for ES according to National Comprehensive Cancer Network (NCCN) guidelines are summarized in Table 8.11.

8.3.4 Treatment Planning

8.3.4.1 Simulation
Ewing's sarcoma can arise from any part of the body. Simulation for RT planning should be done with the affected part being stabilized properly. Intravenous contrast use is recommended.

8.3.4.2 Contouring
Historically, the entire bone was irradiated; however, the randomized trial of Pediatric Oncology Group (POG) 8346 reported no benefit of this approach showing the fact that LF usually occurs within the high-dose volume [105]. The RT fields are currently more limited. The still open COG trial recommendations for the target volumes are shown in Table 8.12.

Table 8.11 NCCN guidelines version 2.2018 (https://www.nccn.org/professionals/physician_gls/pdf/bone.pdf)

Primary treatment	Re-staging	Response evaluation	Local therapy			In case of progression
Multiagent CHT (≥9 weeks)	X-rays, MRI ± CT of the primary, chest CT, ± PET/CT or bone scan	Improved/ stable disease	Wide excision	SM+	CHT + RT RT + CHT	CHT ± RT
				SM−	CHT	
			Definitive RT + CHT			
			Amputation	CHT ± RT		
		Progressive disease	RT and/or surgery to the primary for local control or palliation			CHT or BSC

Abbreviations: *CHT* chemotherapy, *MRI* magnetic resonance imaging, *CT* computed tomography, *PET/CT* positron emission tomography/CT, *SM* surgical margin, *RT* radiotherapy, *BSC* best supportive care

Table 8.12 COG contouring recommendations for the primary tumor of Ewing's sarcoma

Volume	Definition
GTV-1	pre-chemotherapy tumor volume including all T1-contrast enhancing tumor, all T2 signal abnormality, and all bone abnormalities
CTV-1[a]	GTV-1 + 1 cm
PTV-1[b]	CTV-1 + 0.5–1 cm[a]
GTV-2	Residual soft-tissue mass after induction chemotherapy and all bone abnormalities that were present before chemotherapy
CTV-2[a]	GTV-2 + 1 cm
PTV-2[b]	CTV-2 + 0.5–1 cm[a]

Abbreviations: *GTV* gross tumor volume, *CTV* clinical target volume, *PTV* planning target volume

[a]CTVs should be modified for anatomic pushing borders such as the abdominal cavity and lung or to be restricted to fascial planes if there is no evidence of infiltration. All surgically contaminated areas, scars, and drainage sites must be included

[b]Depending on tumor location and daily image guidance

In patients with lung metastasis, both lungs down to the diaphragmatic recess should be irradiated from the anterior and posterior with 15–20 Gy in 1.5-Gy fractions. If possible, breath-hold technique should be used to reduce the volume of irradiated liver, stomach, and upper kidneys. The best timing for WLI is after conventional CHT is completed. During WLI, doxorubicin and actinomycin-D must be avoided to decrease the risk of pneumonitis, actinomycin-D should also be avoided after WLI because of the risk of 'recall' phenomenon, and WLI should not be administered at all in patients using a busulfan-containing regimen because of the risk of significant lung toxicity.

For a limited number of bone metastasis, definitive RT is recommended to all initially involved sites. In patients with multiple bone metastases, RT can be administered at the end of whole therapy to all involved sites or bulky, slowly-responding, or residual sites can be selected to be irradiated in order to avoid myelosupression.

8.3.4.3 Case Contouring

In the first phase, the left hemipelvis of the patient was irradiated with 45 Gy in 1.8-Gy fractions. Then, the residual soft tissue mass with a 1-cm margin was administered a boost dose of 5.4 Gy in 1.8 Gy fractions (Fig. 8.17). The total dose applied was 50.4 Gy (Fig. 8.18). After the completion of RT to the primary site, CHT was continued. The solitary lung lesion disappeared after CHT and 15 Gy WLI was administered in 1.5-Gy fractions (Fig. 8.19).

8.3.4.4 Prescription Dose and Dose Constraints for Critical Structures

Dose Recommendations

The Intergroup Ewing Sarcoma Study (IESS-I) trial reported no benefit of 65 Gy over 30 Gy in terms of LC [77]. However, in St. Jude Hospital series, the LC rate

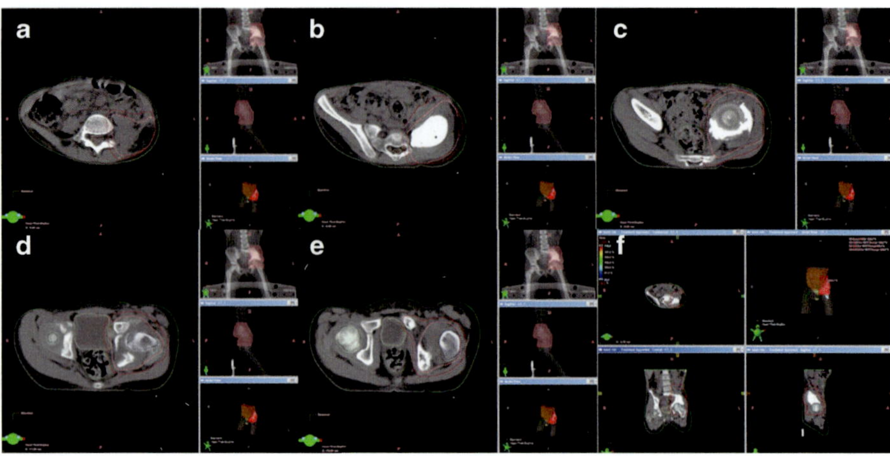

Fig. 8.17 The contouring of the case. (**a–e**). The first phase, (**f**). The second phase (pink = GTV, red = CTV)

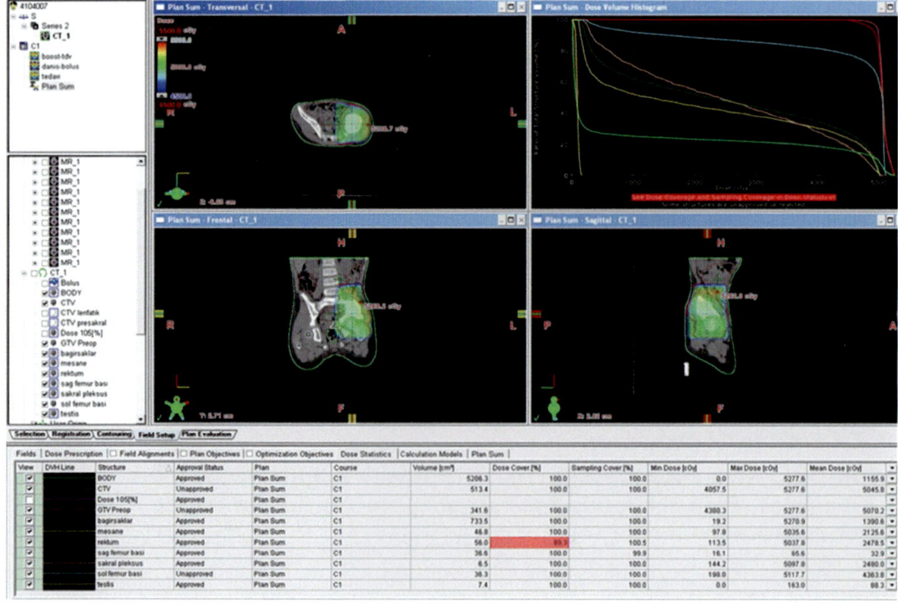

Fig. 8.18 Final plan of the case

was reported to be lower with doses <40 Gy [106]. The recommended dose for definitive RT is 55–60 Gy. For neoadjuvant or adjuvant RT, the doses range between 45 Gy and 55 Gy. In the adjuvant setting, the recommended dose in AEWS 1031 trial is 45 Gy to pre-CHT CTV, 50.4 Gy for microscopic positive margins, and 55.8 Gy to post-CHT residual disease in 1.8-Gy fractions [81]. Hyperfractionated RT regimens did not result in LC benefit [99].

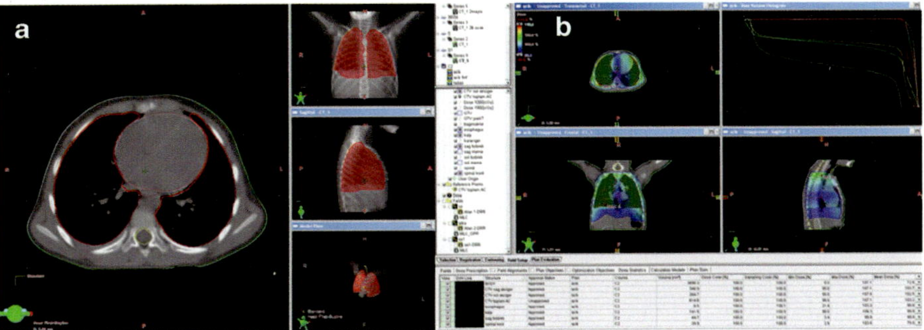

Fig. 8.19 Whole lung irradiation contouring (**a**) and plan (**b**) of the case

Patients with chest wall tumors often present with pleural effusion, and even the tumor is resected, hemithorax irradiation is recommended with a total dose of 15 Gy for patients <14 years and 20 Gy for older patients. The 7-year EFS was reported 63% in patients that underwent hemithorax irradiation compared to 46% in patients that did not in the EICESS 92 trial [84].

For vertebral lesions, 45 Gy is the standard dose but it is not clear whether this dose is adequate for LC. The average dose used in the CESS 81, CESS 86, and EICESS 92 trials was 49.6 Gy [101]. Sacral lesions should be treated to the full dose.

Dose Constraints for Critical Structures

The actuarial complication rate related to the treatment of ES was reported 70% at 35 years [107]. The most common complications of RT are on the skeletal system. Abnormal growth and development of the skeletal system due to premature closure of active epiphyses may occur. The degree of growth discrepancy depends on the patient's age, the location of the epiphysis irradiated, and RT dose. Another skeletal complication of RT is pathologic fractures which is observed in 10% of patients. It usually occurs within 24 h after RT, and the most affected site is the proximal femur. Doses of <40 Gy in conventional fractionation and hyperfractionated schemes carry a lower risk of bone fractures [108, 109]. Radiotherapy can also cause decreased range of motion, weakness and pain in the extremity, and discoloration of the skin.

As the risk of lymphedema is increased, particularly in tumors of the leg, circumferential irradiation of the extremities should be avoided by sparing at least a 1- to 2-cm strip of tissue. Besides, growth plates and vertebral bodies should be either fully irradiated or not be included at all in growing children in order to prevent asymmetric growth and functional deficits.

In patients that receive high doses of cyclophosphamide or ifosfamide, the risk of radiation cystitis increases, even at doses as low as 20 Gy. Pelvic tumors do not usually invade to the tissues in the vicinity of the urinary bladder, but push them aside; therefore, neoadjuvant CHT allows sparing the bladder better if good tumor shrinkage is obtained. A 1-cm medial margin on the residual disease at the time of treatment is adequate from the beginning of RT.

The most frightening complication of RT in children is the increased risk of secondary malignancies. There is no threshold for the development of secondary malignancies, but the risk increases with increased RT doses. The most common secondary malignancy related to RT is sarcoma, and the risk of sarcoma development was reported 1–4% at 20 years [77, 110, 111].

8.3.5 Follow-Up (F/U) Recommendations

Patients should be followed up with physical exam, plain radiographs, MRI ± CT of the primary site, and chest x-ray or CT every 2–3 months in the first 2 years, every 6 months in years 3–4, and annually thereafter (https://www.nccn.org/professionals/physician_gls/pdf/bone.pdf). Complete blood count and other laboratory studies should be performed as indicated. A PET/CT (head-to-toe) or bone scan can also be considered.

8.4   Rhabdomyosarcoma

Overview

Epidemiology: Soft-tissue sarcomas account for approximately 7% of all pediatric cancers, and rhabdomyosarcoma (RMS) comprises 40% of them. Median age is <5 years, but there is a second incidence peak in the mid-teens. The etiology is unknown but some genetic mutations have been defined.

Pathology: Rhabdomyosarcoma is one of the small, round, blue cell malignancies of childhood. The most common histological subtype is embryonal RMS with the best prognosis, and it has spindle cell and botryoid variants. Alveolar RMS comprises approximately 25% of all RMS, and the least favorable subtype is the undifferentiated sarcoma. Loss of heterozygosity in chromosome 11p and RAS/NF1 pathway mutations were identified in patients with embryonal RMS, whereas t(2;13) or t(1;13) translocations result in PAX-FKHR fusion protein in 80% of all patients with alveolar RMS. Besides, RMS can also occur in patients with neurofibromatosis type-1, Li-Fraumeni syndrome, and Beckwith-Wiedemann syndrome.

Diagnosis: Patients present with symptoms related to tumor location and extent of disease. The head and neck (H&N) region is the most frequent site of involvement. In general, lymph node (LN) involvement is <5% in RMS; however, the rate can be up to 25% in paratesticular and extremity tumors. Distant metastasis (DM) is present in 20% of all patients at the time of diagnosis. For the exact diagnosis, a magnetic resonance imaging (MRI) of the primary tumor site, computed tomography (CT) of the chest and abdomen (for infradiaphragmatic tumors), and a bone scintigraphy should be performed. A biopsy of the primary tumor and/or metastasis is warranted. As the rate of LN metastasis is high, LN sampling is recommended for paratesticular and extremity lesions. For H&N lesions, cerebrospinal fluid cytology; and for genitourinary lesions, examination under anesthesia should also be performed.

Treatment: For all RMS, an upfront surgery is the first line of therapy. Adjuvant chemotherapy (CXT) and radiotherapy (RT) are indicated in most cases. The standard CXT regimen is vincristine, actinomycin-D, and cyclophosphamide (VAC)–based CXT, resulting in a 5-year event-free survival (EFS) rate of 90%, 70%, and <30% in patients with low-risk, intermediate risk, and high risk, respectively. The recommended doses for adjuvant RT are 36 Gy for microscopic disease, 41.4 Gy for microscopic residual disease, and 50.4 Gy for gross residual disease with local failure rates of approximately 10%.

Key Words: Rhabdomyosarcoma; Radiotherapy

8.4.1 Case Presentation

An 8-year old girl was brought to the emergency room by her parents with abdominal pain lasting for 10 days in November 2016. Abdominal ultrasonography (USG) revealed an 87 × 75 × 85-mm heterogeneous, solid mass with cystic areas and central vascularization in the left adnexal region. The uterus and ovaries could not be visualized separately from the mass. On abdominal MRI, the lesion was 92 × 77 × 89 mm, filling the whole bony pelvis. The uterus was not separately visualized, and there was suspicious invasion to the pelvic muscles at the posterior (Fig. 8.20). The rectum and sigmoid colon were pushed to the right and the urinary bladder to the anterior and superior because of the mass. Fine needle aspiration cytology included a small number of cells resembling mesenchymal tissue fragments and a small round cell malignant tumor. Tru-cut biopsy also revealed a round cell malignant tumor. After immunohistochemical examination, embryonal RMS was diagnosed. The Ki-67 proliferation index was 80%. Thorax CT showed no lung metastasis.

VAC chemotherapy was initiated. After 3 cycles, the size of the tumor diminished to 60 × 55 × 80 mm, and after 6 cycles it was 42 × 36 × 55 mm on abdominal USG. The MRI in April 2017 revealed a significant reduction in size (49 × 27 × 51 mm), the uterus could be visualized separately but not the left ovary (Fig. 8.21). Besides, the left internal iliac artery was in close proximity to the lesion

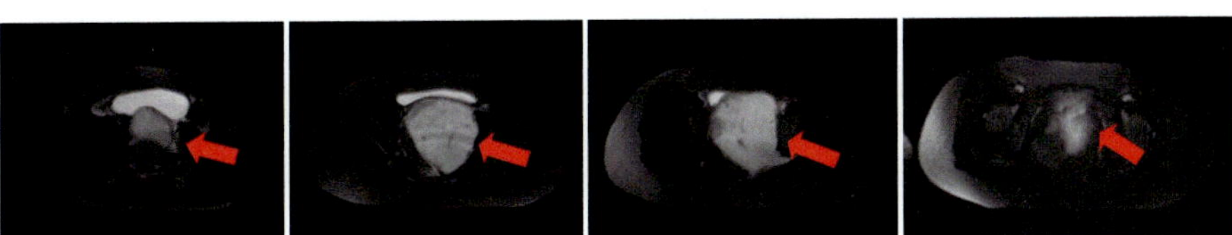

Fig. 8.20 The diagnostic T2-weighted MRI images of the case

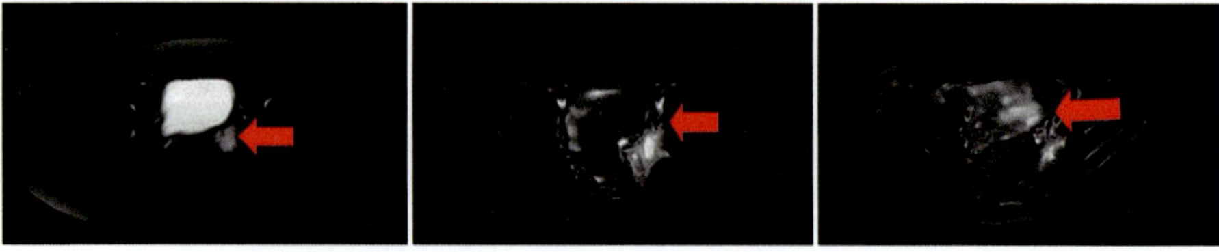

Fig. 8.21 T2-weighted MRI images of the case after the completion of chemotherapy

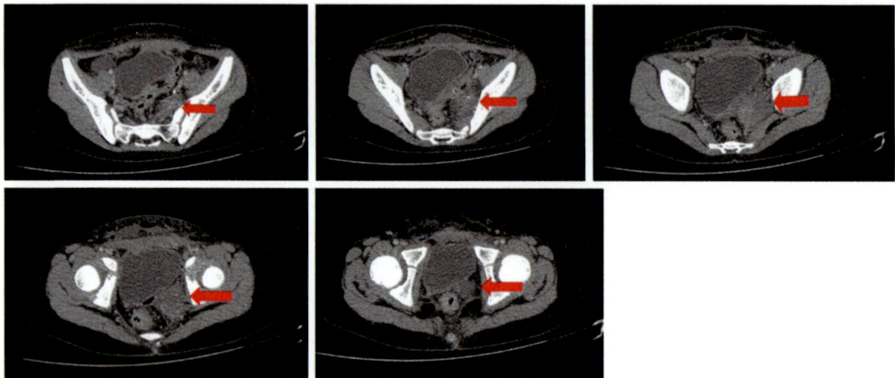

Fig. 8.22 Postoperative CT images of the case prior to radiotherapy

Table 8.13 Favorability of RMS according to tumor site

Characteristic	Site
Favorable	Orbit Non-parameningeal H&N (scalp, parotid, oropharynx, oral cavity, larynx) Nonbladder-prostate genitourinary (paratestes, vagina, vulva, uterus) Biliary tract
Unfavorable	Parameningeal H&N (nasopharynx, nasal cavity, paranasal sinuses, middle ear, mastoid, pterygopalatine fossa, infratemporal fossa) Urinary bladder and prostate Extremity Other (trunk, retroperitoneum)

Abbreviations: *RMS* rabdomyosarcoma, *H&N* head and neck

and some of its branches were within it. In May 2017, the patient underwent excisional biopsy. During the operation, the mass was seen to have a venous plexus inside and massive hemorrhage had occurred; therefore, total excision was not possible. The final pathology revealed RMS infiltration in the lesion resected from the posterior of the bladder and on the internal iliac artery. On postoperative abdominal CT, the mass was $43 \times 32 \times 60$ mm, and there was invasion in the left internal iliac vessels (Fig. 8.22). In the tumor board, the patient was accepted as intermediate risk (favorable site, T2bN0M0, stage I, group IIIA, embryonal) (Tables 8.13, 8.14, 8.15, 8.16, and 8.17), and adjuvant RT was planned.

Table 8.14 TNM classification of rhabdomyosarcoma

Primary tumor (T)	
T category	T criteria
T1	Tumor is confined to site/organ of origin
T1a	$\leq$5 cm
T1b	>5 cm
T2	Tumor extends beyond site/organ of origin
T2a	$\leq$5 cm
T2b	>5 cm
Regional lymph nodes (N)	
N category	N criteria
N0	No regional lymph node involvement
N1	Regional lymph node involvement
Distant metastasis (M)	
M category	M criteria
M0	No distant metastasis
M1	Distant metastasis

Table 8.15 Intergroup rhabdomyosarcoma study (IRS) preoperative staging system

Stage	Site	T stage	N stage	M stage
I	Favorable	Any T	N0–1	M0
II	Unfavorable	T1a/T2a	N0	M0
III	Unfavorable	T1b/T2b	N0	M0
	Unfavorable	Any T	N1	M0
IV	Any site	Any T	N0–1	M0

Table 8.16 Intergroup rhabdomyosarcoma study (IRS) surgical-pathological grouping system

Group	Definition
I	Localized disease, completely resected
Ia	Confined to organ or muscle of origin
Ib	Involvement outside organ or muscle of origin (contiguously)
II	Gross total resection
IIa	Microscopic residual disease, no regional lymph node involvement
IIb	Regional nodal involvement without microscopic residual disease
IIc	Regional nodal involvement with microscopic residual disease
III	Incomplete resection with gross residual disease
IIIa	After biopsy
IIIb	After gross major resection (>50% of disease)
IV	Distant metastasis at diagnosis

Table 8.17 Intergroup rhabdomyosarcoma study (IRS) risk groups

Risk group	Definition
Low-risk	– Localized embryonal/botyroid histology at favorable sites (stage I, groups I–III)
	– Localized embryonal/botyroid histology at unfavorable sites with completely resected or microscopic residual disease (stages II–III, groups I–II)
Intermediate-risk	– Embryonal/botyroid histology at unfavorable sites with gross residual disease (stages II–III, group III)
	– Patients 2–10 years with metastatic embryonal histology (stage IV)
	– Nonmetastatic alveolar/undifferentiated histology (stages I–III)
High-risk	– Any stage IV/group IV (except for patients 2–10 years with embryonal histology)

8.4.2 Evidence Based Treatment Recommendations

8.4.2.1 Intergroup RMS Study (IRS) Group Trials

Multimodality approach is performed in patients with RMS. A number of IRS trials have been held since 1972, and each one answered several important questions.

In IRS-I (1972–1978), 40–45 Gy RT was given to all patients; at the beginning of treatment in groups I and II, but was delayed until the sixth week in groups III and IV [112]. All patients also underwent VAC chemotherapy for 2 years. The results were:

1. In group I, postoperative RT is unnecessary if the patient is given 2 years of VAC. The 5-year relapse-free survival (RFS) and overall survival (OS) rate was 80% and 81–93%, respectively, in these patients. However, postoperative RT can be beneficial in patients in this group with alveolar or undifferentiated histology [113].
2. In group II, VAC is not superior to intensive VA if the patient receives RT. The 5-year RFS and OS was 65–72% and 72% in these patients, respectively.
3. In groups III and IV, VACA (VAC + Adriamycin) is not superior to VAC if the patient receives RT. The complete remission rate was 69% and 50% in group III and IV, respectively. The chance of staying in remission after complete remission was 60% and 30%, and the 5-year OS rate was 52% and 20% in the respective groups.
4. The 5-year OS rate was 55% in all patients.
5. After relapse, the 1- and 2-year OS rate was 32% and 17%, respectively.
6. The risk of DM is higher than the risk of local recurrence (LR).
7. The sites with best prognosis are the orbit and genitourinary tract, and the worst is the retroperitoneum.
8. Patients with alveolar histology have a poor prognosis, especially if the lesion is in the extremities.

Based on the findings of IRS-I, IRS-II was held (1978–1984) [114]. The results were:

1. In group I (excluding alveolar histology in the extremity), VAC is superior to VA in terms of disease-free survival (DFS) (82% vs. 68%) with similar 5-year OS rates (82% vs. (8%). Therefore, VAC is standard if the patient does not receive RT.
2. In group II, intensive VA has similar results with VAC if the patient receives postoperative RT. The 5-year OS rate was 77% and 90%, and 5-year DFS rate was 68% and 75% in patients that received VA and VAC, respectively.
3. In group III, 2 years of repetitive pulse CXT (doxorubicin or dactinomycin) increased the survival rate, but not in group IV. Patients in group III and IV had a complete remission rate of 72%, and this remained in 70% at 5 years with a survival rate of 64%.

4. The 5-year OS was increased to 62% in the whole group (7% improvement over IRS-I).
5. The 5-year OS rate after relapse was 17%.
6. In IRS-I, patients with parameningeal tumors with high-risk factors such as cranial nerve palsy, erosion of the skull base, or intracranial extension had a high incidence of central nervous system (CNS) relapse. In IRS-II, whole brain RT +/- intrathecal CXT decreased the rate of meningeal recurrence and increased survival in these patients.
7. VAC did not reduce the frequency of total cystectomy or produce durable bladder salvage in genitourinary tumors, and the survival was not compromised.

The results of IRS-III (1984–1991) are below [115]:

1. In group I with favorable histology, the efficacy of 1-year of VA was similar to VAC with 5-year progression-free survival (PFS) rate of 83% and 76%, respectively.
2. In group II with favorable histology (excluding orbit, H&N, and paratesticular tumors), VAD (VA + doxorubicin) was not superior to 1-year of VA + RT.
3. In group III (excluding genitourinary, orbit, and non-parameningeal H&N tumors), better results were achieved with a more intensive treatment with CXT (VAC + D + P[cisplatin] + E[etoposide]) + RT and second-look surgery compared to IRS-II with 5-year PFS rates of 62% and 52%, respectively.
4. In group IV, the aggressive therapy of IRS-III did not result in any benefit.
5. The 5-year OS for all patients was increased to 71% (9% improvement over IRS-II). The 5-year PFS rate was 65% (10% improvement over IRS-II).
6. In groups I and II with unfavorable histology, the combination of VADR-VAC + P and RT improved the outcome compared to IRS-II with VA or VAC + RT.
7. In group II with favorable-histology in the paratesticular regions and groups II and II with favorable-histology in the orbit and H&N, the addition of cyclophosphamide is unnecessary if the patient receives 1-year of VA + RT.
8. In group III with tumors of the bladder, vagina, and central pelvis, the outcomes were significantly improved compared to IRS-II. This was attributed to the early administration of RT, which increased the rate of bladder preservation to 60% from 25% of IRS-II.
9. In patients with parameningeal H&N tumors with cranial nerve palsy or skull base erosion, whole-brain RT was omitted, and the risk of CNS relapse and survival were not compromised. However, patients with intracranial extension still received whole-brain RT.

IRS-IV (1991–1997) introduced the presurgical staging [116]. The results were:

1. A prognostic classification was made based on histologic subtype, stage, and group: Low-risk disease included all groups of stage I embryonal histology and group I–II of stage II–III embryonal histology. All other patients with locoregional disease were accepted intermediate risk.

2. In group I–II orbit or eyelid tumors, VA led to excellent results, and so did RT in group II disease.
3. In group III, standard RT of 50.4 Gy in 1.8 Gy daily fractions were compared to hyperfractionated RT of 59.4 Gy in 1.1 Gy twice daily fractions, and no difference was observed between the two schemes in terms of failure-free survival (FFS) (73% vs. 73%) and local failure (LF) (15% vs. 12%) [117].
4. In patients with embryonal histology, the 3-year FFS was increased compared to IRS-III (83% vs. 74%); however, the rate did not differ for alveolar or undifferentiated histologies.
5. In non-metastatic disease survival rates were similar between patients that received VAC, VAI (VA + ifosfamide), and VIE.
6. In metastatic disease, IE resulted in increased OS rate compared to V + melphalan.
7. In this study, whole-brain RT was omitted in all patients with parameningeal H&N tumors but the ones with cytologic evidence of cerebrospinal fluid involvement. Survival was not compromised by this approach.
8. In group I paratesticular disease, the retrospective comparison to IRS-III revealed that patients <10 years of age could be evaluated by CT for retroperitoneal (RP) LN involvement without the need for RPLN dissection (RPLND) with a FFS rate of 90%. On the other hand, RPLND provided a FFS advantage over CT alone (100% vs. 63%) in patients ≥10 years of age benefited in terms of defining nodal involvement and the need for subsequent lymphatic RT [118].

IRSG V (1997–2005) is the last of the IRS trials. The results are below:

1. In group II, RT dose was reduced from 41.4 Gy–36 Gy in case of positive microscopic surgical margins. For orbital tumors the dose was reduced to 45 Gy. These doses were safe and effective in low-risk disease, especially if the patient received cyclophosphamide in the CXT regimen [119, 120].
2. In intermediate-risk disease, VAC and VAC alternated with VTC (topotecan instead of actinomycin-D) were compared, and the 4-year FFS was similar (73% vs. 68%, respectively) [121].
3. In intermediate- and high-risk disease, V + irinotecan demonstrated a 70% response rate with a low 2-year FFS rate (26%).

The ARST0331 trial reported the results of a tailored therapy for low-risk disease with embryonal histology groups I and II stages I–III, and group III stage I disease [122]. The RT dose was 36 Gy for microscopic disease and 41.4 Gy for nodal disease. In group III vaginal tumors, RT was delayed or completely omitted but the 2 year-FFS rate was 42% in these patients demonstrating that RT is necessary for improving local control (LC). The results of ARST0531 trial which compares VAC and VAC/V + irinotecan in intermediate-risk disease with embryonal histology group III stages II–III, and alveolar RMS group I–III stages I–III; ARST0431 trial on multiple-agent systemic therapy in high-risk disease; and ARST08P1 trial which incorporates an insulin-like growth factor-1 receptor inhibitor and temozolomide are awaited.

8.4.2.2 International Society of Pediatric Oncology (SIOP) Trials

The French SIOP began multi-institutional trials for RMS in 1975 and has reported results from three studies to date. These studies mainly focus on using risk-adapted intensification of CXT, minimizing local therapy at the first place and saving them for salvage. In the first SIOP study (RMS-75), VACD was used in group III patients and early local therapy was compared to delayed local therapy after maximal CXT response [123]. Surgery was preferred over RT as the local therapy. Although the OS rate was only 40%, two arms were similar in terms of survival. In the second SIOP study (MMT-84), RT was administered only in patients with residual tumor after CXT and surgery [124]. The 5-year OS and EFS was reported 68% and 53%, respectively, with an isolated LR rate of 29%. The third SIOP study (MMT-89), showed that alkylating agents can be omitted in patients with the most favorable prognosis [125]. Radiotherapy was used in a few patients, and the LF rate was 34%.

The difference of the aim of SIOP and IRS trials is that in IRS studies early introduction of RT is encouraged in patients with residual tumor after surgery, but in SIOP studies RT is avoided in most patients but the ones with residual tumor after CXT and surgery. The comparison of IRS and SIOP studies revealed that in some patients, cure can be achieved without the addition of RT; however, in the presence of residual tumor after initial surgery, RT yields higher survival rates in most subsets of patients [126].

8.4.2.3 Cooperative Weichteilsarkom Studiengruppe (CWS) Trials

Another group that studied on RMS is the German-based CWS. In the CWS-81 trial; no, 40 Gy or 50 Gy RT was applied based on the response to CXT and second-look surgery [127]. The authors reported that prognosis is similar in patients with a complete response to CXT and in patients with an initial complete tumor resection. On the other hand, patients without a complete response to CXT by week 9 should undergo early surgery or RT. In non-metastatic patients, the 5-year DFS rate was found 68%, and the most common cause of failure was LR. In the CWS-86 study, all patients received ifosfamide but in patients with favorable prognosis the CXT scheme was shortened [128]. Hyperfractionated accelerated RT was used in most patients; 32 Gy after a good response and 54.4 Gy after a poor response to CXT in 1.6 Gy twice daily fractions concurrently with ifosfamide and doxorubicin. In case of complete response to CXT, no RT was administered. The study concluded that in most favorable patients, the duration of CXT can be reduced to 16 weeks, response rates are improved with the use of ifosfamide compared to cyclophosphamide, and hyperfractionated accelerated RT concurrent with CXT can easily be tolerated providing satisfactory LC rates. Most failures were again local in this trial, especially in patients with group II and III disease that did not receive RT. In the CWS-91 study, induction CXT and second-look surgery was encouraged in all patients, and RT was not applied in case of a complete resection and no high-risk features [129]. Other patients received 32 or 48 Gy RT in 1.6 Gy twice daily fractions depending on the response to initial CXT and risk factors. When compared to historical controls from the CWS-86 study, the rates of LC and EFS were improved with RT, lower doses of 32 or 48 Gy resulted in similar outcomes with higher doses in the

CWS-86 study, and in group I-II disease with favorable risk factors, less intensive CXT yielded similar results compared to the more intensive regimen in CWS-86.

8.4.3 Treatment Recommendations

Multimodality approach is applied in patients with RMS. A non-morbid surgical resection should be performed if applicable. Otherwise, RT should be chosen because it offers equivalent rates of LC with organ preservation. Radiotherapy can be administered after multiple weeks of CXT to allow reduction in tumor size and to give a chance to a second-look surgery. However, in patients with parameningeal disease and intracranial extension, RT should be initiated within the first few weeks of the start of CXT [130].

Radiotherapy is used to eradicate microscopic disease after resection, treat gross disease, and consolidate visible sites of metastatic involvement. In patients with group I disease, based on the IRS I-III trials, RT should be applied in case of alveolar histology as it increases the rates of FFS and OS, but unnecessary for patients with embryonal histology [113]. For all patients in groups II, III and IV, RT is indicated in different doses based on surgical margins and residual tumor bulk. Besides these general concepts, specific treatment approaches are present based on tumor location.

1. Orbital tumors are one of the favorable sites; the histology is embryonal in most tumors, and lymphatic involvement and DM are very rare. Surgery is not recommended in orbital tumors to preserve vision. Biopsy is adequate for diagnosis. Treatment starts with VAC or VA CXT, and local RT begins between the third and twelfth week of treatment. 45 Gy RT is sufficient when cyclophosphamide-containing regimens are used, otherwise 50 Gy RT can be more adequate [120]. Adding RT to CXT resulted in >90% cure rates [115]. The LC and EFS rates are lower with CXT alone, and although salvage RT can still be curative, vision is generally impaired in this setting [131].
2. In parameningeal tumors of the H&N, RT is essential for maximizing the chance of cure [114, 115]. The most important point for these tumors are that they have a propensity for invading the skull base, causing cranial nerve palsy, and directly extending into the CNS, which can be seen up to 41% of patients [130]. Complete resection is usually not possible, and can delay the initiation of CXT. Historically, whole-brain RT was applied to all patients with parameningeal tumors for CNS prophylaxis. However, based on the results of IRS trials, the current approach is to avoid whole-brain RT, even in patients with direct intracranial tumor extension because multi-agent CXT and adequate irradiation of the primary tumor and adjacent meninges is sufficient. On the other hand, in patients with known meningeal dissemination, craniospinal irradiation should be applied. Based on the IRS studies, RT should be started within 2 weeks of diagnosis in the presence of intracranial tumor extension to improve LC [130]. In non-parameningeal H&N

tumors, the prognosis is better and they require a less-intensive CXT regimen [115, 116]. Complete surgical resection is more possible for these tumors, and RT is indicated based on surgical margins. The rate of regional LN metastasis is 15% in these tumors; however, prophylactic irradiation of lymphatic sites is not necessary.

3. In bladder and prostate tumors, anterior pelvic exenteration was performed together with CXT historically, and RT was indicated in case of microscopic or gross residual disease with a survival rate of approximately 70% [132]. However, recent approach is to preserve the bladder. In the IRS-II trial, more conservative surgical approaches resulted in inferior DFS; however, with an intensified CXT regimen and routine RT in the proceeding IRS trials, survival rates were similar to aggressive surgery [133].

4. Patients with paratesticular tumors generally present with early-stage disease that is amenable to complete resection with a cure rate of approximately 90%. Inguinal orchiectomy is recommended; however, RPLND is still controversial, and some authors prefer intensified CXT instead and salvage RT, if necessary. In the IRS trials, on the other hand, ipsilateral RPLND is recommended for children ≥10 years of age [118].

5. In gynecologic tumors, the most common site is the vagina. Vaginal RMS is often diagnosed before the age of 3, and botyroid histology is common. Initial treatment requires surgery but because of cosmetic and functional deformities, total resection is not always possible. These tumors are generally sensitive to CXT; however, CXT alone results in high rates of LF [120, 122]. The Children's Oncology Group (COG) recommends adjuvant RT in case of microscopic or gross residual tumor. For uterine, cervical, and vulvar tumors, initial surgery continues with CXT and RT based on surgical margins. Brachytherapy (BRT) is a good alternative to external beam RT (EBRT) with fewer complications and excellent LC rates.

6. Extremity tumors have poor prognosis with alveolar or undifferentiated histology, large tumor bulk, deep invasive, and a high probability of LN involvement and DM. Complete surgical resection is difficult to achieve, and RT with multi-agent CXT provides excellent LC rates.

The timing of RT depends on the risk groups and presence of any urgent situation. In low- and intermediate-risk disease, RT is performed after 12 weeks of CXT. However, patients with parameningeal tumors and intracranial extension should receive RT within 2 weeks of the treatment scheme. In high-risk disease, aggressive CXT is required and local therapies can be considered at week 20. If symptomatic metastasis is present, urgent RT can be administered. In asymptomatic patients with metastatic disease, these sites are irradiated with similar doses at the end of systemic therapy. Vincristine, cyclophosphamide, and irinotecan can be administered concurrently with RT. However, actinomycin-D should not be applied concurrently with RT because of its potential for increased skin and mucosal toxicities.

8.4.4 Treatment Planning

8.4.4.1 Simulation

Simulation for RT planning should be done with the affected part being stabilized properly. Intravenous contrast use is recommended.

8.4.4.2 Contouring

Imaging studies at the time of diagnosis and after CXT should be used to define the extent of disease. An MRI is essential for better visualization of the soft tissue component. In the first phase of RT planning, the gross tumor volume (GTV)-1 is the tumor at the time of diagnosis. Clinical target volume (CTV)-1 is formed by adding 1 cm to the GTV1, and should not extend beyond anatomic barriers without tumor involvement. The planning target volume (PTV)-1 is generally formed by adding a 0.5-cm margin to CTV1. This volume is prescribed 36 Gy and if the surgical margins are negative, it is the only phase. If surgical margins are positive, in the second phase, GTV2 is the residual tumor after CXT and surgery including the whole surgical bed, clips and biopsy tracts; CTV2 is GTV2+1 cm; and PTV2 is CTV2+0.5 cm. Prophylactic LN irradiation is not necessary if the patient will be receiving combination CXT.

Although the bony orbit and the adjacent globe are very thin and fragile, they are not involved by orbital RMS and should not be included in the CTV. If the tumor extends through these structures, parameningeal involvement should be considered. In these patients, and also in patients with parameningeal H&N tumors, the adjacent meninges should be covered in the RT field. For orbital tumors, irradiation of the entire orbit is not necessary. For parameningeal H&N tumors, the skull base should also be included in the CTV to cover the possible intracranial extension.

For paratesticular tumors, irradiation of the periaortic and ipsilateral iliac LNs is recommended if there is LN involvement. In case the scrotum was surgically violated or invaded by the tumor, hemiscrotectomy or, less commonly, scrotal irradiation is indicated. If scrotal irradiation is to be performed, orchiopexy should be considered prior to treatment. Similarly, oophoropexy should be considered prior to RT for girls with pelvic tumors.

8.4.4.3 Case Contouring

In our case, GTV1 was the pre-CXT tumor volume. By adding a 0.5 cm margin to GTV1, CTV1 was formed and 36 Gy was prescribed to this volume. The reason for the 0.5 cm margin was the anatomical borders that were not invaded by the tumor. The post-CXT and postsurgical volume with all surgical clips was contoured as GTV2. A 1-cm margin was added to GTV2 to form the CTV2, and a 14.4 Gy boost dose was prescribed to this volume (Figs. 8.23 and 8.24). 0.5-cm margin was added to both CTVs to form PTVs, and the total dose was 50.4 Gy (Fig. 8.25).

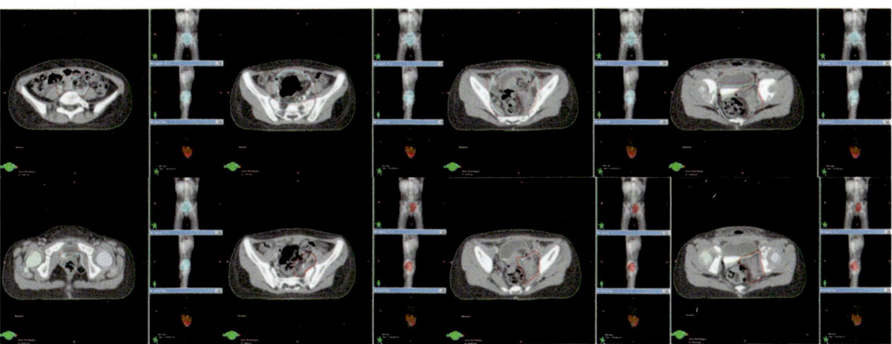

Fig. 8.23 The delineation of the case. Cyan = GTV1, red = CTV1, pink = GTV2, magenta = CTV2

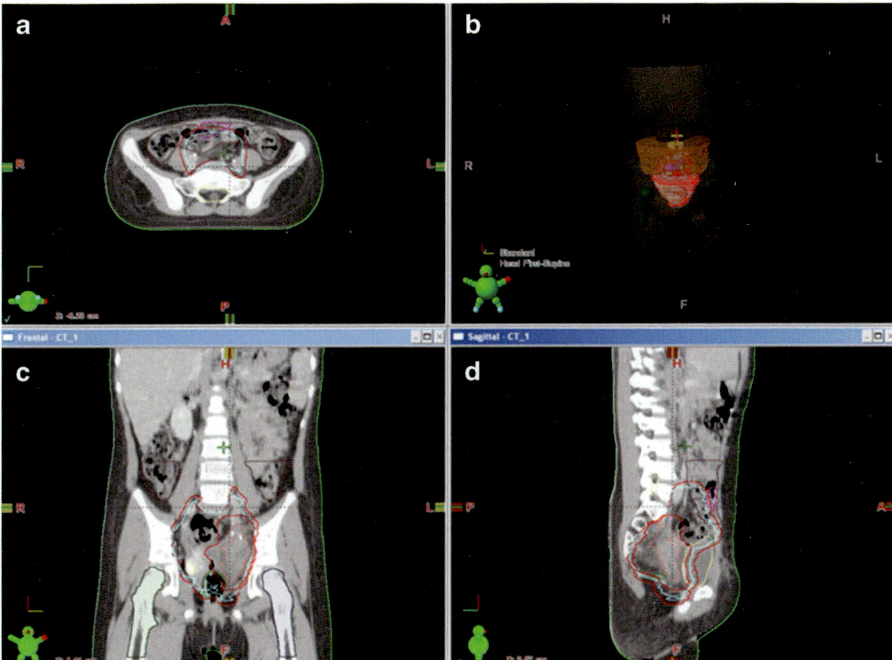

Fig. 8.24 Transverse (**a**), coronal (**c**), and sagittal (**d**) views of contouring the case. (**b**) shows all target volumes and critical organs in coronal view

8.4.4.4 Prescription Dose

Radiotherapy doses differ according to the surgical margin status and histological subtype. If the surgical margins are negative, RT is not indicated for embryonal histology, but 36 Gy RT is indicated for alveolar histology. If the surgical margins are microscopically positive, tumors of both histology should receive

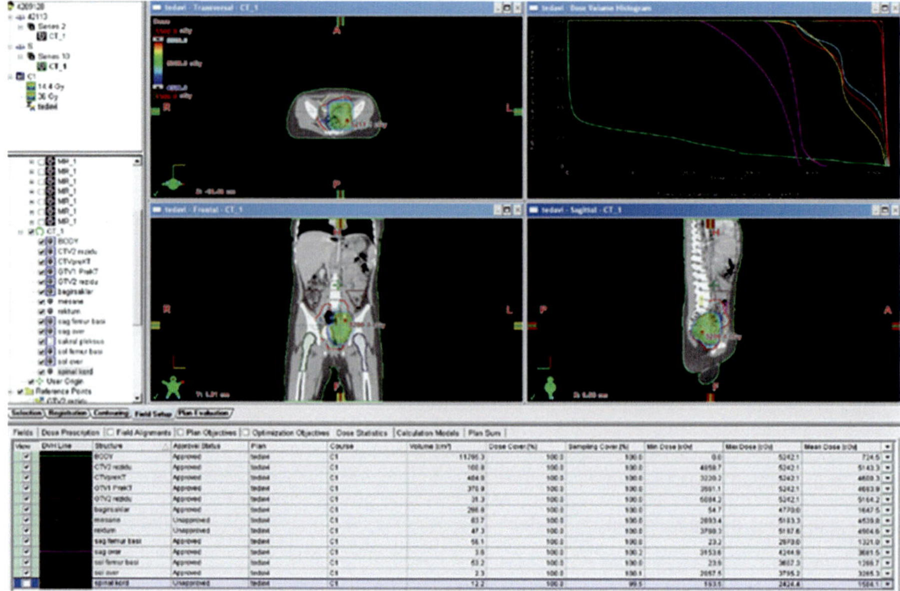

Fig. 8.25 Treatment plan of the case

36 Gy. If there is LN involvement, the involved regional LN area should receive 41.4 Gy in both histological subtypes. If there is gross residual disease, 50.4 Gy is prescribed for both histologies. Doses are delivered at 1.8 Gy per fraction daily.

For orbital tumors, a definitive RT dose of 45 Gy RT in 1.8 Gy daily fractions yields excellent local control. For parameningeal H&N tumors, 50.4 Gy in 28 fractions to the primary site is commonly used.

8.4.4.5 Dose Constraints for Critical Structures

Dose constraints for organs at risk of certain tumor locations can be found in related chapters.

8.4.5 Follow-Up (F/U) Recommendations

Patients are followed up with physical examination, laboratory studies, MRI of the primary area, CT of the chest and other metastatic imaging every 3 months in the first year; physical examination, laboratory studies, MRI of the primary area, CT of the chest and other metastatic imaging every 4 months in the second and third years; physical examination, MRI of the primary area and chest radiograph every 6 months in the fourth and fifth years, and annually thereafter.

References

1. Fletcher CDM, Unni K, Mertens F. World Health Organization classification of tumours: pathology and genetics of tumours of soft tissue and bone. Lyon: IARC Press; 2002.
2. Burningham Z, Hashibe M, Spector L, Schiffman JD. The epidemiology of sarcoma. Clin Sarcoma Res. 2012;2(1):14.
3. Lawrence W Jr, Donegan WL, Natarajan N, Mettlin C, Beart R, Winchester D. Adult soft tissue sarcomas. A pattern of care survey of the American College of Surgeons. Ann Surg. 1987;205(4):349–59.
4. Simon MA, Enneking WF. The management of soft-tissue sarcomas of the extremities. J Bone Joint Surg Am. 1976;58(3):317–27.
5. Enneking WF, Spanier SS, Malawer MM. The effect of the Anatomic setting on the results of surgical procedures for soft parts sarcoma of the thigh. Cancer. 1981;47(5):1005–22.
6. Daigeler A, Klein-Hitpass L, Stricker I, Muller O, Kuhnen C, Chromik AM, et al. Malignant fibrous histiocytoma—pleomorphic sarcoma, NOS gene expression, histology, and clinical course. A pilot study. Langenbeck's Arch Surg. 2010;395(3):261–75.
7. Coindre JM, Terrier P, Guillou L, Le Doussal V, Collin F, Ranchere D, et al. Predictive value of grade for metastasis development in the main histologic types of adult soft tissue sarcomas: a study of 1240 patients from the French Federation of Cancer Centers Sarcoma Group. Cancer. 2001;91(10):1914–26.
8. Pisters PW, Leung DH, Woodruff J, Shi W, Brennan MF. Analysis of prognostic factors in 1041 patients with localized soft tissue sarcomas of the extremities. J Clin Oncol. 1996;14(5):1679–89.
9. Zagars GK, Ballo MT, Pisters PW, Pollock RE, Patel SR, Benjamin RS, et al. Prognostic factors for patients with localized soft-tissue sarcoma treated with conservation surgery and radiation therapy: an analysis of 1225 patients. Cancer. 2003;97(10):2530–43.
10. Parsons HM, Habermann EB, Tuttle TM, Al-Refaie WB. Conditional survival of extremity soft-tissue sarcoma: results beyond the staging system. Cancer. 2011;117(5):1055–60.
11. Gutierrez JC, Perez EA, Franceschi D, Moffat FL Jr, Livingstone AS, Koniaris LG. Outcomes for soft-tissue sarcoma in 8249 cases from a large state cancer registry. J Surg Res. 2007;141(1):105–14.
12. Canter RJ, Beal S, Borys D, Martinez SR, Bold RJ, Robbins AS. Interaction of histologic subtype and histologic grade in predicting survival for soft-tissue sarcomas. J Am Coll Surg. 2010;210(2):191–8.e2.
13. Rosenberg SA, Tepper J, Glatstein E, Costa J, Baker A, Brennan M, et al. The treatment of soft-tissue sarcomas of the extremities: prospective randomized evaluations of (1) limb-sparing surgery plus radiation therapy compared with amputation and (2) the role of adjuvant chemotherapy. Ann Surg. 1982;196(3):305–15.
14. Baldini EH, Goldberg J, Jenner C, Manola JB, Demetri GD, Fletcher CD, et al. Long-term outcomes after function-sparing surgery without radiotherapy for soft tissue sarcoma of the extremities and trunk. J Clin Oncol. 1999;17(10):3252–9.
15. Pisters PW, Pollock RE, Lewis VO, Yasko AW, Cormier JN, Respondek PM, et al. Long-term results of prospective trial of surgery alone with selective use of radiation for patients with T1 extremity and trunk soft tissue sarcomas. Ann Surg. 2007;246(4):675–81; discussion 81-2.
16. Cahlon O, Spierer M, Brennan MF, Singer S, Alektiar KM. Long-term outcomes in extremity soft tissue sarcoma after a pathologically negative re-resection and without radiotherapy. Cancer. 2008;112(12):2774–9.
17. Fabrizio PL, Stafford SL, Pritchard DJ. Extremity soft-tissue sarcomas selectively treated with surgery alone. Int J Radiat Oncol Biol Phys. 2000;48(1):227–32.
18. Zagars GK, Ballo MT, Pisters PW, Pollock RE, Patel SR, Benjamin RS. Surgical margins and reresection in the management of patients with soft tissue sarcoma using conservative surgery and radiation therapy. Cancer. 2003;97(10):2544–53.

19. Lewis JJ, Leung D, Espat J, Woodruff JM, Brennan MF. Effect of reresection in extremity soft tissue sarcoma. Ann Surg. 2000;231(5):655–63.

20. Pisters PW, Harrison LB, Leung DH, Woodruff JM, Casper ES, Brennan MF. Long-term results of a prospective randomized trial of adjuvant brachytherapy in soft tissue sarcoma. J Clin Oncol. 1996;14(3):859–68.

21. Yang JC, Chang AE, Baker AR, Sindelar WF, Danforth DN, Topalian SL, et al. Randomized prospective study of the benefit of adjuvant radiation therapy in the treatment of soft tissue sarcomas of the extremity. J Clin Oncol. 1998;16(1):197–203.

22. O'Sullivan B, Davis AM, Turcotte R, Bell R, Catton C, Chabot P, et al. Preoperative versus postoperative radiotherapy in soft-tissue sarcoma of the limbs: a randomised trial. Lancet. 2002;359(9325):2235–41.

23. Alektiar KM, Leung D, Zelefsky MJ, Healey JH, Brennan MF. Adjuvant brachytherapy for primary high-grade soft tissue sarcoma of the extremity. Ann Surg Oncol. 2002;9(1):48–56.

24. Nag S, Shasha D, Janjan N, Petersen I, Zaider M, American Brachytherapy Society. The American Brachytherapy Society recommendations for brachytherapy of soft tissue sarcomas. Int J Radiat Oncol Biol Phys. 2001;49(4):1033–43.

25. Fein DA, Lee WR, Lanciano RM, Corn BW, Herbert SH, Hanlon AL, et al. Management of extremity soft tissue sarcomas with limb-sparing surgery and postoperative irradiation: do total dose, overall treatment time, and the surgery-radiotherapy interval impact on local control? Int J Radiat Oncol Biol Phys. 1995;32(4):969–76.

26. Dickie CI, Griffin AM, Parent AL, Chung PW, Catton CN, Svensson J, et al. The relationship between local recurrence and radiotherapy treatment volume for soft tissue sarcomas treated with external beam radiotherapy and function preservation surgery. Int J Radiat Oncol Biol Phys. 2012;82(4):1528–34.

27. Kim B, Chen YL, Kirsch DG, Goldberg SI, Kobayashi W, Kung JH, et al. An effective preoperative three-dimensional radiotherapy target volume for extremity soft tissue sarcoma and the effect of margin width on local control. Int J Radiat Oncol Biol Phys. 2010;77(3):843–50.

28. Mendenhall WM, Indelicato DJ, Scarborough MT, Zlotecki RA, Gibbs CP, Mendenhall NP, et al. The management of adult soft tissue sarcomas. Am J Clin Oncol. 2009;32(4):436–42.

29. Baldini EH, Lapidus MR, Wang Q, Manola J, Orgill DP, Pomahac B, et al. Predictors for major wound complications following preoperative radiotherapy and surgery for soft-tissue sarcoma of the extremities and trunk: importance of tumor proximity to skin surface. Ann Surg Oncol. 2013;20(5):1494–9.

30. Cheng EY, Dusenbery KE, Winters MR, Thompson RC. Soft tissue sarcomas: preoperative versus postoperative radiotherapy. J Surg Oncol. 1996;61(2):90–9.

31. Davis AM, O'Sullivan B, Turcotte R, Bell R, Catton C, Chabot P, et al. Late radiation morbidity following randomization to preoperative versus postoperative radiotherapy in extremity soft tissue sarcoma. Radiother Oncol. 2005;75(1):48–53.

32. Holt GE, Griffin AM, Pintilie M, Wunder JS, Catton C, O'Sullivan B, et al. Fractures following radiotherapy and limb-salvage surgery for lower extremity soft-tissue sarcomas. A comparison of high-dose and low-dose radiotherapy. J Bone Joint Surg Am. 2005;87(2):315–9.

33. Al-Absi E, Farrokhyar F, Sharma R, Whelan K, Corbett T, Patel M, et al. A systematic review and meta-analysis of oncologic outcomes of pre- versus postoperative radiation in localized resectable soft-tissue sarcoma. Ann Surg Oncol. 2010;17(5):1367–74.

34. Alektiar KM, Brennan MF, Healey JH, Singer S. Impact of intensity-modulated radiation therapy on local control in primary soft-tissue sarcoma of the extremity. J Clin Oncol. 2008;26(20):3440–4.

35. Folkert MR, Singer S, Brennan MF, Kuk D, Qin LX, Kobayashi WK, et al. Comparison of local recurrence with conventional and intensity-modulated radiation therapy for primary soft-tissue sarcomas of the extremity. J Clin Oncol. 2014;32(29):3236–41.

36. Alektiar KM, Brennan MF, Singer S. Local control comparison of adjuvant brachytherapy to intensity-modulated radiotherapy in primary high-grade sarcoma of the extremity. Cancer. 2011;117(14):3229–34.

37. O'Sullivan B, Griffin AM, Dickie CI, Sharpe MB, Chung PW, Catton CN, et al. Phase 2 study of preoperative image-guided intensity-modulated radiation therapy to reduce wound and combined modality morbidities in lower extremity soft tissue sarcoma. Cancer. 2013;119(10):1878–84.
38. Wang D, Zhang Q, Eisenberg BL, Kane JM, Li XA, Lucas D, et al. Significant reduction of late toxicities in patients with extremity sarcoma treated with image-guided radiation therapy to a reduced target volume: results of radiation therapy oncology group RTOG-0630 trial. J Clin Oncol. 2015;33(20):2231–8.
39. Sarcoma Meta-analysis Collaboration. Adjuvant chemotherapy for localised resectable soft-tissue sarcoma of adults: meta-analysis of individual data. Lancet. 1997;350(9092):1647–54.
40. Pervaiz N, Colterjohn N, Farrokhyar F, Tozer R, Figueredo A, Ghert M. A systematic meta-analysis of randomized controlled trials of adjuvant chemotherapy for localized resectable soft-tissue sarcoma. Cancer. 2008;113(3):573–81.
41. Woll PJ, Reichardt P, Le Cesne A, Bonvalot S, Azzarelli A, Hoekstra HJ, et al. Adjuvant chemotherapy with doxorubicin, ifosfamide, and lenograstim for resected soft-tissue sarcoma (EORTC 62931): a multicentre randomised controlled trial. Lancet Oncol. 2012;13(10):1045–54.
42. Gortzak E, Azzarelli A, Buesa J, Bramwell VH, van Coevorden F, van Geel AN, et al. A randomised phase II study on neo-adjuvant chemotherapy for 'high-risk' adult soft-tissue sarcoma. Eur J Cancer. 2001;37(9):1096–103.
43. Kraybill WG, Harris J, Spiro IJ, Ettinger DS, DeLaney TF, Blum RH, et al. Long-term results of a phase 2 study of neoadjuvant chemotherapy and radiotherapy in the management of high-risk, high-grade, soft tissue sarcomas of the extremities and body wall: Radiation Therapy Oncology Group Trial 9514. Cancer. 2010;116(19):4613–21.
44. DeLaney TF, Spiro IJ, Suit HD, Gebhardt MC, Hornicek FJ, Mankin HJ, et al. Neoadjuvant chemotherapy and radiotherapy for large extremity soft-tissue sarcomas. Int J Radiat Oncol Biol Phys. 2003;56(4):1117–27.
45. Wang D, Bosch W, Roberge D, Finkelstein SE, Petersen I, Haddock M, et al. RTOG sarcoma radiation oncologists reach consensus on gross tumor volume and clinical target volume on computed tomographic images for preoperative radiotherapy of primary soft tissue sarcoma of extremity in Radiation Therapy Oncology Group studies. Int J Radiat Oncol Biol Phys. 2011;81(4):e525–8.
46. White LM, Wunder JS, Bell RS, O'Sullivan B, Catton C, Ferguson P, et al. Histologic assessment of peritumoral edema in soft tissue sarcoma. Int J Radiat Oncol Biol Phys. 2005;61(5):1439–45.
47. Devisetty K, Kobayashi W, Suit HD, Goldberg SI, Niemierko A, Chen YL, et al. Low-dose neoadjuvant external beam radiation therapy for soft tissue sarcoma. Int J Radiat Oncol Biol Phys. 2011;80(3):779–86.
48. Alektiar KM, Velasco J, Zelefsky MJ, Woodruff JM, Lewis JJ, Brennan MF. Adjuvant radiotherapy for margin-positive high-grade soft tissue sarcoma of the extremity. Int J Radiat Oncol Biol Phys. 2000;48(4):1051–8.
49. Holloway CL, Delaney TF, Alektiar KM, Devlin PM, O'Farrell DA, Demanes DJ. American Brachytherapy Society (ABS) consensus statement for sarcoma brachytherapy. Brachytherapy. 2013;12(3):179–90.
50. Porter GA, Baxter NN, Pisters PW. Retroperitoneal sarcoma: a population-based analysis of epidemiology, surgery, and radiotherapy. Cancer. 2006;106(7):1610–6.
51. Anaya DA, Lahat G, Wang X, Xiao L, Pisters PW, Cormier JN, et al. Postoperative nomogram for survival of patients with retroperitoneal sarcoma treated with curative intent. Ann Oncol. 2010;21(2):397–402.
52. Pacelli F, Tortorelli AP, Rosa F, Papa V, Bossola M, Sanchez AM, et al. Retroperitoneal soft tissue sarcoma: prognostic factors and therapeutic approaches. Tumori. 2008;94(4):497–504.
53. Schwarzbach MH, Hohenberger P. Current concepts in the management of retroperitoneal soft tissue sarcoma. Recent Results Cancer Res. 2009;179:301–19.

54. Stoeckle E, Coindre JM, Bonvalot S, Kantor G, Terrier P, Bonichon F, et al. Prognostic factors in retroperitoneal sarcoma: a multivariate analysis of a series of 165 patients of the French Cancer Center Federation Sarcoma Group. Cancer. 2001;92(2):359–68.

55. Lewis JJ, Leung D, Woodruff JM, Brennan MF. Retroperitoneal soft-tissue sarcoma: analysis of 500 patients treated and followed at a single institution. Ann Surg. 1998;228(3):355–65.

56. Hassan I, Park SZ, Donohue JH, Nagorney DM, Kay PA, Nasciemento AG, et al. Operative management of primary retroperitoneal sarcomas: a reappraisal of an institutional experience. Ann Surg. 2004;239(2):244–50.

57. Catton CN, O'Sullivan B, Kotwall C, Cummings B, Hao Y, Fornasier V. Outcome and prognosis in retroperitoneal soft tissue sarcoma. Int J Radiat Oncol Biol Phys. 1994;29(5):1005–10.

58. Gronchi A, Casali PG, Fiore M, Mariani L, Lo Vullo S, Bertulli R, et al. Retroperitoneal soft tissue sarcomas: patterns of recurrence in 167 patients treated at a single institution. Cancer. 2004;100(11):2448–55.

59. Singer S, Antonescu CR, Riedel E, Brennan MF. Histologic subtype and margin of resection predict pattern of recurrence and survival for retroperitoneal liposarcoma. Ann Surg. 2003;238(3):358–70; discussion 70-1.

60. Ferrario T, Karakousis CP. Retroperitoneal sarcomas: grade and survival. Arch Surg. 2003;138(3):248–51.

61. Baldini EH, Wang D, Haas RL, Catton CN, Indelicato DJ, Kirsch DG, et al. Treatment guidelines for preoperative radiation therapy for retroperitoneal sarcoma: preliminary consensus of an international expert panel. Int J Radiat Oncol Biol Phys. 2015;92(3):602–12.

62. Mori S, Hara R, Yanagi T, Sharp GC, Kumagai M, Asakura H, et al. Four-dimensional measurement of intrafractional respiratory motion of pancreatic tumors using a 256 multi-slice CT scanner. Radiother Oncol. 2009;92(2):231–7.

63. Wysocka B, Kassam Z, Lockwood G, Brierley J, Dawson LA, Buckley CA, et al. Interfraction and respiratory organ motion during conformal radiotherapy in gastric cancer. Int J Radiat Oncol Biol Phys. 2010;77(1):53–9.

64. Langen KM, Jones DT. Organ motion and its management. Int J Radiat Oncol Biol Phys. 2001;50(1):265–78.

65. Fein DA, Corn BW, Lanciano RM, Herbert SH, Hoffman JP, Coia LR. Management of retroperitoneal sarcomas: does dose escalation impact on locoregional control? Int J Radiat Oncol Biol Phys. 1995;31(1):129–34.

66. Sindelar WF, Kinsella TJ, Chen PW, DeLaney TF, Tepper JE, Rosenberg SA, et al. Intraoperative radiotherapy in retroperitoneal sarcomas. Final results of a prospective, randomized, clinical trial. Arch Surg. 1993;128(4):402–10.

67. Alektiar KM, Hu K, Anderson L, Brennan MF, Harrison LB. High-dose-rate intraoperative radiation therapy (HDR-IORT) for retroperitoneal sarcomas. Int J Radiat Oncol Biol Phys. 2000;47(1):157–63.

68. Jones JJ, Catton CN, O'Sullivan B, Couture J, Heisler RL, Kandel RA, et al. Initial results of a trial of preoperative external-beam radiation therapy and postoperative brachytherapy for retroperitoneal sarcoma. Ann Surg Oncol. 2002;9(4):346–54.

69. Gieschen HL, Spiro IJ, Suit HD, Ott MJ, Rattner DW, Ancukiewicz M, et al. Long-term results of intraoperative electron beam radiotherapy for primary and recurrent retroperitoneal soft tissue sarcoma. Int J Radiat Oncol Biol Phys. 2001;50(1):127–31.

70. Petersen IA, Haddock MG, Donohue JH, Nagorney DM, Grill JP, Sargent DJ, et al. Use of intraoperative electron beam radiotherapy in the management of retroperitoneal soft tissue sarcomas. Int J Radiat Oncol Biol Phys. 2002;52(2):469–75.

71. Ahrens S, Hoffmann C, Jabar S, Braun-Munzinger G, Paulussen M, Dunst J, et al. Evaluation of prognostic factors in a tumor volume-adapted treatment strategy for localized Ewing sarcoma of bone: the CESS 86 experience. Cooperative Ewing Sarcoma Study. Med Pediatr Oncol. 1999;32(3):186–95.

72. Marcus RB Jr, Berrey BH, Graham-Pole J, Mendenhall NP, Scarborough MT. The treatment of Ewing's sarcoma of bone at the University of Florida: 1969 to 1998. Clin Orthop Relat Res. 2002;397:290–7.

73. Oberlin O, Patte C, Demeocq F, Lacombe MJ, Brunat-Mentigny M, Demaille MC, et al. The response to initial chemotherapy as a prognostic factor in localized Ewing's sarcoma. Eur J Cancer Clin Oncol. 1985;21(4):463–7.

74. Bacci G, Ferrari S, Longhi A, Donati D, Barbieri E, Forni C, et al. Role of surgery in local treatment of Ewing's sarcoma of the extremities in patients undergoing adjuvant and neoadjuvant chemotherapy. Oncol Rep. 2004;11(1):111–20.

75. Schuck A, Ahrens S, Paulussen M, Kuhlen M, Konemann S, Rube C, et al. Local therapy in localized Ewing tumors: results of 1058 patients treated in the CESS 81, CESS 86, and EICESS 92 trials. Int J Radiat Oncol Biol Phys. 2003;55(1):168–77.

76. Schuck A, Hofmann J, Rube C, Hillmann A, Ahrens S, Paulussen M, et al. Radiotherapy in Ewing's sarcoma and PNET of the chest wall: results of the trials CESS 81, CESS 86 and EICESS 92. Int J Radiat Oncol Biol Phys. 1998;42(5):1001–6.

77. Nesbit ME Jr, Gehan EA, Burgert EO Jr, Vietti TJ, Cangir A, Tefft M, et al. Multimodal therapy for the management of primary, nonmetastatic Ewing's sarcoma of bone: a long-term follow-up of the First Intergroup study. J Clin Oncol. 1990;8(10):1664–74.

78. Burgert EO Jr, Nesbit ME, Garnsey LA, Gehan EA, Herrmann J, Vietti TJ, et al. Multimodal therapy for the management of nonpelvic, localized Ewing's sarcoma of bone: intergroup study IESS-II. J Clin Oncol. 1990;8(9):1514–24.

79. Grier HE, Krailo MD, Tarbell NJ, Link MP, Fryer CJ, Pritchard DJ, et al. Addition of ifosfamide and etoposide to standard chemotherapy for Ewing's sarcoma and primitive neuroectodermal tumor of bone. N Engl J Med. 2003;348(8):694–701.

80. Granowetter L, Womer R, Devidas M, Krailo M, Wang C, Bernstein M, et al. Dose-intensified compared with standard chemotherapy for nonmetastatic Ewing sarcoma family of tumors: a Children's Oncology Group Study. J Clin Oncol. 2009;27(15):2536–41.

81. Womer RB, West DC, Krailo MD, Dickman PS, Pawel BR, Grier HE, et al. Randomized controlled trial of interval-compressed chemotherapy for the treatment of localized Ewing sarcoma: a report from the Children's Oncology Group. J Clin Oncol. 2012;30(33):4148–54.

82. Jurgens H, Exner U, Gadner H, Harms D, Michaelis J, Sauer R, et al. Multidisciplinary treatment of primary Ewing's sarcoma of bone. A 6-year experience of a European Cooperative Trial. Cancer. 1988;61(1):23–32.

83. Paulussen M, Ahrens S, Dunst J, Winkelmann W, Exner GU, Kotz R, et al. Localized Ewing tumor of bone: final results of the cooperative Ewing's Sarcoma Study CESS 86. J Clin Oncol. 2001;19(6):1818–29.

84. Paulussen M, Craft AW, Lewis I, Hackshaw A, Douglas C, Dunst J, et al. Results of the EICESS-92 Study: two randomized trials of Ewing's sarcoma treatment—cyclophosphamide compared with ifosfamide in standard-risk patients and assessment of benefit of etoposide added to standard treatment in high-risk patients. J Clin Oncol. 2008;26(27):4385–93.

85. Craft AW, Cotterill SJ, Bullimore JA, Pearson D. Long-term results from the first UKCCSG Ewing's Tumour Study (ET-1). United Kingdom Children's Cancer Study Group (UKCCSG) and the Medical Research Council Bone Sarcoma Working Party. Eur J Cancer. 1997;33(7):1061–9.

86. Craft A, Cotterill S, Malcolm A, Spooner D, Grimer R, Souhami R, et al. Ifosfamide-containing chemotherapy in Ewing's sarcoma: The Second United Kingdom Children's Cancer Study Group and the Medical Research Council Ewing's Tumor Study. J Clin Oncol. 1998;16(11):3628–33.

87. Rosen G, Caparros B, Mosende C, McCormick B, Huvos AG, Marcove RC. Curability of Ewing's sarcoma and considerations for future therapeutic trials. Cancer. 1978;41(3):888–99.

88. Kushner BH, Meyers PA, Gerald WL, Healey JH, La Quaglia MP, Boland P, et al. Very-high-dose short-term chemotherapy for poor-risk peripheral primitive neuroectodermal tumors, including Ewing's sarcoma, in children and young adults. J Clin Oncol. 1995;13(11):2796–804.

89. Kolb EA, Kushner BH, Gorlick R, Laverdiere C, Healey JH, LaQuaglia MP, et al. Long-term event-free survival after intensive chemotherapy for Ewing's family of tumors in children and young adults. J Clin Oncol. 2003;21(18):3423–30.

90. Hayes FA, Thompson EI, Meyer WH, Kun L, Parham D, Rao B, et al. Therapy for localized Ewing's sarcoma of bone. J Clin Oncol. 1989;7(2):208–13.

91. Meyer WH, Kun L, Marina N, Roberson P, Parham D, Rao B, et al. Ifosfamide plus etoposide in newly diagnosed Ewing's sarcoma of bone. J Clin Oncol. 1992;10(11):1737–42.

92. Marina NM, Pappo AS, Parham DM, Cain AM, Rao BN, Poquette CA, et al. Chemotherapy dose-intensification for pediatric patients with Ewing's family of tumors and desmoplastic small round-cell tumors: a feasibility study at St. Jude Children's Research Hospital. J Clin Oncol. 1999;17(1):180–90.

93. Bacci G, Mercuri M, Longhi A, Bertoni F, Barbieri E, Donati D, et al. Neoadjuvant chemotherapy for Ewing's tumour of bone: recent experience at the Rizzoli Orthopaedic Institute. Eur J Cancer. 2002;38(17):2243–51.

94. Oberlin O, Deley MC, Bui BN, Gentet JC, Philip T, Terrier P, et al. Prognostic factors in localized Ewing's tumours and peripheral neuroectodermal tumours: the third study of the French Society of Paediatric Oncology (EW88 study). Br J Cancer. 2001;85(11):1646–54.

95. Gaspar N, Rey A, Berard PM, Michon J, Gentet JC, Tabone MD, et al. Risk adapted chemotherapy for localised Ewing's sarcoma of bone: the French EW93 study. Eur J Cancer. 2012;48(9):1376–85.

96. Elomaa I, Blomqvist CP, Saeter G, Akerman M, Stenwig E, Wiebe T, et al. Five-year results in Ewing's sarcoma. The Scandinavian Sarcoma Group experience with the SSG IX protocol. Eur J Cancer. 2000;36(7):875–80.

97. Ladenstein R, Potschger U, Le Deley MC, Whelan J, Paulussen M, Oberlin O, et al. Primary disseminated multifocal Ewing sarcoma: results of the Euro-EWING 99 trial. J Clin Oncol. 2010;28(20):3284–91.

98. Enneking WF. A system of staging musculoskeletal neoplasms. Clin Orthop Relat Res. 1986;204:9–24.

99. Dunst J, Jurgens H, Sauer R, Pape H, Paulussen M, Winkelmann W, et al. Radiation therapy in Ewing's sarcoma: an update of the CESS 86 trial. Int J Radiat Oncol Biol Phys. 1995;32(4):919–30.

100. Bacci G, Longhi A, Briccoli A, Bertoni F, Versari M, Picci P. The role of surgical margins in treatment of Ewing's sarcoma family tumors: experience of a single institution with 512 patients treated with adjuvant and neoadjuvant chemotherapy. Int J Radiat Oncol Biol Phys. 2006;65(3):766–72.

101. Schuck A, Ahrens S, von Schorlemer I, Kuhlen M, Paulussen M, Hunold A, et al. Radiotherapy in Ewing tumors of the vertebrae: treatment results and local relapse analysis of the CESS 81/86 and EICESS 92 trials. Int J Radiat Oncol Biol Phys. 2005;63(5):1562–7.

102. Ozaki T, Hillmann A, Hoffmann C, Rube C, Blasius S, Dunst J, et al. Significance of surgical margin on the prognosis of patients with Ewing's sarcoma. A report from the Cooperative Ewing's Sarcoma Study. Cancer. 1996;78(4):892–900.

103. Donaldson S, Shuster J, Andreozzi C. The Pediatric Oncology Group (POG) experience in Ewing's sarcoma of bone. Med Pediatr Oncol. 1989;17:283.

104. Paulussen M, Ahrens S, Burdach S, Craft A, Dockhorn-Dworniczak B, Dunst J, et al. Primary metastatic (stage IV) Ewing tumor: survival analysis of 171 patients from the EICESS studies. European Intergroup Cooperative Ewing Sarcoma Studies. Ann Oncol. 1998;9(3):275–81.

105. Donaldson SS, Torrey M, Link MP, Glicksman A, Gilula L, Laurie F, et al. A multidisciplinary study investigating radiotherapy in Ewing's sarcoma: end results of POG #8346. Pediatric Oncology Group. Int J Radiat Oncol Biol Phys. 1998;42(1):125–35.

106. Krasin MJ, Rodriguez-Galindo C, Billups CA, Davidoff AM, Neel MD, Merchant TE, et al. Definitive irradiation in multidisciplinary management of localized Ewing sarcoma family of tumors in pediatric patients: outcome and prognostic factors. Int J Radiat Oncol Biol Phys. 2004;60(3):830–8.

107. Fuchs B, Valenzuela RG, Inwards C, Sim FH, Rock MG. Complications in long-term survivors of Ewing sarcoma. Cancer. 2003;98(12):2687–92.

108. Bolek TW, Marcus RB Jr, Mendenhall NP, Scarborough MT, Graham-Pole J. Local control and functional results after twice-daily radiotherapy for Ewing's sarcoma of the extremities. Int J Radiat Oncol Biol Phys. 1996;35(4):687–92.

109. Wagner LM, Neel MD, Pappo AS, Merchant TE, Poquette CA, Rao BN, et al. Fractures in pediatric Ewing sarcoma. J Pediatr Hematol Oncol. 2001;23(9):568–71.

110. Kuttesch JF Jr, Wexler LH, Marcus RB, Fairclough D, Weaver-McClure L, White M, et al. Second malignancies after Ewing's sarcoma: radiation dose-dependency of secondary sarcomas. J Clin Oncol. 1996;14(10):2818–25.

111. Tucker MA, D'Angio GJ, Boice JD Jr, Strong LC, Li FP, Stovall M, et al. Bone sarcomas linked to radiotherapy and chemotherapy in children. N Engl J Med. 1987;317(10):588–93.

112. Maurer HM, Beltangady M, Gehan EA, Crist W, Hammond D, Hays DM, et al. The Intergroup Rhabdomyosarcoma Study-I. A final report. Cancer. 1988;61(2):209–20.

113. Wolden SL, Anderson JR, Crist WM, Breneman JC, Wharam MD Jr, Wiener ES, et al. Indications for radiotherapy and chemotherapy after complete resection in rhabdomyosarcoma: a report from the Intergroup Rhabdomyosarcoma Studies I to III. J Clin Oncol. 1999;17(11):3468–75.

114. Maurer HM, Gehan EA, Beltangady M, Crist W, Dickman PS, Donaldson SS, et al. The Intergroup Rhabdomyosarcoma Study-II. Cancer. 1993;71(5):1904–22.

115. Crist W, Gehan EA, Ragab AH, Dickman PS, Donaldson SS, Fryer C, et al. The Third Intergroup Rhabdomyosarcoma Study. J Clin Oncol. 1995;13(3):610–30.

116. Crist WM, Anderson JR, Meza JL, Fryer C, Raney RB, Ruymann FB, et al. Intergroup Rhabdomyosarcoma Study-IV: results for patients with nonmetastatic disease. J Clin Oncol. 2001;19(12):3091–102.

117. Donaldson SS, Meza J, Breneman JC, Crist WM, Laurie F, Qualman SJ, et al. Results from the IRS-IV randomized trial of hyperfractionated radiotherapy in children with rhabdomyosarcoma—a report from the IRSG. Int J Radiat Oncol Biol Phys. 2001;51(3):718–28.

118. Wiener ES, Anderson JR, Ojimba JI, Lobe TE, Paidas C, Andrassy RJ, et al. Controversies in the management of paratesticular rhabdomyosarcoma: is staging retroperitoneal lymph node dissection necessary for adolescents with resected paratesticular rhabdomyosarcoma? Semin Pediatr Surg. 2001;10(3):146–52.

119. Raney RB, Walterhouse DO, Meza JL, Andrassy RJ, Breneman JC, Crist WM, et al. Results of the Intergroup Rhabdomyosarcoma Study Group D9602 protocol, using vincristine and dactinomycin with or without cyclophosphamide and radiation therapy, for newly diagnosed patients with low-risk embryonal rhabdomyosarcoma: a report from the Soft Tissue Sarcoma Committee of the Children's Oncology Group. J Clin Oncol. 2011;29(10):1312–8.

120. Breneman J, Meza J, Donaldson SS, Raney RB, Wolden S, Michalski J, et al. Local control with reduced-dose radiotherapy for low-risk rhabdomyosarcoma: a report from the Children's Oncology Group D9602 study. Int J Radiat Oncol Biol Phys. 2012;83(2):720–6.

121. Arndt CA, Stoner JA, Hawkins DS, Rodeberg DA, Hayes-Jordan AA, Paidas CN, et al. Vincristine, actinomycin, and cyclophosphamide compared with vincristine, actinomycin, and cyclophosphamide alternating with vincristine, topotecan, and cyclophosphamide for intermediate-risk rhabdomyosarcoma: Children's Oncology Group study D9803. J Clin Oncol. 2009;27(31):5182–8.

122. Walterhouse DO, Meza JL, Breneman JC, Donaldson SS, Hayes-Jordan A, Pappo AS, et al. Local control and outcome in children with localized vaginal rhabdomyosarcoma: a report from the Soft Tissue Sarcoma committee of the Children's Oncology Group. Pediatr Blood Cancer. 2011;57(1):76–83.

123. Rodary C, Rey A, Olive D, Flamant F, Quintana E, Brunat-Mentigny M, et al. Prognostic factors in 281 children with nonmetastatic rhabdomyosarcoma (RMS) at diagnosis. Med Pediatr Oncol. 1988;16(2):71–7.

124. Flamant F, Rodary C, Rey A, Praquin MT, Sommelet D, Quintana E, et al. Treatment of non-metastatic rhabdomyosarcomas in childhood and adolescence. Results of the second study of the International Society of Paediatric Oncology: MMT84. Eur J Cancer. 1998;34(7):1050–62.

125. Stevens MC, Rey A, Bouvet N, Ellershaw C, Flamant F, Habrand JL, et al. Treatment of non-metastatic rhabdomyosarcoma in childhood and adolescence: third study of the International Society of Paediatric Oncology—SIOP Malignant Mesenchymal Tumor 89. J Clin Oncol. 2005;23(12):2618–28.

126. Donaldson SS, Anderson JR. Rhabdomyosarcoma: many similarities, a few philosophical differences. J Clin Oncol. 2005;23(12):2586–7.

127. Koscielniak E, Jurgens H, Winkler K, Burger D, Herbst M, Keim M, et al. Treatment of soft tissue sarcoma in childhood and adolescence. A report of the German Cooperative Soft Tissue Sarcoma Study. Cancer. 1992;70(10):2557–67.

128. Koscielniak E, Harms D, Henze G, Jurgens H, Gadner H, Herbst M, et al. Results of treatment for soft tissue sarcoma in childhood and adolescence: a final report of the German Cooperative Soft Tissue Sarcoma Study CWS-86. J Clin Oncol. 1999;17(12):3706–19.

129. Dantonello TM, Int-Veen C, Harms D, Leuschner I, Schmidt BF, Herbst M, et al. Cooperative trial CWS-91 for localized soft tissue sarcoma in children, adolescents, and young adults. J Clin Oncol. 2009;27(9):1446–55.

130. Michalski JM, Meza J, Breneman JC, Wolden SL, Laurie F, Jodoin M, et al. Influence of radiation therapy parameters on outcome in children treated with radiation therapy for localized parameningeal rhabdomyosarcoma in Intergroup Rhabdomyosarcoma Study Group trials II through IV. Int J Radiat Oncol Biol Phys. 2004;59(4):1027–38.

131. Rousseau P, Flamant F, Quintana E, Voute PA, Gentet JC. Primary chemotherapy in rhabdomyosarcomas and other malignant mesenchymal tumors of the orbit: results of the International Society of Pediatric Oncology MMT 84 Study. J Clin Oncol. 1994;12(3):516–21.

132. Rodary C, Gehan EA, Flamant F, Treuner J, Carli M, Auquier A, et al. Prognostic factors in 951 nonmetastatic rhabdomyosarcoma in children: a report from the International Rhabdomyosarcoma Workshop. Med Pediatr Oncol. 1991;19(2):89–95.

133. Raney RB Jr, Gehan EA, Hays DM, Tefft M, Newton WA Jr, Haeberlen V, et al. Primary chemotherapy with or without radiation therapy and/or surgery for children with localized sarcoma of the bladder, prostate, vagina, uterus, and cervix. A comparison of the results in Intergroup Rhabdomyosarcoma Studies I and II. Cancer. 1990;66(10):2072–81.

Lymphoma

9

Yasemin Bolukbasi, Duygu Sezen, Yucel Saglam,
and Ugur Selek

9.1 Hodgkin Lymphoma

Overview

Epidemiology: Hodgkin lymphoma (HL) is a curable malignancy that shows a bimodal age distribution in economically developed countries with peaks in young adulthood and after 50 years of Males slightly greater incidence than females (1.3:1) [1]. First-degree relatives of patients have five times higher risk for HL. Epstein–Barr virus is associated with mixed cellularity HL [2].

Histology: HL had been categorized into two general histologic categories as Classic type (95%) and Nodular lymphocyte predominant (5%) [1]. Blood test: blood count, Sedimentasyon rate, LDH, albumin are a part of initial diagnosis. PET/CT is valuable for initial, interim, and posttreatment staging [3].

Y. Bolukbasi (✉)
Department of Radiation Oncology, Faculty of Medicine, Koç University, Istanbul, Turkey

Department of Radiation Oncology, The University of Texas MD Anderson Cancer Center, Houston, TX, USA
e-mail: yaseminb@ameriaknhastanesi.org

D. Sezen · Y. Saglam
Department of Radiation Oncology, School of Medicine, Koç University, Istanbul, Turkey
e-mail: yucels@amerikanhastanesi.org

U. Selek
Department of Radiation Oncology, The University of Texas MD Anderson Cancer Center, Houston, TX, USA

Department of Radiation Oncology, Koç University, Istanbul, Turkey

© Springer Nature Switzerland AG 2019
G. Ozyigit, U. Selek (eds.), *Radiation Oncology*,
https://doi.org/10.1007/978-3-319-97145-2_9

Treatment: Selection of initial treatment for HL is usually based upon presenting stage and prognostic factors. The EORTC defines the limited stage favorable prognostic group as patients age 50 or under; without large mediastinal adenopathy; with an ESR of less than 50 mm/h and no B symptoms (or with an ESR of less than 30 mm/h in those who have B symptoms); and disease limited to three or fewer regions of involvement [4]. The GHSG defines the limited stage favorable prognostic group as patients with no more than two sites of disease; no extranodal extension; no mediastinal mass measuring one-third the maximum thoracic diameter or greater; and ESR less than 50 mm/h (less than 30 mm/h if B symptoms present). Patients with early stage disease are treated with a combination of chemotherapy plus radiation therapy. The amount of chemotherapy and dose of radiation differs for patients with favorable and unfavorable prognosis disease. ABVD (doxorubicin, bleomycin, vinblastine, and dacarbazine) remains the "gold standard" chemotherapy for these patients [5]. Four to six monthly cycles of ABVD are usually required for patients with bulky disease and advanced stage HL [4]. Escalated BEACOPP (bleomycin, etoposide, doxorubicin, cyclophosphamide, vincristine, procarbazine, and prednisone and Stanford V (doxorubicin, vinblastine, mechlorethamine, vincristine, bleomycin, etoposide, and prednisone) in combination radiation therapy. Radiation fields can be safely limited to involved regions as determined by CT scan and PET imaging [6, 7]. HL survivors are at risk of developing therapy-related complications that may present years after treatment (e.g., second malignancies, cardiac disease, radiation-induced hypothyroidism). Follow-up includes physical examination and monitoring for long term side effects [8, 9].

Keywords: Hodgkin lymphoma, Radiotherapy

9.1.1 Case Presentation

A 28-year-woman presented with swelling nodes at bilateral neck for 3 weeks. The patient also complained of a productive cough but denied fever or weight loss. The patient had a history of allergic rhinitis and having a smoking history of 4 pack/year. On physical examination, the patient had clinically palpable lymphadenopathy in bilateral neck but no evident organomegaly.

Laboratory finding showed an elevated level of C-reactive protein and eosinophilia. The remainder of the physical and laboratory examination was unremarkable. Upon admission, chest radiography revealed a widening of the aortopulmonary stripe. 18F-fluoro-2-deoxyglucose positron emission tomography (FDGPET)/ CT showed heterogeneous hypermetabolic lesions in the anterior mediastinum, right upper lobe, and sternum in addition to the enlarged lymph nodes to bilateral neck (Fig. 9.1) an ultrasound-guided needle biopsy of the sternal lesion and supraclavicular lymph node was performed Hematoxylin and eosin staining of the tumor tissue

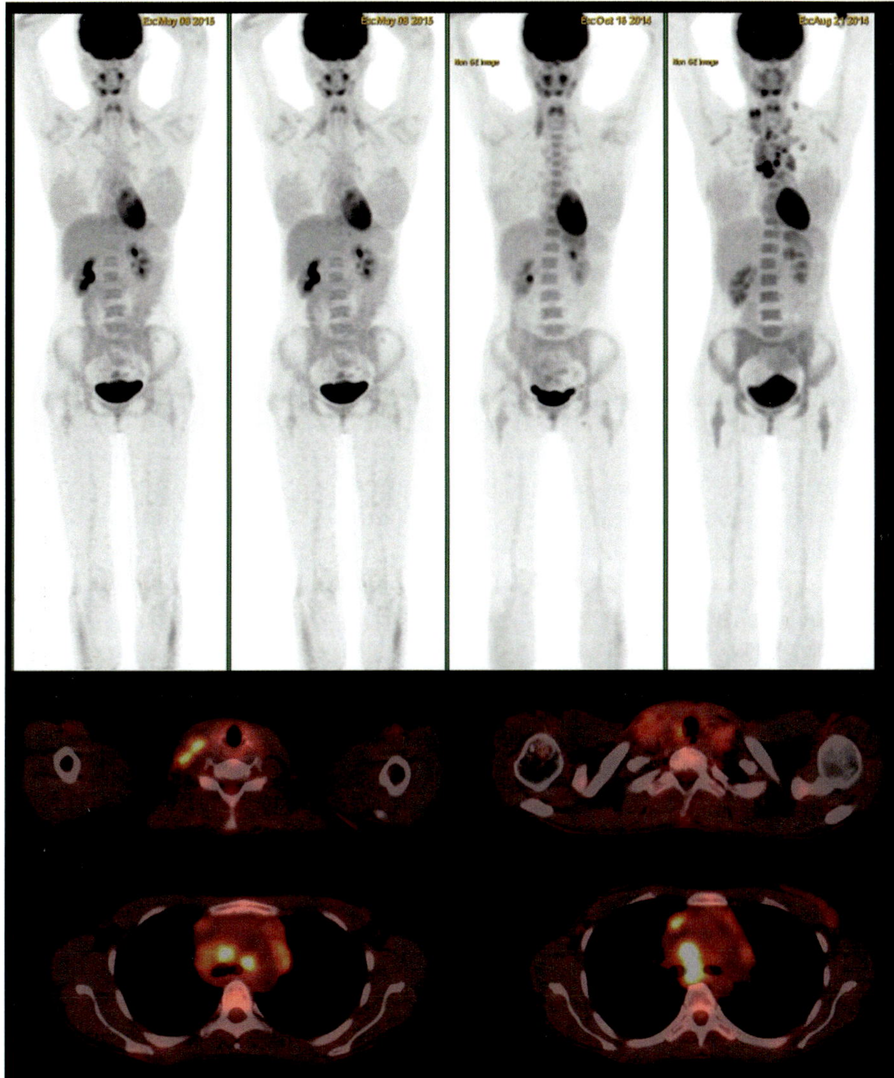

Fig. 9.1 CT and PET/CT images of a 28-year-old woman with Hodgkin lymphoma. A PET/CT scan demonstrates heterogeneous hypermetabolic lesions in the right anterior mediastinum, and bilateral supraclavicular enlarged lymph nodes. *CT* computed tomography, *PET* positron emission tomography

showed characteristic broad collagen bands surrounding nodules composed of a highly variable number of Reed–Sternberg cells, lymphocytes, and other inflammatory cells, which is a typical pattern for nodular sclerosis HL. Immunohistochemistry of these atypical cells was positive for CD-15 and CD-30 and negative for CD-3, CD-20, and ALK. The in-situ hybridization test for Epstein–Barr virus was negative. The patient was staged as having IIB HL and was started treatment with 4 cycles of doxorubicin, bleomycin, vincristine, and dacarbazine (ABVD) regimen. After chemotherapy, the patient had shown a complete response to the treatment in PET-CT evaluation.

9.1.1.1 Patient Evaluation

- At the time of diagnosis, patient's most common presentation is non-tender lymphadenopathy (cervical 80%, mediastinal 50%), usually with supradiaphragmatic lymphadenopathy. Complete lymph node exam has to be completed [9].
- Axillary or inguinal adenopathy are less frequently seen.
- If the patient present with large mediastinal mass, shortness of breath, chest pain, cough or vena cava superior syndrome could be questioned.
- Even HL involves contiguous lymph node groups, HL could also involve extranodal tissues (spleen, lungs, liver and bone marrow) by hematologus spread [10].
- B symptoms (fever $\geq$38 °C, >10% weight loss in $\leq$6 months, drenching sweats) occur in 15–20% of stage I–II, 33% overall.
- Alcohol induced pain at a specific site, could be a sign of bony involvement or enlarged lymph node of that area.
- Lab works could be listed as CBC with differential, LFTs, BUN, /Cr, ESR, chemistries, alkaline phosphatase, LDH, albumin. Pregnancy test. HIV test (if risk factors)
- Fine needle aspiration or core needle biopsies are not adequate as to provide diagnose, pathologist has to see the architectural design of the lymph node so excisional LN biopsy is preferred [11].
- Bone marrow biopsy is always a part of staging work flow for patients with B symptoms, stage III–IV, bulky disease, recurrent disease.
- Diagnostic imaging has to include CT chest, abdomen and pelvis, more importantly Fluorodeoxyglucose positive emission tomography (FDGPET) scanning has served as an important tool in the staging of patients with HL, gathering treatment information and guidance with interim PET-CT provided compared to other imaging modalities [12].

9.1.1.2 Diagnosis

More than 170 years ago, Thomas Hodgkin first described the disease named after him with specific the malignant Reed-Sternberg cell, which is of follicular center B-cell origin within the appropriate cellular environment of normal reactive lymphocytes, eosinophils and histiocytes [9, 10]. The bi- or multinucleated Reed-Sternberg cells most likely originate from the mononuclear Hodgkin cells during cytokinesis. HL is composed of two distinct disease entities; the more commonly diagnosed classical HL and the rare nodular lymphocyte predominant HL (Table 9.1) [4]. Nodular sclerosis, mixed cellularity, lymphocyte depletion, and lymphocyte-rich HL are subgroups of classical HL. HL cells have largely lost their B-cell phenotype and express a very unusual expression of many markers of other hematopoietic

Table 9.1 Characteristics of Hodgkin lymphoma subtypes

WHO classification	Nodular lymphocyte predominant (NLPHL)	Classic HL (CHL) nodular sclerosis	Mixed cellularity	Lymphocyte rich	Lymphocyte depleted
Incidence/epidemiology	5% of all HL More common age > 40	70% cHL more common in adolescents and young adults	20% cHL more common young children	15% cHL	<5% cHL
Presentation	Often early stage	Mediastinum often involved One third have B symptom	Often advanced disease	Usually early stage	Rare, mostly advanced B symptoms
Prognosis	Best occasional late relapse	Intermediate between LR and LD cHL	Intermediate between LR and LD cHL	Good	Worst
CD15	–	+	+	+	+
CD30	–	+	+	+	+
CD20	+	±	±	±	±
CD45	+	–	–	–	–

cell lineages, which supports in the differential diagnosis between classical HL (cHL) and NLPHL and differentiates cHL from all other hematopoietic malignancies [1].

9.1.1.3 Classical Hodgkin Lymphoma

The presence of malignant multinucleated giant Reed-Sternberg cells within the characteristic reactive cellular background is the pathologic hallmark of classical HL. In most of the cases CD 45 antigen is absent whereas CD30 and CD 15 were present although they are normally cannot be detected in normal B or T cells. The immunophenotypic and genetic features of the malignant cell of four histological subtypes of classical HL is similar except nature of surrounding reactive cells, association of EBV and clinical presentation [13].

Nodular sclerosis, accounts for almost 70% of cHL, commonly seen in adolescent and young adults and usually presents with localized disease involving cervical, supraclavicular and mediastinal regions [14]. Mixed cellularity HL is more frequently seen in developing countries and accounts for 25% of CHL. It is more affecting pediatric group as well as older age groups. In the clinic presentation, it is commonly diagnose at a more advanced stage of disease and have a poorer prognosis. The incidence of lymphocyte depletion HL is almost 5% of the whole group [14]. This subtype seen mainly in older age patients and often the patients had a type of immune deficiency syndrome. Characteristically, symptomatic extensive disease without peripheral lymphadenopathy is the clinical scenario of presentation and the prognosis is known to be slightly better than the rest of the subgroup [4].

The last subgroup is Lymphocyte rich classical Hl and the architectural structure is similar to nodular lymphocyte predominant HL on morphologic grounds; but represents by increased number of Reed Stenberg cell and depleted lymphocytes counts [1].

9.1.1.4 Nodular Lymphocyte Predominant Hodgkin Lymphoma

Nodular lymphocyte predominant HL comprises 5% of HL. The unique malign cell also called as popcorn cells is significantly different to classical HL [15]. Popcorn cells are characterized by a neoplastic population of larger cells with folded lobulated nuclei known as lymphocytic and histiocytic cells. Unlike classical HL, these cells are consistently CD20, CD 45 positive and commonly negative for CD30. Pathologically, lymphocyte predominant HL lacks the typical Reed- Sternberg cells [16].

Lymphocyte predominant HL is more frequently seen in men. Clinical presentation is with limited nodal disease usually located at the neck region and extranodal disease are rare. More importantly, it has an indolent course with a tendency for late recurrences [15, 16].

9.1.1.5 Risk Stratification

Early stage HL (Stage I–II) has defined several factor and based on them, it has been divided into Favorable (no risk factors) and unfavorable ($\geq$1 risk factor) (Table 9.2) [17]. These factors can be listed as B symptoms, sedimentation, bulky disease, age and histology. Various groups are used different combination of these factors to define unfavorable characterizes [4, 18] (Table 9.3).

For advanced stage evaluation, International prognostic score was established with a combination of seven and three factors (Tables 9.4 and 9.5) and used to guide trials, patient selection and guiding tailored therapy [19].

9.1.1.6 Fluorodeoxyglucose Positive Emission Tomography (FDG-PET)

Functional imaging using 18-fluorodeoxyglycose ($[^{18}F]FDG$) positron emission tomography combined with computed tomography (PET/CT) has become a major imaging modality in Hodgkin lymphoma [21]. This imaging modality consents for a significant perfection in staging, improved sensitivity, which comprises separating residual tumors from fibrosis during treatment evaluation, and highly influences treatment decisions. At the beginning, the use of PET-CT as part of the staging work up of HL has been demonstrated in numerous studies reporting that the functional image is more accurate than CT alone. In one prospective study, 19% of patients who underwent both PET-CT and CT, PET-CT, upstaged and moreover treatment strategy shift, was demonstrated in 9% of the 99 patients in total [11]. In the Response Adapted Therapy in Advanced Hodgkin Lymphoma (RATHL) trial, the use of PET-CT for staging was confirmed as the standard in HL work-up and reported that using the Deauville criteria to assess response, provides the concordance between expert and community readers. Besides staging, PET evaluation improved the assessment

Table 9.2 HL staging (AJCC 8th edition, 2017)

Stage	Stage descriptions
Limited stage	
I	Involvement of a single lymphatic site (i.e., Nodal region, Waldeyer's ring, thymus, or spleen)
IE	Single extra lymphatic site in the absence of nodal involvement (rare in Hodgkin lymphoma)
II	Involvement of two or more lymph node regions on the same side of the diaphragm
IIE	Contiguous extralymphatic extension from a nodal site with or without involvement of other lymph node regions on the same side of the diaphragm
II Bulky	Bulky Stage II with disease bulk[a, b]
Advanced stage	
III	Involvement of the lymph node regions on both sides of the diaphragm: nodes above the diaphragm with spleen involvement
IV	Diffuse or disseminated involvement of one or more extra lymphatic organs, with or without associated lymph node involvement or noncontiguous extralymphatic organ involvement in conjunction with nodal stage II or any extralymphatic organ involvement in nodal stage III disease stage IV includes any involvement of the CSF, bone marrow, live or lungs)other than by direct extension in Stage II E disease)

Note: Hodgkin lymphoma uses A or B designation with stage group. A/B is no longer used in NHL
Used with permission of the American College of Surgeons, Chicago, Illinois. The original and primary source for this information is the AJCC Cancer Staging Manual, Eighth Edition (2017) published by Springer International Publishing
[a]Stage II bulky may be considered either early or advanced stage based on lymphoma histology and prognostic factors (see discussion of Hodgkin lymphoma prognostic factors)
[b]The definition of disease bulk varies according to lymphoma histology. In the Lugano classification, bulk in Hodgkin lymphoma is defined as a mass greater than one third of the thoracic diameter on CT of the chest or a mass >10 cm. For NHL, the recommended definitions of bulk vary by lymphoma histology. In follicular lymphoma, 6 cm has been suggested based on the follicular lymphoma International Prognostic Index-2 (FLIPI-2) and its validation. In DLBCL, cutoffs ranging from 5 to 10 cm have been used although 10 cm is recommended

Table 9.3 Risk factors for stage I–II HL

Risk factor	GHSB	EORTC	NCIC	NCCN
Age	–	≥50	≥40	–
Histology	–	MC or LD	–	–
ESR or B semptom	50 if A or > 30 if B	>50 if A or > 30 if B	>50 or any B sx	>50 Mor any B sx
Large mediastinal adenopathy	MMR > 0.33 10CM	MMR > 0.35	MMR > 0.33	MMR > 0.33
# Nodal sites	>2	>3	>3	>2
Extranodal lesions	Any	–	–	–
Bulky	–	–	–	10 cm

Mediastinal mass measured on CXR by the mediastinal mass ratio (MMR) maximum width of mass/maximum intrathoracic diameter
Early stage treated with chemo-RT, 5-year FFF 95% and OS >95%
ESR erythrocyte sedimentation rate, LD lymphocyte depletion, MC mixed cellularity

Table 9.4 IPS-7 risk group for advanced stage HL [19]

	IPI score	5-year PFS (%)	5-year OS (%)
1 point per factor for advanced stage HL	0	84	89
Gender male	1	77	90
Age ≥ 45	2	67	81
Stage IV	3	60	78
Albumin <4 g/dL, Hgb < 10.5 g/dL	4	51	61
WBC >15,000/uL, lymphocyte <8% or < 600 uL	>5	42	56

Table 9.5 IPS-3 risk group for advanced stage HL [20]

	IPS score	5-year PFS (%)	5-year OS (%)
1 point per factor	0	83	95
Age ≥ 45	1	74	85
Stage IV	2	68	75
Hgb < 10.5 g/dL	3	63	52

of extranodal disease, especially in bone and organ involvement. As PET was demonstrated almost 90% sensitivity in detecting bone marrow involvement in HL, the need for invasive bone marrow biopsy diminished [22].

The other major role of PET-CT in HL is response evaluation: (1) Interim analysis to distinguish in whom treatment alterations may be needed (iPET) [23] and (2) at the conclusion of treatment (cPET) [24].

During the course of treatment, iFDG-PET scanning now plays a role in decisions to complete therapy as planned, or tailor a risk-adapted therapy. It predicts progression-free survival (PFS) and overall survival (OS) for patients with HL and was a better factor for outcome than stage, extranodal disease, or other prognostic marker [23]. Any post-treatment PET positive mass was advised to be biopsied before further treatment due to risk of false positives including thymic hyperplasia in young patients [25].

The importance of PET CT at follow up was evaluated with an aim to detect relapses and initiate salvage treatment earlier. Interestingly, PET-CT has not shown clear evidence of benefit in this setting. In a follow-up protocol study, 160 HL patients had regular PET scans at 6, 12, 18, and 24 month intervals. PET identified early relapse in only 10% of patients with HL [26]. As s conclusion PET- CT has been used in clinical setting as a gold standard for staging, interim analysis and completion of treatment. But the recent Lugano classification discourages the use of routine surveillance scans, PET or CT, in surveillance of HL [9, 26].

9.1.2 Evidence Based Treatment Recommendation

9.1.2.1 Early-Stage Classical HL

Historically, early stage favorable patients were candidates for extended field's radiation administration alone with curative intent resulting in 90% 10 year overall- survival [10]. These results were excellent in relatively young group of patients, so with the long follow-up, the late term complication as secondary malignancies and cardio-vascular complications has been recognized with high rates [4]. To balance the side effects and excellent survival, the use chemotherapy and radiotherapy in combined fashion has been increased. In addition to the combination strategy, the technique of radiotherapy has evolved in last decades with CT based planning, 3D conformal radiotherapy and more sophisticated planning such as IMRT and VMAT [7]. Besides technical development, radiotherapy target volume has diminished from extended fields such as mantle field to involved field and more over to involved site fields [27].

Trials designed at the beginning of 2000s, report improved PFS with chemo-therapy added to radiotherapy compared to radiotherapy alone. GHSG HD7 study investigated whether combined-modality treatment (CMT) with two cycles of doxo-rubicin, bleomycin, vinblastine, and dacarbazine (ABVD) followed by extended-field radiotherapy (EF-RT) is superior to EF-RT alone in patients with early favorable Hodgkin's lymphoma (HL) [28]. Between 1993 and 1998, 650 patients with newly diagnosed, histology-proven HL in clinical stages IA to IIB without risk factors were enrolled. At a median observation time of 87 months, there was no dif-ference between treatment arms in terms of complete response rate (arm A, 95%; arm B, 94%) and overall survival (at 7 years: arm A, 92%; arm B, 94%; P = .43). However, freedom from treatment failure was significantly different, with 7-year rates of 67% in arm A (95% CI, 61% to 73%) and 88% in arm B (95% CI, 84% to 92%; P ≤ 0.0001). This was due mainly to significantly more relapses after EF-RT only (arm A, 22%; arm B, 3%) [28]. These results were also confirmed by SWOG 9133/CALGB 9391 and EORTC-GELA H8F/U studies [29, 30].

The second important step in early stage HL treatment was to diminish the target volume of radiotherapy as chemotherapy was effective for microscopic disease. Smaller radiotherapy field sizes are questioned to replace extended-field or subtotal nodal irradiation (STNI) fields when combined with chemotherapy. GHSG HD8 [31]. Study randomized 40 Gy extended field (EF) to 40 Gy involved field (IF) after four cycles of chemotherapy. After median 54 months follow-up, survival rates at 5 years after start of radiotherapy revealed no differences for both modality, respec-tively, in terms of FFTF (85.8% and 84.2%) and OS at 5 years (90.8% and 92.4%). There also were no differences in both arms, respectively, in terms of complete remission (98.5% and 97.2%), progressive disease (0.8% and 1.9%), relapse (6.4% and 7.7%), death (8.1% and 6.4%), and secondary neoplasia (4.5% and 2.8%). In contrast, acute side effects including leukopenia, thrombocytopenia, nausea, gastro-intestinal toxicity, and pharyngeal toxicity were more frequent in the EF arm. Depending on the results, radiotherapy volume size reduction from EF to IF after COPP + ABVD chemotherapy for two cycles proven to provide similar results and less toxicity in patients with early-stage unfavorable HD [31].

This finding also confirmed by EORTC H7F, Milan studies [32, 33]. EORTC-GELA H8F/U study compared three cycles of mechlorethamine, vincristine, pro-carbazine, and prednisone (MOPP) combined with doxorubicin, bleomycin, and vinblastine (ABV) plus involved-field radiotherapy with subtotal nodal radiother-apy alone for favorable stage I-II HL patients [30]. In the H8-U trial, similar strategy was tested for unfavorable group (we compared three regimens: six cycles of MOPP-ABV plus involved-field radiotherapy, four cycles of MOPP-ABV plus involved-field radiotherapy, and four cycles of MOPP-ABV plus subtotal nodal radiotherapy). At the 92 months follow-up, H8-F trial established 5-year event-free survival rate was significantly higher after three cycles of MOPP-ABV plus involved-field radiotherapy than after subtotal nodal radiotherapy alone (98% vs. 74%, P < 0.001). The 10-year overall survival estimates were 97% and 92%, respectively (P = 0.001). In the H8-U trial, the estimated 5-year event-free survival rates were similar in the three treatment groups: 84% after six cycles of MOPP-ABV plus involved-field radiotherapy, 88% after four cycles of MOPP-ABV plus involved-field radiotherapy, and 87% after four cycles of MOPP-ABV plus subtotal nodal radiotherapy. The 10-year overall survival estimates were 88%, 85%, and 84%, respectively [30]. After all, chemotherapy plus involved-field radiotherapy announced as the standard treatment for Hodgkin's disease with favorable prognostic features.

Furthermore, the studies have investigated the idea of omitting radiotherapy for early-stage. EORTC H9F randomized 783 patients with favorable IA–IIB randomized to no IFRT, IFRT (20 Gy), or IFRT (36 Gy), after achieving complete response with 6 cycles of EBVP. Four-year event free survival decreased without IFRT (70%) vs. 84% (20 Gy) and 87% (36 Gy). Due to unacceptable failure rate of >20% in the arm designed without radiotherapy, but overall survival were 98% in all three arms. The result also indicated that 20 Gy is sufficient after complete response versus 36 Gy [34]. GHSG HD10 trial randomized to 2 cycle ABVD versus 4 cycle, followed by IFRT 20 versus 30 Gy. The study included 1370 patients with favorable I–II with no risk factors [35]. At medium follow-up 7.5 years, no statistically significant difference between any of the arms. This study 2 cycle ABVD plus 20 Gy IFRT as the standard approach of early stage I-IIA (the absence of adverse risk factors, specifically erythrocyte sedimentation rate >50 or >30 with B symptoms, extranodal disease, more than 2 sites of involvement, or mediastinal bulk disease) [35].

The other important study form Canadian group, NCIC/ECOG HD.6 compared 4 cycle ABVD vs. STNI alone (favorable) or STNI + 2 cycle ABVD × (unfavorable) in a cohort of 405 IA or IIA non-bulky HL patients stratified into favorable or unfavorable [36]. In favorable group, no difference in OS or EFS at 12 years. In unfavorable group, ABVD + STNI improved 12-year freedom from disease progression (94% vs. 86%) but worse 12-year OS (81% vs. 92%) compared to ABVD alone mostly caused by more non-cancer deaths. More secondary cancers (23 vs. 10) and cardiac events (26 vs. 16) reported with STNI [36]. When this study was published, STNI was already accepted as a historical radiotherapy method.

Based on these results NCCN consensus guidelines and European society of medical oncology accepted radiotherapy and chemotherapy combination treatment for stage I-IIA HL with a 5 year progression free survival %90-95%. Selected patients may be treated with chemotherapy alone if radiation is not suitable [9].

Even ABVD (doxorubicin, bleomycin, vinblastine, dacarbazine) is the widely accepted standard chemotherapy schedule, Stanford V and BEACOPP regimes have been also used in clinical trials. The GHSG HD11 trail for patients with large mediastinal adenopathy, elevated ESR, the presence of extra nodal disease or more than 2 sites, stratified to BEACOPP chemotherapy vs. ABVD schema and the involved radiotherapy dose 30 Gy to 20 Gy [37]. The results revealed that 20 Gy IFRT is sufficient in combination with BEACOPP. The other major limitation of BEACOPP was the reported high toxicity rates. 4 cycles of ABVD plus 30 Gy IFRT arm was accepted as the standard approach for stage I-II unfavorable group with 5 year OS of 94%, progression free survival of 87% [37].

Parallel to the success of combination treatment, the importance of PET-CT in lymphoma as an interim evaluation and guidance role for treatment intensification was widely reported in the literature [21, 23]. The new aim is to reduce the treatment by omitting radiotherapy for PET negative patients and intensify chemotherapy by switching to BEACOPP regime. The European Organization for Research and Treatment of Cancer (EORTC) H10 study recruited 1137 favorable and unfavorable early-stage patients. The standard arm received 3 cycles of ABVD + INRT and the experimental arm was 2 cycles of ABVD flowed by FDG-PET, if PET positive, then the chemotherapy schema switch to escalated 2 cycles of BEACOPP and INRT; if PET negative then continue with 2 cycles of ABVD [6]. The response rates were after 2 cycles of ABVD patients were reported as PET negative in 85-88% of favorable and 74-78% of unfavorable cases, respectively. With a median follow-up of just over 1 year, for the PET-negative groups, the no IFRT arm showed significantly inferior PFS in the favorable group (94.9% vs. 100%; HR = 9.36; P = 0.017) and 94.7% versus 97.3% in the unfavorable group (HR = 2.42; P = 0.026) [6]. This suggested that even in the PET negative patients, IFRT has an important role in progression free survival. More follow-up is needed OS.

In United Kingdom, RAPID trial, 602 CS I–IIA treated with 3 cycles of ABVD followed by PET. If the scan was negative (Deauville 1 and 2), patients randomized to IFRT 30 Gy or no further treatment [38]. At a median follow-up time of 48 months, by intent to treat analysis, 3-year PFS 94.6% in RT group vs. 90.8% in ABVD alone arm. However there is a significant trend toward lower survival in the radiotherapy arm (97.1% vs. 99.5%, p = 0.07), in fact the deaths occurred in radiotherapy arm has been occurred prior to radiotherapy [38]. In Meta-analysis evolving randomized controlled trials (RCTs) comparing FDG-PET-adapted therapy to standard treatment in early stage HL patients with a negative PET-scan (N:1480) [39]. Only one trial provided data for OS, without evidence for a difference between both arms (HR 0.51; 95% CI0.15–1.68). Progression free survival was found to be inferior in the PET-adapted Arms without radiotherapy compared to the standard treatment arms (HR 2.40; 95% CI 1.63–3.53). Adverse events were reported similar in both arms. There were no data on long-term adverse events, quality of life and treatment-related mortality available [39].

The treatment for early stage HL is still evolving. Based on the early studies and a met [1] analysis evaluating the omission of radiotherapy, PFS was reported reduced but similar overall survival rates. Two ongoing studies conducted by GHSG are exploring PET response directed treatment options. HD 16 trial randomized patients with low risk early stage disease to two cycles of ABVD followed by 30 Gy IFRT versus two cycles of chemotherapy and IFRT if PET was positive vs. no further therapy if PET was negative. HD 17 trial studies high risk cHL treating with either 2 cycles of de-escalated BEACOPP, 2 cycle of ABVD followed by 30 Gy or same two-two regimen and 30 Gy IFRT depending on the PET response [4].

9.1.2.2 Advanced Stage

Six to eight cycles of ABVD is still considered as standard systemic therapy for locally advanced stage HL. Even dose escalated BEACOPP was shown as superior to ABVD, the accessed toxicity was the most important disadvantage of administrating this regime [1, 9].

Routine use of radiotherapy in this stage HL patient, but several trials assessed the role of radiotherapy as a consolidation where usually improved PFS particularly for patients with bulky disease or poor responders to chemotherapy were reported. EORTC 20884/GPMC H34 trial consists CS III/IV patients who received 6–8 cycles of MOPP-ABV [20]. If CR was achieved, patients were randomized to observation vs. consolidative IFRT (24 Gy). IFRT did not improve RFS or OS but for patients with PR, the use of radiotherapy provided similar oncological outcomes (8-year EFS 76% and OS 84%) to those with CR ± RT (75 and 82%) [20]. The role for RT has been established in PR status of stage III–IV patients.

In the randomized controlled trial from the United Kingdom Lymphoma Group (LY09 trial) that compared ABVD with two other multidrug regimens, IFRT was recommended for incomplete response to chemotherapy or bulk disease at presentation [40]. PFS was superior for patients who received RT (5-year PFS was 71% without RT and 86% with RT) and a similar advantage was seen for OS [40].

A confirming study form India had randomized 179 patients with stage I–IV achieved CR after six cycles ABVD to no RT or consolidation RT. RT improved 8-year EFS (76 vs. 88%) and OS (89 vs. 100%) [41]. GHSG HD12 was another randomized trial of 1670 patients with CS IIB/IIIA and risk factors or stage IIIB/IV randomized to escalated eight cycles of BEACOPP vs. four cycles of escalated BEACOPP + and 4 cycles standard BEACOPP with IFRT to residual vs. no RT to residual for both arms [42]. Second randomization of IFRT (30 Gy) vs. no IFRT to initial bulky or residual enlarged nodes. At 5 years, no statistical difference between any of the four arms. RT improved FFTF (87 vs. 90.4%), but no difference in survival [42].

In PET-CT era, GHSG HD15, 2182 patients with newly diagnosed advanced stage Hodgkin's lymphoma aged 18–60 years were randomly assigned to receive either eight cycles of BEACOPPescalated (8 × Besc group), six cycles of BEACOPPescalated (6 × Besc group), or eight cycles of BEACOPP14 (8 × B14 group) [43]. Patients with a persistent mass after chemotherapy measuring 2·5 cm or larger and positive on PET scan received additional radiotherapy with 30 Gy; the negative predictive value for tumour recurrence of PET at 12 months was an independent endpoint. In the intention-to-treat analysis set, freedom from treatment failure was sequentially non-inferior for the 6 × Besc and 8 × B14 groups as compared with 8 × Besc. 4-year PFS was 92% for PET-negative CT-persistent residual disease and 86% for PET+ PR patients [43]. Treatment with six cycles of BEACOPPescalated followed by PET-guided radiotherapy was more effective in terms of freedom from treatment failure and less toxic than eight cycles of the same chemotherapy regimen.

The Stanford V program includes only 12 weeks of chemotherapy with less doxorubicin and bleomycin dose compared to ABVD. Radiation therapy is routinely added to initially bulky (>5 cm) sites of disease, as well as macroscopic spleen involvement to a total dose of 30-36 Gy [4].

9.1.2.3 Nodular Lymphocyte Predominant Hl

NLPHL has a long term disease free survival after the involved field treatment, different from cHL. The usual dose is 30. In a retrospective study by Eichenauer, 256 patients with stage IA NLPHL treated on GHSG protocols were analyzed and 8-year PFS/OS was IFRT 92/99%, EFRT 84/96%, and combined modality treatment 89/99% [44]. IFRT, for example ipsilateral field for stage IA high cervical lymph node involvement, is considered the standard of care due to the lowest risk of toxic effects. Rituximab alone studies demonstrated inferior 4-year PFS of 81% [4].

9.1.3 Radiation Techniques

9.1.3.1 Simulation

3D simulation (CT, PET/CT, or MRI) is always recommended.

IV contract use has encouraged as accurate identification of vessels are important.

Simulation has to be specific for disease site. If the disease is located at head and neck, the hyperextended neck position and immobilization with mask is helpful for stabilization. If axillary region is involved, the arms preferentially placed above the head or Akimbo position and immobilized using a custom mold to enhance reproducibility and pulling axillary lymph nodes form chest to allow for additional lung sparing (Fig. 9.2).

PTV expansion for setup uncertainty should be determined on a case-by-case and institutional basis. In general 1 cm margin could be considered sufficient, but in the chest and upper abdomen, a larger margin in the superior-inferior direction may be needed to compensate for respiratory motion.

4DCT and breath hold gating could be considered with ITV for locations where internal organ movement is of concern especially in cases with mediastinum involvement (Fig. 9.3).

Treatment with photons, electrons, or protons may all be appropriate, depending upon clinical circumstances to reduce normal tissue toxicity while achieving local control. Using Shielding for testis in men and considering the dose to ovaries for women must keep in mind.

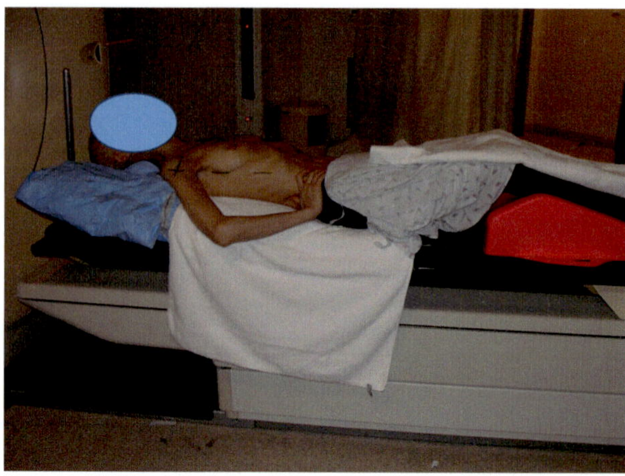

Fig. 9.2 Setup photo of the patient with immobilization performed with blue med-tec and angled board

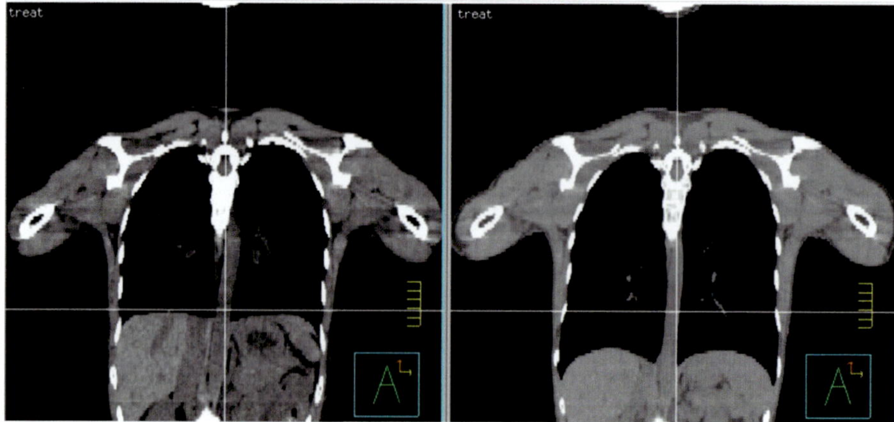

Fig. 9.3 Free breathing and deep breath hold CT scans of a patient with stage II cHL. The volume of lungs increases and the position of heart changes down and elonges

The significant dose-sparing for these OARs is the most important aim of best clinical practice. Achieving highly conformal dose distributions is especially important for patients who are being treated with curative intent or who have long life expectancies following therapy.

An intensity-modulated radiation therapy (IMRT) technique named as "butterfly" IMRT with anterior beams of $300° - 30°$ and posterior beams of $160° - 210°$ has been presented as avoids excess exposure of heart, breast, lung, and spinal cord to doses of 30 or 20 Gy; mildly increases V5 to the breasts; and decreases the V107% (Fig. 9.4) [45].

Deep inspiration breath-hold (DIBH) was evaluated in dosimetric and prospective phase 2 trials. The results have demonstrated that this technique can reduce

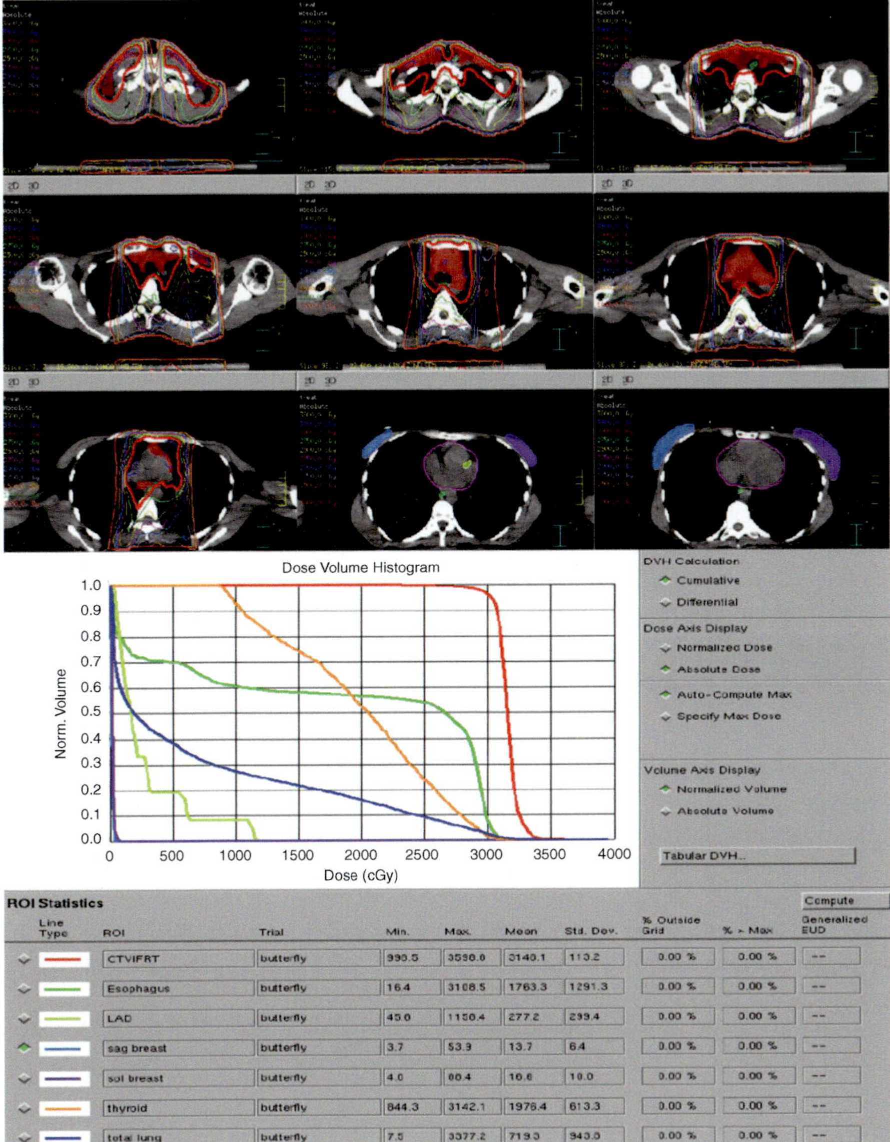

Fig. 9.4 IMRT-field in field planning for stage IIA patient to a total dose of 30 Gy. 95% isodose coverage (red) and Dose-volume histogram. Delineation of treatment volumes for stage IIB with mediastinum involvement. Red: CTV, yellow: thyroid, green: esophagus

radiation doses to the lungs, heart, and cardiac structures without compromising the target dose for patients with mediastinal cHL. In the analysis of plans for 22 patients, DIBH reduced the mean estimated lung dose by 2.0 Gy (median: 8.5 Gy vs. 7.2 Gy) (p < 0.01) and the mean heart dose by 1.4 Gy (6.0 Gy vs. 3.9 Gy) (p < 0.01) compared to FB. The lung and heart V20Gy were reduced with a median of 5.3% and 6.3%. Mean doses to the female breasts were equal with FB and DIBH [46].

Radiotherapy starts 3 to 4 weeks after the completion of chemotherapy.

9.1.3.2 Field Design

International lymphoma international working group published following guidelines [7].

Delineation and field setup depends on the origin of disease and the response to systemic therapy. The historical changes of radiation treatment fields can be listed as.

Extended Field Radiotherapy (EFRT)

Mantle field: Bilateral cervical, supraclavicular, axilla, mediastinal and hilar nodes.
Mini mantle: mantle excluding mediastinum.
Modified mantle: mantle excluding axilla.
Inverted Y: paraaortic, bilateral pelvic nodes ± spleen.
Total lymphoid irradiation: Mantle and inverted Y fields.
Subtotal lymphoid irradiation: TLI excluding pelvis.

Involved Field Radiotherapy

The pre-chemo the lymph node site of the clinically involved lymph node group determines the borders of the field. Lymph node grouping are not clearly defined. Examples of field design are listed below.

Cervical field: includes unilateral or bilateral neck and supraclavicular lymph nodes extending form the base of the skull to clavicles.

Mediastinal region: mediastinum, bilateral hila and supraclavicular lymph nodes.

Definitions of IFRT dependent on bony landmarks without 3D target delineation.

Involved-Site RT (ISRT)

CT-based simulation is essential. The pre-chemo GTV determines CTV. CT scans should be performed before and after chemotherapy and when possible in the treatment position. The goal to target site of originally involved lymph node(s) is to encompass the original volume prior to surgery or chemotherapy while sparing uninvolved organs once lymph node has regressed. An online EORTC-GELA contouring atlas is available at http://groups.eortc.be/lymphoma/final_eortc-gela_notebook.pdf.

GTV: Does not exist if there is complete response.

CTV: includes the initial lymph node volume before chemotherapy. CTV encompasses all re-chemotherapy lymphoma involvement, modified for normal tissue boundaries, tumor shrinkage, and other anatomic changes. The CTV has to cover length of mediastinal mass or lymph node before chemotherapy and with corresponds to the width of them after chemotherapy.

The ITV should be added to the CTV only in situations where internal organ movement is of concern. The CTV (or ITV if used) will be expanded further to create the PTV.

Involved-Node RT (INRT)

INRT for early-stage classic HL was developed by the EORTC to replace the traditional larger IFRT that was used in previous studies by the EORTC and other groups. INRT can therefore be regarded as a special case of ISRT wherein optimal imaging is available. Up-front PET/CT is mandatory for INRT design and should be acquired with the patient in the treatment position and using the same breathing instructions that will be used later for RT. Moreover, the patient should be scanned on a flat couch top, with the use of appropriate immobilization devices, and using markers at skin positions that are visible in the imaging [7].

As a summary, INRT represents a special case of ISRT, in which prechemotherapy imaging is ideal for post chemotherapy treatment planning. When pre-chemo PET/CT imaging is not obtained in the radiotherapy treatment position, ISRT is used with clinical judgment to delineate a larger CTV to take into count the uncertainties in defining the pre- chemo GTV.

If no prechemotherapy imaging is available, the situation is more challenging. The radiation oncologist must obtain as much information as possible from the description of the prechemotherapy physical examination of the patient, the location of scars and scar tissue on the postchemotherapy planning CT scan. The CTV should be contoured taking into account all of this information, making generous allowance for the many uncertainties in the process.

The contouring process is now as follows:

1. The CT images of the prechemotherapy PET/CT and/or CT are used to delineate the initially involved lymphoma volume, the GTVprechemo.
2. The prechemotherapy PET/CT and or CT is fused with the postchemotherapy planning CT scan, and the GTVprechemo is imported to the planning CT images.
3. The postchemotherapy tissue volume (GTVpostchemo (if there is residual disease)/CTV postchemo), which contained the initially involved lymphoma tissue, is contoured using information from both prechemotherapy PET and prechemotherapy CT, taking into account tumor shrinkage and other anatomic changes.

The CTV encompasses all of the initial lymphoma volume while still respecting normal structures that were never involved by lymphoma, such as lungs, chest wall, muscles, and mediastinal normal structures (Fig. 9.5).

Organ at risk-dose constraints are summarized in Table 9.6.

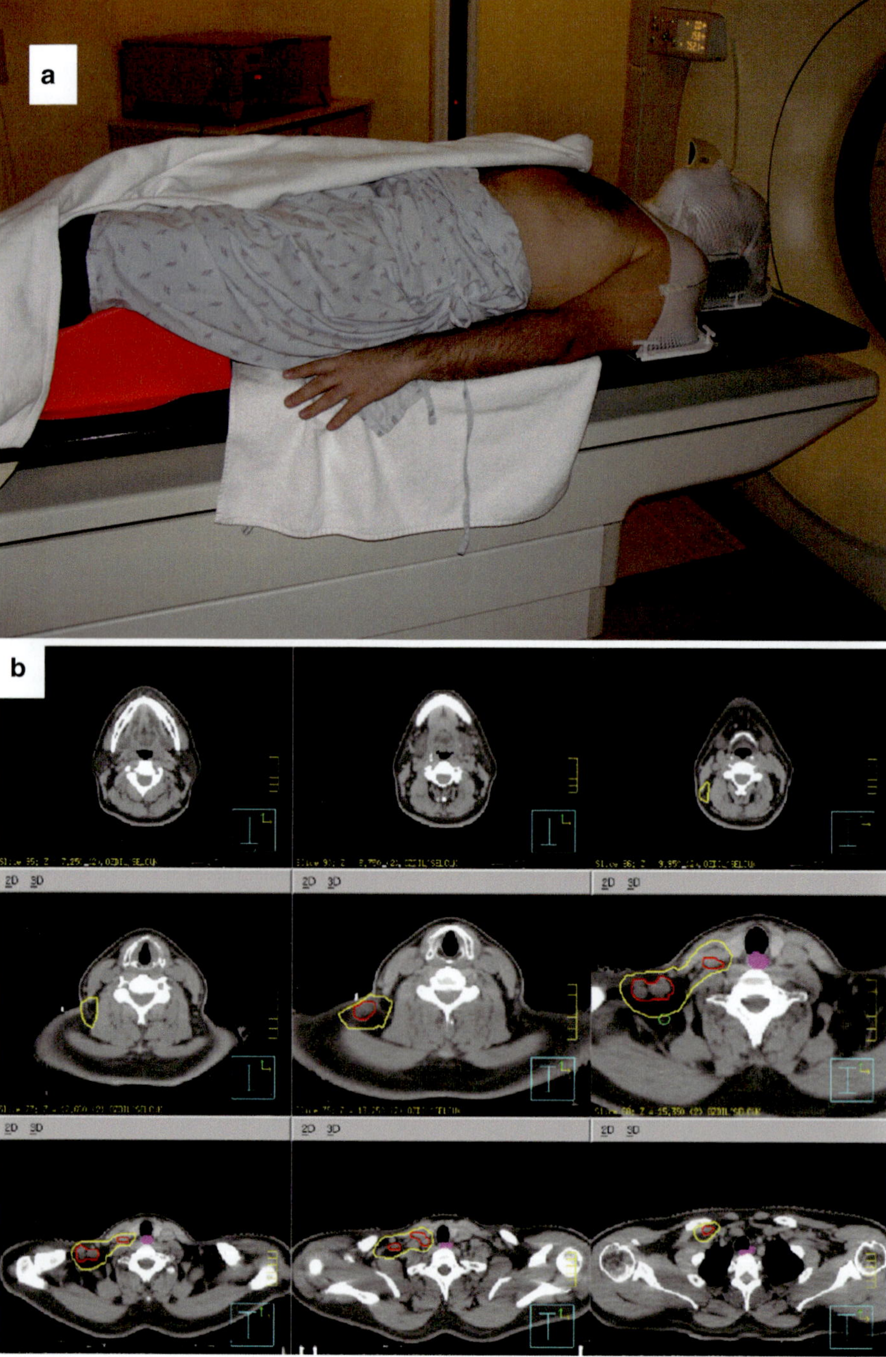

Fig. 9.5 Setup photo of the patient with immobilization performed with blue med-tec and angled board, and the deliniation of target volumes

Table 9.6 Organ at risk-dose constraints

OAR	Constraints
Heart	Mean < 5 Gy ideal, no higher than 15 Gy
Coronaries and left ventricle	V5 < 10% ideal, no hotspots in coronaries
Lungs	Mean < 13.5 Gy, V20 < 30%, V5 < 55%
Breasts	Minimize V4 or ALARA
Parotid	Mean < 5–11 Gy or ALARA
Thyroid	V25 < 63.5%
Kidneys	Minimize V5, ALARA
Spleen	ALARA
Liver	V30 < 30% or ALARA
Submandibular glands	Mean < 11 Gy

The dose to OARs that is achievable varies according to the disease distribution. We always aim for as low as reasonably achievable (ALARA)

Table 9.7 Recommended treatment algorithm Hodgkin lymphoma

Stage/risk	Chemotherapy	Consolidation RT
Classical		
Favorable early Stage I, II nonbulky and no GHSG risk factors (rf)	2 cycles of ABVD	20 Gy (10 fx), ISRT 30 Gy (if treated with Stanford V)
Unfavorable early: Stage I, IIA and ≥1 GHSG rf Stage IIB and ≥1 rf (no ENE or bulky)	4 cycles of A(B)VD	30.6 Gy (17 fx), ISRT
Stage IIB bulky or ENE	4–6 cycles of A(B)VD	*30.6 Gy (17 fx), ISRT*
Advanced: Stage III, IV	6 cycles of A(B)VD	± 30.6–36 Gy (17–20 fx) for pre-chemo bulky supradiaphragmatic sites or residual disease after chemo 30 Gy (if treated with Stanford V)
NLPHL		
Stage IA, contiguous IIA	None	30.6 Gy ISRT[a] (17 fx) 36 Gy (20 fx) if bulky
Stage III, IV or B symptoms	R-CHOP	24 or 30.6 (12 or 17 fx) Gy ISRT

ABVD—doxorubicin, bleomycin, vinblastine, dacarbazine. (B)leomycin held for 2 cycles if using 6 cycles. *ISRT* involved site radiation therapy
[a]More generous involved site is permitted in patients who do not receive chemotherapy

9.1.4 Recommended Treatment Algorithm

Recommended treatment algorithm is summarized in Table 9.7.

9.1.5 Follow-Up

- Routine follow up is recommended for every 3–6 months for 1–2 years, then every 6–12 months until year 3, and then annually with H&P, labs (ESR, albumin) as indicated. Given the very low risk of relapse in Hodgkin lymphoma, no more detailed routine imaging is recommended.
- PET/CT if previous Deauville 4–5
- Radiation pneumonitis occurs within 6–12 months
- Monitor patients for secondary cancers
- Advice smoke secession programs
- Follow thyroid function yearly
- Late cardiovascular toxicities: consider Cardiology follow-up to aggressively manage cardiac risk factors, consider echocardiogram/stress and carotid ultrasound
- Secondary malignancies: Start annual breast screening the earlier of 8–10 years after therapy or age 40. Add MRI to mammography, if chest radiation given at ≤30 year of age [9, 47]
- Late risks of particular concern gastric ulcer, pulmonary toxicity, and infertility

9.2 Non-Hodgkin's Lymphoma

Overview

Epidemiology: The non-Hodgkin lymphomas (NHL) are a heterogeneous group of lymphoproliferative malignancies with divergent patterns of behavior and responses to treatment [48] (https://www.nccn.org/professionals/physician_gls/pdf/b-cell_blocks.pdf). NHL usually initiates in lymphoid tissues and can spread to extranodal sites. The prognosis was determined by on the histologic type, stage, and treatment [49]. The median age 60–65 years at diagnose [49, 50].

Pathology: NHL can be divided into two prognostic groups: the indolent lymphomas and the aggressive lymphomas [51]. The majority of NHLs are of B-cell origin, with more than 90% of patients expressing CD20 antigen [51].

Diagnosis: Diagnosis is based on histology of preferably a biopsy of a lymph node. Follicular lymphoma (FL) is characterized by diffuse lymphadenopathy, bone marrow involvement, splenomegaly and less commonly other extranodal sites of involvement. Aggressive NHL Patients most often present with a rapidly growing tumor mass in single or multiple, nodal or extranodal sites. PET/CT is the most important diagnostic imaging for staging interim analyses and at the completion of the treatment [52].

> ***Treatment***: Indolent NHL types have a relatively good prognosis with a median survival as long as 20 years, but they usually are not curable in advanced clinical stages [53]. Early-stage (stage I and stage II) indolent NHL can be effectively observe or treated with radiation therapy alone. The aggressive type of NHL has a shorter natural history, but a significant number of these patients can be cured with intensive combination chemotherapy regimens. R-CHOP (rituximab plus cyclophosphamide, doxorubicin, vincristine, and prednisone) remains the "gold standard," despite all of our insights into cell-of-origin and other subgroups. In general, with modern treatment of patients with NHL, overall survival at 5 years is over 60%. Of patients with aggressive NHL, more than 50% can be cured [51].
>
> **Keywords**: Non-Hodgkin lymphoma, Radiotherapy

9.2.1 Case Presentation

A 42 year's old man has admitted to hospital with swelling lymph node in neck 2 months ago. He used antibiotics and had no clinical response. He denied night sweats, fevers or weight loss. There is no history of comorbidities and medication use, smoking and alcoholism. In the neck palpation, there was a cervical lymph node in right level IV about 2 cm size, it was moveable, soft and painless. The Waldeyer ring was clinically normal. The flexible nasofibrolaryngoscopy, and laboratory tests did not show changes in peripheral blood and the serology for Cytomegalovirus, Epstein Barr virus, rubella, syphilis, HIV and toxoplasmosis were all negative. Computed tomography imaging noted a cervical lymph nodes at right level IV-V measuring 2.4 × 1.4 × 2.2 cm. A PET-CT was performed showing only neck lymph nodes at right supraclavicular, posterior cervical (Fig. 9.6). He underwent neck excisional biopsy. Fragmented tissue biopsies measuring 0.5 × 0.5 cm in diameter were received. Histologically, the tumor resulted in non-Hodgkin's follicular lymphoma (positive for CD19, CD20, CD22, HILA-DR, CD10) grad 1–2.

The patient was referred to the hematology service for specific treatment. Options such as observation, radiotherapy, rituximab was discussed with the patient and his family. He decided to undergo radiotherapy of 24 Gy in 12 fractions. In control examination, there were no signals of the lesion and no complains. A neck ultrasound has been performing every 6 months after treatment and there were no more lesions.

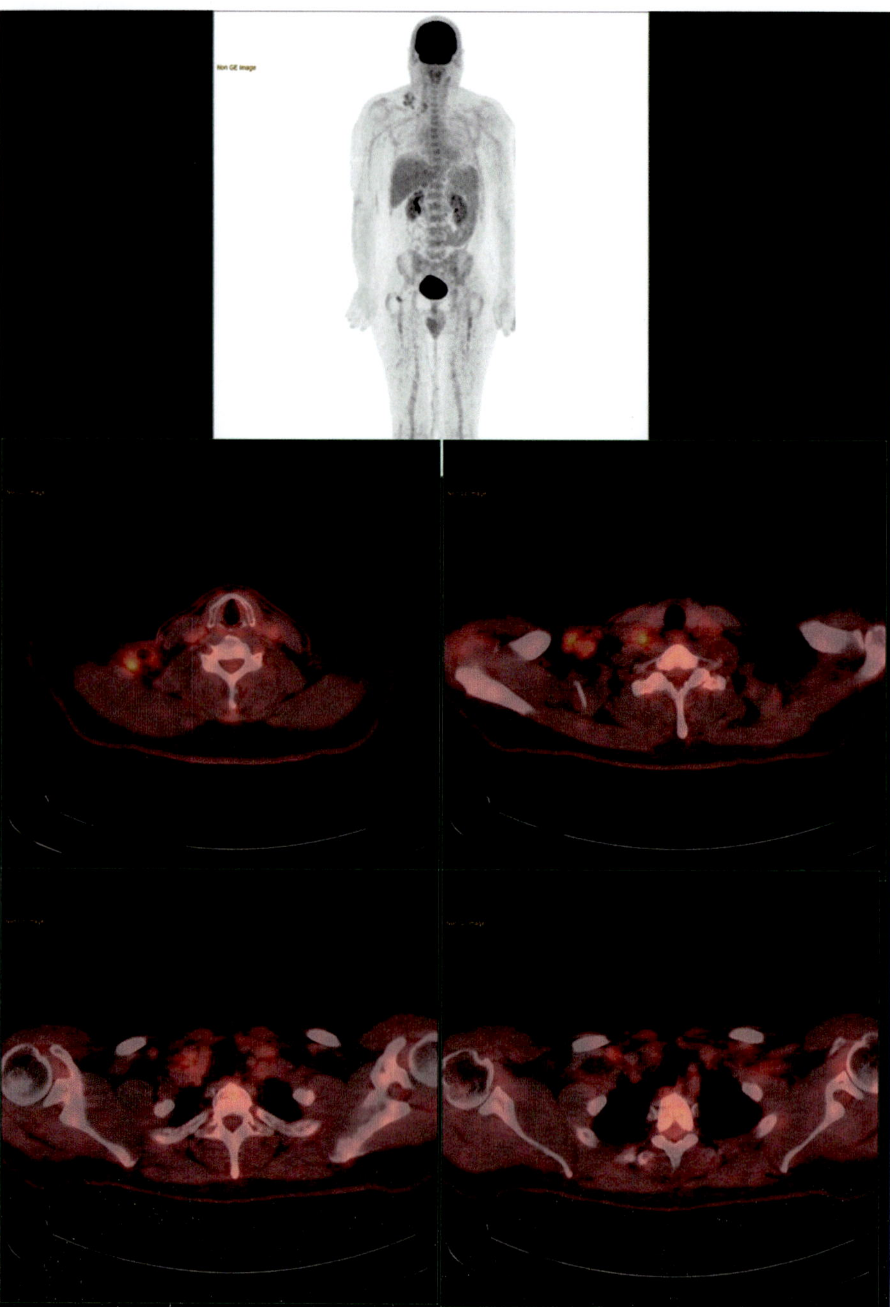

Fig. 9.6 PET/CT images of a patient with non- Hodgkin lymphoma enlarged lymph nodes. CT = computed tomography, PET = positron emission tomography

9.2.1.1 Patient Evaluation

Non Hodgkin lymphoma are a heterogeneous group of malignancies of the lymphoid system characterized by an abnormal clonal proliferation of B cells, T cell or both [54].

Several immunodeficiency disease, environmental agents and infections agents have been associated with the development of lymphoma (https://www.nccn.org/professionals/physician_gls/pdf/b-cell_blocks.pdf).

Immunodeficiency: The frequency of NHL the second most common cancer among patients with HIV infections and solid organ transplant recipients. Also autoimmune and chronic inflammatory diseases also have a higher risk of NHL [55].

Environmental and occupational exposures

Farmers, teachers, dry cleaners, butchers, wood workers and mechanic have the higher risk for developing NHL could be related to the expose of arsenic, lead, Pesticide, hair dyes, organic solvents [55].

Infectious disease [56]:

EBV—Burkitt lymphoma

HTLV-1—Adult T cell lymphoma

Helicobacter Pylori—Gastric MALT

Human Herpes virus 8—Kaposi sarcoma

Patients could be presented with a very divert clinical appearance as symptoms depend on what area of the body is affected by the cancer and grade effects the symptom duration related to growing rate of cancer. Symptoms may include: night sweats, Fever and chills that come and go, itching, swollen lymph nodes in the neck, underarms, groin, or other areas, weight loss, coughing or shortness of breath if the cancer affects the thymus gland or lymph nodes in the chest, abdominal pain or swelling, leading to loss of appetite, constipation, nausea, and vomiting, headache, concentration problems, personality changes, or seizures if the cancer affects the brain. A detailed generalized physical is examination has to be completed. Depending on the symptoms, an ophthalmology and Otolaryngology consultations are needed.

Lab tests including protein levels, liver function, kidney function, uric acid level, complete blood count (CBC), creatinine, alkaline phosphatase, LDH, Beta 2 microglobulin, HBsAg, HCV Ab, and HIV is important for evaluation [48].

CT scans of the chest, abdomen and pelvis or PET-CT scan provides information about the extent of the dissemination. Incisional or fine needle aspiration is not demonstrating the structure of the lymph node so Excisional LN biopsy is needed for a diagnose with H&E, immunophenotyping, genotyping, and molecular profiling.

Bone marrow biopsy and CSF cytology if indicated (CNS, epidural or testicular lymphoma) [57, 58].

Disease Extent Is Determined by PET/CT for FDG Avid Lymphomas and CT for FDG Non-avid Lymphomas Tonsils, Waldeyer Ring, and Spleen are Considered Nodal Tissues, Not Extranodal Sites.

9.2.1.2 Pathology

The WHO modification of the REAL classification recognizes three major categories of lymphoid malignancies based on morphology and cell lineage: B-cell neoplasms, T-cell/natural killer (NK)-cell neoplasms, and Hodgkin lymphoma (HL) (https://www.nccn.org/professionals/physician_gls/pdf/b-cell_blocks.pdf). Both lymphomas and lymphoid leukemias are included in this classification because both solid and circulating phases are present in many lymphoid neoplasms and distinction between them is artificial. Within the B-cell and T-cell categories, two subdivisions are recognized: precursor neoplasms, which correspond to the earliest stages of differentiation, and more mature differentiated neoplasms [57, 59].

> **Updated REAL/WHO Classification**
> **B-cell neoplasms**
> Precursor B-cell neoplasm: precursor B-acute lymphoblastic leukemia/lymphoblastic lymphoma (LBL).
> Peripheral B-cell neoplasms.
> B-cell CLL/small lymphocytic lymphoma.
> B-cell prolymphocytic leukemia.

Lymphoplasmacytic lymphoma/immunocytoma.
Mantle cell lymphoma.
Follicular lymphoma.
Extranodal marginal zone B-cell lymphoma of mucosa-associated lymphatic tissue (MALT) type.
Nodal marginal zone B-cell lymphoma (± monocytoid B-cells).
Splenic marginal zone lymphoma (± villous lymphocytes).
Hairy cell leukemia.
Plasmacytoma/plasma cell myeloma.
Diffuse large B-cell lymphoma.
Burkitt lymphoma.

T-Cell and Putative NK-Cell Neoplasms
Precursor T-cell neoplasm: precursor T-acute lymphoblastic leukemia/LBL.
Peripheral T-cell and NK-cell neoplasms.
T-cell CLL/prolymphocytic leukemia.
T-cell granular lymphocytic leukemia.
Mycosis fungoides (including Sézary syndrome).
Peripheral T-cell lymphoma, not otherwise characterized.
Hepatosplenic gamma/delta T-cell lymphoma.
Subcutaneous panniculitis-like T-cell lymphoma.
Angioimmunoblastic T-cell lymphoma.
Extranodal T-/NK-cell lymphoma, nasal type.
Enteropathy-type intestinal T-cell lymphoma.
Adult T-cell lymphoma/leukemia (human T-lymphotrophic virus [HTLV] 1+).
Anaplastic large cell lymphoma, primary systemic type.
Anaplastic large cell lymphoma, primary cutaneous type.
Aggressive NK-cell leukemia.

9.2.2 Staging

Ann Arbor staging classification for Hodgkin Lymphoma is used (Table 9.8) [48] (https://www.nccn.org/professionals/physician_gls/pdf/b-cell_blocks.pdf). Commonly used prognostic score indexes are summarized in Table 9.9. Lymphoma Staging according to the Lugano Classification is also given in Table 9.10.

Table 9.8 Ann Arbor staging classification for Hodgkin Lymphoma is used

Stage	Description
I	Involvement of a single lymphatic site (i.e., nodal region, Waldeyer's ring, thymus, or spleen) (I); or localized involvement of a single extralymphatic organ or site in the absence of any lymph node involvement (IE)
II	Involvement of two or more lymph node regions on the same side of the diaphragm (II); or localized involvement of a single extralymphatic organ or site in association with regional lymph node involvement with or without involvement of other lymph node regions on the same side of the diaphragm (IIE)
III	Involvement of lymph node regions on both sides of the diaphragm (III), which also may be accompanied by extralymphatic extension in association with adjacent lymph node involvement (IIIE) or by involvement of the spleen (IIIS) or both (IIIE,S)
IV	Diffuse or disseminated involvement of one or more extralymphatic organs, with or without associated lymph node involvement; or isolated extralymphatic organ involvement in the absence of adjacent regional lymph node involvement, but in conjunction with disease in distant site(s). Stage IV includes any involvement of the liver or bone marrow, lungs (other than by direct extension from another site), or cerebrospinal fluid
Designations applicable to any stage	
A	No symptoms
B	Fever (temperature >38 °C), drenching night sweats, unexplained loss of >10% of body weight within the preceding 6 months
E	Involvement of a single extranodal site that is contiguous or proximal to the known nodal site
S	Splenic involvement

[a]Reprinted with permission from AJCC: Hodgkin and non-Hodgkin lymphomas. In: Edge SB, Byrd DR, Compton CC, et al., eds.: AJCC Cancer Staging Manual. 7th ed. New York, NY: Springer, 2010, pp 607–11. Sites that are extranodal (E): Waldeyer's ring, thymus, and spleen

Table 9.9 Commonly used prognostic score indexes

Index	Aim	Adverse factors	Scoring
International Prognostic Index [60]	Aggressive NHL	Age $\geq$ 60 years, stage III/IV, elevated LDH, reduced performance status (e.g., ECOG $\geq$2), and more than one site of extranodal involvement	Low risk (0-1 risk factors) Low-intermediate (2), intermediate-high (3), high-risk (4–5)
Follicular lymphoma international prognostic Index-2 [61]	Folliculer lymphoma	Beta-2 microglobulin > upper limit of normal, bone marrow involvement, nodes >6 cm in greatest diameter, number of involved nodal and extra nodal sites, B-symptoms, age (>60 years), stage III/IV, hemoglobin level (<120 g/L), number of nodal areas (>4), and elevated LDH	Low risk (0–1 risk factor), intermediate risk (2), and high-risk (3–5)
Mantle cell lymphoma international prognostic index (MIPI) [62]	Mantle cell lymphoma	Age (<50 = 0, 50–59 = 1, 60–69 = 2, $\geq$70 = 1), performance status (ECOG $\geq$2 = 2), lactate dehydrogenase (<0.67, upper limit of normal (ULN) = 0, 0.67– 0.99, ULN = 1, 1–1.49, ULN = 2, $\geq$1.5, ULN = 3), and leukocyte count (<6.7 = 0, 6.7–9.9 = 1, 10–14.9 = 2, $\geq$15 = 3)	Low (<5.70) Intermediate (5.70–6.20) High risk ($\geq$6.20)

Table 9.10 Lymphoma staging according to the Lugano classification [63]

Stage		Nodal disease	Extranodal disease
Limited	I	One node or a group of adjacent node	Single extranodal lesions without nodal involvement
	II	Two or more nodal groups on either side of the diaphragm	Stage I or II with limited contiguous extranodal involvement
	II bulky	II as above with bulky disease	
Advanced	III	Nodes on both sides of the diaphragm; nodes above the diaphragm with spleen involvement	Not applicable, because nodal stage III plus extranodal involvement constitutes stage IV disease
	IV	Additional noncontiguous extra lymphatic involvement	Not applicable

9.2.3 Treatment Recommendations

9.2.3.1 Indolent NHL

Indolent non-Hodgkin lymphoma (NHL) includes the following subtypes: Follicular lymphoma, Lymphoplasmacytic lymphoma (Waldenström macroglobulinemia), Marginal zone lymphoma, Splenic marginal zone lymphoma, Primary cutaneous anaplastic large cell lymphoma.

9.2.3.2 Follicular Lymphoma

Follicular lymphoma consist of 20% of all NHL and almost 70% of the indolent lymphomas reported [64]. Most patients with follicular lymphoma are age 50 years and older and present with widespread disease at diagnosis. Nodal involvement is most common and is often accompanied by splenic and bone marrow disease [53]. Diagnosis is based on histology of preferably a biopsy of a lymph node. Immunohistochemical staining is positive in virtually all cases for cell surface CD19, CD20, CD10, and monoclonal immunoglobulin, as well as cytoplasmic expression of bcl-2 protein [65]. The overwhelming majority of cases have the characteristic t(14;18) translocation involving the IgH/bcl-2 genes [66]. As a result of indolent natural behavior, despite the advanced stage, the median survival ranges from 8 to 15 years. Watchful waiting, defined as postponing the treatment until the patient becomes symptomatic, is an option for patients with advanced-stage follicular lymphoma [65]. FLIPI and FLIPI-2 are the prognostic indexes to predict progression-free survival (PFS) and OS developed for follicular lymphoma, but the scores are not recommended to individualize the need for therapy, nor to predict response [61]. The aim to use FLIPI or FLIPI-2 is to guarantee a stability of prognostic factors in randomized clinical trials [48]. Currently, no randomized trials have mature results to guide clinicians about the initial choice of rituximab, nucleoside analogs, alkylating agents, combination chemotherapy, radiolabeled monoclonal antibodies, or combinations of these options [64]. Patients with indolent lymphoma may present a relapse with a more aggressive histology, if possible, a biopsy should be performed in case of relapse. The risk of histologic transformation was 30% by 10 years in a retrospective review of 325 patients [67]. Radiotherapy is a preferred treatment approach for stage I–II patients. In British Columbia study reported the results of 237 patients with stage I–II FL treated with RT alone [68]. Ten-year PFS/OS were 49% and 66%. Also using INRT did not differ in PFS or OS and only 1% developed regional-only recurrence [68]. The radiotherapy dose was evaluated in prospective randomized UK FORT trial. Two different radiotherapy schema: 4 Gy in 2 fx vs. 24 Gy in 12 fx were compared for patients with follicular or marginal zone lymphoma [64]. The response rates were higher response rate with 24 Gy (overall 91% vs. 81%; CR 68% vs. 49%) but similar OS reported. Analyses of the national cancer data base 35,961 patients with follicular lymphoma in National Cancer Database (NCDB). Radiotherapy was showed to improve 5/10-year OS vs. those who did not (86%/68% vs. 74%/54%) [69].

9.2.3.3 Marginal Zone Lymphoma

Marginal zone lymphomas were previously included among the diffuse, small lymphocytic lymphomas. When marginal zone lymphomas involve the nodes, they are called monocytoid B-cell lymphomas or nodal marginal zone B-cell lymphomas, and when they involve extranodal sites (e.g., gastrointestinal tract, thyroid, lung, breast, orbit, and skin), they are called mucosa-associated lymphatic tissue (MALT) lymphomas [70].

9.2.3.4 Gastric MALT

Patients with gastric malt usually have a history of autoimmune disease, such as Hashimoto thyroiditis or Sjögren syndrome, or of Helicobacter gastritis [70]. Most patients present with stage I or stage II extranodal disease, limited to the stomach. First action is to treat *Helicobacter pylori* infection and after standard antibiotic regimens, in the endoscopic evaluation, 50% of patients show resolution after 3 months [70, 71]. The response can be detected up to 12 to 18 months of observation. Translocation t(11;18) in patients with gastric MALT predicts for poor response to antibiotic therapy. At the time of progression, radiation therapy, rituximab, chemotherapy or combined–modality therapy could be advised [71]. The use of endoscopic ultrasonography may help clinicians to follow responses in these patients [70].

9.2.3.5 Extragastric MALT

Localized involvement of other sites can be treated with radiation or surgery. Patients with extragastric MALT lymphoma have a higher relapse rate than patients with gastric MALT lymphoma in some series, with relapses many years and even decades later [72].

9.2.3.6 Primary Cutaneous Anaplastic Large Cell Lymphoma

Primary cutaneous anaplastic large cell lymphoma presents in the skin only with no pre-existing lymphoproliferative disease and no extracutaneous sites of involvement. Patients with localized disease usually undergo radiation therapy. With more disseminated involvement, watchful waiting or doxorubicin-based combination chemotherapy is applied [73].

9.2.3.7 Aggressive Lymphoma

Diffuse Large B Cell Lymphoma

Diffuse large B-cell lymphoma (DLBCL) is the most common subtype of non-Hodgkin lymphoma (NHL) [51]. There are two major biologically distinct molecular subtypes of DLBCL are defined: germinal center B-cell (GCB) and activated B-cell (ABC) [74]. These entities share a number of other features such as the MHC class II gene expression. There was a striking difference in survival between these subgroups of patients, with overall survival at 5 years of 76% for GCB and 16% for ABC DLBCL patients [75, 76]. The ABC subtype is characterized by chronic active B-cell receptor (BCR) signaling, which stimulates NF-κB activity via Bruton tyrosine kinase [76]. Different from ABCDLBCL, The GCB DLBCL subgroup present the t(14;18) translocation affecting the *BCL2* gene, overexpression of *C-REL* from chromosome 2p, as well as upregulation of *LMO2* suggesting that GCB DLBCL cells originate from normal GC B cells [77]. In addition to GCB and ABC subtypes, double-hit lymphomas (approximately 5% to 10% of patients) and double-expressor lymphomas, which overexpress MYC and BCL2 protein, are aggressive DLBCLs and are also associated with a poor prognosis [77]. Double-hit lymphomas have concurrent chromosomal rearrangements of MYC plus BCL2 (or less likely, BCL6). Molecular classification of DLBCL is the major prognostic factor, but encourages the studies directed to the personalization of therapy for DLBCL [74, 77]. The optimal combination of chemotherapy and radiotherapy has been the major topic for the studies. SWOG 8736 randomized intermediate-grade, stage I/IE/II/IIE, or bulky stage I lymphoma patients to 3 cycles of CHOP + IFRT (40–50 Gy) or 8 cycles CHOP alone. Five-year results showed improved OS and FFS with CHOP-IFRT, but in the longer follow up to 12 years, this difference has been lost [78].

Another study from ECOG E1484, evaluated the use of IFRT(30–40 Gy) after 8 cycles of CHOP in 352 patients with intermediate-grade, bulky or extranodal stage I, nonbulky stage II/IIE disease. IFRT resulted in improved 6-year DFS (73 vs. 56%), but this did not turn into a OS difference [79]. GELA LNH93-1 and GELA LNH93-4 also investigated the use of IFRT CHOP and no additional benefit was demonstrated [80].

In Rituximab era, there is only retrospective series and cancer database analysis exploring the use of radiotherapy. A retrospective analysis from MDACC revealed that use of selective RT after R-CHOP resulted in improved 5-year OS/PFS for stage I/II patients (92%/82% vs. 73%/68%) and stage III/IV patients (89%/76% vs. 66%/55%) [81]. NCDB database with 59,255 stage I-II DLBCL patients demonstrated that adding RT improved 5/10-year OS form 75%/55% to 82%/64%, respectively [82]. The same year published SEER-Medicare database reported similar OS with additional RT, more importantly RT use lowered risk of second-line therapy and febrile neutropenia than 6–8 cycles R-CHOP [83].

Studies of advanced DLBCL had usually evaluated patients in two age categories (cut off: 60 years). RICOVER-60 evaluated 6 vs. 8 cycles of CHOP-14 (given at 2-week intervals) ± rituximab in 1222 patients 61–80 years with stage I–IV DLBCL

[84]. Patients with initial bulky disease (diameter ≥ 7.5 cm) or extranodal involvement received 36 Gy RT. 6-cycle R-CHOP improved 3-year EFS (47 vs. 66%) and OS (68 vs. 78%) vs. CHOP alone. In subgroup analysis, RT administration for bulky or extranodal involvement had improved 3-year EFS (80% vs. 54%), PFS (88% vs. 62%), and OS (90% vs. 65%) [84]. As PET-CT was not available at the time of this study, questions of the role of PET-CT were evaluated in ongoing trials with an aim of selecting more effective patients with obtaining an end treatment PET-CT.

The other radiotherapy indication is irradiate the skeletal involvement as Rituximab failed to improve the outcome of skeletal involvement. Held et al. performed a secondary analysis of the patients with skeletal involvement in MiNT and RICOVER-60 trials. Importantly, the use of consolidative RT to skeletal involvement improved 3-year EFS form 36% to 75% with trend for improved OS (86% vs. 71%) [85].

9.2.3.8 Primary Mediastinal B-Cell Lymphoma

Primary mediastinal B-cell lymphoma (PMBCL) is recognized as a distinct clinico-pathologic entity that predominantly affects young female adults and median age at diagnose is 37 [86]. Histologically, it arises from thymus medullary B cells and comprises 2.4% of all NHL. In addition to the absence of BCL2 and BCL6 rearrangements, *PDL2* (programmed death ligand 2), which is located on chromosome 9p overlapping significantly with Hodgkin lymphoma, are characteristic changes [86, 87]. Most cases occurring in young women as mediastinal disease, with better five-year overall survival compared to DLBCL (64 vs. 46%) [87]. Treatment with dose-adjusted EPOCH (etoposide, doxorubicin, cyclophosphamide, vincristine, prednisone) chemotherapy and rituximab (DA-EPOCH-R) has become the standard of care for primary mediastinal B-cell lymphoma (PMBCL) at many institutions, but combination of chemotherapy and radiotherapy could be an option for treatment approach [86].

9.2.3.9 CNS Lymphoma

Most patients with PCNSL have DLBCL. RT is primarily used as consolidative therapy after high-dose methotrexated based chemotherapy. Historically, 45 Gy have been shown to decrease the risk of progression or relapse after chemotherapy but at the cost of significant neurotoxicity, particularly in patients older than 60 years. Ferreri et al. have not found a benefit for increasing the dose beyond 36 Gy, and the role of additional boost remains questionable in the era of effective chemotherapy. Recently, Memorial Sloan-Kettering Cancer Center has reported long-term follow-up of a prospective combined modality program using WBRT of 23.4 Gy after chemotherapy-induced CR. Higher doses (36 Gy) are required when RT is used as a single modality therapy, either in patients who cannot receive chemotherapy or as salvage treatment after chemotherapy failure. The whole brain treatment is the standard. A retrospective study from Japan analyzed the relapse patterns and reported that margins smaller than 4 cm around the lesion(s) were associated with a higher failure rate and decreased survival. The optic nerve and the retina are considered part of the CNS, PCNSL whole brain field design always includes the posterior part of the orbits even no disease was evident. Detailed examination of the eyes by an ophthalmologist should be performed as if the eyes are involved at diagnose, the WBRT should be include the entire globe to a dose of 30 to 36 Gy.

9.2.4 Recommended Treatment Algorithm

Stage	Standard treatment options
Indolent, stage I and contiguous stage II adult NHL	Radiation therapy
	ISRT (24–30 Gy at 1.5–2 Gy/fx)
	Rituximab with or without chemotherapy
	Watchful waiting
	Other therapies as designated for patients with advanced-stage disease
Indolent, noncontiguous stage II/III/IV adult NHL	Watchful waiting for asymptomatic patients
	Rituximab
Symptomatic: decision to treat based on international criteria (GELF or FLIPI), which consider symptoms, threatened end-organ dysfunction, cytopenias, bulky disease at presentation, steady progression of disease, or patient preference	Obinutuzumab
	Purine nucleoside analogs
	Alkylating agents (with or without steroids)
	Combination chemotherapy
	Yttrium Y 90-ibritumomab tiuxetan
	Maintenance rituximab
	4 Gy × 1 or 2 Gy × 2
Indolent, recurrent adult NHL	Chemotherapy (single agent or combination)
	Rituximab
	Lenalidomide
	Radiolabeled anti-CD20 monoclonal antibodies
	Palliative radiation therapy
Aggressive, stage I and contiguous stage II adult NHL	R-CHOP with or without IF-XRT
	Favorable (nonbulky <7.5 cm; stage I; <60 years, PS 0–1, normal LDH)
	R-CHOP (rituximab, cyclophosphamide, doxorubicin, vincristine, prednisone) × 3c, then ISRT (30–36 Gy)
	R-CHOP × 6c
	Unfavorable (bulky; stage II; >60 years; PS ≥2; elevated LDH) R-CHOP × 6 ± ISRT (30–36 Gy)
	Alternative: R-CHOP × 3c + ISRT (30–36 Gy)
Aggressive, noncontiguous stage II/III/IV adult NHL	R-CHOP
	Other combination chemotherapy
	If not a candidate for further chemo, RT alone (40–55 Gy)
Adult lymphoblastic lymphoma	Intensive therapy
	Radiation therapy
Diffuse, small, noncleaved-cell/Burkitt lymphoma	Aggressive multidrug regimens
	Central nervous system (CNS) prophylaxis
Aggressive, recurrent adult NHL	Bone marrow or stem cell transplantation
	Re-treatment with standard agents
	Palliative radiation therapy

Stage	Standard treatment options
Gastric malt Stage I–II	For H. pylori positive patients, 3–4 drug current antibiotic regimen with proton pump inhibitor for 2 weeks t(11:18) is a predictor for lack of response to antibiotic therapy and these patients should be considered for RT. if disease persists despite antibiotic therapy or if H. Pylori negative, RT to entire stomach and perigastric nodes (30 Gy in 20 fractions) Rituximab
Gastric malt stage III–IV	Chemotherapy Rituximab

CNS central nervous system, *CHOP* cyclophosphamide, doxorubicin, vincristine, and prednisone, *IF-XRT* involved-field radiation therapy, *NHL* non-Hodgkin lymphoma, *R-CHOP* rituximab, an anti-CD20 monoclonal antibody

9.2.4.1 The Role of PET-CT

Limited number of studies consisting mixed lymphoma populations have focused on PET(/CT) in the staging of patients with aggressive NHL alone. A prospective cohort of patients with diffuse large B-cell lymphoma (DLBCL), demonstrated that PET/CT has higher sensitivity than CT alone, providing upstaging of 15% of the patients [88]. In case of indolent lymphomas, PET(/CT) seems to be a promising for staging as well as directing biopsy in patients with indolent NHL suspected of transformation into aggressive disease. The literature to evaluate the importance of an interim FDG-PET for diffuse large B-cell lymphoma is still controversy [52].

The experiences with FDG-PET-guided consolidative irradiation in DLBCL after R-CHOP were reported from the analysis of a treatment policy in British Columbia established since 2005 [89]. In this treatment scheme, residual masses that remained PET positive were irradiated when feasible, whereas patients with a negative PET scan were observed. Finally, of 262 patients, 167 (64%) were PET negative, 82 (31%) were PET positive, and 13 (5%) had an indeterminate PET. The 4-year OS was comparable for PET-positive patients who underwent consolidative irradiation (85%) and PET negative patients (83%) and was poorer in PET-positive patients who were not irradiated (30%). These results points a possible indication of a PET/CT to guide the selected use of consolidative irradiation [89]. In the interim analysis of the OPTIMAL > 60 trial, The PET-guided strategy resulted in a 42% decrease of radiotherapy administration without compromising the oncological outcomes [90]. The results suggest that a negative postinduction PET reduces the need for consolidation radiotherapy of bulky sites. Several retrospective reviews reported that routine surveillance scans after obtaining clinical complete remission for diffuse large B-cell lymphoma has no additional gain for early detection or treatment outcomes. Full publication of the both study could alter the practical treatment approach in this issue, but until we have more published evidence, treatment tailoring depending on PET/CT out of clinical studies, is not a standard approach.

9.2.5   Radiation Technique

The International Lymphoma Radiation Oncology Group (ILROG) guidelines provides a consensus on the modern approach to radiation therapy (RT) delivery in the treatment of NHL. Historic approach for lymphoma RT identify fields to cover (gross) disease and subclinical sites. In the era of modern radiotherapy and sophisticated imaging techniques, using anatomic landmarks and encompassing adjacent uninvolved lymph nodes are no longer appropriate in the light of increasing evidence to suggest effective local control with such reduced field sizes.

Historically radiation therapy is the only treatment and to cure, more generous fields and higher doses were prescribed. Radiation dose used in the definitive radiotherapy treatment lowered by UK multicenter trial Prospective randomized trial comparing RT to 40–45 Gy in 20–23 fx vs. 24 Gy in 12 fx (indolent) or 30 Gy in 15 fx (aggressive) [91]. This study includes both indolent lymphoma and aggressive lymphoma with almost all indications as definitive RT alone, consolidative RT following chemotherapy, or palliation. In indolent group, lowering the dose from 30 Gy to 24 Gy did showed no difference in LC at 5 years. (79% high dose vs. 76% low dose). Parallel to this, LC at 5 years (84% high dose vs. 82% low dose) for aggressive lymphomas by two different RT dose schedule was found to be similar also [91]. With having similar PFS or OS at 5 years for both indolent and aggressive NHL, the results reset the new rules for standard RT dose for lymphomas.

9.2.5.1 Treatment Volume Principles

In daily practice, ESMO and ILROG had published delineation, target definition, simulation and dose guidelines for NHL. We will be summarizing these clinical guidelines that is often used in practice [54, 57–59].

9.2.5.2 Simulation

3-dimensional (3D) simulation study using either a CT simulator, a positron emission tomography (PET)-CT simulator, 4DCT simulator or an MRI simulator is highly recommended (Fig. 9.7). If PET and/or CT information has been obtained separately or before simulation, it should be fused electronically with the CT simulation study [57, 59].

Prechemotherapy (or presurgery) GTV: Imaging abnormalities suggestive of lymphomatous involvement obtained before any intervention.

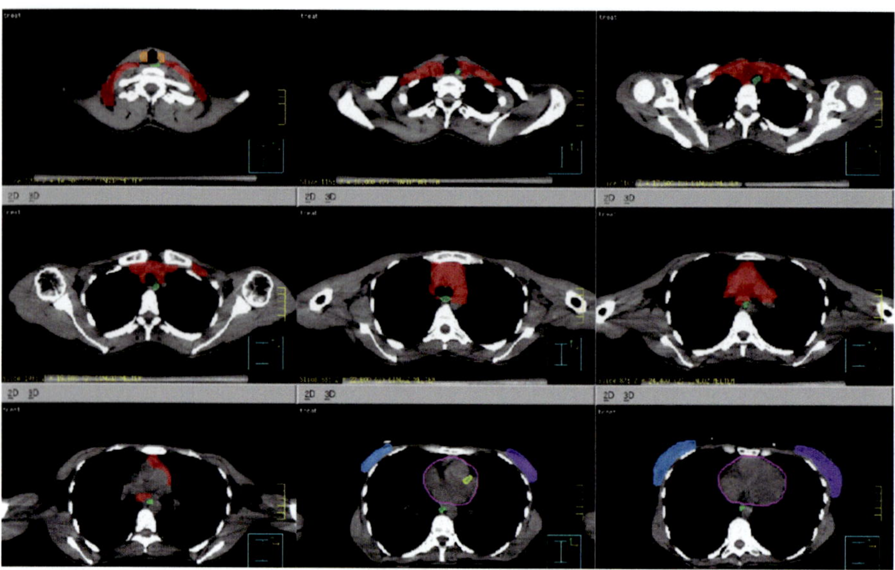

Fig. 9.7 Deliniation of treatment volumes for stage II NHLRed: GTV, Blue: right breast, purple: left breast

Postchemotherapy GTV: The primary of treated lesions with chemotherapy.

CTV: GTV + microscopic disease, even if extended beyond the involved tissue or organ (Fig. 9.8). Normal structures such as lungs, kidneys, and muscles that were clearly uninvolved, should be excluded from the CTV. If case nodal volumes are <5 cm apart, they can potentially be included in the same CTV [57, 59].

Internal target volume (ITV): is defined in ICRU report 62 as the CTV plus a margin taking into account uncertainties in size, shape, and position of the CTV within the patient. The ITV is most commonly defined in the chest and upper abdomen with respiratory movements. The optimal way is to use 4-dimensional (4D) CT simulation to obtain the ITV margins. Alternatively, the ITV may be determined by fluoroscopy or estimated by an experienced clinician. In sites that are unlikely to change shape or position during or in between treatments (e.g., the head and neck), outlining the ITV is not required.

For extranodal lymphomas; Many organs (such as stomach, salivary glands, thyroid gland, and the CNS), of lymphoma is multifocal, and the organ is often treated totally, even if the disease is demonstrated only in one part. When adjacent tissue/structures have been involved, some or all of the invaded structure/organ may be included in the CTV. Uninvolved lymph nodes are not routinely included in the CTV. However, first echelon nodes of uncertain status close to the primary organ may be included, and if part of a nodal group/chain is included in the CTV as part of the volume delineation, it may be prudent to encompass that part of the chain adequately.

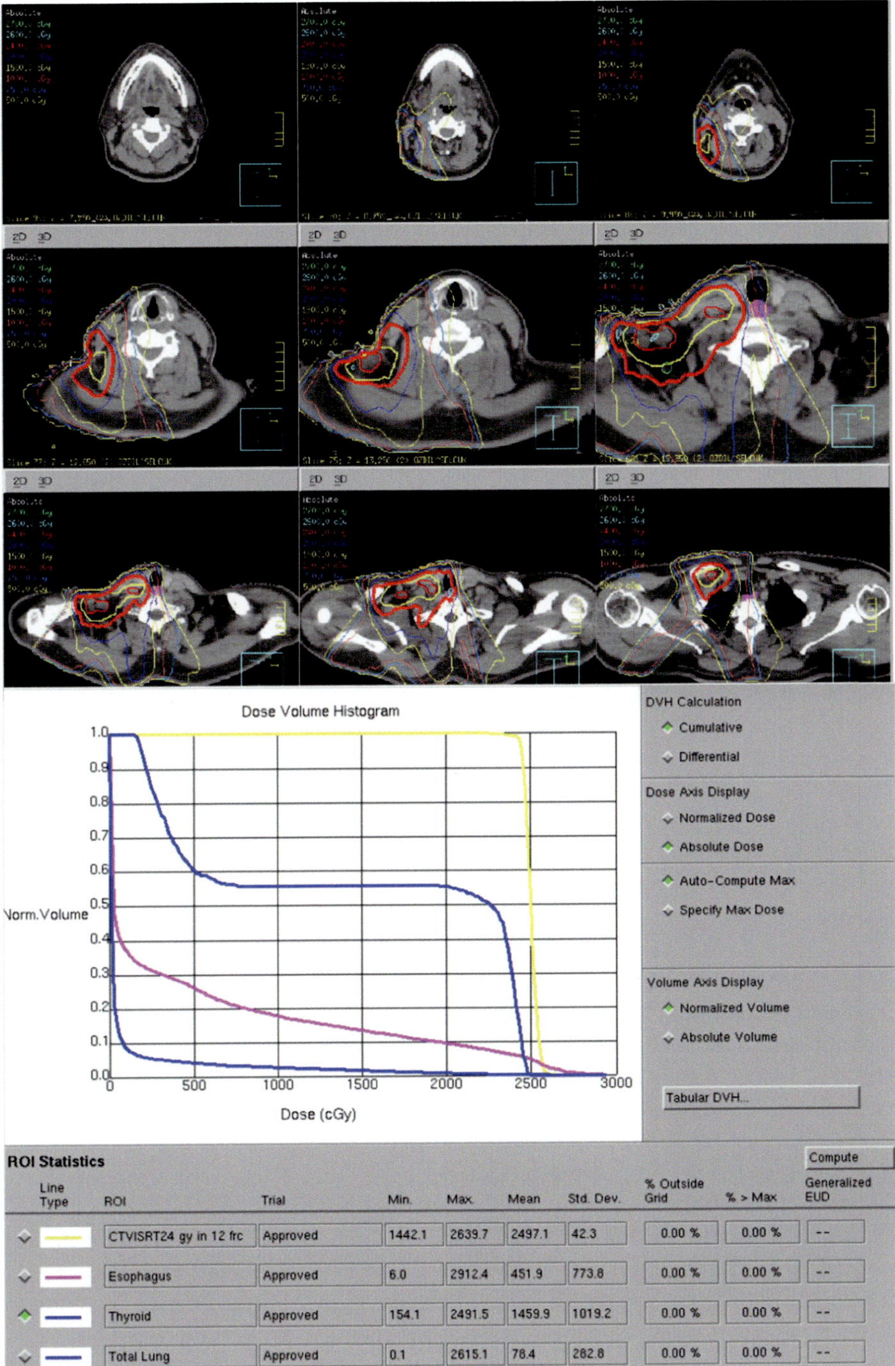

Fig. 9.8 IMRT- Field in field planning for stage I patient to a total dose of 24 Gy. (**b**) 24 Gy iso-dose coverage (red) (**c**) Dose –volume histogram are presented

Determination of PTV: The practice of determining the PTV varies across institutions depending on estimated setup variations that are a function of immobilization device, body site, internal organ motion, and patient cooperation.

> **Involved-Site RT**
>
> This concept assumes that chemotherapy eradicates adjacent or regional microscopic disease, and ISRT targets the identifiable prechemotherapy disease. In the situation in which prechemotherapy imaging (e.g., CT, PET, or MRI) of all the initially involved lymphoma sites of disease is available.
>
> The role of larger-field RT is now limited essentially to salvage treatment in patients who fail chemotherapy and are unable to embark upon more-intensive salvage treatment schedules. Such salvage cases are usually addressed on a case-by-case basis, and it is not feasible to produce guidelines given the diversity of individual cases. A dose of 30–40 Gy to sites of residual disease is recommended.

9.2.5.3 Organs at Risk

The planner should contour all the normal tissue (salivary gland, heart, thyroid, etc..) in the vicinity of the lymph nodes to see dose-volume histograms, and the plan should be evaluated in consideration of the expected normal tissue complication probability.

9.2.5.4 Radiation Treatment Planning

Diagnostic contrast use is recommended to help to delineate nodal stations and differentiate nodes from vessels at the time of simulation. Also for abdominal and pelvic locations, oral contrast should be used. Four-dimensional CT imaging as part of the simulation may be helpful in determining the ITV for sites that move with respiration.

9.2.5.5 Immobilization

A planning CT should be taken with the patient having site specific immobilization. Contiguous slices with a slice thickness of 3–5 mm should be taken through the regions at least 2 cm above and below of interest. Exp: Head and neck regions: a customized thermoplastic mask.

9.2.5.6 Treatment Techniques

The most appropriate treatment technique usually depends on the based on site, volume nor normal tissue in the vicinity for example, conventional anteroposterior-posteroanterior techniques may be preferred, because the smallest volume of normal tissue would be irradiated with this technique. More-conformal techniques, such as intensity modulated RT (IMRT), arc therapy, or tomotherapy, may offer significantly better sparing of critical normal structures, usually with a larger low dose of normal tissue irradiated. The clinician has to consider potential benefits and risks to offer the lowest risk of significant late toxicity for that patient. In some clinical situations such as bulky mediastial mass, sparing lung and heart, IMRT in combination with breath-hold techniques, and image guided RT may offer significant and clinically relevant advantages for especially dealing with young generation [92]. In selected patients, IMRT shown to reduce pulmonary toxicity parameters in DVH evaluation (lower values for Dmean and V20) and allows for superior protection of the heart and coronary arteries. This dosimetric gain is normally more apparent in situations in which a large PTV involves the anterior mediastinum. As tightly conformal doses and steep gradient next to normal tissues in IMRT required very careful target definition and delineation and treatment delivery verification to avoid the risk of tumor geographic miss [92].

Localized Indolent Lymphoma
Stage IA/IIA disease.
  Dose: 24–30 Gy in 12–15 fractions.

Advanced-Stage Indolent Lymphoma
Dose: 4 Gy in 2 fractions (Prospective, randomized trial in the United Kingdom comparing 4 Gy with 24 Gy for follicular lymphoma).
  If there is bulky disease, hard to monitor such as retroperitoneum: 24–30 Gy to provide durable long term local disease control.

Extranodal Lymphoma
FL, MZL, and small lymphocytic lymphomas:
  Dose: 20–30 Gy.
  Palliation dose: 4 Gy.

Diffuse Large B-Cell Lymphoma (DLBCL)
Dose: 30–36 Gy is an appropriate dose after a complete response 40–45 Gy for gross residual disease benefit from a higher dose.

Refractory and Recurrent Aggressive NHL
Dose: 30–40 Gy before or after ASCT is recommended.
  Timing: Within 6–8 weeks after stem cell infusion.
  Field: Encompass the known site(s) of disease recurrence, without prophylactic inclusion of adjacent lymph nodal stations.

Peripheral T-Cell Lymphoma (PTCL)

Dose: 30–36 Gy is an appropriate dose after a complete response 40–45 Gy for gross residual disease benefit from a higher dose.

Primary CNS Lymphoma

CTV=Whole brain including 1 or 2 upper cervical vertebrae and the posterior aspect of the eyes.

If the eyes were originally involved, both eyes should be included in their entirety in the WBRT field.

Dose: 24 Gy-CR after chemotherapy.

36 Gy to 45 Gy (1.5 to 1.8 Gy/fraction) after incomplete response.

40 to 50 Gy (1.5 to 1.8 Gy/fraction) as primary treatment for noncandidates for chemotherapy: 30 to 36 Gy in 10 or 15 for palliation.

Primary Intraocular Lymphoma

CTV: the globe of the eye(s), optic nerve (s) to the level of the chiasm.

Dose is 36 Gy.

Preplanning studies includes: Full ophthalmologic evaluation and brain/orbital MRI and cerebrospinal fluid evaluation.

Dura Matter Lymphoma

CTV: Whole brain to 24 Gy and boosting the involved sites with additional 12 Gy. A single lesion may be treated with the presurgical/biopsy MRI volume (GTV) plus margins constituting the CTV.

Dose: 30 to 36 Gy.

Orbital (Ocular Adnexal) Lymphomas

Indolent disease.

CTV: for most cases of indolent NHL, the entire bony orbit including definite or suspected extraorbital extensions.

When disease is limited to the conjunctiva, the CTV includes the entire conjunctival sac and local extensions to eyelid.

Dose: indolent disease.

Dose: 24 to 25 Gy in 1.5- to 2-Gy fractions.

DLBCL

CTV: The entire orbit should be included. In the presence of residual disease after chemotherapy, a GTV should be defined for a boost dose. When DLBCL involves the lacrimal gland alone, the CTV for consolidation RT (after CR to chemotherapy) may be limited to the lacrimal gland.

Dose: Consolidation after chemotherapy CR: 30 Gy.

After partial response (PR) or relapse, or for use of RT alone, consider 30 to 36 Gy to whole orbit and extensions, shielding lacrimal gland and avoiding full dose on ocular surface if appropriate. Residual GTV should be treated to a dose of 40 to 45 Gy depending on the volume and proximity to critical structures.

Lymphomas of the Head and Neck

CTV: determined by the prechemotherapy GTV, but often the entire involved structure is included because of uncertainty about the exact extent of initial involvement.

Uninvolved sinuses are not included in the CTV, and neck nodes are treated only if involved.

Doses: 30 Gy consolidation after CR to chemotherapy, 40 Gy for residual (PR) or uncertain CR.

In the rare cases of indolent lymphomas, the dose is 24 to 30 Gy.

Lymphomas of the Pharynx.

Field: CTV is determined by the prechemotherapy GTV, but often the entire involved structure (e.g., the whole tonsillar fossa from the level of the soft palate to the level of the vallecula) is included because of uncertainty about the exact extent of initial involvement. Uninvolved structures are not included in the CTV, and neck nodes are treated only if involved.

Dose: 30 Gy consolidation after CR to chemotherapy; 40 Gy for residual (PR) or uncertain CR. In the rare cases of indolent lymphomas, the dose is 24 to 30 Gy.

Lymphomas of the Oral Cavity, Larynx, and Hypopharynx

CTV: determined by the prechemotherapy or prebiopsy GTV, with margins determined by the quality of prechemotherapy/surgery information. Often the entire involved structure (larynx, hypopharynx, or subsite of the oral cavity) is included because of uncertainty about the exact extent of initial involvement. Uninvolved structures are not included in the CTV, and neck nodes are treated only if involved.

Doses: 30 Gy consolidation after CR to chemotherapy; 40 Gy for residual (PR) or uncertain CR. For indolent and mantle cell lymphoma, 24–30 Gy is adequate.

Lymphomas of the Parotid and Other Salivary Glands
CTV: the whole unilateral salivary gland.

Thyroid Lymphoma
CTV: primary or consolidation RT is the whole thyroid and should include the prechemotherapy or preresection GTV.

Extranodal NK/T-Cell Lymphoma, Nasal Type
Nasal NKTCL
   CTV: Limited stage IE (confined to unilateral, anterior or middle nasal cavity without extension into adjacent organs):
   CTV covers the bilateral nasal cavity, ipsilateral maxillary sinus, bilateral anterior ethmoid sinuses, and hard palate.
   Bilateral nasal cavity involvement: CTV covers the bilateral nasal cavity, bilateral maxillary sinus, bilateral anterior ethmoid sinuses, and hard palate.
   Nasal tumor located near the posterior nasal aperture extending into the nasopharynx: CTV should include the nasopharynx.
   For disease extending into anterior ethmoid sinuses: CTV should cover the posterior ethmoid sinuses.
   For disease extending into adjacent structures (extended stage I) or with cervical lymph node involvement (stage IIE): CTV should include involved paranasal organs/tissues or cervical lymph nodes.
   Prophylactic nodal irradiation is not necessary for patients with nasal NKTCL.
   Dose: Primary treatment: standard dose is 50 Gy with a boost to the residual primary of 5 to 10 Gy. If RT is given as consolidation after CR to chemotherapy, the dose is reduced to 45 to 50 Gy.

Breast Lymphoma
CTV: primary or consolidation RT is the whole breast. Uninvolved lymph nodes need not be included.

Lymphoma of the Lung
GTV/CTV: GTV that is expanded by clinical judgement to accommodate imaging uncertainties and suspected adjacent microscopic infiltration.

Gastric Lymphoma

Changes in stomach position induced by respiration are detected by 4D CT simulation or by fluoroscopy to determine the ITV, and an additional margin of approximately 1 cm is often added to the CTV. Patients are always simulated and treated with an empty stomach after a fast of at least 4 h or overnight. Patients should be simulated supine with arms up using customized immobilization device. A small volume (<50 mL) of oral contrast medium should be used in all cases; intravenous contrast medium is recommended if there are suggestive lymph nodes. Images should be acquired before and after oral contrast medium is given because even small volumes of ingested contrast medium may lead to stomach dilatation and a CTV that is not representative of the CTV during treatment. Respiratory motion should be assessed with 4D CT Or fluoroscopy.

Volumes.

GTV: Gross disease (if visualized on PET, CT, or both) and pathologically enlarged lymph nodes.

CTV: GTV + stomach volume outlined from gastroesophageal junction to beyond the duodenal bulb; the whole wall is included (perigastric nodes are encompassed, if visible).

ITV is determined by 4D CT or by fluoroscopy to track variation of stomach position during respiration. An additional margin of at least 1–2 cm is added to the CTV to accommodate stomach movement.

PTV is influenced by setup variation; in the abdomen, 1 cm over final ITV is advised.

Organs at risk volumes for consideration in planning include kidneys, liver, heart, lungs, bowel, cord.

Rarely, the duodenum is also involved. In this case, duodenal volume is included in the CTV.

Testicular Lymphoma

Setup: With the patient supine in a frog-leg position, the penis is lifted and taped to the abdominal wall, and the scrotum is supported and immobilized with bolus under and around the scrotum.

Volume: An anterior electron field with energy calculated according the thickness of the scrotum/testis is set; bolus may be required.

Dose: 25–30 Gy in 1.5–2 Gy per fraction.

References

1. Ansell SM. Hodgkin lymphoma: 2016 update on diagnosis, risk-stratification, and management. Am J Hematol. 2016;91(4):434–42.
2. Salati M, et al. Epidemiological overview of Hodgkin lymphoma across the Mediterranean Basin. Mediterr J Hematol Infect Dis. 2014;6(1).
3. Amitai I, et al. PET-adapted therapy for advanced Hodgkin lymphoma—systematic review. Acta Oncol. 2018:1–8.
4. Ansell SM. Hodgkin lymphoma: 2018 update on diagnosis, risk-stratification, and management. Am J Hematol. 2018;93(5):704–15.
5. Ferme C, et al. ABVD or BEACOPP baseline along with involved-field radiotherapy in early-stage Hodgkin lymphoma with risk factors: results of the European Organisation for Research and Treatment of Cancer (EORTC)-Groupe d'Etude des Lymphomes de l'Adulte (GELA) H9-U intergroup randomised trial. Eur J Cancer. 2017;81:45–55.
6. Andre MPE, et al. Early positron emission tomography response-adapted treatment in stage I and II Hodgkin lymphoma: final results of the randomized EORTC/LYSA/FIL H10 trial. J Clin Oncol. 2017;35(16):1786–94.
7. Specht L, et al. Modern radiation therapy for Hodgkin lymphoma: field and dose guidelines from the international lymphoma radiation oncology group (ILROG). Int J Radiat Oncol Biol Phys. 2014;89(4):854–62.
8. Bartlett NL. Limited-stage Hodgkin lymphoma: optimal chemotherapy and the role of radiotherapy. In American Society of Clinical Oncology educational book; 2013. p. 374–80.
9. Hoppe RT, et al. Hodgkin lymphoma version 1.2017, NCCN clinical practice guidelines in oncology. J Natl Compr Cancer Netw. 2017;15(5):608–38.
10. Hoskin PJ, et al. Long-term results of a randomised trial of involved field radiotherapy vs extended field radiotherapy in stage I and II Hodgkin lymphoma. Clin Oncol (R Coll Radiol). 2005;17(1):47–53.
11. Maraldo MV, et al. Radiation therapy planning for early-stage Hodgkin lymphoma: experience of the International Lymphoma Radiation Oncology Group. Int J Radiat Oncol Biol Phys. 2015;92(1):144–52.
12. Hutchings M, Eigtved AI, Specht L. FDG-PET in the clinical management of Hodgkin lymphoma. Crit Rev Oncol Hematol. 2004;52(1):19–32.
13. Levin LI, et al. Atypical prediagnosis Epstein-Barr virus serology restricted to EBV-positive Hodgkin lymphoma. Blood. 2012;120(18):3750–5.
14. Shanbhag S, Ambinder RF. Hodgkin lymphoma: a review and update on recent progress. CA Cancer J Clin. 2018;68(2):116–32.
15. Lee AI, LaCasce AS. Nodular lymphocyte predominant Hodgkin lymphoma. Oncologist. 2009;14(7):739–51.
16. Goel A, et al. Nodular lymphocyte predominant Hodgkin lymphoma: biology, diagnosis and treatment. Clin Lymphoma Myeloma Leuk. 2014;14(4):261–70.
17. Blank O, et al. Chemotherapy alone versus chemotherapy plus radiotherapy for adults with early stage Hodgkin lymphoma. Cochrane Database Syst Rev. 2017;4:CD007110.
18. Nguyen VT, et al. Early stage, bulky Hodgkin lymphoma patients have a favorable outcome when treated with or without consolidative radiotherapy: potential role of PET scan in treatment planning. Br J Haematol. 2017;179(4):674–6.
19. Hasenclever D, Diehl V. A prognostic score for advanced Hodgkin's disease. International prognostic factors project on advanced Hodgkin's disease. N Engl J Med. 1998;339(21):1506–14.
20. Aleman BM, et al. Involved-field radiotherapy for patients in partial remission after chemotherapy for advanced Hodgkin's lymphoma. Int J Radiat Oncol Biol Phys. 2007;67(1):19–30.
21. Hutchings M, et al. Clinical impact of FDG-PET/CT in the planning of radiotherapy for early-stage Hodgkin lymphoma. Eur J Haematol. 2007;78(3):206–12.
22. Oner AO, et al. Efficacy of (18)F-2-fluoro-2-deoxy-D-glucose positron emission tomography/computerized tomography for bone marrow infiltration assessment in the initial staging of lymphoma. Mol Imaging Radionucl Ther. 2017;26(2):69–75.

23. Kanoun S, Rossi C, Casasnovas O. [(18)F]FDG-PET/CT in Hodgkin lymphoma: current usefulness and perspectives. Cancers (Basel). 2018;10(5). pii: E145.
24. Karls S, Shah H, Jacene H. PET/CT for lymphoma post-therapy response assessment in other lymphomas, response assessment for autologous stem cell transplant, and lymphoma follow-up. Semin Nucl Med. 2018;48(1):37–49.
25. Kasamon YL, Wahl RL. FDG PET and risk-adapted therapy in Hodgkin's and non-Hodgkin's lymphoma. Curr Opin Oncol. 2008;20(2):206–19.
26. Buchpiguel CA. Current status of PET/CT in the diagnosis and follow up of lymphomas. Rev Bras Hematol Hemoter. 2011;33(2):140–7.
27. Specht L, Yahalom J. The concept and evolution of involved site radiation therapy for lymphoma. Int J Clin Oncol. 2015;20(5):849–54.
28. Engert A, et al. Two cycles of doxorubicin, bleomycin, vinblastine, and dacarbazine plus extended-field radiotherapy is superior to radiotherapy alone in early favorable Hodgkin's lymphoma: final results of the GHSG HD7 trial. J Clin Oncol. 2007;25(23):3495–502.
29. Press OW, et al. Phase III randomized intergroup trial of subtotal lymphoid irradiation versus doxorubicin, vinblastine, and subtotal lymphoid irradiation for stage IA to IIA Hodgkin's disease. J Clin Oncol. 2001;19(22):4238–44.
30. Fermé C, et al. Chemotherapy plus involved-field radiation in early-stage Hodgkin's disease. New Engl J Med. 2007;357(19):1916–27.
31. Engert A, et al. Involved-field radiotherapy is equally effective and less toxic compared with extended-field radiotherapy after four cycles of chemotherapy in patients with early-stage unfavorable Hodgkin's lymphoma: results of the HD8 trial of the German Hodgkin's Lymphoma Study Group. J Clin Oncol. 2003;21(19):3601–8.
32. Noordijk EM, et al. Combined-modality therapy for clinical stage I or II Hodgkin's lymphoma: long-term results of the European Organisation for Research and Treatment of Cancer H7 randomized controlled trials. J Clin Oncol. 2006;24(19):3128–35.
33. Bonadonna G, et al. ABVD plus subtotal nodal versus involved-field radiotherapy in early-stage Hodgkin's disease: long-term results. J Clin Oncol. 2004;22(14):2835–41.
34. Eghbali H, Brice P, Creemers GY, Marwijk Kooij M, Carde P, Van't Veer MB. Comparison of three radiation dose levels after EBVP regimen in favorable supradiaphragmatic clinical stages (CS) I-II Hodgkin's lymphoma (HL): preliminary results of the EORTC-GELA H9-F trial. In ASH annual meeting abstracts; 2005. p. 814.
35. Engert A, et al. Reduced treatment intensity in patients with early-stage Hodgkin's lymphoma. New Engl J Med. 2010;363(7):640–52.
36. Meyer RM, et al. ABVD alone versus radiation-based therapy in limited-stage Hodgkin's lymphoma. New Engl J Med. 2012;366(5):399–408.
37. Eich HT, et al. Intensified chemotherapy and dose-reduced involved-field radiotherapy in patients with early unfavorable Hodgkin's lymphoma: final analysis of the German Hodgkin Study Group HD11 trial. J Clin Oncol. 2010;28(27):4199–206.
38. Radford J, et al. Results of a trial of PET-directed therapy for early-stage Hodgkin's lymphoma. New Engl J Med. 2015;372(17):1598–607.
39. Sickinger MT, et al. PET-adapted omission of radiotherapy in early stage Hodgkin lymphoma—a systematic review and meta-analysis. Crit Rev Oncol Hematol. 2016;101:86–92.
40. Johnson PW, et al. Consolidation radiotherapy in patients with advanced Hodgkin's lymphoma: survival data from the UKLG LY09 randomized controlled trial (ISRCTN97144519). J Clin Oncol. 2010;28(20):3352–9.
41. Laskar S, et al. Consolidation radiation after complete remission in Hodgkin's disease following six cycles of doxorubicin, bleomycin, vinblastine, and dacarbazine chemotherapy: is there a need? J Clin Oncol. 2004;22(1):62–8.
42. Borchmann P, et al. Eight cycles of escalated-dose BEACOPP compared with four cycles of escalated-dose BEACOPP followed by four cycles of baseline-dose BEACOPP with or without radiotherapy in patients with advanced-stage Hodgkin's lymphoma: final analysis of the HD12 trial of the German Hodgkin Study Group. J Clin Oncol. 2011;29(32):4234–42.

43. Engert A, et al. Reduced-intensity chemotherapy and PET-guided radiotherapy in patients with advanced stage Hodgkin's lymphoma (HD15 trial): a randomised, open-label, phase 3 non-inferiority trial. Lancet. 2012;379(9828):1791–9.

44. Eichenauer DA, et al. Long-term course of patients with stage IA nodular lymphocyte-predominant Hodgkin lymphoma: a report from the German Hodgkin Study Group. J Clin Oncol. 2015;33(26):2857–62.

45. Voong KR, et al. Dosimetric advantages of a "butterfly" technique for intensity-modulated radiation therapy for young female patients with mediastinal Hodgkin's lymphoma. Radiat Oncol. 2014;9:94.

46. Petersen PM, et al. Prospective phase II trial of image-guided radiotherapy in Hodgkin lymphoma: benefit of deep inspiration breath-hold. Acta Oncol. 2015;54(1):60–6.

47. Maraldo MV, et al. Estimated risk of cardiovascular disease and secondary cancers with modern highly conformal radiotherapy for early-stage mediastinal Hodgkin lymphoma. Ann Oncol. 2013;24(8):2113–8.

48. Horwitz SM, et al. NCCN guidelines insights: non-Hodgkin's lymphomas, version 3. J Natl Compr Cancer Netw. 2016;14(9):1067–79.

49. Brittinger G. Histopathology and clinical problems in non-Hodgkin lymphomas. Blut. 1981;43(3):139–41.

50. Gospodarowicz M. Radiotherapy in non-Hodgkin lymphomas. Ann Oncol. 2008;19(Suppl 4):iv47–50.

51. Li S, Young KH, Medeiros LJ. Diffuse large B-cell lymphoma. Pathology. 2018;50(1):74–87.

52. Barrington SF, Kluge R. FDG PET for therapy monitoring in Hodgkin and non-Hodgkin lymphomas. Eur J Nucl Med Mol Imaging. 2017;44(Suppl 1):97–110.

53. Fowler N. Indolent and mantle cell NHL: the future is BRIGHT. Blood. 2014;123(19):2905–6.

54. Vitolo U, et al. Extranodal diffuse large B-cell lymphoma (DLBCL) and primary mediastinal B-cell lymphoma: ESMO clinical practice guidelines for diagnosis, treatment and follow-up. Ann Oncol. 2016;27(Suppl 5):v91–v102.

55. Wang SS, et al. Medical history, lifestyle, family history, and occupational risk factors for peripheral T-cell lymphomas: the InterLymph non-Hodgkin Lymphoma Subtypes Project. J Natl Cancer Inst Monogr. 2014;2014(48):66–75.

56. Ascari E, Gobbi PG. Prognostic factors in malignant lymphomas (Hodgkin and non-Hodgkin). Acta Haematol. 1987;78(Suppl 1):146–50.

57. Yahalom J, et al. Modern radiation therapy for extranodal lymphomas: field and dose guidelines from the International Lymphoma Radiation Oncology Group. Int J Radiat Oncol Biol Phys. 2015;92(1):11–31.

58. Ng AK, et al. Role of radiation therapy in patients with relapsed/refractory diffuse large B-cell lymphoma: guidelines from the International Lymphoma Radiation Oncology Group. Int J Radiat Oncol Biol Phys. 2018;100(3):652–69.

59. Illidge T, et al. Modern radiation therapy for nodal non-Hodgkin lymphoma-target definition and dose guidelines from the International Lymphoma Radiation Oncology Group. Int J Radiat Oncol Biol Phys. 2014;89(1):49–58.

60. A predictive model for aggressive non-Hodgkin's lymphoma. N Engl J Med. 1993;329(14):987–94.

61. Federico M, et al. Follicular lymphoma international prognostic index 2: a new prognostic index for follicular lymphoma developed by the international follicular lymphoma prognostic factor project. J Clin Oncol. 2009;27(27):4555–62.

62. Hoster E, et al. A new prognostic index (MIPI) for patients with advanced-stage mantle cell lymphoma. Blood. 2008;111(2):558–65.

63. Cheson BD, et al. Recommendations for initial evaluation, staging, and response assessment of Hodgkin and non-Hodgkin lymphoma: the Lugano classification. J Clin Oncol. 2014;32(27):3059–67.

64. Hoskin PJ, et al. 4 Gy versus 24 Gy radiotherapy for patients with indolent lymphoma (FORT): a randomised phase 3 non-inferiority trial. Lancet Oncol. 2014;15(4):457–63.

65. Tang T, Martin P. When indolent follicular lymphoma is not indolent. Leuk Lymphoma. 2014;55(11):2417–8.
66. Brem EA, Davids MS. Is Bcl-2 a valid target in the treatment of indolent non-Hodgkin lymphoma? Leuk Lymphoma. 2014;55(12):2675–7.
67. Lossos IS, Gascoyne RD. Transformation of follicular lymphoma. Best Pract Res Clin Haematol. 2011;24(2):147–63.
68. Campbell BA, et al. Long-term outcomes for patients with limited stage follicular lymphoma: involved regional radiotherapy versus involved node radiotherapy. Cancer. 2010;116(16):3797–806.
69. Vargo JA, et al. What is the optimal management of early-stage low-grade follicular lymphoma in the modern era? Cancer. 2015;121(18):3325–34.
70. Vannata B, Stathis A, Zucca E. Management of the marginal zone lymphomas. Cancer Treat Res. 2015;165:227–49.
71. Juarez-Salcedo LM, et al. Primary gastric lymphoma, epidemiology, clinical diagnosis, and treatment. Cancer Control. 2018;25(1):1073274818778256.
72. Zucca E, et al. Nongastric marginal zone B-cell lymphoma of mucosa-associated lymphoid tissue. Blood. 2003;101(7):2489–95.
73. Kempf W, Kerl K, Mitteldorf C. Cutaneous CD30-positive T-cell lymphoproliferative disorders-clinical and histopathologic features, differential diagnosis, and treatment. Semin Cutan Med Surg. 2018;37(1):24–9.
74. Davies A. Tailoring front-line therapy in diffuse large B-cell lymphoma: who should we treat differently? Hematology Am Soc Hematol Educ Program. 2017;2017(1):284–94.
75. Alizadeh AA, et al. Distinct types of diffuse large B-cell lymphoma identified by gene expression profiling. Nature. 2000;403(6769):503–11.
76. Rosenwald A, et al. The use of molecular profiling to predict survival after chemotherapy for diffuse large-B-cell lymphoma. N Engl J Med. 2002;346(25):1937–47.
77. Frick M, Dörken B, Lenz G. The molecular biology of diffuse large B-cell lymphoma. Ther Adv Hematol. 2011;2(6):369–79.
78. Stephens DM, et al. Continued risk of relapse independent of treatment modality in limited-stage diffuse large B-cell lymphoma: final and long-term analysis of Southwest Oncology Group Study S8736. J Clin Oncol. 2016;34(25):2997–3004.
79. Horning SJ, et al. Chemotherapy with or without radiotherapy in limited-stage diffuse aggressive non-Hodgkin's lymphoma: Eastern Cooperative Oncology Group study 1484. J Clin Oncol. 2004;22(15):3032–8.
80. Reyes F, et al. ACVBP versus CHOP plus radiotherapy for localized aggressive lymphoma. New Engl J Med. 2005;352(12):1197–205.
81. Phan J, et al. Benefit of consolidative radiation therapy in patients with diffuse large B-cell lymphoma treated with R-CHOP chemotherapy. J Clin Oncol. 2010;28(27):4170–6.
82. Vargo JA, et al. Treatment selection and survival outcomes in early-stage diffuse large B-cell lymphoma: do we still need consolidative radiotherapy? J Clin Oncol. 2015;33(32):3710–7.
83. Odejide OO, et al. Limited stage diffuse large B-cell lymphoma: comparative effectiveness of treatment strategies in a large cohort of elderly patients. Leuk Lymphoma. 2015;56(3):716–24.
84. Pfreundschuh M, et al. Six versus eight cycles of bi-weekly CHOP-14 with or without rituximab in elderly patients with aggressive CD20+ B-cell lymphomas: a randomised controlled trial (RICOVER-60). Lancet Oncol. 2008;9(2):105–16.
85. Held G, et al. Impact of rituximab and radiotherapy on outcome of patients with aggressive B-cell lymphoma and skeletal involvement. J Clin Oncol. 2013;31(32):4115–22.
86. Dabrowska-Iwanicka A, Walewski JA. Primary mediastinal large B-cell lymphoma. Curr Hematol Malig Rep. 2014;9(3):273–83.
87. Tai WM, et al. Primary mediastinal large B-cell lymphoma: optimal therapy and prognostic factors in 41 consecutive Asian patients. Leuk Lymphoma. 2011;52(4):604–12.
88. Fuertes S, et al. Interim FDG PET/CT as a prognostic factor in diffuse large B-cell lymphoma. Eur J Nucl Med Mol Imaging. 2013;40(4):496–504.

89. Sehn LH, Klasa R, Shenkier T, et al. Long-term experience with PET-guided consolidative radiation therapy (XRT) in patients with advanced stage diffuse large B-cell lymphoma (DLBCL) treated with R-CHOP. Oral presentation. Hematol Oncol. 2013;31(Suppl. I):96–150. [Abstract]. End-of-therapy PET scan to guide consolidation radiotherapy in aggressive B-cell lymphoma.
90. Pfreundschuh M, Christofyllakis K, Altmann B, et al. Radiotherapy to bulky disease PET-negative after immunochemotherapy in elderly DLBCL patients: results of a planned interim analysis of the first 187 patients with bulky disease treated in the OPTIMAL>60 study of the DSHNHL. J Clin Oncol. 2017;35:abstr 7506.
91. Lowry L, et al. Reduced dose radiotherapy for local control in non-Hodgkin lymphoma: a randomised phase III trial. Radiother Oncol. 2011;100(1):86–92.
92. Aristophanous M, et al. Deep-inspiration breath-hold intensity modulated radiation therapy to the mediastinum for lymphoma patients: setup uncertainties and margins. Int J Radiat Oncol Biol Phys. 2018;100(1):254–62.

Printed by Printforce, the Netherlands